MAKING EYE HEALTH A POPULATION HEALTH IMPERATIVE

VISION FOR TOMORROW

Steven M. Teutsch, Margaret A. McCoy, R. Brian Woodbury, and Annalyn Welp, *Editors*

Committee on Public Health Approaches to Reduce Vision Impairment and Promote Eye Health

Board on Population Health and Public Health Practice

Health and Medicine Division

A Report of

The National Academies of
SCIENCES · ENGINEERING · MEDICINE

THE NATIONAL ACADEMIES PRESS
Washington, DC
www.nap.edu

THE NATIONAL ACADEMIES PRESS 500 Fifth Street, NW Washington, DC 20001

This activity was supported by American Academy of Ophthalmology; American Academy of Optometry; American Optometric Association; Association for Research in Vision and Ophthalmology; National Alliance for Eye and Vision Research; National Center for Children's Vision and Eye Health; Prevent Blindness; Research to Prevent Blindness; Contract No. 200-2011-38807, TO#32 with the U.S. Department of Health and Human Services [Centers for Disease Control and Prevention]; and Contract No. HHSN2632012000741, TO#61 with the U.S. Department of Health and Human Services [National Institutes of Health]. Any opinions, findings, conclusions, or recommendations expressed in this publication do not necessarily reflect the views of any organization or agency that provided support for the project.

International Standard Book Number-13:   978-0-309-43998-5
International Standard Book Number-10:   0-309-43998-1
Digital Object Identifier: 10.17226/23471
Library of Congress Control Number: 2016956972

Additional copies of this publication are available for sale from the National Academies Press, 500 Fifth Street, NW, Keck 360, Washington, DC 20001; (800) 624-6242 or (202) 334-3313; http://www.nap.edu.

Suggested citation: National Academies of Sciences, Engineering, and Medicine. 2016. *Making Eye Health a Population Health Imperative: Vision for Tomorrow.* Washington, DC: The National Academies Press. doi: 10.17226/23471.

COMMITTEE ON PUBLIC HEALTH APPROACHES TO REDUCE VISION IMPAIRMENT AND PROMOTE EYE HEALTH

Reviewers

This report has been reviewed in draft form by individuals chosen for their diverse perspectives and technical expertise. The purpose of this independent review is to provide candid and critical comments that will assist the institution in making its published report as sound as possible and to ensure that the report meets institutional standards for objectivity, evidence, and responsiveness to the study charge. The review comments and draft manuscript remain confidential to protect the integrity of the deliberative process. We wish to thank the following individuals for their review of this report:

SUSAN A. COTTER, Southern California College of Optometry
JORGE CUADROS, University of California, Berkeley
DAVID S. FRIEDMAN, Johns Hopkins University
MARSHA GOLD, Mathematica Policy Research, Inc.
EMMETT B. KEELER, Pardee RAND Graduate School
RICARDO MARTINEZ, Adeptus Health Inc.
GLEN MAYS, University of Kentucky
DAVID O. MELTZER, The University of Chicago
ALAN R. MORSE, Lighthouse Guild International
CYNTHIA OWSLEY, University of Alabama at Birmingham
ROBERT M. PESTRONK, Ruth Mott Foundation
LOUISE POTVIN, Université de Montréal
SUSAN A. PRIMO, Emory University School of Medicine
DEJURAN RICHARDSON, Lake Forest College

BETSY SLEATH, University of North Carolina Eshelman School of
    Pharmacy
FRANK A. SLOAN, Duke University
ALFRED SOMMER, Johns Hopkins University
JOHN C. TOWNSEND, Veterans Health Administration
M. ROY WILSON, Wayne State University

Although the reviewers listed above have provided many constructive comments and suggestions, they were not asked to endorse the conclusions or recommendations nor did they see the final draft of the report before its release. The review of this report was overseen by **BOBBIE BERKOWITZ,** Columbia University School of Nursing and Columbia University Medical Center, and **BRADFORD H. GRAY,** Urban Institute. They were responsible for making certain that an independent examination of this report was carried out in accordance with institutional procedures and that all review comments were carefully considered. Responsibility for the final content of this report rests entirely with the authoring committee and the institution.

Contents

APPENDIXES

Acronyms and Abbreviations

AAMC	Association of American Medical Colleges
AAN	American Academy of Neurology
AAO	American Academy of Ophthalmology
AAP	American Academy of Pediatrics
AAPOS	American Association for Pediatric Ophthalmology and Strabismus
ACA	Patient Protection and Affordable Care Act of 2010
ACF	Administration for Children and Families
ACO	accountable care organization
ACVREP	Academy for Certification of Vision Rehabilitation and Education Professionals
ADA	Americans with Disabilities Act of 1990
ADL	activity of daily living
AER	Association for Education and Rehabilitation of the Blind and Visually Impaired
AFB	American Foundation for the Blind
AHRQ	Agency for Healthcare Research and Quality
AMD	age-related macular degeneration
APHA	American Public Health Association
ASPPH	Association of Schools and Programs of Public Health
AOA	American Optometric Association
AOTA	American Occupational Therapy Association
AUPO	Association of University Professors of Ophthalmology
AWV	annual wellness visit

BLS	Bureau of Labor Statistics
BPEDS	Baltimore Pediatric Eye Disease Study
BPHC	Bureau of Primary Health Care
BRFSS	Behavioral Risk Factor Surveillance System
BROS	Blind Rehabilitation Outpatient Specialist
CCG	categorical condition group
CCTV	closed caption television
CDC	Centers for Disease Control and Prevention
CEA	Cost-Effectiveness Analysis
CED	coverage with evidence development
CHC	community health center
CHIP	Children's Health Insurance Program
CHNA	community health needs assessment
CLVT	certified low vision therapist
CMS	Centers for Medicare & Medicaid Services
COMS	certified orientation and mobility specialist
CQI	continuous quality improvement
CVRT	certified vision rehabilitation therapist
DME	diabetic macular edema
DoD	U.S. Department of Defense
DOL	U.S. Department of Labor
DOT	U.S. Department of Transportation
DSI	dual sensory impairment
ED	U.S. Department of Education
EEOC	Equal Employment Opportunity Commission
EHR	electronic health record
EPA	U.S. Environmental Protection Agency
EPSDT	early and periodic screening, diagnostic, and treatment
FDA	U.S. Food and Drug Administration
FEDVIP	Federal Employees Dental and Vision Insurance Program
FPL	federal poverty level
FQHC	federally qualified health center
FSA	flexible spending account
HEED	Health Economics Evaluations Database
HHS	U.S. Department of Health and Human Services
HRA	health risk assessment
HRSA	Health Resources and Services Administration
HSA	health savings account

HUD	U.S. Department of Housing and Urban Development
ICD	*International Classification of Diseases*
IDEA	Individuals with Disabilities Education Act
IHS	Indian Health Service
ILVS	interdisciplinary low vision service
IPPE	initial preventive physical exam
IOL	intraocular lens
IOM	Institute of Medicine
IOP	intraocular pressure
KAP	Knowledge, Attitudes, and Practices
LALES	Los Angeles Latino Eye Study
LCD	local coverage determination
LCIF	Lions Club International Foundation
LHD	local health department
MCBS	Medicare Claims Beneficiary Survey
MCHB	multicultural health broker
MEPEDS	Multi-Ethnic Pediatric Eye Disease Study
MEPS	Medicare Expenditure Panel Survey
NAAL	National Assessment of Adult Literacy
NACCHO	National Association of County and City Health Officials
NACDD	National Association of Chronic Disease Directors
NAMCS	National Ambulatory Medical Care Survey
NAPVI	National Association for Parents of Children with Vision Impairments
NBEO	National Board of Examiners in Optometry
NCD	national coverage determination
NCQA	National Committee for Quality Assurance
NEHEP	National Eye Health Education Program
NEI	National Eye Institute
NEOS	New England Ophthalmological Society
NHAMC	National Hospital Ambulatory Medical Care Survey
NHANES	National Health and Nutrition Examination Survey
NHIS	National Health Interview Survey
NHS EED	National Health Service Economic Evaluation Database
NHSC	National Health Service Corps
NIDDK	National Institute of Diabetes and Digestive and Kidney Diseases
NIH	National Institutes of Health

NIOSH	National Institute for Occupational Safety and Health
NQF	National Quality Forum
NRT	nicotine replacement therapy
OHPDP	Office of Health Promotion and Disease Prevention
OSHA	Occupational Safety and Health Administration
PACT	Patient Aligned Care Team
PBA	Prevent Blindness America
PCMH	patient-centered medical home
PEP	protective eyewear promotion
PHAB	Public Health Accreditation Board
PHD	public health department
QALY	quality-adjusted life year
QOL	quality of life
RCT	randomized controlled trial
RLSB	Royal London Society for Blind People
ROC	Resuscitations Outcomes Consortium
SES	socioeconomic status
TAYE	Think About Your Eyes
USDA	U.S. Department of Agriculture
USPSTF	U.S. Preventive Services Task Force
UV	ultraviolet
VA	U.S. Department of Veterans Affairs
VEGF	vascular endothelial growth factor
VHI	Vision Health Initiative
VHIPP	Vision Health Integration and Preservation Program
VISOR	Vision Impairment Services in Outpatient Rehabilitation
VPUS	Vision Problems in the U.S.
VSP	Vision Service Plan
WHO	World Health Organization

Preface

Losing one's eyesight, at any age, is frightening. That fear has merit: compared to their peers, people with vision loss have reduced independence and quality of life, lower performance in school, lower wages and job attainment, and higher health costs. Fortunately, two of the most common causes of vision loss among adults (i.e., refractive errors and cataracts) can be readily treated with proper access to, and utilization of, currently available care. This report estimates that undiagnosed or untreated refractive error alone affects between 8.2 and 15.9 million people in the United States. Uncorrectable vision impairment affects another 6.4 million people. The toll of correctable vision loss among children who do not received adequate detection, follow-up, and treatment is troubling. Ensuring that people receive proper visual acuity screenings and preventive eye care services and adhere to effective eye protection practices would eliminate thousands of preventable or correctable cases of vision impairment that result each year from amblyopia and eye injuries. Success in simply applying current knowledge would reduce significant health care disparities, because avoidable vision loss disproportionately affects minorities and the poor. Failure of the United States to address these sources of preventable suffering and disparity is simply not acceptable.

But the population health imperative for eye health does not end with eliminating avoidable vision loss. Even if all vision impairment due to refractive errors, cataracts, or avoidable conditions vanished, millions of people would still be visually impaired. Although recent advances in eye care are impressive and have reduced the vision loss that results from genetic conditions and common, age-related eye diseases (e.g., age-related macular degeneration, glaucoma, diabetic retinopathy), there remains no cure. Due to the aging of our population and the strongly age-related incidence of many eye diseases, we project a near doubling, by 2050, in the prevalence of "chronic vision impairment." The good news for people living with vision impairment and blindness is that vision impairment is a surmountable obstacle. With proper training, equipment, and accommodations, people with vision impairment can lead independent, productive, joyful lives. The problem is that many individuals today do not receive the full complement of resources they need to overcome vision-related disability.

An important and immediate population health need is to bolster our ability as a nation to manage the rising challenge of chronic vision impairment. Despite enormous potential costs for individuals, caregivers, and society, chronic vision impairment receives little emphasis in most national and public health agendas focused on chronic conditions. Chronic vision impairment frequently co-occurs with, and may be a risk factor for, many comorbid conditions including other sensory impairments, depression, anxiety, and cognitive impairment. Comorbidities add to the challenge of living with and accommodating vision loss, and in turn, vision impairment complicates one's ability to manage other health conditions. Due to its prevalence and potential interference with other health domains, chronic vision impairment must not only receive greater attention as a chronic condition in its own right, but also be a part of all dialogues and action plans geared toward maximizing health and well-being in an aging society.

The primary goal of this Committee was to outline population health strategies to promote eye health and reduce vision impairment and its consequences in the United States. The ultimate objective is straight-forward: (1) no person should live with vision impairment that could have been avoided or could be treated and (2) every person with chronic vision impairment should have access to community and health services that minimize the impact of vision loss on overall health and life. Making this objective a reality will be complicated. It will require action from national, state, and local stakeholders. It will require practical changes to policies and systems as well as cultural changes that involve shifts in paradigms and ways of thinking.

This report represents the collective conclusions and recommendations of a diverse group of experts, each of whom brought their expertise and perspectives. The Committee recognizes and salutes the many devoted people across the nation already working tirelessly to promote eye and vision health and lessen the burden of vision impairment. This report emphasizes the need to address the underlying social and environmental conditions that contribute to unacceptable health disparities as well as to make quality clinical eye care and support services available to everyone. To accomplish this will take the concerted action of eye professionals, payers, clinical care systems, public health, and community organizations. We can eliminate preventable vision loss and ensure that each person with chronic vision impairment has every opportunity to live a full and productive life. We need to do so.

Steven M. Teutsch, *Chair*
Committee on Public Health Approaches to
Reduce Vision Impairment and Promote Eye Health

Summary

Avoidable vision impairment occurs too frequently in the United States and is the logical result of a series of outdated assumptions, missed opportunities, and manifold shortfalls in public health policy and health care delivery. Eyesight affects how human beings perceive and interpret the world and is used for everyday communication, social activities, educational and professional pursuits, the care of others, and the maintenance of personal health, independence, and mobility. Vision loss in adults is associated with increased risk of falls and injuries, social isolation, depression, and other psychological problems and can amplify the adverse effects of other chronic illnesses, increasing the risk for all-cause and injury-related mortality (Christ et al., 2014; Crews et al., 2016; Lam et al., 2008; Lee et al., 2003; Lord, 2006; McKean-Cowdin et al., 2007). Similarly, undiagnosed or uncorrected refractive errors and other visual disorders in children can lead to developmental, academic, and social challenges, and in some cases permanent vision loss, which has lifelong implications (Birch, 2013; Davidson and Quinn, 2011). Moreover, the economic and social costs of vision impairment and eye disease to patients, the health care system, and society are considerable (Koberlein et al., 2013; Wittenborn et al., 2013). Yet, as a chronic condition, vision impairment remains notably absent from many public health agendas and community programs. Rather, vision is often regarded as a given—until it is not.

The vast majority of individuals in the United States who reach average life expectancy are at risk for some form of vision loss and impairment during their lifetimes, given current knowledge about effective prevention strategies, injury rates, barriers to accessing appropriate health care, and the aging process itself. *Vision loss* can affect any one at any time. It is the process by which physiological changes or damage to the structure of the eye or visual information processing structures in the brain occurs, resulting in compromised subclinical or clinical function of the eye or visual processing system.[1] Vision loss may occur suddenly and completely, for example from injury, or may subtly evolve over time, with permanent structural damage leading to progressive changes in eye function until more pronounced deficits become noticeable. *Vision impairment*, defined in this report as a measure of the functional limitation of the eye or visual system that results from vision loss, remains an unmet and important public health threat and is largely attributable to a few conditions or diseases in the United States.

No reliable data exist on the number of people affected by all causes of vision impairment in the United States. One model, based on a review of 12 major epidemiological studies applied to the 2010 U.S. Census population, estimates that approximately 90 million of the 142 million adults over the age of 40 in the United States experienced vision problems attributable to vision impairment, blindness, refractive error (i.e., myopia and hyperopia), age-related macular degeneration (AMD),[2] cataracts, diabetic retinopathy, and glaucoma (Prevent Blindness, 2012).[3] Presbyopia, an age-related condition that affects the ability to focus clearly on near objects, affects almost everyone entering the middle-age years (Petrash, 2013). Other measures of eye and vision health have different but significant implications for broad population health strategies to reduce the burden of vision impairment. For example, *uncorrectable vision impairment* (i.e., the amount of vision impairment that remains after appropriate treatment or intervention) can range from mild to severe and affects an estimated 6.4 million people, including adults and children, in the United States.[4] *Uncorrected vision impairment* (i.e., the proportion of overall vision impairment that could be improved through currently available treatments) affects millions more people in the United States, with estimates for uncorrected refractive error alone ranging from 8.2 million (Varma et al., 2016) to 11.0 million (CDC,

---

[1] The committee adopted these definitions of vision loss and vision impairment to help facilitate discussion of eye and vision health in the context of population health. Justifications for these definitions are discussed in Chapter 1.

[2] The estimate for AMD includes individuals ages 50 and older.

[3] This statistic was corrected following release of the prepublication copy of the report.

[4] This figure was determined by combining the estimates of 4.24 million U.S. adults ages 40 and older (Varma et al., 2016) and 2.155 million U.S. children, adolescents, and young adults through age 39 (Wittenborn and Rein, 2013). Both studies define uncorrectable vision impairment and blindness separately and as a measure of visual acuity.

2015c) to 15.9 million (Wittenborn and Rein, 2016).[5] As the baby boomer generation ages, older adults will account for an ever larger proportion of the total population, and the prevalence of age-related eye diseases and conditions is projected to increase accordingly (Varma et al., 2016; Wittenborn and Rein, 2016). Actions to evaluate, monitor, and protect eye and vision health should begin early in life, but the systems and policies to encourage these behaviors in a fair and equitable manner are lacking.

The prevalence and impact of vision loss, as well as the severity of vision impairment, varies across geographic areas by etiology, age, race and ethnicity, and gender, putting certain populations at higher risk for specific types of vision loss (Congdon et al., 2004; Kirtland et al., 2015; Qiu et al., 2014; Zhang et al., 2012). The probability of vision impairment increases with age among all populations, particularly among people older than 60 years (Varma et al., 2016). Increased risk for poor eye health is also associated with social, economic, cultural, health, and environmental conditions, which further contribute to overall health disparities (Ulldemolins et al., 2012; Zambelli-Weiner et al., 2012; Zhang et al., 2012). Identifying populations at high risk for certain types of vision loss can help target limited resources, tailor effective interventions, and promote policies that better achieve eye and vision health and improve population health equity.

Some of the most notable successes in preventing vision loss have been anchored in population health strategies (CDC, 2015b; Kumaresan, 2005; Rao, 2015). Preventing vision-threatening injury, infection, and underlying chronic disease could have substantial effects on protecting or maintaining eye and vision health before treatment is needed. Promoting optimal conditions for eye and vision health can also alleviate many other social ills, including poverty, other health inequities, increasing health care costs, and avoidable mortality and morbidity (Christ et al., 2014; Kirtland et al., 2015; Lee et al., 2003; Rahi et al., 2009; Rein, 2013). Short- and long-term population health strategies should address broad determinants of health, including policies that influence individual behaviors, healthy environments and social conditions, and their potential impact on eye and vision health. Some strategies may be simpler and accomplished more quickly, such as

---

[5] The committee commissioned an analysis, which was not available in the current literature, to establish the preventable burden of vision impairment in the United States from five conditions (diabetic retinopathy, glaucoma, refractive error, cataracts, and AMD). Estimates are based on a variety of sources (including population surveys and compilations of population-based studies) and reflect the best available public data. The committee presents only the results related to cataracts and uncorrected refractive error in this report because the analyses are most robust for these conditions. Chapter 3 provides a more in-depth description of the study's assumptions and limitations, which are also documented in the commissioned paper itself (Wittenborn and Rein, 2016). This citation was added post release.

implementing policies that encourage using protective eyewear in hazardous work environments and during some recreational activities (CDC, 2013, 2015d; NEI/NIH, 2016). Other strategies will require more concerted and coordinated efforts to support social and built environments that promote eye-healthy behaviors or improved access to health care.

Early diagnosis and appropriate access to high-quality treatment could improve the trajectory of modifiable, correctable, and uncorrectable vision impairment by either slowing the progression of specific diseases or conditions, correcting the vision impairment itself, or improving the functionality, independence, and quality of life of populations with uncorrectable vision impairment. For example, estimates suggest that vision impairment caused by uncorrected refractive error and cataracts—both largely treatable— accounts for a substantial portion of undiagnosed vision impairment every year in the United States (CDC, 2015c; Wittenborn and Rein, 2016). Many public and private health insurance coverage policies, including Medicare, exclude eye examinations for initially asymptomatic or low-risk patients, corrective lenses, and visual assistive devices. Thus, in many cases, people must purchase additional vision insurance or shoulder costs out of pocket. Moreover, interventions exist to improve or maintain the functioning of people with vision impairment, but information about, and access to, these services is often limited (Overbury and Wittich, 2012; Pollard et al., 2003). These factors contribute to inequities that already affect populations with lower socioeconomic status and poor health (DeVoe et al., 2007; Levin et al., 2013).

Coordinated efforts are needed to expand public health capacities and to encourage policies and programmatic emphases that recognize improved eye and vision health as an important population health outcome and as a strategy to achieve better health equity. This will require federal and state support, coupled with public–private partnerships, to enhance local health department capabilities and energize other local institutions and organizations, families, and individuals to respond to community needs and goals (CDC, 2007).

This report proposes a population health action framework to guide action and coordination among various—and sometimes competing— stakeholders in pursuit of improved eye and vision health and health equity in the United States. This report also introduces a model for action that highlights different levels of prevention activities across a range of stakeholders and provides specific examples of how population health strategies can be translated into cohesive areas for action at federal, state, and local levels. Initial public- and private-sector investment has helped identify some of the chief information gaps and has led to a more nuanced understanding of the connection between eye and vision health and other measures of overall health, but more is needed. Implementing a coherent and comprehensive response to address vision loss will be challenging. Establishing conditions and policies that promote population eye and vision health and that minimize preventable and correctable vision impairment is an essential, timely, and achievable objective—one that is necessary to improve the overall quality of life, functioning, and productivity of individuals.

STATEMENT OF TASK AND REPORT OVERVIEW

In 2014, the Health and Medicine Division of the National Academies of Sciences, Engineering, and Medicine convened a multidisciplinary committee to "examine the core principles and public health strategies to reduce visual impairment and promote eye health in the United States," including short- and long-term strategies to prioritize eye and vision health through collaborative actions across a variety of topics, settings, community stakeholders, and levels of government. The committee reviewed the relevant literature and held five meetings, including two public workshops and one public session to obtain input from an array of experts and stakeholders. To further inform its deliberations, the committee also commissioned a paper on the costs and preventable burden of vision impairment for select eye conditions.

A POPULATION HEALTH APPROACH TO IMPROVE EYE AND VISION HEALTH

A population health approach involves multiple actors who work separately and cooperatively to "[focus] on interrelated conditions and factors that influence the health of populations over the life course, identif[y] systematic variations in their patterns of occurrence, and appl[y] the resulting knowledge to develop and implement policies and actions to improve the health and well-being of those populations" (Kindig and Stoddart, 2003, p. 380). The health of individuals and populations is affected by multiple determinants, including (1) individual traits; (2) behaviors; (3) social, family, and community networks; (4) living and working conditions; and (5) broad social, economic, cultural, health, and environmental conditions and policies, which are each part of larger social and physical environments (IOM, 2003a). Health care services are an important component of the "living and working conditions" that affect health. The vast majority of health determinants exists outside the clinical care delivery system (Braveman and Gottlieb, 2014; McGinnis et al., 2002), which provides a wide range of opportunities and environments in which to influence eye and vision health. As this report documents, eye and vision health is also affected by factors within each health determinant category. Figure S-1 provides an example of how multiple determinants of health could be used to target various factors

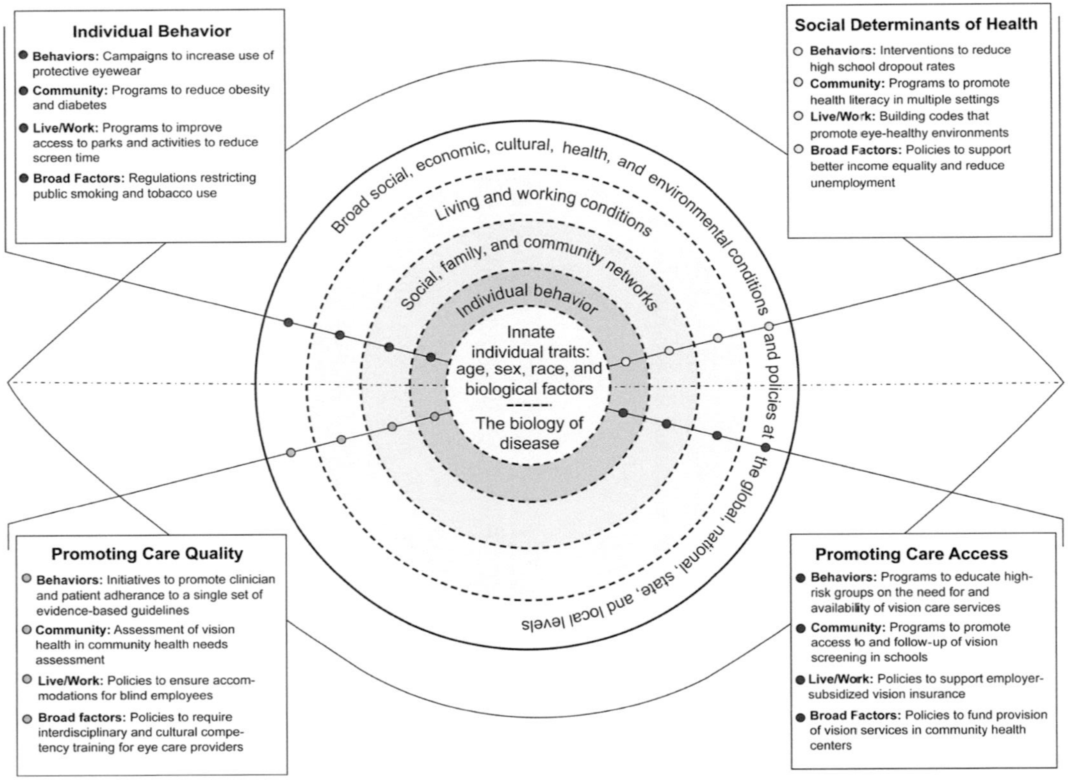

FIGURE S-1 Examples of factors that could be part of a population health approach to eye and vision health. SOURCE: Adapted from IOM, 2003a, p. 52.

within each health determinant category as part of a broad population health approach to improve eye and vision health. These targets, which are included in four separate boxes, include both risk and protective factors for vision loss. The inclusion of these targets should not be interpreted as a prioritization of relevant research topics or as a conclusion that individual targets are each supported by the same strength of evidence.

The three functions of a population health approach are assessment (i.e., monitoring communities to identify and characterize public health needs and priorities); policy development (i.e., the use of scientific evidence to guide the design and implementation of programs and policies to address public health issues); and assurance (i.e., policy development and enforcement, ensuring that health and public health systems have the resources to implement programs, and evaluating the health impacts of interventions) (CDC, 2007; IOM, 1988). In the context of eye and vision health and the committee's charge, these actions include short- and long-term strategies to address overarching determinants of health (primordial prevention) as well as efforts to support, educate, and promote healthy eye and vision behaviors (primary prevention); facilitate pre-symptomatic identification of eye diseases and treatments (secondary prevention); and preserve and enhance the health and functioning of individuals with vision impairment (tertiary prevention). Anchoring eye and vision health promotion in terms of the stages of prevention will allow the nation to reevaluate eye and vision health improvement more broadly as not only a valued outcome in and of itself, but also a potential public health tool to promote health equity among populations.

TRANSLATING A CONCEPTUAL FRAMEWORK INTO ACTION: RECOMMENDATIONS

The long-term goal of a population health approach for eye and vision health should be to transform vision impairment from a common to a rare condition, reducing associated health inequities. Given the genetic and biological components of many eye diseases and conditions, the occurrence of eye injuries, and the aging process itself, populations will never be without vision impairment. Nevertheless, this long-term goal establishes a new platform from which to identify important players, define influential behaviors, and allocate resources in a manner that will preserve and protect the eye and vision health of different populations.

Achieving the twin goals of improving eye and vision health and increasing health equity will require actions that reinforce each other. Figure S-2 identifies five core action areas that provide focus for the committee's recommendations and support the ultimate outcome—improved population eye and vision health and health equity. These actions should

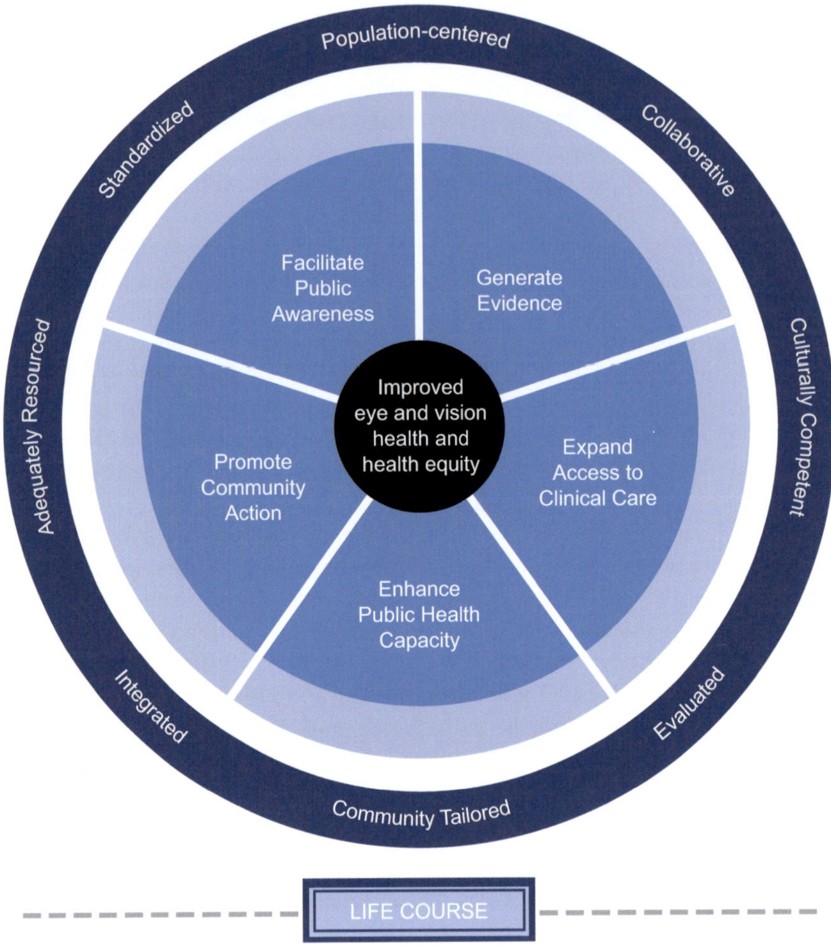

FIGURE S-2 Components of a population health model for action to improve eye and vision health across the lifespan.

be population-centered, collaborative, culturally competent, community-tailored, evidence-based, integrated, standardized, and adequately resourced. Many of the following nine recommendations are broadly framed but are critical to establish conditions that will support a sustainable population health initiative that will effectuate a long-term reduction in vision impairment and its ramifications. These recommendations provide the foundational support for other, more specific actions by stakeholder groups, as described throughout this report.

Facilitate Public Awareness Through Timely Access to Accurate and Locally Relevant Information

> The public should have accessible, transparent, and easily understood information about eye and vision health prevalence, incidence, and impact (on both an individual and community level) and also information about the stakeholders that influence eye and vision health locally and nationally.

According to a recent online poll, 88 percent of the 2,044 respondents surveyed identified good vision as vital to maintaining overall health, and 47 percent rated losing their vision compared to loss of limb, memory, hearing, or speech as "potentially having the greatest effect on their day-to-day life" (Scott et al., 2016, p. E3). Despite the public's perception of the importance of good vision, millions of people continue to grapple with undiagnosed or untreated vision impairment (CDC, 2015c; Varma et al., 2016; Wittenborn and Rein, 2016). Moreover, eye and vision health remain relatively absent from national health priority lists, including efforts to stem the impact of chronic diseases. A number of factors, including the segregation of eye care from the rest of medicine, fragmentation within the eye care community, and a lack of coordination within or across federal entities, contribute to the absence of focused and sustained programmatic investment that would translate into widespread action.

A Call to Action "is a science-based document to stimulate action nationwide to solve a major public health problem" (U.S. Surgeon General, n.d.). The U.S. Department of Health and Human Services (HHS), most often through the Office of the Surgeon General, uses calls to action to draw attention to important public health issues, such as promoting walkable communities and oral health, preventing skin cancer and suicide, improving the health and wellness of persons with disabilities, and reducing underage drinking (Surgeon General, n.d.). These documents, along with other reports, are often used to establish a baseline from which to measure improvement (e.g., Anstev et al., 2011; Mertz and Mouradian, 2009; U.S. Surgeon General, 2014). Vision loss and impairment qualify as public health problems in that they (1) affect a large number of people; (2) impose large morbidity, quality-of-life, and cost burdens; (3) are increasing in severity and are predicted to continue increasing; (4) are perceived by the public to be a threat; and (5) are feasibly addressed by community or public health-level interventions (CDC, 2009). Similarly, the NEI, the U.S. Preventive Services Task Force, and the World Health Organization have identified vision impairment in various populations as national or global public health problems (HHS, 2015; NEI/NIH, 2004; WHO, 2015).

Moreover, like other chronic diseases, most causes of vision impairment require ongoing management over the lifespan of an individual to maintain the activities of daily living. A call to action is needed to stimulate nation-wide discussion of eye and vision health as an essential health outcome and launch measured and directed actions that will reduce the burden of vision impairment in the United States.

<u>**Recommendation 1**</u>
The Secretary of the U.S. Department of Health and Human Services should issue a call to action to motivate nationwide action toward achieving a reduction in the burden of vision impairment across the lifespan of people in the United States. Specifically, this call to action should establish goals to:

- **Eliminate correctable and avoidable vision impairment by 2030,**
- **Delay the onset and progression of unavoidable chronic eye diseases and conditions,**
- **Minimize the impact of chronic vision impairment, and**
- **Achieve eye and vision health equity by improving care in underserved populations.**

Enhancing public knowledge about a health threat is a fundamental first step in informing discussions that promote behavior change across multiple determinants of health and aligning health policies with general public health interests. Unfortunately, lack of awareness of vision and eye health issues remains a major public health concern, especially in the context of linking patients to care and attempting to make population-level changes in behavior and health practice (Bailey et al., 2006; Zhang et al., 2012). Individuals are often unaware of what the most common risks to vision are, how the physiological progression of many eye diseases occurs, early signs of vision loss, and what steps can be taken to reduce the risk of vision-threatening eye disease, conditions, and events and the impact of subsequent vision loss (Alexander et al., 2008; Chou et al., 2014; Lam and Leat, 2015; NEI/LCIF, 2008; Varano et al., 2015). Combined with the asymptomatic nature of many eye diseases and conditions, this lack of awareness can have significant ramifications on overall health.

Although rarely adequate by themselves, public awareness campaigns can be an effective tool for improving knowledge about key messages related to health within populations (Bray et al., 2015; Oto et al., 2011) and are one essential part of an effective population health strategy. Achieving the goals outlined in recommendation 1 will require having reliable, consistent, evidence-based information that is available and accessible by a variety of stakeholders to increase overall knowledge and encourage policies, practices, and behaviors that promote good eye and vision health, support appropriate care to correct or slow progression of a vision-threatening disease or condition, or improve function when vision impairment is uncorrectable. This approach must target various audiences and consider a wide range of factors affecting eye and vision health in communities, including individual-directed strategies, mass media campaigns, and environmental and policy changes across multiple settings within defined geographic areas (e.g., city, state, province, or country).

<u>Recommendation 2</u>
The Secretary of the U.S. Department of Health and Human Services, in collaboration with other federal agencies and departments, nonprofit and for-profit organizations, professional organizations, employers, state and local public health agencies, and the media, should launch a coordinated public awareness campaign to promote policies and practices that encourage eye and vision health across the lifespan, reduce vision impairment, and promote health equity. This campaign should target various stakeholders, including the general population, care providers and caretakers, public health practitioners, policy makers, employers, and community and patient liaisons and representatives.

Generate Evidence to Guide Policy Decisions and Evidence-Based Actions

> Evidence-based decision making should guide population health actions. Without data, population health tools cannot characterize affected populations, identify risk and protective factors (including health care access), establish evidence-based guidelines, or quantify the effectiveness of health care systems and community-based interventions. True accountability requires good data, but less than perfect data should not be an excuse for inaction.

Vision impairment and blindness are appropriate targets for surveillance because they adversely affect a large portion of the population, affect populations unequally, can be improved by treatment and preventive efforts, and will become an increasing burden as the population ages (Saaddine et al., 2003). A comprehensive, nationally representative surveillance system for eye and vision health is needed to better understand the epidemiological patterns, risk factors, comorbidities, and costs associated with vision loss. Such data will allow health care professionals and public health decision makers to better characterize the nature and extent of the public health burden; risk factors and at-risk populations; disparities in access, care, and outcomes; and successful interventions (West and Lee, 2012).

<u>Recommendation 3</u>
The Centers for Disease Control and Prevention (CDC) should develop a coordinated surveillance system for eye and vision health in the United States. To advise and assist with the design of the system, the CDC should convene a task force comprising government, nonprofit and for-profit organizations, professional organizations, academic researchers, and the health care and public health sectors. The design of this system should include, but not be limited to:

- Developing and standardizing definitions for population-based studies, particularly definitions of clinical vision loss and functional vision impairment;
- Identifying and validating surveillance and quality-of-care measures to characterize vision-related outcomes, resources, and capacities within different communities and populations;
- Integrating eye-health outcomes, objective clinical measures, and risk/protective factors into existing clinical-health and population-health data collection forms and systems (e.g., chronic disease questionnaires, community health assessments, electronic health records, national and state health surveys, Medicare's health risk assessment, and databases); and
- Analyzing, interpreting, and disseminating information to the public in a timely and transparent manner.

Understanding the factors that affect the risk of vision impairment for different populations, the barriers to accessing care, interventions to prevent visual impairment and maintain eye function, and ways to improve the quality of care is fundamental to designing and identifying opportunities that minimize vision loss now and that will result in new knowledge and strategies to further reduce the long-term impact of vision impairment. HHS supports a number of federal programs and institutes that focus on vision loss and fund various activities to combat the effects of poor eye and vision health on at-risk populations (CDC, 2015a). Despite these activities, eye and vision health is insufficiently represented as a programmatic focus in federal government programs overall, and existing research programs lack coordination within and across federal agencies and institutes. Establishing a unified research agenda with larger financial and programmatic support to develop and advance knowledge about eye and vision health can maximize efficiencies and build on the strengths of established programs across a broad portfolio of topics and programs, which must include more than basic and clinical research.

<u>Recommendation 4</u>
The U.S. Department of Health and Human Services should create an interagency workgroup, including a wide range of public, private, and community stakeholders, to develop a common research agenda and coordinated eye and vision health research and demonstration grant programs that target the leading causes, consequences, and unmet needs of vision impairment. This research agenda should include, but not be limited to:

- Population-based epidemiologic and clinical research on the major causes and risks and protective factors for vision impairment, with a special emphasis on longitudinal studies of the major causes of vision impairment;
- Health services research, focused on patient-centered care processes, comparative-effectiveness and economic evaluation of clinical interventions, and innovative models of care delivery to improve access to appropriate diagnostics, follow-up treatment, and rehabilitation services, particularly among high-risk populations;
- Population health services research to reduce eye and vision health disparities, focusing on effective interventions that promote eye healthy environments and conditions, especially for underserved populations; and
- Research and development on emerging preventive, diagnostic, therapeutic, and treatment strategies and technologies, including efforts to improve the design and sensitivity of different screening protocols.

Expand Access to Appropriate Clinical Care

> Timely, appropriate, and equitable access to and delivery of effective care in all settings is an important component of a population health approach to improve eye and vision health. Inequitable barriers to effective treatments and therapies should be eliminated. Heightened attention is needed to reduce vision loss and cement its importance in relation to other chronic conditions and overall health.

Professional guidelines are an important tool for advancing policies and practices that promote high-quality care for everyone. They are often used to educate the public and public health and health care professionals and serve as foundational elements of value-driven payment policies and as baselines from which to measure quality improvement and enhanced accountability for care processes and patient health outcomes. No single set of clinical practice guidelines or measures in eye and vision care exists. Although eye and vision guidelines are consistent for the most part, there are some important differences. Differences may reflect the absence of robust data and political tensions within the field of eye and vision health. Available guidelines may provide inconsistent recommendations concerning essential measures, such as the frequency with which different age groups and at-risk populations should receive comprehensive eye exams[6] (e.g., AAO, 2015; AOA, 2015). Health insurance coverage for basic examinations, preventive services and treatments (including corrective lenses), and rehabilitation (including assistive devices) should reflect these guidelines. Particular attention needs to be paid to assuring that essential services and treatments are affordable, particularly for the most vulnerable populations.

<u>Recommendation 5</u>
The U.S. Department of Health and Human Services should convene one or more panels—comprising members of professional organizations, researchers, public health practitioners, patients, and other stakeholders— to develop a single set of evidence-based clinical and rehabilitation practice guidelines and measures that can be used by eye care professionals, other care providers, and public health professionals to prevent, screen for, detect, monitor, diagnose, and treat eye and vision problems. These guidelines and supporting evidence should be used to drive payment policies, including coverage determinations for corrective lenses and visual assistive devices following a diagnosed medical condition (e.g., refractive error).

To cultivate professional relationships and collaboration that advances eye and vision health across medicine and beyond clinical care, it is important to establish a set of common expertise that can align overarching objectives and action among health professionals. The CDC has noted the need to elevate ophthalmic education in medical curricula (CDC, 2007; Shah et al., 2014). With a greater focus on population health in clinical care (Berwick et al., 2008), new skills will be needed to ensure that health care professionals understand the types of patient experiences and data that are relevant to population health activities, including the moral imperative to reduce inequities in both health and health care. Moreover, public health practitioners should be familiar with eye and vision health, its risk factors, and the relationship between vision loss and other chronic health conditions. Translating this knowledge into meaningful patient interactions will

---

[6] The committee defines a comprehensive eye examination as a dilated eye examination that may include a series of other tests, in addition to the dilation of the pupil.

require cultivating trust among different patient populations, providers, and public health practitioners.

<u>Recommendation 6</u>
To enable the health care and public health workforce to meet the eye care needs of a changing population and to coordinate responses to vision-related health threats, professional education programs should proactively recruit and educate a diverse workforce and incorporate prevention and detection of visual impairments, population health, and team care coordination as part of core competencies in applicable medical and professional education and training curricula. Individual curricula should emphasize proficiency in culturally competent care for all populations.

Enhance Public Health Capacities to Support Vision-Related Activities

---

Eye and vision health is a critical part of population health and a valuable public health tool with which to assess the quality, effectiveness, and efficiencies of health care systems and population health programs and initiatives. Improving eye and vision health requires that comparable services, information, and healthy environments are accessible to all populations. Public health departments serve as key community conveners to coordinate responses that address multiple determinants of health and chronic conditions, such as vision impairment.

Integrating public health and local health care systems is an important strategy for improving community health (CDC, 2007). A well-functioning medical care system can expand delivery of appropriate eye and vision care services, allowing public health agencies to focus on preventive policies and action and assurance. Such preventive actions include linking people to needed care, assessing care quality, and promoting community support and policy and environmental conditions that maximize health (IOM, 2003b). Public health agencies and departments can also extend the reach of health care services through vision-specific programs. There has been insufficient partnering to coordinate existing and emerging programs, policies, and quality improvement activities that either directly or indirectly influence eye and vision health.

<u>Recommendation 7</u>
State and local public health departments should partner with health care systems to align public health and clinical practice objectives, programs, and strategies about eye and vision health to:

- Enhance community health needs assessments, surveys, health impact assessments, and quality improvement metrics;
- Identify and eliminate barriers within health care and public health systems to eye care, especially comprehensive eye exams, appropriate screenings and follow-up services, and items and services intended to improve the functioning of individuals with vision impairment;
- Include public health and clinical expertise related to eye and vision health on oversight committees, advisory boards, expert panels, and staff, as appropriate;
- Encourage physicians and health professionals to ask and engage in discussions about eye and vision health as part of patients' regular office visits; and
- Incorporate eye health and chronic vision impairment into existing quality improvement, injury and infection control, and behavioral change programs related to comorbid chronic conditions, community health, and the elimination of health disparities.

Local public health departments are designed to promote health across a wide range of policies, activities, programs, and efforts to improve accountability. In the face of declining public investment, current state and local public health agencies and departments struggle to meet state mandates and requirements (Jacobson et al., 2015). Public health strategies to promote eye and vision health are rarely supported as a categorical focus or even as part of chronic disease programs in state and local health departments due to limitations in resources and other shifting priorities. Moreover, flexibility in how state and local governments use federal grant funds varies (CBO, 2013). In the absence of federal directives and programs to advance eye and vision health, state and local public health departments are hard pressed to incorporate reduction of vision impairment as a categorical programmatic focus.

<u>Recommendation 8</u>
To build state and local public health capacity, the Centers for Disease Control and Prevention should prioritize and expand its vision grant program, in partnership with state-based chronic disease programs and other clinical and nonclinical stakeholders, to:

- Design, implement, and evaluate programs for the primary prevention of conditions leading to visual impairment, including policies to reduce eye injuries;
- Develop and evaluate policies and systems that facilitate access to, and utilization of, patient-centered vision care and rehabilitation services, including integration and coordination among care providers; and
- Develop and evaluate initiatives to improve environments and socioeconomic conditions that underpin good eye and vision health and reduce eye injuries in communities.

Promote Community Actions That Encourage Eye- and Vision-Healthy Environments

> Eye and vision health is affected by a wide range of health determinants within communities, including individual and collective behaviors, the built environment, social conditions, and the health care system. Populations should participate collectively in decision making about population health priorities, which affect and are affected by the eye and vision health of their communities.

Eye and vision health is a community issue—the needs, adequacy of resources, and priorities will vary based on population characteristics, cultures, and values. The impact that vision loss has on function and quality of life varies according to numerous factors, including the built environment, social support, access to health care and rehabilitation services, attitude, preferences, and socioeconomic factors. How these factors affect the occurrence, severity, and impact of vision loss differs for individuals and communities. It is important that community stakeholders (businesses, advocacy organizations, neighborhood groups, local health and public health departments, religious organizations, professional organizations, school boards and faculty, parent support groups, health care providers, eye care providers, etc.) be actively consulted and engaged in options to translate and implement national goals into workable community action plans to reduce the burden of vision loss and the functioning of populations with vision impairment across different community settings.

Recommendation 9
Communities should work with state and local health departments to translate a broad national agenda to promote eye and vision health into well-defined actions. These actions should encourage policies and conditions that improve eye and vision health and foster environments to minimize the

impact of vision impairment, considering the community's needs, resources, and cultural identity. These actions should:

- Improve eye and vision health awareness among different social groups within communities;
- Engage community organizations and groups to promote eye and vision health awareness in daily activities;
- Establish and enforce laws and policies intended to promote eye safety and the functioning of people with vision impairment;
- Identify the need for, and community-level barriers to, vision-related services and resources in their communities; and
- Adopt policies and create community networks that support the design of built environments and the establishment of social environments that promote eye and vision health and independent functioning.

REFERENCES

AAO (American Academy of Ophthalmology). 2015. *Policy statement: Frequency of ocular examinations.* San Francisco, CA: AAO.

Alexander, Jr., R. L., N. A. Miller, M. F. Cotch, and R. Janiszewski. 2008. Factors that influence the receipt of eye care. *American Journal of Health Behavior* 32(5):547.

Anstev, E. H., C. A. MacGowan, and J.A. Allen. 2011. Five-year progress update on the Surgeon General's call to action to support breastfeeding. *Journal of Women's Health* 25(8):768–776.

AOA (American Optometric Association). 2015. Comprehensive eye and vision examination. http://www.aoa.org/patients-and-public/caring-for-your-vision/comprehensive-eye-and-vision-examination?sso=y (accessed March 29, 2016).

Bailey, R. N., R. W. Indian, X. Zhang, L. S. Geiss, M. R. Duenas, and J. B. Saaddine. Visual impairment and eye care among older adults–five states, 2005. 2006. *Morbidity Mortality Weekly Report* 55(49):1321–1325.

Berwick, D. M., T. W. Nolan, and J. Whittington. 2008. The triple aim: Care, health, and cost. *Health Affairs* 27(8):759–769.

Birch, E. E. 2013. Amblyopia and binocular vision. *Progress in Retinal and Eye Research* 33:67–84.

Braveman, P., and L. Gottlieb. 2014. The social determinants of health: It's time to consider the causes of the causes. *Public Health Reports* 129(Suppl 2):9–31.

Bray, J. E., L. Straney, B. Barger, and J. Finn. 2015. Effect of public awareness campaigns on calls to ambulance across Australia. *Stroke* 46(5):1377–1380.

CBO (Congressional Budget Office). 2013. Federal grants to state and local governments. Washington, DC: CBO.

CDC (Centers for Disease Control and Prevention). 2007. *Improving the nation's vision health: A coordinated public health approach.* Atlanta, GA: CDC.

———. 2009. Why is vision loss a public health problem? http://www.cdc.gov/visionhealth/basic_information/vision_loss.htm (accessed October 7, 2015).

———. 2013. Eye safety. http://www.cdc.gov/niosh/topics/eye (accessed March 30, 2016).

———. 2015a. About us. http://www.cdc.gov/visionhealth/about/index.htm (accessed March 30, 2016).

———. 2015b. Conjunctivitis (pink eye) in newborns. http://www.cdc.gov/conjunctivitis/newborns.html (accessed March 30, 2016).

———. 2015c. National data. http://www.cdc.gov/visionhealth/data/national.htm (accessed March 30, 2016).

———. 2015d. The work-related injury statistics query system. http://wwwn.cdc.gov/wisards/workrisqs (accessed April 4, 2016).

Chou, C. F., C. E. Sherrod, X. Zhang, L. E. Barker, K. M. Bullard, J. E. Crews, and J. B. Saaddine. 2014. Barriers to eye care among people aged 40 years and older with diagnosed diabetes, 2006–2010. *Diabetes Care* 37(1):180–188.

Christ, S. L., D. Zheng, B. K. Swenor, B.L. Lam, S. K. West, S. L. Tannenbaum, B. E. Munoz, and D. J. Lee. 2014. Longitudinal relationships among visual acutiy, daily functional status, and mortality: The Salisbury Eye Evaluation Study. *Journal of Ophthalmology.* 132(12):1400–1406.

Congdon, N., B. O'Colmain, C. C. Klaver, R. Klein, B. Munoz, D. S. Friedman, J. Kempen, H. R. Taylor, and P. Mitchell. 2004. Causes and prevalence of visual impairment among adults in the United States. *Archives of Ophthalmology* 122(4):477–485.

Crews, J. E., C.-F. Chiu-Fung Chou, J. A. Stevens, and J. B. Saadine. 2016. Falls among persons aged > 65 years with and without severe vision impairment—United States, 2014. *Morbidity and Mortality Weekly Report* 65(17):433–437.

Davidson, S., and G. E. Quinn. 2011. The impact of pediatric vision disorders in adulthood. *Pediatrics* 127(2):334–339.

DeVoe, J. E., A. Baez, H. Angier, L. Krois, C. Edlund, and P. A. Carney. 2007. Insurance + access ≠ health care: Typology of barriers to health care access for low-income families. *Annals of Family Medicine* 5(6):511–518.

HHS (U.S. Department of Health and Human Services). 2015. Healthy people 2020 topics and objectives: Vision. http://www.healthypeople.gov/2020/topics-objectives/topic/vision (accessed October 7, 2015).

IOM (Institute of Medicine). 1988. *The future of public health.* Washington, DC: National Academy Press.

———. 2003a. *The future of the public's health in the 21st century.* Washington, DC: The National Academies Press.

———. 2003b. *Unequal treatment: Confronting racial and ethnic disparities in health care.* Washington, DC: The National Academies Press.

Jacobson, P. D., J. Wasserman, H. W. Wu, and J. R. Lauer. 2015. Assessing entrepreneurship in governmental public health. *American Journal of Public Health* 105(S2):S318–S322.

Kindig, D., and G. Stoddart. 2003. What is population health? *American Journal of Public Health* 93(3):380–383.

Kirtland, K. A., J. B. Saaddine, L. S. Geiss, Thompson, T. J., Cotch, M. F., and Lee, P. P. 2015. Geographic disparity of severe vision loss—United States, 2009–2013. *Morbidity and Mortality Weekly Report* 64(19):513–517.

Koberlein, J., K. Beifus, C. Schaffert, and R. P. Finger. 2013. The economic burden of visual impairment and blindness: A systematic review. *British Medical Journal Open* 3: 1–14.

Kumaresan, J. 2005. Can blinding trachoma be eliminated by 20/20? *Eye* 19(10):1067–1073.

Lam, B. L., S. L. Christ, D. J. Lee, D. D. Zheng, and K. L. Arheart. 2008. Reported visual impairment and risk of suicide: The 1986–1996 National Health Interview Surveys. *Archives of Ophthalmology* 126(7):975–980.

Lam, N., and S. J. Leat. 2015. Reprint of: Barriers to accessing low-vision care: The patient's perspective. *Canadian Journal of Ophthalmology/Journal Canadien d'Ophtalmologie* 50:S34–S39.

Lee, D. J., O. Gomez-Marin, B. L. Lam, and D. D. Zheng. 2003. Visual impairment and unintentional injury mortality: The National Health Interview Survey 1986–1994. *American Journal of Ophthalmology* 136(6):1152–1154.

Levin, A. V., L. T. Pizzi, M. Snitzer, and K. M. Prioli. 2013. Barriers to follow up care in children with vision diseases: Development of a conceptual framework and parent/caregiver survey through the children's eye care adherence project. *Value in Health* 16(3):A38.

Lord, S. R. 2006. Visual risk factors for falls in older people. *Age and Ageing* 35(Suppl 2): ii42–ii45.

McGinnis, J. M., P. Williams-Russo, and J. R. Knickman. 2002. The case for more active policy attention to health promotion. *Health Affairs* 21(2):78–93.

McKean-Cowdin, R., R. Varma, J. Wu, R. D. Hays, S. P. Azen, for the Los Angeles Latino Eye Study Group. 2007. Severity of vision field loss and health-related quality of life. *American Journal of Ophthalmology* 143(6):1013–1023.

Mertz, E., and W. Mouradian. 2009. Addressing children's oral health in the new millennium: Trends in the dental workforce. *Academic Pediatrics* 9(6):433.

NEI/LCIF (National Eye Institute/Lions Club International Foundation). 2008. 2005 survey of public knowledge, attitudes, and practices related to eye health and disease. https:// nei.nih.gov/kap (accessed October 7, 2015).

NEI/NIH (National Eye Institute/National Institutes of Health). 2004. Vision statement and mission—National plan for eye and vision research [NEI strategic planning]. https://nei nih.gov/strategicplanning/np_vision (accessed February 4, 2016).

———. 2016. About sports eye injury and protective eyewear. https://nei.nih.gov/sports (accessed February 12, 2016).

Oto, M. A., O. Ergene, L. Tokgozoglu, Z. Ongen, O. Kozan, M. Sahin, M. K. Erol, T. Tezel, and M. Ozkan. 2011. Impact of a mass media campaign to increase public awareness of hypertension. *Turk Kardiyoloji Dernegi Ars* 39(5):355–364.

Overbury, O., and W. Wittich. 2012. Barriers to low vision rehabilitation: The Montreal Barriers Study. 2011. *Investigative Ophthalmology & Visual Science* 52(12):8933–8938.

Petrash, J. M. 2013. Aging and age-related diseases of the ocular lens and vitreous body. *Investigative Ophthalmology & Visual Science* 54(14):ORSF54–ORSF59.

Pollard, T. L., J. A. Simpson, E. L. Lamoureux, and J. E. Keefe. 2003. Barriers to accessing low vision sevices. *Ophthalmic and Phsyiological Optics* 23(4):321–327.

Prevent Blindness. 2012. Vision problems in the U.S. http://www.visionproblemsus.org (accessed June 5, 2016).

Qiu, M., S. Y. Wang, K. Singh, and S. C. Lin. 2014. Racial disparities in uncorrected and undercorrected refractive error in the United States. *Investigative Ophthalmology & Visual Science* 55(10):6996–7005.

Rahi, J. S., P. M. Cumberland, and C. S. Peckham. 2009. Visual function in working-age adults: Early life influences and associations with health and social outcomes. *Ophthalmology* 116(10):1866–1871.

Rao, G. 2015. The Barrie Jones Lecture—Eye care for the neglected population: Challenges and solutions. *Eye* 29(1):30–45.

Rein, D. B. 2013. Vision problems are a leading source of modifiable health expenditures. *Investigative Ophthalmology & Visual Science* 54(14):ORSF18–ORSF22.

Saaddine, J. B., K. Venkat Narayan, and F. Vinicor. 2003. Vision loss: A public health problem? *Ophthalmology* 110(2):253–254.

Scott, A. W., N. M. Bressler, S. Ffolkes, J. S. Wittenborn, J. Jorkavsky. 2016. Public attitudes about eye and vision health. *JAMA Ophthalmology* 134(10):1111–1118.

Shah, M., D. Knoch, and E. Waxman. 2014. The state of ophthalmology medical student education in the United States and Canada, 2012 through 2013. *Ophthalmology* 121(6):1160–1163.

Ulldemolins, A. R., V. C. Lansingh, L. Guisasola Valencia, M. J. Carter, K. A. Eckert. 2012. Social inequalities in blindness and visual impairment: A review of social determinants. *Indian Journal of Ophthalmology* 60(5):368–375.

U.S. Surgeon General. 2014. *The health consequences of smoking—50 years of progress: A report of the Surgeon General, 2014.* Rockville, MD: U.S. Department of Health and Human Services.

———. n.d. Surgeon General's Calls to Action. http://www.surgeongeneral.gov/library/calls (accessed August 23, 2016).

Varano, M., N. Eter, S. Winyard, K. U. Wittrup-Jensen, R. Navarro, and J. Heraghty. 2015. Current barriers to treatment for wet age-related macular degeneration (WAMD): Findings from the WAMD patient and caregiver survey. *Journal of Clinical Ophthalmology* 9:2243–2250.

Varma, R., T. S. Vajaranant, B. Burkemper, S. Wu, M. Torres, C. Hsu, F. Choudhury, R. McKean-Cowdin. 2016. Visual impairment and blindness in adults in the United States: Demographic and geographic variations from 2015 to 2050. *JAMA Ophthalmology*. May 19 [Epub ahead of print].

West, S. K., and P. Lee. 2012. Vision surveillance in the United States: Has the time come? *American Journal of Ophthalmology* 154(6):S1–S2, e2.

WHO (World Health Organization). 2015. Blindness: Vision 2020—the global initiative for the elimination of avoidable blindness. http://www.who.int/mediacentre/factsheets/fs213/en (accessed October 7, 2015).

Wittenborn, J., and D. Rein. 2013. *Cost of vision problems: The economic burden of vision loss and eye disorders in the United States.* New York: Prevent Blindness America.

———. 2016. *The potential costs and benefits of treatment for undiagnosed eye disorders.* Paper prepared for the Committee on Public Health Approaches to Reduce Vision Impairment and Promote Eye Health. http://www.nationalacademies.org/hmd/~/media/Files/Report%20Files/2016/UndiagnosedEyeDisordersCommissionedPaper.pdf (accessed September 15, 2016).

Wittenborn, J. S., X. Zhang, C. W. Feagan, W. L. Crouse, S. Shrestha, A. R. Kemper, T. J. Hoerger, and J. B. Saaddine. 2013. The economic burden of vision loss and eye disorders among the United States population younger than 40 years. *Ophthalmology* 120(9):1728–1735.

Zambelli-Weiner, A., J. E. Crews, D. S. Friedman. 2012. Disparities in adult vision health in the United States. *American Journal of Ophthalmology* 154(Suppl):S23–S30, e1.

Zhang, X., M. F. Cotch, A. Ryskulova, S. A. Primo, P. Nair, C.-F. Chou, L. S. Geiss, L. Barker, A. F. Elliott, J. E. Crews, and J. B. Saaddine. 2012. Vision health disparities in the United States by race/ethnicity, education, and economic status: Findings from two nationally representative surveys. *American Journal of Ophthalmology* 154(6 Suppl):S53–S62, e51.

1

Introduction

Avoidable vision impairment occurs too frequently in the United States and is the logical result of a series of outdated assumptions, missed opportunities, and manifold shortfalls in public health policy and health care delivery. The ability to see affects how human beings perceive and interpret the world. The sense of sight is critically important to an individual's communication, physical health, independence and mobility, social engagement, educational and employment opportunities, socioeconomic status, and performance of daily activities, such as reading, driving a car, and caring for family members (Alberti et al., 2014; Bowers et al., 2009; Bronstad et al., 2013; Brown et al., 2014; Rahi et al., 2009; Sengupta et al., 2014; Whitson et al., 2007, 2014; Wood et al., 2012). Uncorrectable vision impairment can lead to a progressive inability to participate in family, social, and community activities and is associated with a higher prevalence of chronic health conditions, death, falls and injuries, social isolation, depression, and other psychological problems (Court et al., 2014; Crewe et al., 2013; Crews et al., 2016a,b; Kulmala et al., 2008, 2012; Lord, 2006; Rees et al., 2010; van Landingham et al., 2014). In early childhood, any condition that prevents an eye from focusing clearly (e.g., misalignment of the eyes, pronounced differences in refractive error between the two eyes, or obstruction or deformation of the light into the eye) may result in physiological alterations to the visual pathway that can lead to ongoing visual impairments (Birch, 2013; Davidson and Quinn, 2011). This can significantly affect an infant's or child's development and health, restricting participation in social, physical, and educational activities and, later, employment opportunities (Davidson and Quinn, 2011).

Vision loss,[1] the process by which physiological changes or damage to the structure of the eye or visual information processing structures in the brain occurs, results in compromised subclinical or clinical function of the eye or visual processing system. Vision loss may occur suddenly and completely, for example from injury, or may subtly evolve over time, with permanent structural damage leading to progressive changes in eye function until more pronounced deficits become noticeable. *Vision impairment,* defined in this report as a measure of the functional limitation of the eye or visual system that results from vision loss, remains an unmet and important public health threat and is largely attributable to a few conditions or diseases in the United States.

No reliable data exist on the number of people affected by all causes of vision impairment in the United States. One model, based on a review of 12 major epidemiological studies and the 2010 U.S. Census population, estimates that approximately 90 million of the 142 million adults over the age of 40 in the United States experienced vision problems attributable to vision impairment, blindness, refractive error (i.e., myopia and hyperopia), age-related macular degeneration (AMD),[2] cataract, diabetic retinopathy, and glaucoma (Prevent Blindness, 2012a).[3] Refractive error alone affected more than 48 million people over age 12 in the United States (Prevent Blindness, 2012c). Presbyopia, an age-related condition that affects the ability to focus clearly on near objects, affects almost everyone entering the middle-age years (Petrash, 2013). As demographic trends change (i.e., the "silver tsunami") in the United States, the prevalence of all forms of vision impairment is also projected to increase (Varma et al., 2016). Actions to evaluate, monitor, and protect eye and vision health should begin early in life, but the systems and policies to encourage these behaviors in a fair and equitable manner are lacking.

The prevalence of vision loss, as well as the severity of subsequent vision impairment, varies across geographic areas by etiology, age, race and ethnicity, and gender, putting certain populations at higher risk for specific types of vision loss (Congdon et al., 2004; Kirtland et al., 2015; Qiu et al., 2014; Zhang et al., 2012). Increased risk for poor eye and vision health is also associated with broader social, economic, cultural, health, and environmental conditions, which may contribute to greater overall health disparities (Cumberland et al., 2016; Ulldemolins et al., 2012; Zambelli-Weiner et al., 2012; Zhang et al., 2012). Conversely, the promotion of

---

[1] The committee adopted these definitions of vision loss and vision impairment to help facilitate discussion of eye and vision health in the context of population health. Justifications for these definitions are discussed in this chapter.

[2] The estimate for AMD includes individuals age 50 and older.

[3] This statistic was corrected following release of the prepublication copy of the report.

eye and vision health may positively influence many other social ailments, including poverty, increasing health care costs, and avoidable mortality and morbidity (Christ et al., 2014; Kirtland et al., 2015; Lee, 2003; Rahi et al., 2009; Rein, 2013). Identifying high-risk populations for certain types of vision loss can help target limited resources, tailor effective interventions, and promote policies that better achieve eye and vision health and improve population health equity.

The economic impact of chronic vision loss on individuals and society is substantial. One national study commissioned by Prevent Blindness found that direct medical expenses, other direct expenses, loss of productivity and other indirect costs for visual disorders across all age groups were approximately $139 billion in 2013 dollars (Wittenborn and Rein, 2013), with direct costs for the under-40 population reaching $14.5 billion dollars (Wittenborn et al., 2013). Time spent by caregivers also increases substantially as vision decreases, averaging between 5.8 hours per week and 94.1 hours per week for persons with vision impairment, depending on the severity of vision loss (Köberlein et al., 2013). Moreover, chronic vision loss can amplify the adverse effects of other chronic illnesses and is associated with an increased risk for all-cause and injury-related mortality (Christ et al., 2014; Crews et al., 2006; Lee et al., 2002, 2003). Yet as a chronic condition, vision impairment is rarely supported as a categorical focus or even as part of chronic disease programs (e.g., a single eye health metric) in most state and local health departments because of resource limitations and competing priorities.

Some of the most notable successes in preventing vision loss have been anchored in population health strategies (e.g., CDC, 2015b; Kumaresan, 2005; Rao, 2015). Preventing injury, infection, and underlying chronic disease could have substantial effects on protecting or maintaining eye and vision health. For example, estimates suggest implementing policies that better encourage the use of protective eyewear could reduce work- and sports-related eye injuries by as much as 90 percent (Dang, 2016). Similarly, programs designed to reduce the prevalence of diabetes would also necessarily reduce the prevalence and incidence of diabetic retinopathy.

Early diagnosis and appropriate access to high-quality treatment could improve the trajectory of modifiable or correctable vision impairment by either slowing the progression of specific diseases or conditions or correcting the vision impairment itself. *Uncorrected vision impairment* (i.e., the proportion of overall vision impairment that could be improved through currently available treatments) may represent the clearest opportunity to improve eye and vision health in the United States based on current knowledge and the relative effectiveness of specific treatments. Millions of people over the age of 12 years live with uncorrected refractive error in the United States, with estimates ranging anywhere from 8.2 million (Varma et al.,

2016) to 11.0 million (CDC, 2015d) to 15.9 million (Wittenborn and Rein, 2016).[4] Similarly, cataracts are largely treatable, yet vision impairment from uncorrected cataracts remains problematic, especially for certain minority populations (Shahbazi et al., 2015; Sommer et al., 1991; Wittenborn and Rein, 2016). Programs and payment policies targeting access to appropriate screenings, comprehensive eye examinations,[5] and follow-up care (including coverage of corrective lenses) could improve eye and vision health, especially among populations with lower economic status and poor health.

Uncorrectable vision impairment (i.e., the amount of vision impairment that remains after appropriate treatment or intervention)[6] affects approximately 4.2 million adults over the age of 40 (Prevent Blindness, 2012a; Varma et al., 2016) and another 2.155 million children and adults under age 39 each year in the United States (Wittenborn et al., 2013).[7] Prevalence in the over-40 population is projected to rise to 8.96 million by 2050, as demographic trends change (i.e., the coming of the "silver tsunami") in the United States (Varma et al., 2016). Information about, and access to, interventions that can improve or maintain the function of people with vision impairment are often limited (Overbury and Wittich, 2011; Walter et al., 2004). Population health approaches targeting uncorrectable vision impairment often focus on improving functionality, productivity, and independence through access to visual assistive devices, vision rehabilitation services, and reasonable accommodations—although earlier access to effective treatments may prevent the progression of modifiable to uncorrectable vision impairment for certain conditions and diseases.

This report proposes a conceptual framework to advance eye and vision health as a population health priority among various—and sometimes competing—stakeholders in pursuit of improved eye and vision health

---

[4] The committee commissioned an analysis, which was not available in the current literature, to establish the preventable burden of vision impairment in the United States from five conditions (diabetic retinopathy, glaucoma, refractive error, cataracts, and AMD). Estimates are based on a variety of sources (including population surveys and compilations of population-based studies) and reflect the best available public data. The committee presents only the results related to cataracts and uncorrected refractive error in this report because the analyses are most robust for these conditions. Chapter 3 provides a more in-depth description of the study's assumptions and limitations, which are also documented in the commissioned paper itself (Wittenborn and Rein, 2016). This citation was added post release.

[5] For this report, the committee defines a comprehensive eye examination as a dilated eye examination that may include other tests.

[6] Uncorrectable vision impairment is often defined in terms of visual acuity (e.g., Prevent Blindness, 2012b; Varma et al., 2016).

[7] These figures combine estimates for vision impairment and blindness. Each of these studies defines vision impairment and blindness separately and in terms of visual acuity in the best corrected and better seeing eye (Prevent Blindness, 2012b; Varma et al., 2016, p. E3; Wittenborn and Rein, 2016).

and health equity in the United States. This report also introduces a model for action that highlights different activities that a range of stakeholders must undertake and provides specific examples of how population health strategies can be translated into cohesive action at federal, state, and local levels. Initial public- and private-sector investment has helped identify the chief information gaps and provided a more nuanced understanding of the connection between eye and vision health and other measures of overall health, but more is needed. Implementing a coherent and comprehensive response to address the burden of vision loss will be challenging, but it is achievable.

STATEMENT OF TASK AND SCOPE OF STUDY

In 2014, the Centers for Disease Control and Prevention (CDC) and the National Eye Institute (NEI), along with the American Academy of Ophthalmology, the American Academy of Optometry, the American Optometric Association, the Association for Research in Vision and Ophthalmology, the National Alliance for Eye and Vision Research, the National Center for Children's Vision and Eye Health, Prevent Blindness, and Research to Prevent Blindness asked the National Academies of Sciences, Engineering, and Medicine to conduct a consensus study on the current and potential roles of public health in addressing the burden of blindness and vision impairment, and the conditions, diseases, and injuries that cause them. Specifically, the Committee on Public Health Approaches to Reduce Vision Impairment and Promote Eye Health was asked to characterize the public health burden of major eye diseases, as well as the state of surveillance systems used to measure this burden; to examine existing models of vision care and eye disease prevention; to identify evidence-based health promotion interventions for vision care and encourage their development and utilization; and to develop strategies to promote collaboration among stakeholders in vision care in order to reduce the burden of low vision through the coordinated deployment of public health resources (see Box 1-1).

To respond to this task, the National Academies convened a committee of 15 experts with experience in population health and epidemiology, ophthalmology, optometry, health economics, gerontology, pediatrics, health disparities and behaviors, health law and policy, public policy and public–private partnerships, consumer and research advocacy, vision rehabilitation, and the care of complex, chronic disability (see Appendix A for the committee biographies). In addition to reviewing relevant literature, the committee held five meetings, including two public workshops and one public session (see Appendix B for the workshop agendas) to obtain input from an array of experts and stakeholders who informed the committee's deliberations and final report. Throughout the course of this study, report

---

BOX 1-1
Statement of Task for the Committee on
Public Health Approaches to Reduce Vision
Impairment and Promote Eye Health

The Institute of Medicine will conduct a consensus study to examine the core principles and public health strategies to reduce visual impairment and promote eye health in the United States. The study will describe limitations and opportunities to improve vision and eye health surveillance; reduce vision and eye health disparities; promote evidence-based strategies to improve knowledge, access, and utilization to eye care; identify comorbid conditions and characterize their impact; and promote health for people with vision impairment. The study will also examine the potential for public and private collaborations at the community, state, and national levels to elevate vision and eye health as a public health issue.

Specifically, the committee will examine and make recommendations on the following:

- **Characterizing the Public Health Burden.** Describe and characterize the public health significance of eye disease (e.g., glaucoma, macular degeneration, diabetic retinopathy, and cataract) and vision loss, and the relationship between vision loss and quality of life, health disparities, and comorbid conditions. Identify opportunities to improve surveillance, monitoring, and data integration strategies and to define metrics to support a more accurate assessment of the public health burden of eye diseases and vision loss.
- **Prevention and Care.** Explore innovative models of care, innovative technologies, their application to eye disease/vision impairment detection and management, as well as barriers to their development and use. Examine and explore current and future areas of research on public health interventions that target prevention; access to, and utilization of, vision and eye care; and improved patient outcomes.
- **Evidence-Based Health Promotion Interventions.** Identify strategies to develop, test, and encourage the implementation of health promotion interventions that are evidence based for people with vision impairment.
- **Eye Health and Vision Loss as a Public Health Priority.** Categorize and discuss the possible short- and long-term collaborative strategies to promote vision and eye health as a public health priority, including (1) the role of public–private partnerships (e.g., improving public awareness; improving vision and eye care through federal, state, and community-based partnerships, and enhancing professional education); (2) the role of federal government and state and local communities in integrating vision and eye health interventions into existing public health programs (including systems and policy changes that support vision and eye health) that are both implementable and sustainable; and (3) engagement of key national partners to form collaborations for research, service delivery, outreach, and community-based studies to successfully improve access and quality to vision and eye care.

sponsors provided substantial cooperation, support, and responsiveness as the committee sought additional information for its deliberations.

Given the broad range of activities and partnerships explicitly mentioned in its charge, the wide array of current practices in eye care delivery, and the range of factors that can influence eyesight, the committee interpreted its statement of task as requesting it to target "population health" approaches, and the committee uses this term throughout this report. The term "public health," which is often interpreted as being restricted to the actions of federal, state, and local health departments, is used in the context of governmental public health agencies.

It is important to note that the committee was not charged with defining appropriate scope of practice for various eye care professionals or endorsing specific clinical practice guidelines for various diseases and conditions. The report discusses these topics only in the context of needing consensus when ambiguity or inconsistency affects clear communication and makes it unclear what care should be provided, when, and by whom. The topic is also discussed when identifying key areas where additional evidence is needed.

CORE PRINCIPLES

To respond to its statement of task and anchor its analysis, the committee identified eight core principles to guide sustainable actions that can improve eye and vision health and health equity in the United States:

- *Adequately Resourced.* Resources must be available to allow communities to translate clinical and population health research findings into evidence-based practice in communities.
- *Collaborative.* The promotion of eye and vision health and environments outcomes will require cooperation, participation, and responsibility on the part of the public and institutional stakeholders (government, business, employers, the public, health care providers, and others).
- *Community Tailored.* Eye and vision health is local. The priorities and interventions related to vision impairment and population health must be assessed according to individual communities needs, resources, and values.
- *Culturally Competent.* The clinical and public health workforces must be adequately educated and trained to support eye and vision health in culturally diverse communities.
- *Evidence-based.* Community-based and clinical interventions to improve eye and vision health must be evidence-based in order

to establish efficacy as well as to gather information with which to guide other communities.

- *Integrated.* Eye and vision health should be integrated into current and future population health initiatives.
- *Population-centered.* In order to be effective policies and actions to improve population eye and vision health should support and respect the needs, identity, dignity, and circumstances of those populations being served.
- *Standardized.* Efforts to improve eye and vision health must be based on a common language that can help to unite stakeholders and make it easier to aggregate surveillance and research datasets.

DEFINITION OF KEY TERMS IN EYE AND VISION HEALTH

Various terms are used throughout the literature to signal different types and severities of vision impairment. Inconsistent definitions make it difficult to search for and compare relevant literature, and they also create confusion in trying to explain the nature, scope, impact, and treatment of eye and vision health. In fact, when conducting literature searches related to eye and vision health, the committee had to include a wide array of terms such as vision loss, vision impairment, visual impairment, blindness, eye health, vision health, and low vision (in addition to specific diseases or conditions) in an attempt to capture all relevant studies.

Even specific terms may not be defined or measured consistently. For example, although historically the term "low vision" has referred to some presentation of the visual system or range of vision outside of what may be considered "normal," the term continues to be used in many different ways by different stakeholders. The NEI defines low vision as a visual impairment that is not correctable by standard eyeglasses, contact lenses, medication, or surgery and that interferes with the ability to perform everyday activities (NEI/NIH, 2008). In the context of rehabilitation services, the Centers for Medicare & Medicaid Services defines "low vision" as a best-corrected visual acuity of less than 20/60 in the better-seeing eye, including diagnosis codes ranging from "moderate visual impairment" (less than 20/60) to "total blindness" (no perception of light) as well as visual field defects, such as hemianopsias, generalized constriction, and central scotomas, as listed in the *International Classification of Diseases, 9th Edition–Clinical Modification Manual* (ICD-9) (AHRQ, 2004). During the past decade, the term "vision impairment" was introduced with the intention of replacing the term "low vision" to better describe the continuum of eye and vision problems and subsequent vision loss (Dandona and Dandona, 2006).

Similarly, some studies define "blindness" as the "total loss of sight," or the inability to perceive any light (i.e., no light perception) (e.g., Bastable,

2016, p. 307; Joseph and Robinson, 2012, p. 21). However, "statutory blindness" under U.S. Social Security laws is defined as "central visual acuity of 20/200 or less in the better eye with the use of a correcting lens" and/or when the "widest diameter of the [eye's] visual field subtends an angle no greater than 20 degrees."[8] The World Health Organization defines blindness as best corrected visual acuity of less than 20/400 in the better-seeing eye (WHO, n.d.). Regardless of the differences in the acuity threshold, many studies and organizations have criticized both approaches because defining blindness in terms of "best corrected" means that policy makers, public health officials, and health care leaders may overlook a large number of persons with vision impairment who technically could correct their vision problems, such as refractive error, but may not practically be able to do so for various socioeconomic reasons (WHO, n.d.). Another group that may be overlooked are persons whose vision is significantly compromised in other aspects that do not affect visual acuity (e.g., visual processing), described later in this chapter. The committee agrees with the argument that these definitions of blindness leave out many people with visual impairments who should be considered as blind, and it supports efforts to revise this definition under the ICD-10.

To provide greater clarity and consistency in its analysis and recommendations throughout this report, the committee defined specific key terms, which are provided in Table 1-1 along with functional descriptions. The committee chose to define "vision loss" as a process because it emphasizes the importance of approaching vision impairment as the result of a series of decisions, exposures, or circumstances—many of which can potentially be altered to affect the trajectory of the severity of vision impairment across the lifespan. This definition is meant to encourage people to step back and consider the promotion of eye and vision health, rather than simply the treatment of observable eye conditions and diseases. Similarly, vision impairment was defined broadly as a measure of the type and severity of vision loss, which includes blindness. As a general matter, optimizing the eye and vision health of a population should not be based on artificial segmentations of populations as defined by observed outcomes. When analyzing the impact and severity of vision impairment by race, ethnicity, gender, age, and geographic unit, among other risk factors, it is important to track and consider the full range of vision impairment (including uncorrectable and uncorrected) associated with a disease, condition, or event because it can reveal opportunities to reduce inequities. Moreover, categorizing populations based on the severity of vision impairment unnecessarily divides a constituency that must be united to advocate for necessary changes to

---

[8] Social Security Act § 216(i)(1)(B).

TABLE 1-1 Definitions of Key Terms Related to Eye and Vision Health

Term	Clinical Definition	Functional Description
Chronic vision impairment	A vision impairment that is present and must be managed over the lifespan to maintain the activities of daily living.	A vision impairment whose causes or effects cannot be reversed or eliminated by corrective lenses,[a] medication, or surgery. As a result, health care interventions will be necessary over the course of a person's life.
Comprehensive eye examination	A dilated eye examination that may include a series of assessments and procedures to evaluate the eyes and visual system, assess eye and vision health and related systemic health conditions, characterize the impact of disease or abnormal conditions on the function and status of the visual system, and provide treatment and follow-up options.	An in-person clinical encounter between an eye doctor and an individual intended to diagnose and treat any eye disease or condition that might lead to visual impairment, reduce visual function or eye discomfort, and connect the person with other needed clinical and nonclinical services to improve or maximize personal independence and promote health. The dilated eye examination may lead to referrals for other health care and non-clinical services or suggest future eye and vision care to avoid or slow progression of vision impairment.
Eye and vision health	Creating the conditions where people can have the fullest capacity to see and that enable them to achieve their full potential.	
Legal blindness (as defined in the United States)	Visual acuity of 20/200 or less in the better eye with the best possible correction and/or a visual field of 20 degrees or less.[b]	A person sees at 20 feet what a person with normal vision sees at 200 feet, and/or a person sees a visual field of 20 degrees or less in the better field.
Total blindness	Total loss of sight	The inability to perceive any light; e.g., total visual impairment.
Vision impairment	A measure of the type and severity of clinical or functional limitation of one or both eyes or visual information processing structures in the brain.	A measure of the type and severity of limitations in vision, including blindness. Vision impairment can range from mild to total (blindness) and can range from impairments in visual acuity to visual field to other aspects of the eyes and/or visual system.

TABLE 1-1 Continued

Term	Clinical Definition	Functional Description
Vision loss	The process by which physiological changes or structural, neurological, or acquired damage to the structure or function of one or both eyes or visual information processing structures in the brain occurs, resulting in vision impairment.	The process by which eyesight deteriorates. A loss of sight can be affected by many different structures or functions within the eye or brain (see Chapter 2), which can affect one or more dimensions of eye and vision health. In many cases, individuals do not notice the changes that occur until their inability to see begins to affect every day activities. Vision loss is often chronic, progressive, and/or irreversible.
Vision screenings	A tool that allows for the possible identification, but not diagnosis, of eye disease and conditions.	A method to identify potential problems or irregularities with the visual system so that a referral can be made to an appropriate eye care professional for further evaluation and treatment.
Visual acuity	A number that indicates the sharpness or clarity of vision, measured by the ability to discern objects at a given distance according to a fixed standard.	A measure reflecting the distance between the eye and an object at which the object becomes blurry. Visual acuity is a term used to describe the quality of the image perceived.
Visual field	The total area an individual can see off to the side without moving the eye.	Visual field is a term used to describe the "window" that each eye provides to see the world. Visual field describes the extent of the visual system's window on our environment. It can be used to describe partial or total impairments within the window through which we see the world, and is a component of the visual system that is used in determining legal (statutory) blindness and, often, driver's licensure eligibility.

[a] The committee has defined a corrective lens as "a lens worn in front of the eye, usually to correct a refractive error. Examples of corrective lenses include glasses (which include lenses and frames) and contact lenses" (see Appendix C).
[b] Social Security Act § 216(i)(1)(B).

advance eye and vision health and reduce the impact of different types and severities of vision impairment, as described throughout this report.

The committee recognizes that it is necessary to distinguish between individuals with less severe vision impairment from those who are blind (however this is defined) for the enforcement of specific regulations and policies, such as disability law and Medicare payment policies, and for specific surveillance purposes and programmatic emphasis. The committee did not attempt to define the contexts in which specific clinical definitions of specific diseases or severity of vision loss should be used, although the committee notes that inconsistencies across policies, programs, and studies require additional attention.

The continuum of eye and vision health (see Figure 1-1) includes the maintenance of good eye and vision health, as well as the prevention or mitigation of vision loss. It is a continuum that highlights subclinical and observable processes to yield important points of intervention for population health strategies that are aimed at reducing or delaying a wide range of vision impairments and related consequences.

The most effective policies and interventions take into account the specific etiology and causation of vision loss as well as the availability of treatments or therapies for resulting vision impairment. It is worth noting that the term "vision loss" has been applied to the circumstances in which an individual has experienced a deleterious change from some previous visual ability and that it implicitly recognizes the sense of "loss" associated with such a decline in vision. By contrast, an individual with congenital or very early-life blindness may not perceive vision impairment as a loss, which will affect that individual's level of interest in—and willingness to accept—treatments meant to reverse or treat vision impairment. It is important to note that when the committee uses "vision loss" it does not imply that the impairment has been acquired (as opposed to congenital), but rather the committee equates vision loss with the underlying physiological processes associated with sight.

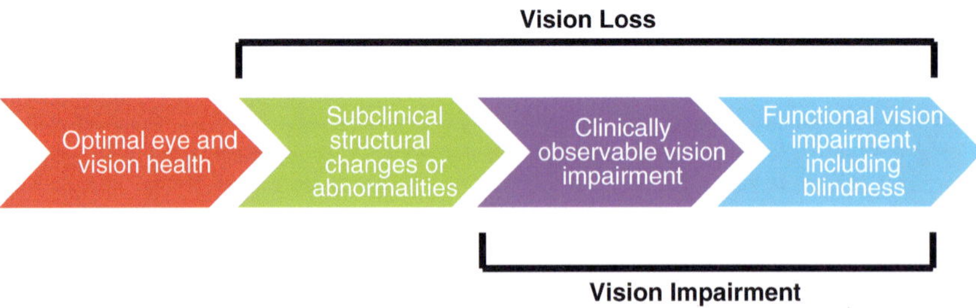

FIGURE 1-1 Continuum of eye and vision health.

Types of Vision Impairment

The degree of vision impairment is characterized by a variety of diagnostic measures, which are affected by numerous diseases and conditions described in greater detail in Chapter 2. The public is probably most familiar with visual acuity tests, which are often associated with identifying letters or symbols on a chart (e.g., a Snellen chart) that become progressively smaller until the letters or symbols are no longer legible to the patient. The resulting fraction (e.g., 20 over 20, 20 over 600) compares the vision of a given individual with that of a person with normal vision; an individual has 20/50 vision, for example, if he or she can make out an object at a distance of 20 feet that a person with normal vision can make out from 50 feet; the ratio is representative of the clarity of a visual image perceived by that individual (NLM, 2016). Table 1-2 provides a description and examples of how different visual acuities could affect functional ability. These interpretations are not standardized across populations and should not be interpreted to mean that two people with the same measured acuity will see the same thing. However, it is important to have a general understanding of how visual acuity loosely translates into measures of function and the population health burden of vision impairment, especially in the context of uncorrected refractive error.

Serious vision impairments can also manifest as problems with contrast sensitivity, visual field loss (i.e., loss of part of the usual visual field), seeing two images (i.e., double vision), extreme sensitivity to light (i.e., photophobia), visual distortion (e.g., blind spots, haloing around an object or light), color blindness, visual perceptual difficulties, or any combination of these conditions. The impact that different aspects of vision have on daily function varies. For example, color blindness affects one's ability to select matching clothes, distinguish different driving signs and signals, or join the Air Force. Significant visual acuity problems make it difficult to see objects in one's house or to navigate city streets or sidewalks safely. Decreasing peripheral vision can result in tunnel vision, which can affect the ability to see things around a person and can create problems with driving or cause one to run into stationary obstacles (e.g., doorframes) while walking. Problems with contrast sensitivity can make it difficult to interpret the significance of different types of shading (e.g., shadows versus stairs), read poorly contrasted text on posters or classroom slides, to move comfortably from a bright to a dark environment or vice versa, or to perceive the presence of an object in front of a similarly shaded background. For a vast majority of people with these conditions, the resulting vision impairment is continuously present and must be managed over the lifespan, which has important implications for public policies concerning health care delivery, community

TABLE 1-2 Description of Functional Ability Based on the Snellen Chart

Snellen ("Customary") Distance Visual Acuity	Level of Vision Impairment	How Might My Vision Change If Uncorrectable?[a]	Examples of Patient Outcomes at This Level[b]
20/10 to 20/25	Range of normal vision	NA	NA
20/30 to 20/60[b,c]	Near-normal vision	• Reduced detail and/or contrast discrimination • After acuity is worse than 20/40, normal newspaper print is less legible, and the inability to recognize usual and customary visual detail becomes apparent	• Street signs not easily read • People or objects across the room lose detail • Regular size print found in newspaper, school books, utility bills, and magazines becomes difficult to read • Skips letters or words when reading • Must sit closer to the computer or television to see image details • Holds phone, tablet, reading materials closer to face • Restrictions may be placed on driver's licensure (e.g., driving in daylight only) • Need for intense lighting/increased illumination • Some difficulty maneuvering stairs, sidewalks, and/or unfamiliar environments, especially in dusk conditions • Labels on food packaging, medication difficult to discern
20/70 to 20/160	Moderate visual impairment	*In addition to the above…* • Continued loss of detail and/or contrast discrimination • Increased delay in response to adapting from bright to dark settings and vice versa • With acuity worse than 20/70, large print (e.g., twice the size of normal size print) becomes less legible, and loss of distinguishing facial details and distant targets is pronounced	*In addition to the above…* • Loss of facial feature discrimination • Highway signage, distance details in low lighting, scrolling television screen information is not discernable • Large print text becomes difficult to read, medication labels not discernable, handwriting is inconsistent, signing one's name on checks/forms very difficult

TABLE 1-2 Continued

Snellen ("Customary") Distance Visual Acuity	Level of Vision Impairment	How Might My Vision Change If Uncorrectable?[a]	Examples of Patient Outcomes at This Level[b]
		• Loss of additional color discrimination; high contrast becomes necessary	• Maximum illumination becomes required for near tasks • Loss or restriction of driver's licensure • Moderate to severe limitations in safely maneuvering changing terrain or unfamiliar environments, especially in dusk conditions
20/200 to 20/400 *(and/or visual field limitation of 20 degrees or less in better eye)*	Severe visual impairment; includes "legal blindness"	*In addition to the above…* • Large print text not discernable • Customary technology like phone buttons and computer keyboards are not distinguishable • Headlines from the newspaper may be the only text recognizable without magnification	*In addition to the above…* • Large print text becomes difficult to read • Ambulation without assistance becomes difficult • Majority of people in this range have remaining useful vision and capacity for improved function with vision rehabilitation
20/500 to 20/1,000	Profound visual impairment	*In addition to the above…* • Customarily available text of any size, and the majority of distance images are not discernable without magnification • Largest available "off-the-shelf" television or computer monitor does not provide large enough image to discern visual detail • Visual field restriction results in severe loss of peripheral vision (i.e., tunnel vision)	*In addition to the above…* • Outlines of shapes (e.g., the head) may be only remaining discernable component of the human form • Loss of recognition of facial features, fingernails • Inability to apply make-up; extreme difficulty with shaving, personal maintenance • Shopping for groceries, cooking becomes extremely difficult • Sensory substitution technology (i.e., talking watch, books on tape, GPS) important adjunct to remaining visual input

continued

TABLE 1-2 Continued

Snellen ("Customary") Distance Visual Acuity	Level of Vision Impairment	How Might My Vision Change If Uncorrectable?[a]	Examples of Patient Outcomes at This Level[b]
Acuity less than 20/1,000 Includes hand motion, light projection, and light perception *(and/or visual field of 5 degrees or less in better eye)*	Near total visual impairment	*In addition to the above...* • Remaining vision may only allow for discerning a moving hand or light, or only the recognition of a light source • Visual field restriction results in profound loss of peripheral vision (i.e., tunnel vision)	*In addition to the above...* • Impaired ability to distinguish light from dark • Loss of the majority of visual input • Sensory substitution technology (speech synthesis from print material and video imagery) is a primary strategy to replacing visual input
No light perception	Total visual impairment; i.e., blindness	• Unable to recognize any visual stimuli • Loss of vision as a sensory input	• Without sight • Cannot discern light

[a] Changes in vision and function are common examples, but may not be the same across individual patients.

[b] Early changes and/or fluctuations in visual acuity in this range are often ignored and may go unnoticed.

[c] Changing customary spectacle or contact lens prescriptions, as well as surgical and/or pharmaceutical intervention(s), does not fully restore visual acuity to the normal range normal range. Exceptions include prescription of lenses for uncorrected refractive error and surgical removal of cataract, both of which customarily provide improvements in visual acuity.

SOURCE: Adapted from AOA, 2007.

design, messaging for public awareness and education campaigns, health professional education, and research prioritization and support.

A POPULATION HEALTH APPROACH TO IMPROVE EYE AND VISION HEALTH AND REDUCE VISION IMPAIRMENT

It is easy to overlook (and perhaps forget) that some of the most notable successes in preventing vision loss have been anchored in population health strategies. International blindness prevention programs have significantly reduced blindness from diseases such as vitamin A deficiency and onchocerciasis (i.e., river blindness) (Rao, 2015). In the United States, the enforcement of regulations aimed at promoting safe workplaces by the

Occupational Safety and Health Administration and efforts to improve the standardization of personal protective equipment (including safety glasses) through such federal entities as the National Personal Protective Technology Lab have vastly reduced occupational eye injuries, although more improvement is needed (BLS, 2012; CDC, 2015e). Trachoma, once widespread and a reason for denying entry to infected immigrants, is now virtually eliminated in the United States (Kumaresan, 2005). Gonococcal conjunctivitis is also now rarely seen in newborns, as most hospitals are required by state law to apply antibiotic drops or ointment to a newborn's eyes to prevent the disease (CDC, 2015b). Still, eye and vision health remains important in the context of some communicable diseases, such as the Ebola or rubella viruses, which can, respectively, remain in the eye for significant periods of time or affect the developing vision system of unborn children (CDC, 2015c; Varkey et al., 2015). Beyond vision loss itself, eye and vision health can also serve as an indicator for other chronic conditions, such as diabetes or multiple sclerosis, and of brain tumors, particularly those affecting the pituitary gland (Crews et al., 2016b; Frohman et al., 2008; Prasad, 2013). Unfortunately, many health-related policies and practices still reflect antiquated positions that do not adequately reflect the connection between eye and vision health (along with other sensory organs) and the promotion of overall health.

During the past few decades, many experts and policy makers have argued for a broader approach to improving the eye and vision health of the nation. The U.S. Department of Health and Human Services (HHS), the NEI, the U.S. Preventive Services Task Force (USPSTF), and the World Health Organization (WHO) have defined vision impairment and blindness as national or global public health problems.[9] The CDC has also identified vision loss as a public health problem, funding a variety of activities to combat the effects of poor eye and vision health on at-risk populations.[10] In 2007 the CDC published the report *Improving the Nation's Vision Health: A Coordinated Public Health Approach*, which identified three key public health activities: assessment (surveillance and epidemiology), application

---

[9] Healthy People 2020, a project of HHS through the Office of Disease Prevention and Health Promotion, lists vision loss as a major public health concern (HHS, 2015). The NEI has called vision loss a major public health problem (NEI/NIH, 2004). WHO identifies blindness and vision impairment, and the diseases that cause them, as public health problems (WHO, 2015a). The USPSTF identifies impairment of visual acuity as a serious public health problem among older adults (USPSTF, 2009).

[10] Per the CDC, there are five definitional features of a public health problem: (1) the problem affects a large number of people; (2) the problem imposes large morbidity, quality of life, and cost burdens; (3) the severity of the problem is increasing and is predicted to continue increasing; (4) the public perceives the problem to be a threat; (5) community or public health-level interventions to the problem are feasible (CDC, 2009b).

(applied public health research), and action (integrating vision health into programs and policy) (CDC, 2007). The report also proposed eight core elements to improve the nation's health: engaging key national partners, collaborating with state and local health departments, implementing vision surveillance and evaluation systems, eliminating eye health disparities by focusing on at-risk populations, integrating vision health interventions into existing public health programs including systems and policy changes that support vision health, addressing the role of behavior in protecting and optimizing vision health, assuring professional workforce development, and establishing an applied public health research agenda for vision. Following the release of that report, the CDC launched the Vision Health Initiative (VHI) to promote vision health and quality of life for all populations, throughout all life stages, by preventing and controlling eye disease, eye injury, and vision loss resulting in disability (CDC, 2015a). Many of the recommendations and actions included in the 2007 report and in various VHI activities are discussed in this report—these are important concepts.

Despite these efforts, eye and vision health remain notably absent as a population health priority in the overarching public health and health care systems. It is also underrepresented in strategic plans that address the impact of chronic diseases and conditions within the United States. This has resulted in having insufficient evidence to guide decisions about policies that affect resource allocation to advance research, health care and rehabilitation service delivery, public health priorities and interventions. It has also impeded opportunities to emphasize efficiency, value, and the role of collaboration in improving the eye and vision health—a critical aspect of overall health—for general and patient populations.

Multiple Determinants of Eye and Vision Health

Eye and vision health of individuals and populations are affected by multiple determinants, including (1) innate individual traits (e.g., age, sex, race, and biological factors); (2) individual behaviors; (3) social, family, and community networks; (4) living and working conditions; and (5) broad social, economic, cultural, health, and environmental conditions and policies, which are each part of larger social and physical environments (IOM, 2003). Some of these determinants are modifiable, whereas others are not. For example, in the context of eye and vision health, genetics and the aging process itself may predispose populations to specific types of eye diseases and conditions. Conversely, exposure to ultraviolet sunlight, which is associated with an increased risk of cataracts, can be mitigated through the use of protective eyewear or window tinting.

Interactions among determinants of health may have impacts at the community or individual level, and understanding the relationships among these determinants is important to achieving the greatest benefit. Lower socioeconomic status can limit access to healthy living environments and also to health care services. Food policies may contribute to the obesity epidemic, which is linked to the other chronic conditions, such as diabetes, which affect the eyes. It is important to note that, within this approach, health care services are only one component of the "living and working conditions" that affect health. The majority of health determinants exist outside the clinical care system (Braveman and Gottlieb, 2014; McGinnis et al., 2002), which provides a wide range of opportunities and environments in which vision health can be influenced. Figure 1-2 provides examples of specific risk and protective factors by health determinant category, which may be the targets of a broad population health approach to improving eye and vision health across the lifespan. Many other examples are provided throughout this report.

A Conceptual Framework to Bridge Public Health and Clinical Approaches to Eye and Vision Health

"[Public health's] purpose is to monitor and evaluate health status as well as to devise strategies and interventions designed to ease the burden of injury, disease, and disability and, more generally, to promote the public's health and safety" (Gostin et al., 2007, p. 7). More generally, the purpose of public health is to create the conditions whereby people can be healthy and achieve their full potential (WHO, 1986). This purpose is advanced through three population health functions: (1) assessment (i.e., monitoring communities to identify and characterize public health needs and priorities), (2) policy development (i.e., the use of scientific evidence to guide the design and implementation of programs and policies to address public health issues), and (3) assurance (i.e., policy development and enforcement, ensuring that health and public health systems have the resources to implement programs, and evaluating the health impacts of interventions) (CDC, 2007; IOM, 1988). Each function comprises 10 essential public health services, as developed by the Core Public Health Functions Steering Committee more than two decades ago (CDC, 2014). Box 1-2 presents these services in the context of eye and vision health. These services represent a full spectrum of activities and are part of a continuous process, which is centered around ongoing research to generate new knowledge that informs decision making and future iterations of interventions and initiatives.

In contrast to clinical care, which focuses on treating individual patients, population health systems concentrate on health risks to populations, addressing underlying determinants of health that affect not only specific health outcomes but also the circumstances that allow populations to make healthy choices and live in healthy environments. Because population

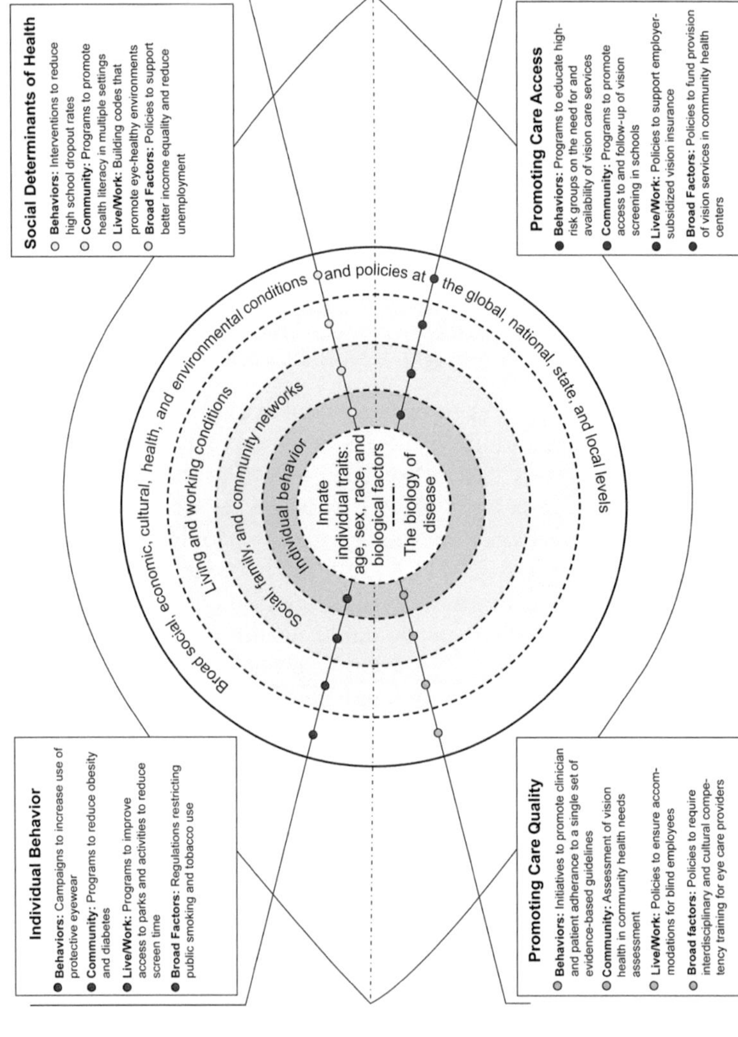

FIGURE 1-2 Examples of factors that could be part of a population health approach to eye and vision health.
SOURCE: Adapted from IOM, 2003, p. 52.

BOX 1-2
10 Essential Population Health Services
to Improve Eye and Vision Health

1. Monitor eye and vision health status to identify and solve community health problems.
2. Diagnose and investigate eye and vision health problems and health hazards in the community.
3. Inform, educate, and empower people about eye and vision health issues.
4. Encourage community partnerships and action to identify and solve eye and vision health problems.
5. Develop policies and plans that support individual and community eye and vision health efforts.
6. Enforce laws and regulations that protect eye and vision health and safety and the function of visually impaired populations.
7. Link people to needed eye and vision health services and ensure the provision of health care when otherwise unavailable.
8. Ensure a competent public and personal health care workforce.
9. Evaluate the effectiveness, accessibility, and quality of personal and population-based eye and vision health care and community services.
10. Research new insights and innovative solutions to eye and vision health problems.

SOURCE: Adapted from CDC, 2014.

---

health focuses on all determinants of health, the responsibility for improving population health has never been the sole province of any one actor or stakeholder. Implementing a population health approach for eye and vision health requires a robust effort and collaboration from multiple stakeholders, including government agencies, businesses, the community, health care providers, the media, and academia (IOM, 2003, 2011).

In the context of eye and vision health, a large amount of attention has focused on the access to and utilization of health care services, which is not typical of many other population health initiatives, such as efforts to combat obesity or reduce tobacco use. However, early and appropriate access to eye care and rehabilitation services will be an important component of any comprehensive population health approach to reduce the severity of vision impairment and the impact of vision impairment on quality of life. For example, comprehensive eye examinations may help identify eye and vision diseases and conditions before a patient notices symptoms (CDC, 2009a; Li et al., 2013). Differences in professional guidelines and medical insurance coverage related to who should receive what service at what frequency present a significant barrier to developing a systematic approach to ensuring that those who need services receive them. Vision acuity screenings in community settings can identify school-aged children who have uncorrected refractive error, but the odds of receiving inadequate refractive correction remain significantly higher for Mexican Americans and non-Hispanic blacks than for whites, with the greatest disparities observed for the 12- to 19-year-old age group (Qiu et al., 2014). Although clinical care interventions and rehabilitation are available to improve or maintain the function of people living with vision impairment, knowledge about and access to these services is limited (Lam and Leat, 2015; Overbury and Wittich, 2011). Many public and private health insurance policies, including Medicare, do not cover periodic eye examinations for functionally asymptomatic or low-risk patients, corrective lenses, and visual assistive devices. In many cases, members of the public must purchase additional insurance or pay out of pocket for these services and items. These policies and circumstances contribute to inequities that already affect populations with lower socioeconomic status and poor health (DeVoe et al., 2007; Yip et al., 2014; Zhang et al., 2013).

The committee noted that the relative success of clinical treatments, combined with the exclusion of eye and vision health from general health policy discussions and the resulting relative lack of shared expertise between public health professionals and eye care providers, has contributed to miscommunications and misconceptions about what represents a population health approach and how this approach relates to clinical care in eye and vision health. Even in its statement of work, the committee was asked to focus on mitigating the effects of vision impairment, a critical but downstream effect of vision loss that is not typically the focus of prevention efforts, which characteristically focus on more upstream determinants of health. As a result, it became important for the committee to develop a conceptual framework that illustrated the relationship between more traditional population health focuses and eye care.

Figure 1-3 presents a diagram of a cylinder, which can be used to conceptualize a comprehensive population health approach to improving eye and vision health and achieving health equity. The cylinder, which consists of the core public health functions, spans four sequential stages of prevention. *Primordial prevention* addresses broad health determinants and behaviors to minimize future health threats by targeting the environmental, economic, social, physical, and cultural factors that increase the risk of poor eye health. It may include such considerations as health literacy, housing, education, income, the availability of health care insurance, or policies to support healthy diets. *Primary prevention* seeks to support, educate, and promote healthy eye and vision behaviors that decrease the risk of poor eye and vision health. Examples in vision impairment include

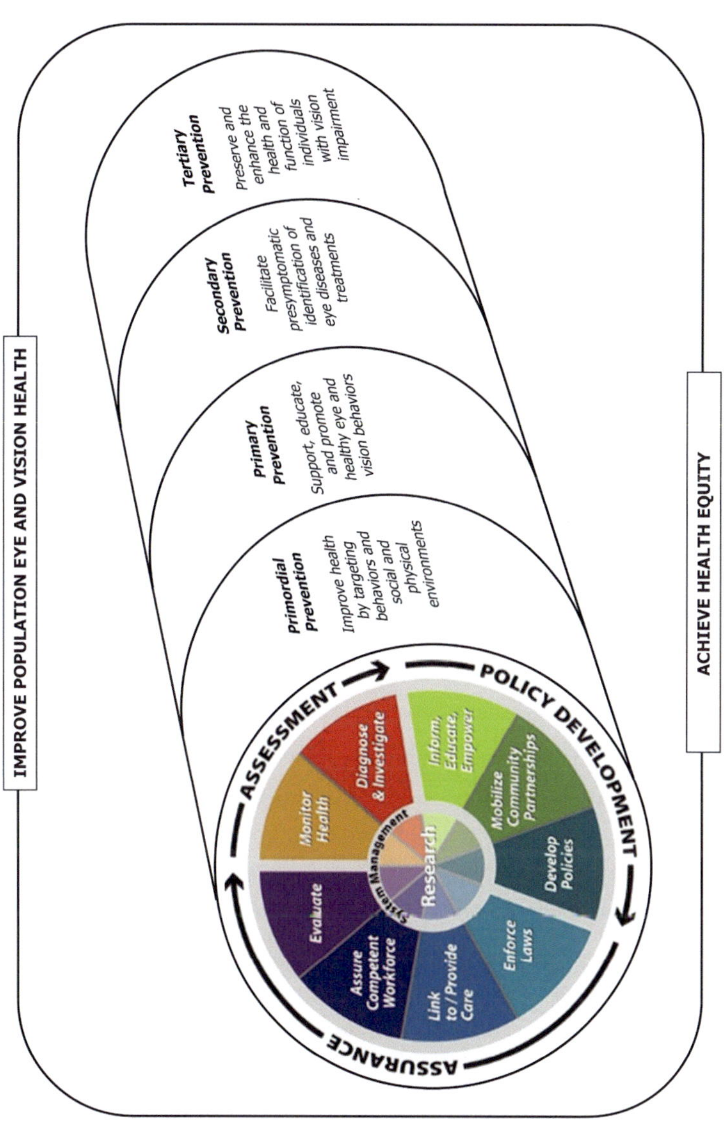

FIGURE 1-3 A conceptual framework to advance eye and vision health.
SOURCE: Adapted from CDC, 2014.

using protective eyewear, spending adequate time outdoors, preventing and managing chronic conditions that predispose populations to vision loss, and ensuring adequate levels of light indoors for near-work activity. *Secondary prevention* facilitates the pre-symptomatic identification of eye diseases and treatments in order to slow or stop the progression of a disease or condition. Examples include screenings for children to detect and treat amblyopia and its risk factors and having a comprehensive eye examination to detect subclinical changes in the eye for glaucoma or diabetic retinopathy. *Tertiary prevention* includes activities designed to preserve and enhance the health, function, and quality of life of individuals with vision impairment. Examples include wearing properly corrected eyewear, improving medication adherence for glaucoma, and providing access to rehabilitation services, social support, or assistive devices. In this framework, vision impairment itself, regardless of the disease(s) or injury that caused it, is treated as a chronic condition in its own right.

Anchoring eye and vision health promotion in terms of the stages of prevention allows the nation to reevaluate eye and vision health improvement as not only a valued outcome in and of itself, but also as a potential public health tool with which to promote health equity more broadly among populations. Moreover, because the three public health functions and 10 essential health services address each prevention stage, this conceptual framework inherently creates a checklist from which to populate and evaluate a comprehensive public health approach to eye and vision health. That is, within each prevention stage, there will be actions related to assessment, assurance, and policy development that various stakeholders can pursue as part of a larger effort. This effort will take coordination and collaboration. A key role for governmental public health departments will be to serve as a convener of these stakeholders to develop and implement action plans that best reflect a community's needs and goals.

This framework was also useful in structuring this report. In addition to introducing the committee's statement of task, this chapter provides the committee's guiding principles, defines key terms related to vision health, and proposes a new conceptual model to guide thinking about vision health as a population health priority. Chapter 2 describes the epidemiology of vision loss in the United States. Chapter 3 discusses the impact of vision loss and how that applies to current public health priorities. Chapter 4 explores the strengths and weaknesses of surveillance tools and systems and research databases to track and measure that burden. Chapter 5 examines the impact that individual health behaviors and community environments can have on the eye health and overall health of populations and reviews strategies to encourage collaboration and action at the community level. Chapter 6 examines the access to clinical services in terms of the distribution of the eye and vision workforce, and the coverage of health care services. Chapter 7 describes efforts to improve the quality and efficiency of clinical care. Chapter 8 focuses on efforts to improve the health and independence of individuals with chronic vision impairments and blindness. Finally, Chapter 9 proposes a model for action and recommendations for improving vision eye and vision health.

CONCLUSION

Vision impairment significantly affects the health, finances, and productivity of individuals, families, and society as a whole. Despite evidence that vision impairment increases the risk of mortality and morbidity from other chronic conditions and related injuries and is associated with a reduced quality of life, eye and vision health are not adequately recognized as a population health priority or as a means by which to achieve better health equity. This report attempts to answer "Why not?" by ascertaining what is known about the burden and epidemiology of vision loss, its risk factors, effective treatments and interventions to maintain or improve function, and population health strategies to introduce and sustain the prioritization of eye and vision health across communities. The report also serves as a call to action to make eye and vision health governmental public health and population health priorities.

A population health approach to eye and vision health must take into account the programs, policies, and systems needed to create the conditions where people can have the fullest capacity to see and that enable them to achieve their full potential. The long-term goal of a population health approach in eye and vision health is to transform vision impairment from an exceedingly common to a rare condition, reducing related health inequities. Given the genetic and biological components of many eye diseases and conditions, the occurrence of eye injuries, and the aging process itself, populations will never be without vision impairment. Nevertheless, this goal establishes a new platform from which to identify important players, define influential behaviors, and allocate resources in a manner that sustains and protects the eye and vision health of different populations. Anchoring population health in terms of prevention more broadly also creates an opportunity for the nation to reevaluate how it values eye and vision health and how this can be translated into daily activities, community discussions, and public policy.

Achieving the twin goals of improving eye and vision health and increasing health equity will require action by a wide range of stakeholders at the national, state, and local levels. This chapter proposed guiding principles and a conceptual framework to guide and coordinate these actions. An effective population health approach to eye and vision health must address each of three public health functions (i.e., assessment, policy development, and assurance) across the four stages of prevention, which focus on sequential but narrowing opportunities for intervention across the continuum of eye and vision health. Prevention and early access to effective eye care is critical to avoiding, identifying, monitoring, and treating many eye diseases and conditions that can lead to vision impairment across the lifespan. Short- and long-term population health strategies should also account for the broad determinants of health, including policies that influence individual behaviors, safe and healthy environments and conditions, and their potential impact on eye and vision health. Good eye and vision health can reduce health disparities, but promoting optimal conditions for eye and vision health can alleviate many other social ailments, including poverty, other health inequities, increasing health care costs, and avoidable mortality and morbidity. The evidence provided throughout this report provides important context for the committee's recommendations, which logically flow from the chapter conclusions. Establishing conditions and policies that promote population eye and vision health and minimize preventable and correctible vision impairment is an essential, timely, and achievable objective—an objective that is necessary to fuel broad actions and sustain the overall quality of life, function, and productivity of the nation.

REFERENCES

AHRQ (Agency for Healthcare Research and Quality). 2004. *Vision rehabilitation for elderly individuals with low vision or blindness.* Rockville, MD: AHRQ. https://www.cms.gov/Medicare/Coverage/DeterminationProcess/Downloads/id95TA.pdf (accessed March 29, 2016).

Alberti, C. F., E. Peli, and A. R. Bowers. 2014. Driving with hemianopia: III. Detection of stationary and approaching pedestrians in a simulator. *Investigative Ophthalmology & Visual Science* 55(1):368–374.

AOA (American Optometric Association). 2007. *Care of the patient with visual impairment (low vision rehabilitation).* St. Louis, MO: AOA. http://www.aoa.org/documents/optometrists/CPG-14.pdf (accessed June 1, 2016).

Bastable, S. B. 2016. *Essentials of patient education.* 2nd ed. Burlington, MA: Jones and Bartlett.

Birch, E. E. 2013. Amblyopia and binocular vision. *Progress in Retinal and Eye Research* 33:67–84.

BLS (Bureau of Labor Statistics). 2012. Injuries, illnesses, and fatalities. http://www.bls.gov/iif (accessed June 1, 2016).

Bowers, A. R., A. J. Mandel, R. B. Goldstein, and E. Peli. 2009. Driving with hemianopia, I: Detection performance in a driving simulator. *Investigative Ophthalmology & Visual Science* 50(11):5137–5147.

Braveman, P., and L. Gottlieb. 2014. The social determinants of health: It's time to consider the causes of the causes. *Public Health Reports* 129(Suppl 2):19–31.

Bronstad, P. M., A. R. Bowers, A. Albu, R. Goldstein, and E. Peli. 2013. Driving with central field loss I: Effect of central scotomas on responses to hazards. *JAMA Ophthalmology* 131(3):303–309.

Brown, J. C., J. E. Goldstein, T. L. Chan, R. Massof, P. Ramulu, and the Low Vision Research Network Study Group. 2014. Characterizing functional complaints in patients seeking outpatient low-vision services in the United States. *Ophthalmology* 121(8):1655–1662, e1651.

CDC (Centers for Disease Control and Prevention). 2007. *Improving the nation's vision health: A coordinated public health approach.* Atlanta, GA: CDC.

———. 2009a. Vision Health Initiative—Eye health tips. http://www.cdc.gov/visionhealth/basic_information/eye_health_tips.htm (accessed October 7, 2015).

———. 2009b. Why is vision loss a public health problem? http://www.cdc.gov/visionhealth/basic_information/vision_loss.htm (accessed October 7, 2015).

———. 2014. The public health system and the 10 essential public health services. http://www.cdc.gov/nphpsp/essentialservices.html (accessed March, 2016).

———. 2015a. About us. http://www.cdc.gov/visionhealth/about/index.htm (accessed March 30, 2016).

———. 2015b. Conjunctivitis (pink eye) in newborns. http://www.cdc.gov/conjunctivitis/newborns.html (accessed March 30, 2016).

———. 2015c. *Epidemiology and prevention of vaccine-preventable diseases.* 13th ed. Edited by J. Hamborsky, A. Kroger, and C. Wolfe. Washington, DC: Public Health Foundation.

———. 2015d. National data. http://www.cdc.gov/visionhealth/data/national.htm (accessed May 26, 2016).

———. 2015e. The work-related injury statistics query system. https://wwwn.cdc.gov/wisards/workrisqs (accessed August 5, 2016).

Christ, S. L., D. D. Zheng, B. K. Swenor, B. L. Lam, S. K. West, S. L. Tannenbaum, B. E. Muñoz, and D. J. Lee. 2014. Longitudinal relationships among visual acuity, daily functional status, and mortality: The Salisbury Eye Evaluation Study. *JAMA Ophthalmology* 132(12):1400–1406.

Congdon, N., B. O'Colmain, C. C. Klaver, R. Klein, B. Munoz, D. S. Friedman, J. Kempen, H. R. Taylor, and P. Mitchell. 2004. Causes and prevalence of visual impairment among adults in the United States. *Archives of Ophthalmology* 122(4):477–485.

Court, H., G. McLean, B. Guthrie, S. W. Mercer, and D. J. Smith. 2014. Visual impairment is associated with physical and mental comorbidities in older adults: A cross-sectional study. *BMC Medicine* 12:181.

Crewe, J. M., N. Morlet, W. H. Morgan, K. Spilsbury, A. S. Mukhtar, A. Clark, and J. B. Semmens. 2013. Mortality and hospital morbidity of working-age blind. *British Journal of Ophthalmology* 97(12):1579–1585.

Crews, J. E., G. C. Jones, and J. H. Kim. 2006. Double jeopardy: The effects of comorbid conditions among older people with vision loss. *Journal of Visual Impairment and Blindness* 100.824–848.

Crews, J. E., C.-F. Chiu-Fung Chou, J. A. Stevens, and J. B. Saadine. 2016a. Falls among persons aged > 65 years with and without severe vision impairment—United States, 2014. *Morbidity and Mortality Weekly Report* 65(17):433–437.

Crews, J. E., C. F. Chou, M. M. Zack, X. Zhang, K. M. Bullard, A. R. Morse, and J. B. Saaddine. 2016b. The association of health-related quality of life with severity of visual impairment among people aged 40–64 years: Findings from the 2006–2010 Behavioral Risk Factor Surveillance System. *Ophthalmic Epidemiology* 23(3):145–153.

Cumberland, P. M., J. S. Rahi, for the UK Biobank Eye and Vision Consortium. 2016. Visual function, social position, and health and life changes: The UK Biobank Study. *JAMA Ophthalmology* 134(9):959–966.

Dandona, L., and R. Dandona. 2006. Revision of visual impairment definitions in the International Statistical Classification of Diseases. *BMC Medicine* 4:7.

Dang, S. 2015. Eye injuries at work. http://www.aao.org/eye-health/tips-prevention/injuries-work (accessed February 16, 2016).

Davidson, S., and G. E. Quinn. 2011. The impact of pediatric vision disorders in adulthood. *Pediatrics* 127(2):334–339.

DeVoe, J. E., A. Baez, H. Angier, L. Krois, C. Edlund, and P. A. Carney. 2007. Insurance + access ≠ health care: Typology of barriers to health care access for low-income families. *Annals of Family Medicine* 5(6):511–518.

Frohman, E. M., J. G. Fujimoto, T. C. Frohman, P. A. Calabresi, G. Cutter, and L. J. Balcer. 2008. Optical coherence tomography: A window into the mechanisms of multiple sclerosis. *Nature Clinical Practice Neurology* 4(12):664–675.

Gostin, L. O. 2007. *A theory and definition of public health law.* Washington, DC: Georgetown University Law Center.

HHS (U.S. Department of Health and Human Services). 2015. Healthy people 2020 topics and objectives: Vision. http://www.healthypeople.gov/2020/topics-objectives/topic/vision (accessed October 7, 2015).

IOM (Institute of Medicine). 1988. *The future of public health.* Washington, DC: National Academy Press.

———. 2003. *The future of the public's health in the 21st century.* Washington, DC: The National Academies Press.

———. 2011. *For the public's health: The role of measurement in action and accountability.* Washington, DC: The National Academies Press.

Joseph, M.-A. M., and M. Robinson. 2012. Vocational experiences of college-educated individuals with visual impairments. *Journal of Applied Rehabilitation Counseling* 43(4):21.

Kirtland, K. A., J. B. Saaddine, L. S. Geiss, T. J. Thompson, M. F. Cotch, and P. P. Lee. 2015. Geographic disparity of severe vision loss—United States, 2009–2013. *Morbidity and Mortality Weekly Report* 64(19):513–517.

Köberlein, J., K. Beifus, C. Schaffert, and R. P. Finger. 2013. The economic burden of visual impairment and blindness: A systematic review. *BMJ Open* 3(11):e003471.

Kulmala, J., P. Era, O. Pärssinen, R. Sakari, S. Sipilä, T. Rantanen, and E. Heikkinen. 2008. Lowered vision as a risk factor for injurious accidents in older people. *Aging Clinical and Experimental Research* 20(1):25–30.

Kulmala, J., S. Sipilä, K. Tiainen, O. Pärssinen, M. Koskenvuo, J. Kaprio, and T. Rantanen. 2012. Vision in relation to lower extremity deficit in older women: Cross-sectional and longitudinal study. *Aging Clinical and Experimental Research* 24(5):461–467.

Kumaresan, J. 2005. Can blinding trachoma be eliminated by 20/20? *Eye* 19(10):1067–1073.

Lam, N., and S. J. Leat. 2015. Reprint of: Barriers to accessing low-vision care: The patient's perspective. *Canadian Journal of Ophthalmology/Journal Canadien d'Ophtalmologie* 50:S34–S39.

Lee, D. J., O. Gómez-Marín, B. L. Lam, and D. D. Zheng. 2002. Visual acuity impairment and mortality in U.S. adults. *Archives of Ophthalmology* 120(11):1544–1550.

———. 2003. Visual impairment and unintentional injury mortality: The National Health Interview Survey 1986–1994. *American Journal of Ophthalmology* 136(6):1152–1154.

Li, L.-H., A. Li, J.-Y. Zhao, G.-M. Zhang, J.-B. Mao, and P. J. Rychwalski. 2013. Finding of perinatal ocular examination performed on 3573, healthy full-term newborns. *British Journal of Ophthalmology* 97(5):588–591.

Lord, S. R. 2006. Visual risk factors for falls in older people. *Age and Ageing* 35(Suppl 2):ii42–ii45.

McGinnis, J. M., P. Williams-Russo, and J. R. Knickman. 2002. The case for more active policy attention to health promotion. *Health Affairs (Millwood)* 21(2):78–93.

NEI/NIH (National Eye Institute/National Institutes of Health). 2004. Vision statement and mission—National Plan For Eye and Vision Research [NEI strategic planning]. https://nei.nih.gov/strategicplanning/np_vision (accessed February 4, 2016).

———. 2008. Low vision. http://www.nei.nih.gov/health/lowvision (accessed February 16, 2016).

NLM (U.S. National Library of Medicine). 2016. Visual acuity test. https://medlineplus.gov/ency/article/003396.htm (accessed August 5, 2016).

Overbury, O., and W. Wittich. 2011. Barriers to low vision rehabilitation: The Montreal Barriers Study. *Investigative Ophthalmology & Visual Science* 52(12):8933–8938.

Petrash, J. M. 2013. Aging and age-related diseases of the ocular lens and vitreous body. *Investigative Ophthalmology and VisualScience* 54(14):ORSF54–ORSF59.

Prasad, S. 2013. Visual problems due to pituitary tumors. http://www.brighamandwomens.org/Departments_and_Services/neurology/services/NeuroOphthamology/PituitaryTumor.aspx (accessed April 1, 2016).

Prevent Blindness. 2012a. Vision problems in the U.S. http://www.visionproblemsus.org (accessed February 12, 2016).

———. 2012b. Vision problems in the U.S.: Methods and sources. http://www.visionproblemsus.org/introduction/methods-and-sources.html (accessed July 5, 2016).

———. 2012c. Vision problems in the U.S.: Refractive error. http://www.visionproblemsus.org/refractive-error.html (accessed February 12, 2016).

Qiu, M., S. Y. Wang, K. Singh, and S. C. Lin. 2014. Racial disparities in uncorrected and undercorrected refractive error in the United States. *Investigative Ophthalmology & Visual Science* 55(10):6996–7005.

Rahi, J. S., P. M. Cumberland, and C. S. Peckham. 2009. Visual function in working-age adults: Early life influences and associations with health and social outcomes. *Ophthalmology* 116(10):1866–1871.

Rao, G. 2015. The Barrie Jones Lecture—Eye care for the neglected population: Challenges and solutions. *Eye* 29(1):30–45.

Rees, G., H. W. Tee, M. Marella, E. Fenwick, M. Dirani, and E. L. Lamoureux. 2010. Vision-specific distress and depressive symptoms in people with vision impairment. *Investigative Ophthalmology & Visual Science* 51(6):2891–2896.

Rein, D. B. 2013. Vision problems are a leading source of modifiable health expenditures. *Investigative Ophthalmology & Visual Science* 54(14):ORSF18–ORSF22.

Sengupta, S., S. W. van Landingham, S. D. Solomon, D. V. Do, D. S. Friedman, and P. Y. Ramulu. 2014. Driving habits in older patients with central vision loss. *Ophthalmology* 121(3):727–732.

Shahbazi, S., J. Studnicki, and C. W. Warner-Hillard. 2015. A cross-sectional retrospective analysis of the racial and geographic variations in cataract surgery. *PLoS ONE* 10(11):e0142459.

Sommer, A., J. M. Tielsch, J. Katz, H. A. Quigley, J. D. Gottsch, J. C. Javitt, J. F. Martone, R. M. Royall, K. A. Witt, and S. Ezrine. 1991. Racial differences in the cause-specific prevalence of blindness in East Baltimore. *New England Journal of Medicine* 325(20):1412–1417.

Ulldemolins, A. R., V. C. Lansingh, L. Guisasola Valencia, M. J. Carter, and K. A. Eckert. 2012. Social inequalities in blindness and visual impairment: A review of social determinants. *Indian Journal of Ophthalmology* 60(5):368–375.

USPSTF (U.S. Preventive Services Task Force). 2009. *Final recommendation statement—impaired visual acuity in older adults: Screening.* http://www.uspreventiveservicestaskforce.org/Page/Document/RecommendationStatementFinal/impaired-visual-acuity-in-older-adults-screening (accessed October 7, 2015).

van Landingham, S. W., R. W. Massof, E. Chan, D. S. Friedman, and P. Y. Ramulu. 2014. Fear of falling in age-related macular degeneration. *BMC Ophthalmology* 14:1–10.

Varkey, J. B., J. G. Shantha, I. Crozier, C. S. Kraft, G. M. Lyon, A. K. Mehta, G. Kumar, J. R. Smith, M. H. Kainulainen, S. Whitmer, U. Ströher, T. M. Uyeki, B. S. Ribner, and S. Yeh. 2015. Persistence of Ebola virus in ocular fluid during convalescence. *New England Journal of Medicine* 372(25):2423–2427.

Varma, R., T. S. Vajaranant, B. Burkemper, S. Wu, M. Torres, C. Hsu, F. Choudhury, R. McKean-Cowdin. 2016. Visual impairment and blindness in adults in the United States: Demographic and geographic variations from 2015 to 2050. *JAMA Ophthalmology* 134(7):802–809.

Walter, C., R. Althouse, H. Humble, M. Leys, and J. Odom. 2004. West Virginia survey of visual health: Low vision and barriers to access. *Visual Impairment Research* 6(1):53–71.

Whitson, H. E., S. W. Cousins, B. M. Burchett, C. F. Hybels, C. F. Pieper, and H. J. Cohen. 2007. The combined effect of visual impairment and cognitive impairment on disability in older people. *Journal of the American Geriatric Society* 55(6):885–891.

Whitson, H. E., R. Malhotra, A. Chan, D. B. Matchar, and T. Ostbye. 2014. Comorbid visual and cognitive impairment: Relationship with disability status and self-rated health among older Singaporeans. *Asia Pacific Journal of Public Health* 26(3):310–319.

WHO (World Health Organization). 1986. The Ottawa Charter for Health Promotion. http://www.who.int/healthpromotion/conferences/previous/ottawa/en (accessed October 7, 2015).

———. 2015. Blindness: Vision 2020—the global initiative for the elimination of avoidable blindness. http://www.who.int/mediacentre/factsheets/fs213/en (accessed October 7, 2015).

———. n.d. Change the definition of blindness. http://www.who.int/blindness/Change%20 the%20Definition%20of%20Blindness.pdf (accessed May 18, 2016).

Wittenborn, J., and D. Rein. 2013. *Cost of vision problems: The economic burden of vision loss and eye disorders in the United States.* Chicago, IL: NORC at the University of Chicago.

———. 2016. *The potential costs and benefits of treatment for undiagnosed eye disorders.* Paper prepared for the Committee on Public Health Approaches to Reduce Vision Impairment and Promote Eye Health. http://www.nationalacademies.org/hmd/~/media/ Files/Report%20Files/2016/UndiagnosedEyeDisordersCommissionedPaper.pdf (accessed September 15, 2016).

Wittenborn, J., X. Zhang, C. W. Feagan, W. L. Crouse, S. Shrestha, A. R. Kemper, T. J. Hoerger, J. B. Saaddine, and the Vision Cost-Effectiveness Study Group. 2013. The economic burden of vision loss and eye disorders among the United States population younger than 40 years. *Ophthalmology* 120(9):1728–1735.

Wood, J. M., P. F. Lacherez, and K. J. Anstey. 2012. Not all older adults have insight into their driving abilities: Evidence from an on-road assessment and implications for policy. *Journals of Gerontology Series A: Biological Sciences and Medical Sciences* 68(5):559–566.

Yip, J. L., R. Luben, A. P. Khawaja, D. C. Broadway, N. Wareham, K. T. Khaw, and P. J. Foster. 2014. Area deprivation, individual socioeconomic status and low vision in the Epic-Norfolk Eye Study. *Journal of Epidemiology and Community Health* 68(3):204–210.

Zambelli-Weiner, A., J. E. Crews, and D. S. Friedman. 2012. Disparities in adult vision health in the United States. *American Journal of Ophthalmology* 154(6 Suppl):S23–S30, e21.

Zhang, X., M. F. Cotch, A. Ryskulova, S. A. Primo, P. Nair, C. F. Chou, L. S. Geiss, L. E. Barker, A. F. Elliott, J. E. Crews, and J. B. Saaddine. 2012. Vision health disparities in the United States by race/ethnicity, education, and economic status: Findings from two nationally representative surveys. *American Journal of Ophthalmology* 154(6):53–62.

Zhang, X., G. L. Beckles, C. F. Chou, J. B. Saaddine, M. R. Wilson, P. P. Lee, N. Parvathy, A. Ryskulova, and L. S. Geiss. 2013. Socioeconomic disparity in use of eye care services among U.S. adults with age-related eye diseases: National Health Interview Survey, 2002 and 2008. *JAMA Ophthalmology* 131(9):1198–1206.

2

Understanding the Epidemiology of Vision Loss and Impairment in the United States

The vast majority of individuals in the United States who reach average life expectancy will experience some type and degree of vision loss and impairment[1] during their lifetimes, given current knowledge about effective prevention strategies, barriers to accessing appropriate health care, and the aging process itself. Even mild vision impairment (i.e., near-normal vision) can have a "tangible influence on quality of life" (Cumberland et al., 2016, p. E1). Many eye diseases, conditions, and injuries affect vision, but they do not all contribute equally to the overall burden of vision loss in terms of numbers or populations affected nor the severity or the permanence of subsequent visual impairment. From clinical management and public health perspectives, it is important to understand what the major etiologies of vision loss are, who is most at risk, what risk and protective factors are known and modifiable, and how outcomes may be changed through policy and practice.

There is no peer-reviewed literature on the total population affected by all causes of vision impairment in the United States. Presbyopia, an

---

[1] In Chapter 1, the committee defines *vision loss* as the process by which physiological changes or structural, neurological, or acquired damage to the structure or function of one or both eyes or visual information processing structures in the brain occurs, resulting in vision impairment. *Vision impairment* is defined as a measure of the type and severity of clinical or functional limitation of one or both eyes or visual information processing structures in the brain. These limitations range in severity from mild impairment to total blindness and can affect visual acuity, visual field, and aspects of the eyes or visual system. However, as indicated throughout this chapter, different studies may define vision impairment more narrowly and separately from blindness.

age-related condition that results from the lens losing its ability to change shape and focus clearly on near objects, affects almost everyone entering the middle-age years but can be treated with near-vision lenses (e.g., bifocal, progressive or multifocal lenses, or reading glasses) (Petrash, 2013). One model, based on a review of 12 major epidemiological studies and the 2010 U.S. Census population, estimates that approximately 90 million of the 142 million adults over the age of 40 in the United States experienced vision problems attributable to vision impairment, blindness, refractive error (i.e., myopia and hyperopia), age-related macular degeneration (AMD),[2] cataracts, diabetic retinopathy, and glaucoma (Prevent Blindness, 2012b).[3] Refractive error alone is estimated to affect more than 48 million people ages 12 and older in the United States (Prevent Blindness, 2012g), and between 8.2 and 15.9 million people have undiagnosed or untreated refractive error (Varma et al., 2016; Wittenborn and Rein, 2016).[4] As the baby boomer generation ages, older adults will account for an ever larger proportion of the total population, and age-related eye diseases and conditions are projected to increase accordingly (Varma et al., 2016; Wittenborn and Rein, 2016).

This chapter provides an overview of the epidemiology of eye and vision health in the United States. The first section describes some of the major components of a healthy, functioning visual system. The second section describes the epidemiology of vision impairment and common eye disorders in the United States, including differences by age, gender, and race and ethnicity and current evidence about specific risk and protective factors. The third section proposes four categories of vision impairment by which to frame different population health approaches and provides examples of relevant interventions and treatments. The fourth section describes potential opportunities to reduce the preventable burden of vision impairment from uncorrected refractive error and cataracts in the United States based, in part, on an analysis commissioned by the committee.[5] The chapter concludes with a brief summary of key knowledge and research gaps.

---

[2] The estimate for AMD includes individuals ages 50 and older.

[3] This statistic was corrected following release of the prepublication copy of the report.

[4] The committee commissioned an analysis, which was not available in the current literature, to establish the preventable burden of vision impairment in the United States from five conditions (diabetic retinopathy, glaucoma, refractive error, cataracts, and AMD). Estimates are based on a variety of sources (including population surveys and compilations of population-based studies) and reflect the best available public data. The committee presents only the results related to cataracts and uncorrected refractive error in this report because the analyses are most robust for these conditions. Chapter 3 provides a more in-depth description of the study's assumptions and limitations, which are also documented in the commissioned paper itself (Wittenborn and Rein, 2016).

[5] The number of people ages 65 years and older in the United States is expected to almost double from 44.7 million (14.1 percent) in 2013 to 82.3 million (21.7 percent) in 2040 (AoA, 2014).

ANATOMY OF THE EYE AND FUNCTION
OF THE VISUAL SYSTEM

Good eye and vision health requires a functioning visual system to effectively capture light from an object and translate it into neural impulses that are processed in the brain. The visual system consists of the eye, the pathways that conduct neural impulses from the eye to the brain, and specific areas within the brain to interpret the signals. Figure 2-1 illustrates some of the major parts of the eye, which are referenced throughout this chapter. Light enters the eye through the cornea, which helps refract light. The pupil is the small opening at the center of the iris, which functions like the shutter of a camera to regulate the amount of light entering the pupil and expanding and contracting the opening in response to ambient light. The lens further focuses light on the retina, with muscles controlling the lens shape to differentially focus on objects based on distance from the eye. Between the lens and the retina is the vitreous humor—a clear gel that gives the eye its spherical shape and keeps the retina in place. The retina includes blood vessels and a thin layer of light-sensitive tissue (photoreceptors called cones and rods), which translate light energy into neural impulses. Within the retina, the macula has millions of tightly packed cones that are concentrated at the fovea and are responsible for sharp, detailed central vision and color vision. Surrounding the macula, rods are more sensitive to light and are responsible for night vision, peripheral vision, and the ability to

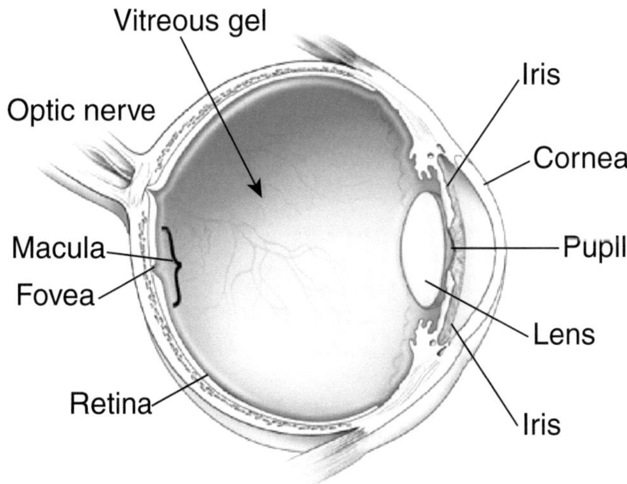

FIGURE 2-1 Anatomy of the human eye.
SOURCE: NEI/NIH, 2012a.

detect motion. Photoreceptors convert light into electrical signals, which are relayed to the brain through the optic nerve. Within the brain, visual information is parsed and relayed along various pathways, and eventually interpreted as a recognizable image.

Vision impairment can result from damage or dysfunction to any part of the visual system, including individual components of the eye. How a person's vision is affected depends on the structures involved and the degree of subclinical and clinical damage or dysfunction to those structures. There are hundreds of diseases, conditions, and injuries to the eye that can negatively affect vision, including various rare diseases, which often have a genetic component and can have substantial impacts on the people affected. However, most cases of vision impairment in the U.S. population are attributable to a small number of causes. Table 2-1 defines and provides

TABLE 2-1 Common Visual System Conditions and Diseases and General Examples of Therapeutic Approaches for Improvement

Disease or Condition	Affected Structure	Definition and General Approaches for Improvement
Age-related macular degeneration (AMD)	Macula	A degenerative eye disease that causes damage to the macula. "Dry" AMD is caused by the breakdown of light-sensitive cells in the macula, where as neovascular or "wet" AMD is caused by fluid leaking from abnormal vessels under the retina, leading to blurred vision, dark areas or distortion in central field of vision, and loss of central vision (NEI/NIH, 2013).
		Treatments are available to slow the progression of neovascular AMD. For late neovasular AMD, eye injections to control edema and the growth of new blood vessels are available. Dry AMD is largely untreatable, although there have been promising discoveries related to nutrition and certain injections.
Amblyopia	Brain	A neurological disorder in children, also referred to as "lazy eye," in which reduced vision in one or both eye occurs due to abnormal interaction or lack of a clear image (Barrett et al., 2013; Pascula et al., 2014).
		Treatments include refractive correction, patching, vision therapy, orthoptics, and eye drops.
Cataracts	Lens	Clouding or discoloration of the lens caused by the clumping of proteins (NEI/NIH, 2010d). Over time the cataracts may grow denser and cloud more of the lens, making it harder to see. Infants may be born with cataracts.
		Treatments include lens removal usually accompanied by lens replacement. Use of eyeglasses, better lighting, and magnifying glasses may help to reduce symptoms.

TABLE 2-1 Continued

Disease or Condition	Affected Structure	Definition and General Approaches for Improvement
Diabetic retinopathy	Blood vessels in retina	Chronically high blood glucose from diabetes causes the blood vessels in the retina to leak fluid and/or hemorrhage, leading to a build-up of fluid in the macula and eventually retinal detachment (NEI/NIH, 2010e). New blood vessels may also form either within the retina or optic nerve. Symptoms include seeing "floating" spots, blurred vision, and permanent vision loss.
		Treatments include control of systemic blood glucose, laser treatment for growth of new blood vessels, and eye injections to control macular edema.
Glaucoma (Open Angle)	Optic nerve	Loss of nerve tissue and axons in the optic nerve associated with elevated intraocular pressure above the level which the eye can tolerate, although normotensive glaucoma occurs in patients without elevated intraocular pressure (NEI/NIH, 2010h).
		Treatments include control of eye pressure through therapeutic eye drops and surgery.
Infection	Different parts of the eye, depending on type of infection	Can include ocular, systemic, and nosocomial infections. Infections can affect the conjunctiva, cornea, and various internal structures of the visual system.
		Prevention includes improved hygiene, up-to-date immunizations, safe sex practices, and other measures.
Injury	The eye or brain	Injuries to the eye, surrounding structures, or damage to visual processing areas within brain.
		Prevention includes use of protective eyewear in workplaces and for sports activities.
Refractive error	Cornea, lens, or eye shape	Irregular shape of cornea, lens, or eyeball prevents light from focusing properly on the retina, causing blurred vision (NEI/NIH, 2010f).
		Treatments include corrective lenses to improve vision and refractive eye surgery.
Strabismus	The accommodative system[a]	A condition in which there is a misalignment of the eyes, such that one eye constantly or intermittently turns in (esotropia), out (exotropia), up, or down as the other eye looks straight ahead (Hatt and Gnanaraj, 2013).
		Treatments include corrective lenses, prism, eye exercises, patching, eye drops, and/or eye muscle surgery.

[a] The accommodative system can be simply described as the lens, eye muscles, and cranial nerves or brainstem that controls eye movement, although the exact pathway and mechanism are more nuanced.

a high-level summary of some of the more common visual system diseases and conditions, which the committee selected based on the number of children and adults affected and to highlight the variety of public health strategies that will be necessary to comprehensively address eye and vision health in the United States.

As a person ages, many physiological changes occur within the eye that affect vision. Over time, virtually every measure of visual function declines to some extent, including but not limited to decreasing visual acuity (the ability to resolve images of various sizes at fixed distances), sensitivity of the visual field (the ability to detect objects of various sizes within visual space), contrast sensitivity (the ability to detect images against decreasingly contrasting backgrounds), slowed visual processing speeds (increasing time to complete visual tasks), tear production and elimination (resulting in dry eye or obscured vision), and dark adaptation (the ability to adjust to low levels of illumination) (Owsley, 2011; Salvi et al., 2006; Sharma and Hindman, 2014). In diseases such as diabetic retinopathy, glaucoma, and AMD, physiological changes related to the aging process alter the physical conditions under which light enters the eye or compromise the cellular function or neural pathways that relay information about the physical environment to the eye or the brain. In their early and intermediate stages, changes in vision may not be noticeable without a dilated eye examination, despite ongoing damage to structures of the visual system.

THE EPIDEMIOLOGY OF VISION IMPAIRMENT IN THE UNITED STATES

Determining the overall burden of vision impairment in the United States is challenging. Several well-designed population-based studies in the United States provide vital epidemiological estimates, but national epidemiological data related to prevalence, incidence, trends, and impact are limited, especially for adults under age 40 and for children and adolescents. (See Chapter 4 for detailed discussion of surveillance and research challenges in eye and vision health.) National prevalence rates of vision impairment by etiology are typically calculated from the results of surveys, often self-reported by respondents, or are an aggregation of smaller studies, usually cross-sectional and not prospective. Studies of specific diseases and conditions may use the history of a medical intervention as a proxy for actual disease prevalence, which likely results in underestimations. Smaller studies of specific diseases and conditions that include comprehensive eye examinations[6] tend to have more accurate measures of prevalence, incidence, and disease severity, but the results may be less generalizable and representative nationally.

Reporting of epidemiological data is further complicated because outcomes are not measured or reported consistently. The differences may seem minor, but they can have substantial implications for which policies and practices are most appropriate, For example, *uncorrectable vision impairment* can be described as the amount of vision impairment that remains after appropriate treatment or intervention. Thus, the public health goal to improve health for individuals with uncorrectable vision impairment is to prevent the impairment, develop new therapies that will further correct or reverse the impairment, or provide services that improve the function of those individuals with the impairment. *Uncorrected vision impairment* refers to the proportion of overall vision impairment that could be improved through currently available and appropriate treatment or intervention. For example, many people have significant refractive error that could easily be corrected through use of prescription glasses or contact lenses. Thus, the public health goal is to either prevent the impairment or to increase access to treatments and interventions that do correct for the vision impairment.

This section presents estimates of overall prevalence for uncorrectable vision impairment only, along with the epidemiology for refractive error, amblyopia and strabismus, visual system injury, glaucoma, diabetic retinopathy, AMD, cataract, vision-threatening infection, and rare eye diseases and conditions. The committee commissioned an analysis to provide current estimates of uncorrected refractive error and cataract in the United States. These results, along with estimates of preventable eye injuries, are discussed in a subsequent section.

Uncorrectable Vision Impairment

Two recent estimates suggest that approximately 4.2 million adults ages 40 years and older in the United States suffer from uncorrectable vision impairment, including blindness (Prevent Blindness, 2012h; Varma et al., 2016). In commissioned work for Prevent Blindness, Wittenborn and colleagues (2013) estimated that another 2.155 million children and adults under age 40 have uncorrectable vision impairment or blindness.[7]

---

[6] The committee defines a comprehensive eye examination as a dilated eye examination that may include a range of other tests, in addition to the dilation of the pupil to see the retinal structures (or back of the eye).

[7] All three studies define "uncorrectable visual impairment" in terms of visual acuity less than 20/40 but better than 20/200 in the better-seeing eye after correction and separate from blindness. Blindness is defined as visual acuity less than or equal to 20/200 in the better-seeing eye after correction (Prevent Blindness, 2012h; Varma et al., 2016; Wittenborn et al., 2013).

This raises questions about how to improve access to treatments to slow progression of vision loss and how to promote function and health within this population.

Vision Impairment in Adults Ages 40 and Older

Most of the data available about overall vision impairment in adults focus on individuals ages 40 and older. The most recent data on the prevalence and total numbers of individuals with uncorrectable visual impairment (20/40 or worse vision with best possible correction) and blindness in adults come from two, separate sources that pool data from a number of studies to calculate national estimates. Varma and colleagues (2016) calculated prevalence rates and the number of individuals with vision impairment by aggregating data from six major U.S. population-based studies that included more detailed data on U.S. minority groups.[8] Prevent Blindness aggregated data from 12 studies that included both U.S. and non-U.S. based studies (Prevent Blindness, 2012e).[9] Both studies have methodological and interpretation limitations due to the pooling of data from diverse studies; however, they are the best estimates available at this time.[10]

Table 2-2 provides prevalence estimates and numbers of persons with uncorrectable vision impairment and blindness from these studies. According to the Varma study, in 2015, the overall estimated prevalence of uncorrectable visual impairment in the U.S. population among individuals ages 40 and older was 2.14 percent, and the overall estimated prevalence of blindness was 0.68 percent. Prevent Blindness estimated the prevalence of uncorrectable visual impairment to be 2.04 percent and the prevalence of blindness to be 0.90 percent based on the 2010 U.S. population (Prevent Blindness

---

[8] Varma and colleagues (2016) pooled prevalence data from U.S.-based studies: Baltimore Eye Survey, Beaver Dam Eye Study, LALES for Asian individuals, Proyecto VER, and the Salisbury Eye Evaluation Study.

[9] Prevent Blindness America pooled data from U.S. and international studies: Baltimore Eye Survey, Beaver Dam Eye Study, Blue Mountains Eye Study, Kongwa Eye Survey, Proyecto VER, Rotterdam Study, Salisbury Eye Evaluation Study, San Antonio Heart Study, San Luis Valley Diabetes Study, Visual Impairment Project, and Wisconsin Epidemiological Study of Diabetic Retinopathy.

[10] Although these studies represent the best available data on the prevalence of vision impairment and blindness in the United States, they are not without limitations. Varma and colleagues (2016) note that their models do not account for changes in treatment or prevention of major causes of vision impairment and blindness, and that the criterion for blindness is based on visual acuity alone. Not accounting for the effects of visual field loss on the prevalence of blindness could lead to an underestimation of the prevalence of vision impairment and blindness. Prevalence data in the Prevent Blindness database are aggregated from 12 studies, including 5 studies on populations outside the United States. Thus, the generalizability to the U.S. general population is limited for this reason.

TABLE 2-2 Estimated Prevalence and Number of Persons with Uncorrectable Vision Impairment and Blindness in the United States

Source	Varma et al. (2016)[a]	Prevent Blindness (2012)[b]
Prevalence estimates (in percentages) for uncorrectable vision impairment	2.14	2.04[c]
Prevalence estimates (in percentages) for blindness	0.68	0.86[d]
Number of persons affected (in millions) for uncorrectable vision impairment	3.22	2.91
Number of persons affected (in millions) for blindness	1.02	1.29
Total number of people with uncorrectable visual impairment and blindness	4.24	4.20

[a] Varma defines uncorrectable vision impairment as best-corrected visual acuity worse than 20/40 but better than 20/200 in the better-seeing eye; Varma defines blindness as best-corrected visual acuity of 20/200 or worse in the better-seeing eye.
[b] Prevent Blindness defines vision impairment as having worse than 20/40 vision in the better eye even with eyeglasses and blindness as visual acuity with best correction in the better eye worse than or equal to 20/200 or a visual field extent of less than 20 degrees in diameter.
[c] Prevalence is calculated by dividing the number of individuals with visual impairment (2,907,691) by the 2010 U.S. Census Population (142,648,393) and multiplying by 100.
[d] Prevalence is calculated by dividing the number of blind individuals (1,288,275) by the 2010 U.S. Census Population (142,648,393) and multiplying by 100.
SOURCES: Prevent Blindness, 2012c,h; Varma et al., 2016, table 5.

2012c,h). Because of continued changes in the size and demographics of the U.S. population and the availability of data on Asians as a separate category, the more recent data from Varma and colleagues (2016), rather than the data from Prevent Blindness, are used to describe current overall prevalence rates for uncorrectable visual impairment and blindness by age, race and ethnicity, and gender.

Table 2-3 provides estimates of uncorrectable vision impairment and blindness by the decades of life, beginning at age 40 for 2015 and projected for 2050; the data are presented for those individuals with uncorrectable vision impairment and blindness. About half of the cases of visual impairment and blindness affect persons ages 40 to 79. The combined total number of persons ages 40 and older who have uncorrectable vision impairment or are blind is projected to more than double from 4.24 million in 2015 to 8.96 million in 2050 (Varma et al., 2016).

Table 2-4 shows the numbers and prevalence of individuals ages 40 and older with uncorrectable visual impairment and blindness by gender and race and ethnicity in the United States for the year 2015 and the projected numbers for 2050. African Americans ages 40 and older have a higher overall age-adjusted prevalence of uncorrectable visual impairment and blindness than people in other racial and ethnic groups. The

TABLE 2-3 The Number of Persons with Uncorrectable Vision Impairment and Blindness in Adults Ages 40 and Older by Age Group in the United States in the Year 2015 and Projected for the Year 2050 (in millions)

	Vision Impairment	Blindness	Total	Vision Impairment	Blindness	Total
Year	2015			2050		
Ages 40–49	0.13	0.11	0.24	0.16	0.13	0.29
Ages 50–59	0.17	0.15	0.32	0.21	0.15	0.36
Ages 60–69	0.52	0.16	0.68	0.70	0.23	0.93
Ages 70–79	0.78	0.17	0.95	1.43	0.32	1.75
Ages 80 and older	1.61	0.43	2.04	4.44	1.18	5.62
All ages 40 and older	3.22	1.02	4.24	6.95	2.01	8.96

SOURCE: Varma et al., 2016, p. E3.

TABLE 2-4 Prevalence and Number of Uncorrectable Visual Impairment and Blindness in Adults Ages 40 and Older by Age Group by Race/Ethnicity and Gender in 2015 and Projected for 2050 in the United States

		Vision Impairment			Blindness		
		Number in Millions		Age-Adjusted Prevalence (%)[a]	Number in Millions		Age-Adjusted Prevalence (%)[a]
Race/Ethnicity	Gender	2015	2050	2015	2015	2050	2015
Non-Hispanic White	Men	0.99	1.78	1.79	0.32	0.46	0.6
	Women	1.29	2.15	2.25	0.37	0.61	0.65
	Total	2.28	3.93	4.04	0.69	1.07	1.25
African American	Men	0.22	0.51	2.84	0.12	0.27	1.47
	Women	0.27	0.62	2.67	0.1	0.20	1.01
	Total	0.49	1.13	5.51	0.21	0.47	2.48
Hispanic/Latino	Men	0.11	0.49	1.12	0.05	0.21	0.52
	Women	0.21	0.92	2.12	0.05	0.21	0.55
	Total	0.32	1.41	3.24	0.10	0.42	1.07
Asian	Men	0.05	0.21	1.38	0.004	0.015	0.18
	Women	0.05	0.2	1.09	0.005	0.018	0.13
	Total	0.1	0.41	2.47	0.009	0.033	0.31
Other Minorities	Men	0.01	0.01	1.83	0.004	0.009	0.62
	Women	0.02	0.02	2.49	0.003	0.008	0.5
	Total	0.03	0.03	4.32	0.007	0.018	1.12
All Races	Men	1.38	3.00	8.96	0.50	0.96	3.39
	Women	1.84	3.91	10.62	0.53	1.05	2.84
	Total	3.22	6.91[b]	19.58	1.03	2.01	6.23

[a] Projections for age-adjusted estimates were not available for 2050.
[b] Slight difference due to rounding.
SOURCE: Varma et al., 2016, p. E3, eTable 2, and eTable 4.

age-adjusted prevalence of uncorrectable vision impairment and blindness is lower among Hispanics and Asians than among other minorities and non-Hispanic whites. Among Hispanics, non-Hispanic whites, and other minorities, uncorrectable vision impairment occurs more frequently in women than in men; among African Americans and Asians, men are at a greater risk of uncorrectable vision impairment than women. Non-Hispanic white women contribute larger numbers to the current and projected burden of uncorrectable vision impairment and blindness than any other group.

Minority populations in the United States are already at risk for poorer overall health (IOM, 2003). Demographic trends in the United States suggest that the burden of uncorrected vision impairment will increasingly affect these populations. By 2020, more than half of all children in the United States will be part of a minority race or ethnic group; by 2044, that will be true of all age groups (U.S. Census Bureau, 2015). These demographic trends will affect the relative prevalence of uncorrectable vision impairment among groups (see Figure 2-2). Women will continue to account for more cases of uncorrectable vision impairment and blindness than men, but this gap will close slightly from 1.33 to 1.3 women for every man in 2015 and

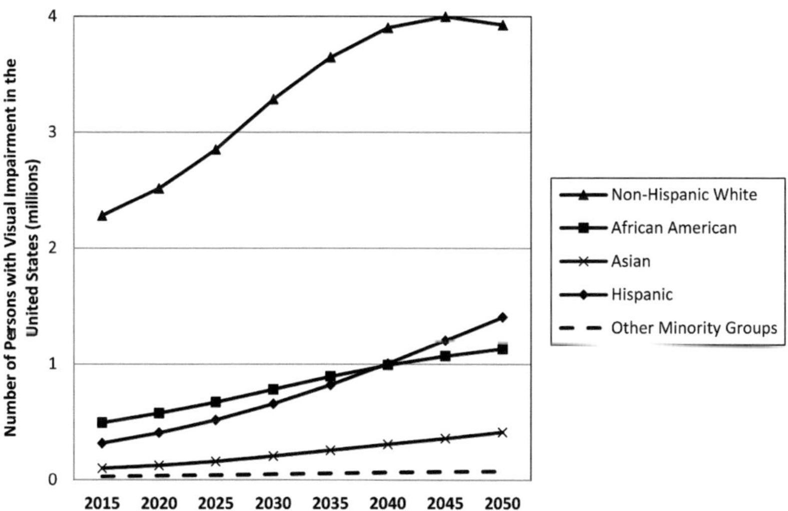

FIGURE 2-2 Estimated numbers of persons with uncorrectable visual impairment (not including blindness) ages 50 and older in the United States by race/ethnicity (all persons) from 2015 to 2050.
SOURCE: Varma et al., 2016, Figure 1.

2050, respectively (Varma et al., 2016). Similarly, non-Hispanic whites will account for the majority of uncorrectable visual impairment cases, but this proportion will decrease from 71 percent in 2015 to 57 percent in 2050. The number of Hispanics, African Americans, and Asians with uncorrectable vision impairment is also predicted to increase from 2015 to 2050, but the number of "other minorities" will remain relatively static. By 2050, Hispanics will surpass the number of African Americans with uncorrectable visual impairment. The estimated number of individuals with blindness follows similar trends; non-Hispanic whites will continue to account for a greater proportion of individuals affected by blindness followed by African Americans and Hispanics. The total number of cases of blindness among people ages 80 and older is projected to increase from 430,000 in 2015 to 1.18 million in 2050.

Vision Impairment in Younger Adults

Data on the visual conditions and disorders affecting younger adults and children are more limited. Wittenborn and colleagues (2013) used data from the 2003 to 2008 Medical Expenditure Panel Surveys (MEPS) to estimate that approximately 2.41 million (2.62 percent) of individuals ages 18 to 39 were affected with 13 medical eye conditions (excluding disorders of refraction and accommodation) in 2012 (see Table 2-5). Injury and burns to the eye and disorders of the conjunctiva were the most prevalent.

Wittenborn and colleagues (2013) also included estimates on the severity of uncorrectable visual impairment based on companion data from the 2005–2008 National Health and Nutrition Examination Study (NHANES). As discussed in Chapter 4, for children ages 12 and older, NHANES has included general questions related to eye and vision health from 2005 to 2008, along with a "vision examination" from 2003 to 2008 (CDC, 2015d). Researchers can impute prevalence for younger ages based on "incidence of blindness adjusted such that predicted prevalence at age 16 equals the observed NHANES prevalence" (Wittenborn et al., 2013, p. 1731). Of the 1.3 million people 39 years old and younger who had some degree of uncorrectable vision impairment, approximately 83 percent (1.1 million) had mild impairment (a visual acuity of worse than 20/40 to 20/80), 10 percent (128,000) had moderate impairment (visual acuity of 20/80 to 20/200), and about 7 percent (92,000) were blind (Wittenborn et al., 2013).[11]

---

[11] The nomenclature of mild and moderate impairment understates the degree to which the impairment can affect one's ability to operate in the wider world; for example, driver's licenses are often restricted for persons with visual acuity worse than 20/40.

TABLE 2-5 Prevalence of Vision Disorder Diagnoses Among Young Adults (Ages 18–39) in the Medical Expenditure Panel Survey, 2003 Through 2008

Condition[a]	Prevalence (%)[b]	Individuals (in thousands)
Disorders of the globe	0.45	417
Injury and burns	0.56	511
Disorders of conjunctiva	0.54	493
Other eye disorders	0.46	422
Strabismus, binocular eye movements	0.03[c]	27
Visual disturbances	0.17	160
Blindness and low vision	0.12	107
Disorders of lacrimal system	0.13	120
Cataract	0.05	48
Retinal detachment, defects, and disorders	0.05	48
Disorders of the eyelids	0.19	174
Glaucoma	0.11	97
Disorders of optic nerve and visual pathways	0.03[c]	24
Total	2.62	2,405

[a] Medical conditions exclude disorders of refraction and accommodation.
[b] Values do not sum because some individuals had multiple conditions.
[c] Not statistically distinguishable from zero.
SOURCE: Adapted from Wittenborn et al., 2013.

Vision Impairment in Children and Adolescents

The epidemiology of visual impairment in children and adolescents differs from that in adults, and far less information is available on the prevalence of visual impairment in this group. Vision impairment in young children is common (Kemper et al., 2004). The U.S. Preventive Services Task Force states that between 1 and 5 percent of preschool-aged children in the United States have vision impairment (USPSTF, 2011). One study found that among U.S. children ages 30 to 72 months, visual impairment due to an underlying eye disease occurred in the worse eye of 3.4 percent of Asian children and 2.6 percent of non-Hispanic white children (Tarczy-Hornoch et al., 2013). The prevalence of visual impairment or amblyopia from uncorrected refractive error was more than 5 percent among African American and Hispanic preschoolers (ages 30 to 72 months) (MEPEDS, 2009). Among 0 to 17-year-olds, Wittenborn et al. (2013) estimated that 857,000 individuals have uncorrectable vision loss (prevalence of 1.16 percent), and parses this group by degree of impairment: 775,000 have mild impairment (visual acuity of less than 20/40 to 20/80), 76,000 have moderate impairment (visual acuity of 20/80 to 20/200), and 6,000 are blind. Table 2-6 lists the prevalence of 13 types of vision problems among

TABLE 2-6 Prevalence of Vision Disorder Diagnoses Among Children (Ages 0–17) in the Medical Expenditure Panel Survey, 2003 Through 2008

Condition[a]	Prevalence (%)[b]	Individuals (in thousands)
Disorders of the globe	0.67	499
Injury and burns	0.38	280
Disorders of conjunctiva	1.76	1,302
Other eye disorders	0.51	377
Strabismus, binocular eye movements	0.24	175
Visual disturbances	0.26	196
Blindness and low vision	0.09	69
Disorders of lacrimal system	0.18	136
Cataract	0.01[c]	11
Retinal detachment, defects, and disorders	0.04	31
Disorders of the eyelids	0.16	121
Glaucoma	0.04[c]	28
Disorders of optic nerve and visual pathways	0.02[c]	14
Total	4.13	3,063

[a] Medical conditions exclude disorders of refraction and accommodation.
[b] Values do not sum because some individuals had multiple conditions.
[c] Not statistically distinguishable from 0.
SOURCE: Adapted from Wittenborn et al., 2013.

U.S. children ages 17 and younger, which does not include refractive error or accommodation disorders.

Geographic Distribution of Uncorrectable Vision Impairment and Blindness

The overall burden of eye disease varies from state to state, and the pattern of highest and lowest prevalence varies by condition. Similarly, the distribution of uncorrectable visual impairment and blindness varies significantly by region and state. Figures 2-3, 2-4, 2-5, and 2-6 depict the estimated per-capita rates of visual impairment and blindness in each state for populations ages 40 and older in 2015 and 2050 (Varma et al., 2016). Per-capita rates (per 100 persons) were highest in the District of Columbia (2.75), Florida (2.56), Mississippi (2.35), Hawaii (2.35), and Pennsylvania (2.29), whereas the lowest per-capita rates were found in Western states—Alaska (1.53), Utah (1.80), Colorado (1.83), Nevada (1.90), and Washington (1.91) (Varma et al., 2016). By 2050, the projected per-capita rates will remain the highest in the District of Columbia (4.29) and Florida (3.98), followed by Hawaii (3.93), South Dakota (3.70), and North Dakota (3.69),

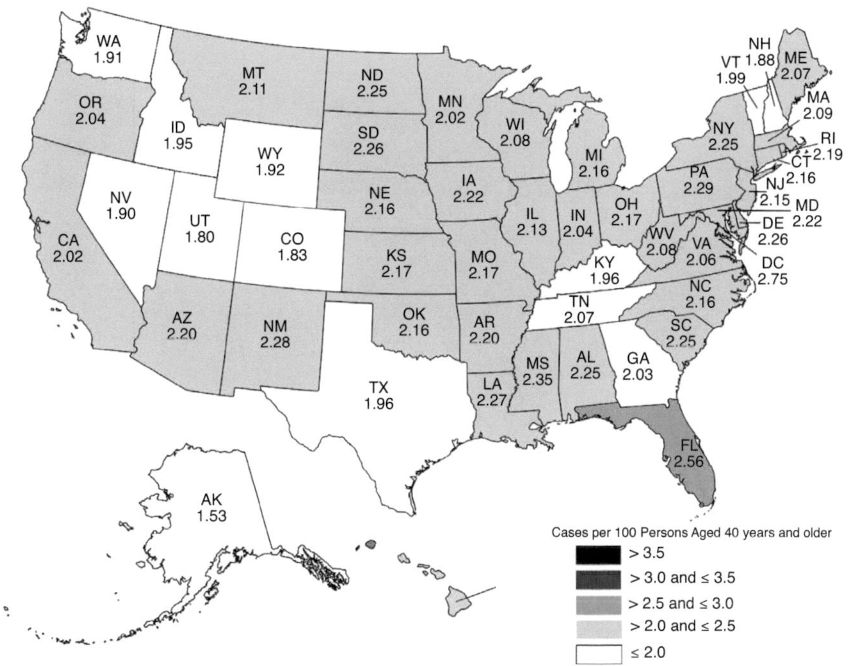

FIGURE 2-3 Per-capita prevalence of uncorrectable visual impairment in the United States in 2015.
SOURCE: Used with permission, Varma et al., 2016.

although per-capita prevalence of uncorrectable visual impairment is projected to rise in every state.

Per-capita rates of blindness in the United States demonstrate similar patterns. In 2015, the District of Columbia (1.07), Mississippi (0.83), Louisiana (0.79), and Florida (0.78), have the highest per-capita rates, followed closely by South Carolina, Alabama, and Maryland (0.77). Hawaii (0.42), Alaska (0.49), Utah (0.56), Colorado (0.58), and Washington (0.58) have the lowest per-capita rates. Projected per-capita rates of blindness in 2050 will remain higher in the East than in the West, with every state projected to have prevalence increases.

Another study by the Centers for Disease Control and Prevention (CDC) collected data from 19 states that fielded a special vision module during the 2006–2008 Behavioral Risk Factor Surveillance System (BRFSS) to estimate prevalence rates based on self-reported data among adults ages 65 and older for cataract, glaucoma, AMD, and diabetic retinopathy (CDC,

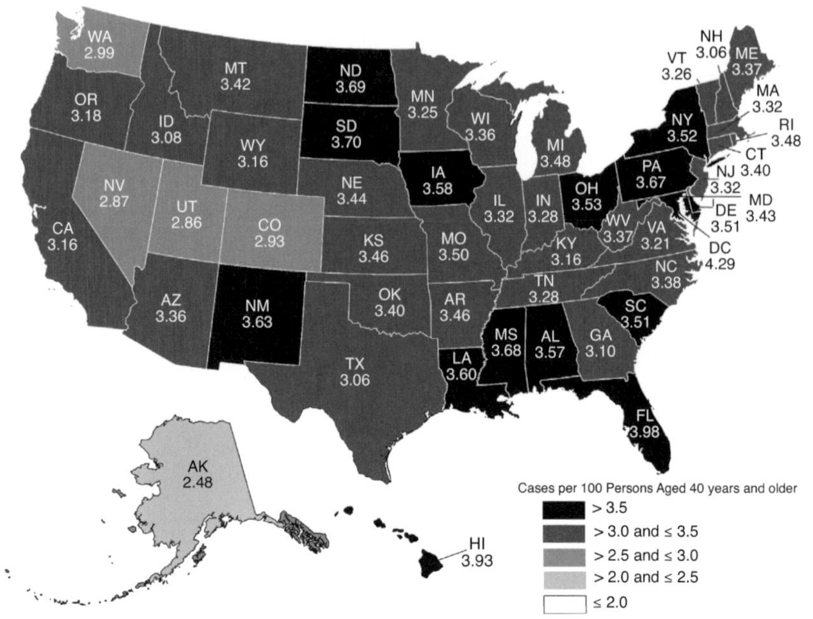

FIGURE 2-4 Per-capita prevalence of uncorrectable visual impairment in the United States in 2050.
SOURCE: Used with permission, Varma et al., 2016.

2011b). Iowa, Missouri, North Carolina, and West Virginia reported the highest prevalence rates for cataract (31.2 to 33.7 percent). New York, North Carolina, Ohio, and Texas reported the highest prevalence rates for glaucoma (10.3 to 12.3 percent). Indiana, Nebraska, New Mexico, and Wyoming reported the highest prevalence rates of age-related macular degeneration (10.6 to 11.5 percent). Alabama, Georgia, Indiana, New York, and North Carolina reported the highest prevalence rates of diabetic retinopathy (4.0 to 5.0 percent).[12]

Even within states there can be substantial variation in severity of vision loss. At the county level, variations in the prevalence of vision loss are dramatic. Data from the American Community Survey from 2009 to 2013 show significant inter-county variation (between less than 1.0 percent to 18.4 percent) in the prevalence of severe vision loss among adults ages

---

[12] Note: BRFSS data can be compared to Prevent Blindness data at www.visionproblems. org/index/state-summaries.html (accessed August 28, 2016).

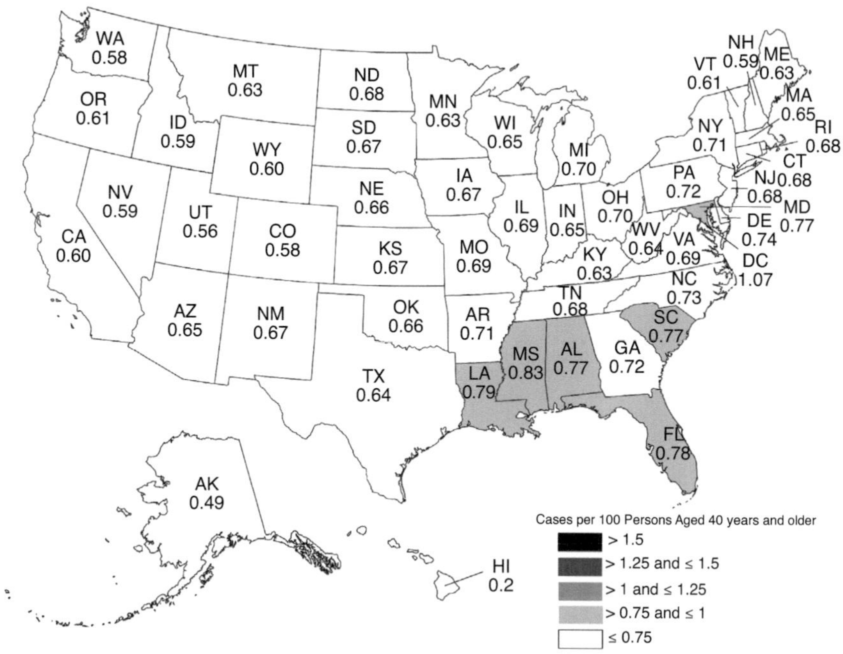

FIGURE 2-5 Per-capita prevalence of blindness in the United States in 2015.
SOURCE: Used with permission, Varma et al., 2016.

18 and older (Kirtland et al., 2015).[13,14] Of counties in the top quartile of severe vision loss prevalence,[15] 77.3 percent are located in Southern states. High prevalence rates have also been significantly correlated with poverty (Kirtland et al., 2015).

Prevalence rates are influenced by characteristics of the population, such as age, race and ethnicity, and socioeconomic status, among other broader determinants of health. Better county-level data would allow for more specific allocation of resources than state-level data. State-level data can mask disparities among and within geographically smaller areas. Smaller geographic areas more closely align with service referral and delivery patterns

---

[13] The survey included people ages 18 and older.

[14] Severe vision loss is defined in the American Community Survey as a positive self-reported response to the question, "Is this person blind or does s/he have serious difficulty seeing even when wearing glasses?"

[15] The top quartile was defined as ≥ 4.2 percent compared with a national median of 3.1 percent.

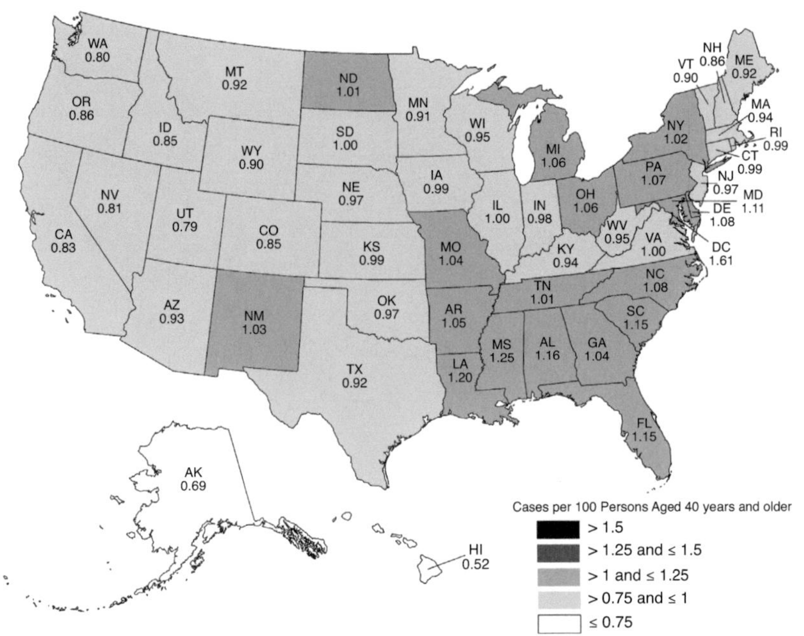

FIGURE 2-6 Per-capita prevalence of blindness in the United States in 2050. SOURCE: Used with permission, Varma et al., 2016.

where interventions can be more easily targeted, but small sample sizes can affect generalizability and raise privacy concerns. Better data from all states and their subdivisions are needed to assist in efforts to target resources. Chapter 4 of this report contains more detail on what additional surveillance activities and vision-related research data are needed.

Socioeconomic Status and the Risk for Vision Impairment

"[S]ocioeconomic status itself is an important determinant of visual impairment" (Tielsch et al., 1991, p. 637). Both nationally and globally, vision impairment and blindness are more prevalent in less affluent regions (Ho and Schwab, 2001; Shweikh et al., 2015; Yip et al., 2014). As noted by Kirtland and colleagues (2015), socioeconomic factors are associated with eye disease burden in a geographical area. Persons of all ages are at greater risk of developing eye disease if they are poor, have less education, or are unemployed (e.g., Ko et al., 2012; Roy, 2000; Roy and Affouf, 2006; Tielsch et al., 1991; Varma et al., 2004b). One study of individuals with age-related eye disease (i.e., AMD, diabetic retinopathy, glaucoma, and cataracts) found that a lower income and a lower level of education attainment were both associated with a decreased likelihood of having an eye care visit in the past 12 months (Zhang et al., 2012). A study of individuals with diabetes also found that minority patients are also more likely to have poor glycemic control and not perceive a need for care (Chou et al., 2014).

Children who live in low-income homes are also at greater risk for various types of vision loss and untreated vision impairment. Being a member of a family who lives below the federal poverty level nearly doubles the likelihood that a child will be visually impaired compared with children from families whose income is greater than or equal to 200 percent of the poverty level (Cotch et al., 2005). In a nationally representative sample of school-age children, those from lower-income families were more likely to have eye conditions that were underdiagnosed or undertreated than children from wealthier families, "placing them at risk for future problems" (Ganz et al., 2006, p. 2298). A citywide screening program in Philadelphia found that 10 percent of the 924 children needed continuous eye care, most notably for amblyopia, 10 children needed ocular surgery for strabismus and other conditions, and 567 needed eyeglasses (Dotan et al., 2015). Similarly, a study of 2,286 first-graders in Southern California schools found that 14 of the 17 students with amblyopia were not receiving treatment at the time the exam was performed, and 45 of the 57 students with clinically meaningful hyperopia lacked eyeglasses (Kodjebacheva et al., 2016). This same study also found that students who were Hispanic or African American or attending a Title 1 school were more likely to have untreated refractive error as well. In a previous MEPEDS project examining African American and Hispanic children living in a less affluent community, none of those with amblyopia had been identified before the study (Tarczy-Hornoch et al., 2007).

Insurance status can have a direct impact on whether populations have access to appropriate eye and vision care. Numerous studies have identified an association between lack of insurance and lower utilization of eye and vision care (Li et al., 2013; Varma et al., 2004c), especially in minority populations (Chou et al., 2014), although some studies did not find insurance to be significant after controlling for other factors (Sloan et al., 2014). Although having insurance can help mitigate the impact associated with lower family income, additional barriers can still affect access to care. For example, Kovarik and colleagues (2016) found that 89 percent of patients at an inner-city hospital in Pittsburgh had insurance, yet 25 percent and 19 percent of this population had undiagnosed retinopathy and advanced sight-threatening retinopathy, respectively, because of barriers such as low income, transportation issues, and physical disabilities associated with diabetes complications (Kovarik et al., 2016). Other factors may include limited physical and cognitive function and distance to an eye care provider (Sloan et al., 2014). The lack of awareness about the causes of eye diseases and what can be done to minimize subsequent vision impairment, which can be another risk factor, is discussed in Chapter 4. Strategies to improve the access and quality of eye and vision care are described in more detail in Chapters 6 and 7, respectively.

UNDERSTANDING THE ETIOLOGY OF VISION IMPAIRMENT IN THE UNITED STATES

Understanding how the etiology of vision impairment and blindness vary among populations can help policy makers and communities tailor interventions and deploy limited resources to best achieve health equity and improve population health. As with overall vision impairment, the prevalence of specific eye disorders varies among individuals age 40 and older. The prevalence of hyperopia, cataract, diabetic retinopathy, glaucoma, and age-related macular degeneration increases with advancing age; in the case of myopia, this trend is reversed. Because an individual can have more than one eye disorder, combining the number of cases of specific diseases represented in Table 2-7 would likely result in higher total than actually exists.

The prevalence and distribution of specific eye diseases also vary by race and ethnicity. Figure 2-7 depicts the extent to which different eye diseases contribute to the prevalence of vision impairment and blindness among different racial and ethnic groups. Glaucoma and diabetic retinopathy account for a greater proportion of vision impairment and blindness among Hispanics and individuals of African ancestry than among non-Hispanic whites. By comparison, age-related macular degeneration accounts for a greater proportion of vision impairment and blindness among non-Hispanic whites than among other racial and ethnic groups. For all represented populations, cataract is the most common cause of vision impairment. Among individuals of African ancestry, cataract is also the most common cause of blindness.

Refractive Error

Refractive error results from an irregular shape of the cornea, lens, or eyeball, which prevents light from focusing properly on the retina. Symptoms of uncorrected refractive error may include blurry vision, headaches, haziness, and eye strain (NEI/NIH, 2010f). Myopia and hyperopia are conditions in which abnormalities in the shape of the cornea, lens, or length of the eye cause light entering the eye to focus at points in front and/or behind the retina (NEI/NIH, 2010f). With myopia (nearsightedness), objects close up appear clear, while objects far away appear blurry. With hyperopia (farsightedness), distant objects appear clear, while objects that are close

TABLE 2-7 Number Affected and Rate of Prevalence for Eye Diseases and Vision Disorders by Age in Adults Ages 40 and Older in the United States in 2010

Disease or Condition	Measure	Total Population Ages 40+	40–49	50–59	60–69	70–79	80+
Hyperopia	Number (in millions)	14.2	1.59	3.13	3.76	3.09	2.62
	Rate per 100 persons[a]	9.95	3.65	7.47	12.84	18.62	23.31
Myopia	Number (in millions)	34.12	15.05	9.61	4.97	2.50	1.98
	Rate per 100 persons[a]	23.92	34.52	22.91	16.88	15.09	17.60
Cataract	Number (in millions)	24.41	1.09	2.96	5.67	7.01	7.67
	Rate per 100 persons[a]	17.11	2.51	7.05	19.40	42.22	68.30
Diabetic retinopathy[b]	Number (in millions)	7.69	1.02	3.24	1.92	1.51	—
	Rate per 100 persons[a]	5.39	2.34	5.50[a]	8.84[a]	8.13[a]	—
Glaucoma	Number (in millions)	2.72	0.30	0.45	0.53	0.56	0.89
	Rate per 100 persons[a]	1.91	0.69	1.07	1.80	3.34	7.89
Age-related macular degeneration	Number (in millions)	2.07	NA	0.16	0.21	0.38	1.32
	Rate per 100 persons[a]	1.45	NA	0.38	0.71	2.30	11.73

[a] The rate per 100 persons is calculated by dividing the number of individuals affected by the 2010 Census population for the specific age group.
[b] Age ranges for diabetic retinopathy include 40–49, 50–64, 65–74, and 75+.
SOURCE: Prevent Blindness, 2012a.

appear blurry. However, younger individuals with hyperopia may be able to accommodate sufficiently to see clearly. Astigmatism occurs when the unequal curvature of one or more refractive surfaces of the eye does not allow for light to focus evenly onto the retina (NEI/NIH, 2010g; Tarczy-Hornock et al., 2010). Uncorrected astigmatism can lead to reductions in visual performance for both distance and near tasks.

Refractive Error in Adults

Refractive error is the most common cause of vision impairment among adults in the United States. One estimate suggests that more than 48 million

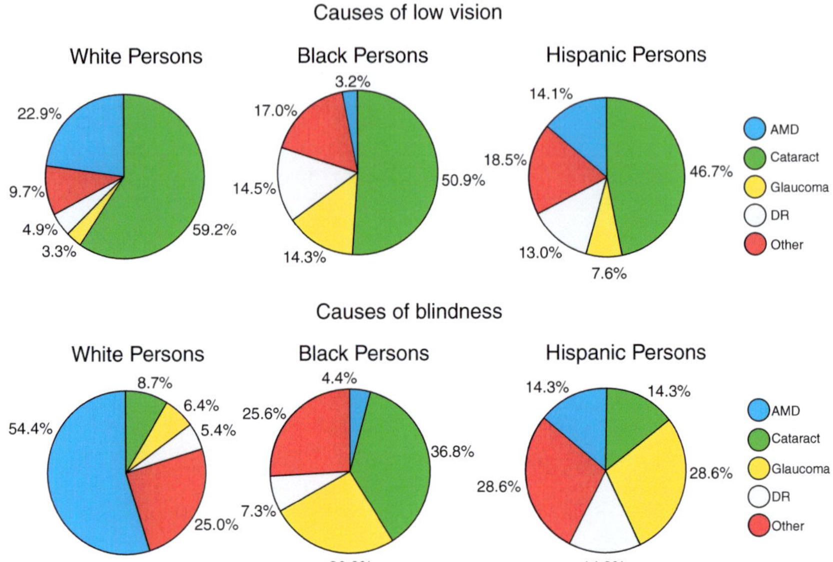

FIGURE 2-7 Causes of vision impairment by race/ethnicity in the United States.
NOTES: Study authors defined "low vision" as best-corrected visual acuity of
20/40 or worse in the better-seeing eye, excluding those who were categorized as
being blind. Blindness refers to best-corrected visual acuity of 20/200 or worse in
the better-seeing eye.
AMD = age-related macular degeneration; DR = diabetic retinopathy.
SOURCE: Adapted from Congdon et al., 2004a.

adults ages 40 and older in the United States—approximately one out of
every three—experienced some degree of myopia (34 million) or hyperopia
(14 million) in 2010 (Prevent Blindness, 2012g). Another estimate based on
NHANES data from 1999 to 2004 found age-standardized prevalences of
3.6 percent, 33.1 percent, and 36.2 percent for hyperopia, myopia, or astigmatism, respectively, in populations over the age of 20 (Vitale et al., 2008).
In older adults, uncorrected refractive error can lead to a greater risk of
mortality, functional decline, social isolation, falls and related hip fractures,
and accidents (Cummings et al., 1995; Klein et al., 1998; Thompson et al.,
1989; West et al., 1997), whereas corrected refractive error can improve
"vision-specific quality of life" and vision-related mental health and well-
being (Coleman et al., 2006). One recent study found that older adults
ages 65 to 84 with uncorrected refractive error and vision impairment[16]

---

[16] Uncorrected refractive error was defined as visual acuity between 20/30 and 20/80 without corrective lenses, and vision impairment was defined as post-refraction best-corrected
visual acuity in both eyes of 20/30 or worse (Zebardast et al., 2015).

walked more slowly, demonstrated slower near-task performance, experienced more frequent driving cessation, and self-reported more visual difficulties compared to individuals with normal vision, although the impact of vision impairment was greater and affected more functional metrics than the impact of uncorrected refractive error (Zebardast et al., 2015).

The prevalence of hyperopia and myopia varies by gender, as well as by race and ethnicity. Prevalence of myopia and hyperopia are slightly higher among women than among men ages 40 and older (Prevent Blindness, 2012d,f). In 2010, the prevalence rate of hyperopia among persons ages 40 and older self-identifying as white was 11.4 percent; African American, 5.2 percent; Hispanic, 6.4 percent; and other minorities, 7.2 percent (NEI/NIH, 2010a). Figure 2-8 shows how hyperopia prevalence increases with age for all racial and ethnic groups. Between 2010 and 2050, the estimated number of cases of hyperopia will increase for all racial and ethnic groups (NEI/NIH, 2010a).

In 2010, the prevalence rate for myopia among persons ages 40 and older self-identifying as white was 26.4 percent; African American, 14.5 percent; Hispanic, 18.3 percent; and other minorities, 20.7 percent (NEI/NIH, 2010b). Figure 2-9 shows that myopia decreases by age group for all races and ethnicities after age 40, although the prevalence of myopia remains higher overall for white and other populations, compared to Hispanic and black populations. Estimates for the projected number of cases of myopia between 2010 and 2050 indicate that, among whites, the number of cases will remain fairly stable, there will be a 1.5-fold increase of cases in African Americans, an almost 3-fold increase in the number of cases among Hispanics, and a 2.5-fold increase in cases among other minority

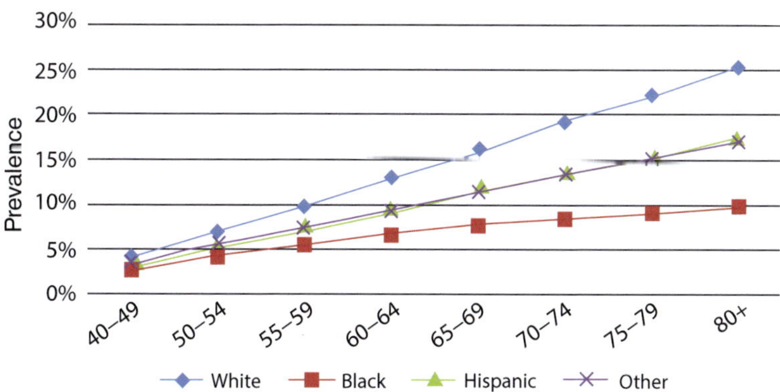

FIGURE 2-8 2010 U.S. age-specific prevalence rates for hyperopia by age (40 years and older), and race/ethnicity (in percent).
SOURCE: NEI/NIH, 2010a.

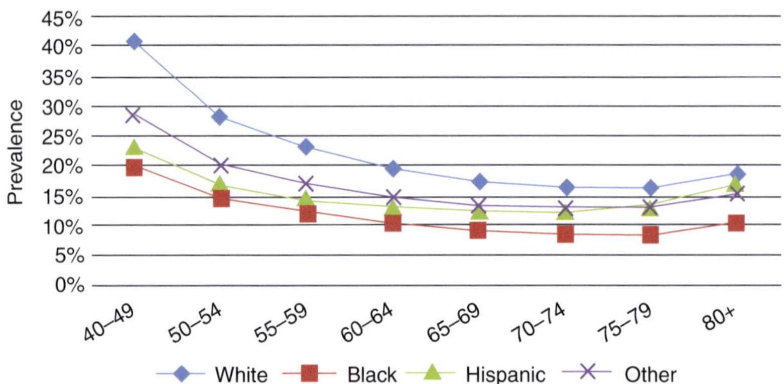

FIGURE 2-9 2010 U.S. age-specific prevalence rates for myopia by age (40 years and older) and race/ethnicity.
SOURCE: NEI/NIH, 2010b.

populations (NEI/NIH, 2010b). Using NHANES data from 1999 to 2004, Vitale and colleagues (2008) found the prevalence of astigmatism was 31 percent among people ages 40 and older in the United States.

Using data from 1999 to 2004 to assess the occurrence of clinically important refractive error[17] in 20- to 39-year-olds, as well as in older age groups, Vitale and colleagues (2008) found that myopia was more prevalent in females than in males (40 versus 33 percent), whereas hyperopia was less prevalent among females than males (0.8 percent versus 1.3 percent). Astigmatism affected 23.1 percent of this age group and 36.2 percent of all participants.

Refractive Error in Children

Uncorrected refractive error can have a substantial impact on children. Uncorrected refractive error in young children can lead to physical, developmental, and academic problems. For example, hyperopia is associated with amblyopia and strabismus, as well as delays in visuomotor and visuocognitive development in children younger than age 7 (Atkinson et al., 2007). As compared to children ages 4 to 5 without hyperopia, those with uncorrected bilateral hyperopia are more likely to underperform on some measures of preschool early literacy, which has been associated with future

---

[17] Clinically important refractive error was defined using data from the eye with a greater absolute spherical equivalent (SphEq) value: hyperopia, SphEq value of 3.0 diopters (D) or greater; myopia, SphEq value of –1.0 D or less; and astigmatism, cylinder of 1.0 D or greater in either eye (Vitale et al., 2008).

performance in learning to read and write (Kulp et al., 2016). Similarly, a recent study found that astigmatism is associated with two measures of reduced academic readiness among at-risk preschool-age children (Orlansky et al., 2015).

Establishing the prevalence of refractive error in the United States for those younger than age 12 is more difficult than for older populations. There is no national database tracking the prevalence or incidence of refractive error in children under age 12, requiring prevalence to be imputed, as discussed earlier. Large population-based studies have been used to estimate national rates for younger age groups. One study found prevalence for myopia of 4.5 percent and 28 percent among 6- to 7-year-olds and 12-year-olds, respectively, in the United States (Zadnik, 1997). The Collaborative Longitudinal Evaluation of Ethnicity and Refractive Error (CLEERE) study, a longitudinal observational study encompassing grades 1 to 8 and four race and ethnicity groups estimated overall population prevalence rates of 9.2 percent for myopia, 12.8 percent for hyperopia, and 28.4 percent for astigmatism in 1997 (Kleinstein et al., 2003). Table 2-8 presents estimates from four studies on the prevalence for different types of refractive errors among children of different age groups.

Racial and socioeconomic disparities have been examined as potential risk factors in uncorrected and undercorrected refractive error in both adult and pediatric populations. Qiu and colleagues (2014) identified high-risk groups among the population ages 12 and older surveyed in the 2005–2008 NHANES. Overall, half of the subjects had refractive errors, and among these individuals the unmet need for proper correction was 11.7 percent. Mexican Americans and non-Hispanic blacks were more likely to have inadequate refractive corrections than non-Hispanic whites across all age groups. This observed disparity was greatest among 12- to 19-year-olds. Other factors that are associated with worse adult access to eye care were low socioeconomic status (low income, low education) and a lack of health insurance. Similarly, a direct assessment of 11,332 first-graders in low-income areas visited by the University of California, Los Angeles, Mobile Eye Clinic found that 95 percent of the students with decreased visual acuity did not have the glasses needed for attaining normal vision (Kodjebacheva et al., 2011). More than 95 percent of the students were identified as being of a minority race or ethnicity. Boys were less likely than girls to have eyeglasses, and African American and Latino students were less likely than non-Hispanic white students to have glasses. The authors noted the importance of early interventions to address this deficit and to prevent problems later in life.

TABLE 2-8 Examples of Studies on the Prevalence of Different Types of Refractive Error Among Children by Race/Ethnicity

Study Age	Population	Myopia (%)	Hyperopia (%)	Astigmatism (%)
Ages 6–72 months (BPEDS)[a]	Non-Hispanic white	1.1[f]	13.2[g]	8.3(WTR)[h] 0.7(ATR)[h] 2.4(OBL)[h]
	African Americans	7.4[f]	6.9[g]	9.0(WTR)[h] 1.0(ATR)[h] 3.1(OBL)[h]
Grades 1–8 (ages 5–17 years)[b]	Non-Hispanic white	4.4[i]	19.3[j]	26.4[k]
	African American	6.6[i]	6.4[j]	20.0[k]
	Hispanic	13.2[i]	12.7[j]	36.9[k]
	Asian	18.5[i]	6.3[j]	33.6[k]
	Groups combined	9.2[i]	12.8[j]	28.4[k]
Ages 6–72 months (MEPEDS)[c,d]	African American	6.6[f]	8.8[g]	12.7[h]
	Hispanic	3.7[f]	12.0[g]	16.8[h]
Ages 6–72 months (MEPEDS)[e]	Non-Hispanic white	1.20[f]	9.13[g]	6.33[h]
	Asian	3.98[f]	4.84[g]	8.29[h]

NOTES: [f] Prevalence of myopic spherical equivalent refractive error of ≤–1.00 D in the eye with the greater refractive error. [g] Prevalence of hyperopic spherical equivalent refractive error of ≥+3.00 D in the eye with the greater refractive error. [h] Prevalence of Astigmatism of ≥1.50 D or greater in the eye with greater refractive error. [i] Prevalence of myopia of ≤–0.75 D in each principal meridian. [j] Prevalence of hyperopia of ≥+1.25 D in each principal meridian. [k] Prevalence of astigmatism of ≥1.00 D difference in refractive error between the two principal meridians.

ATR = against the rule; BPEDS = Baltimore Pediatric Eye Disease Study; MEPEDS = Multi-Ethnic Pediatric Eye Disease Study Group; OBL = oblique; WTR = with the rule.

SOURCES: [a] Giordano et al., 2009; [b] Kleinstein et al., 2003; [c] Fozailoff et al., 2011; [d] MEPEDS, 2010; [e] Wen et al., 2013.

Common Risk Factors for Refractive Error

Risk factors for significant refractive error in childhood include parental history; having had prenatal, perinatal, or postnatal complications; and having had a significant neurodevelopmental condition (Jones-Jordan et al., 2010; O'Donoghue et al., 2015; Parssinen et al., 2014; Zadnik et al., 1994, 2015). For example, the prevalence of myopia in 12-year-old children in Australia was approximately 15 percent and 44 percent for children with one and two myopic parents, respectively, compared with almost 8 percent in children with no myopic parents (Ip et al., 2007). Children with neurodevelopmental diagnoses (e.g., Down syndrome, fragile X, or cerebral palsy, as well as children who are born very low birth weight or preterm) are also at a higher risk for significant refractive errors along with other ocular complications (Salt and Sargent, 2014). Of a study cohort of 1,098 infants born at extremely low birth weight (401–1,000 grams), some vision impairment was present in 9 percent, and vision impairment was increased in infants with lower birth weight. This ranged from 5 percent of infants weighing between 801–900 and 901–1,000 grams exhibiting some degree of vision impairment, to 21 percent of infants weighing between 401–500 grams (Vohr et al., 2000). Another follow-up study evaluating extremely preterm children at the age of 6.5 years found that 37.9 percent of the children had some ophthalmologic abnormality, compared with 6.2 percent of the control cohort (Hellgren et al., 2016). Other risk factors for refractive errors in children may include a sedentary lifestyle and maternal smoking during pregnancy (Borchert et al., 2011; O'Donoghue et al., 2015; Pan et al., 2012).

Environmental factors can also play an important role in the development of myopia. A number of studies have found an inverse association between myopia and the amount of time spent outdoors in school-age children (Dirani et al., 2009; Parssinen et al., 2014; Rose et al., 2008). For example, one cross-sectional study comparing the prevalence of myopia in 6- and 7-year-old children of Chinese ethnicity in Sydney and Singapore found that low levels of outdoor time and high near-work time were significant factors associated with differences in the prevalence of myopia between the two study populations, 3.3 and 29.1 percent, respectively (Rose et al., 2008). A recent randomized controlled trial among 6-year-old school children in China found the addition of 40 minutes of outdoor time resulted in a 9.1 percent decrease in the incidence of myopia over the next 3 years, compared to the control group (He et al., 2015).

Most studies on myopia and near work (e.g., time spent reading, studying, watching television, or playing computer or video games) include self-reported data and are cross-sectional, so they cannot explore the temporal relationship between outcomes and predictors. Studies on near-work and myopia in younger adults have had mixed results, depending on the measure of near work. For example, a study of adolescent students in rural China did not find the length of near-work activity to be significantly different between children with and without myopia (Lu et al., 2009), but another study of 12-year-old Australian school children did find an association between myopia and close reading distance and time spent continuously reading before taking a 5-minute break (Ip et al., 2008). A longitudinal study of non-myopic first-grade students followed through 8th grade found that children who become myopic spend less time outdoors than non-myopic children, which may influence levels of near work (Jones-Jordan et al., 2011). Citing evidence of seasonal effects on myopia progression, the study concluded that less time spent outdoors may have a stronger influence on subsequent development of myopia than near work. Data evaluating myopia in children and cumulative near work, using various measures of near work, did not find a relationship between near-work activities and the onset of myopia (Jones-Jordan et al., 2011).

The biological mechanism that would explain the association between outdoor activity and myopia is not well understood, but the evidence suggests that greater exposure to it may be an opportunity to reduce prevalence rates of myopia (Dirani et al., 2009). The effect of gene–environment interaction on the etiology of myopia is still controversial, with inconsistent findings in different studies (Pan et al., 2012). Longitudinal cohort studies or randomized clinical trials of community-based health behavior interventions should be conducted to further clarify the etiology of myopia (Pan et al., 2012).

Strabismus and Amblyopia

Strabismus and amblyopia are frequent diagnoses associated with monocular vision loss in children, but may also persist or develop during adulthood. Other related conditions, which are not examined in this chapter but are important to acknowledge, include anisometropia (significant differences in refractive error in both eyes), convergence insufficiency (an eye muscle condition in which both eyes do not easily turn inward to see at near distances), or eye tracking problems (e.g., difficultly following words across a page, smoothly following a moving object, or jumping from one object to another), among others.

Strabismus is a condition in which there is a misalignment of the eyes, such that one eye constantly or intermittently turns in (esotropia), out (exotropia), up, or down as the other eye looks straight ahead (Hatt and Gnanaraj, 2013). As a result of the misalignment, a person's eyes do not fixate on the same object in space, and two different signals are sent to the brain. The amount of eye turn, the frequency of the eye turn, and the level of stereoacuity (sensory fusion of images) affects the severity of the strabismus (Hatt and Gnanara, 2015). Strabismus typically will not improve without intervention, which may involve refractive correction, patching, surgery, or pharmacological treatment (PEDIG, 2006).

Amblyopia, also referred to as "lazy eye," is a neurological disorder in children, in which reduced vision in one or both eyes occurs due to abnormal interaction or lack of a clear image (Barrett et al., 2013; Pascual et al., 2014). To develop normal vision, both eyes must receive a clear, single image from both eyes. If one of the images is less clear, then the brain may compensate by inhibiting or suppressing input from the weaker eye, which can eventually result in decreased vision in that eye. Amblyopia can cause persistent deficits in cortical processing, even after normal input to the brain is restored (Hamm et al., 2014). Treatments for amblyopia generally include correcting the underlying condition and reducing or eliminating the suppressive effects of the dominant eye through patching or pharmaceuticals (PEDIG, 2012), although ongoing studies are investigating the effects of refractive correction alone or different combinations of treatments to sustain long-term outcomes for different age groups (Cotter et al., 2014; PEDIG, 2006).

A number of population-based studies provide data on the prevalence of amblyopia and strabismus among children in the United States. The prevalence of amblyopia ranges from 0.8 percent to 2.6 percent in children ages 30 to 71 months, and the prevalence of strabismus ranges from 2.1 percent to 3.5 in children ages 6 to 71 months (Friedman et al., 2009; McKean-Cowdin et al., 2013; MEPEDS, 2008). The Baltimore Pediatric Eye Disease Study (BPEDS) examining white and African American children found a higher rate of strabismus among non-Hispanic white children (3.3 percent) compared to African American children (2.1 percent). The prevalence of amblyopia was also higher in non-Hispanic white children (1.8 percent) compared to African American children (0.8 percent) (Friedman et al., 2009). Strabismus was more prevalent in older children than in younger children, whereas amblyopia prevalence varied little within the narrow age range examined (i.e., 30 to 71 months). Data from the Multi-Ethnic Pediatric Eye Disease Study (MEPEDS) found similar rates of strabismus (3.2 percent and 3.5 percent, respectively) and amblyopia (1.8 percent) in white and Asian children (McKean-Cowdin et al., 2013). Among African American and Hispanic children participating in the same study, the prevalence rate of strabismus was similar (2.5 percent and 2.4 percent, respectively), but a significantly higher rate of amblyopia was found among Hispanic children (2.6 percent) compared to African American children (1.5 percent) (MEPEDS, 2008). Table 2-9 provides a summary of these findings.

Data on the prevalence or incidence of adult-onset strabismus are limited. One study based on claims data from Medicare fee-for-service beneficiaries found a 0.68 percent prevalence rate of adult-onset strabismus and increased with age and specific comorbidities for the period 2008 to 2010 (Repka et al., 2013). The prevalence of adult-onset strabismus also varies by geography with a significantly higher prevalence in the Southern region. Another study, including individuals ages 19 and older residing in Olmstead County, Minnesota, found that the annual incidence rate for adult-onset strabismus was 54.1 cases per 100,000 people and the lifetime risk of adult-onset strabismus was 4 percent after adjusting for age and gender (Martinez-Thompson et al., 2014). The study also found that the risk of developing adult-onset strabismus was similar for men and women and that the incidence peaked during the eighth decade of life. The characteristics

TABLE 2-9 Prevalence of Amblyopia and Strabismus Among Children by Race/Ethnic Group (in percent)

Study	Race/Ethnic Group	Prevalence of Amblyopia (children ages 30–71 months)	Prevalence of Strabismus (children ages 6–71 months)
Friedman et al., 2009 (BPEDS)	Non-Hispanic white	3.3	1.8
	African Americans	2.1	0.08
McKean-Cowdin et al., 2013 (MEPEDS)	Non-Hispanic white	3.2	1.8
	Asian	3.5	1.81
MEPEDS, 2008	African Americans	2.5	1.5
	Hispanics	2.4	2.6

NOTE: BPEDS = Baltimore Pediatric Eye Disease Study Group; MEPEDS = Multi-Ethnic Pediatric Eye Disease Study Group.
SOURCES: Friedman et al., 2009; McKean-Cowdin et al., 2013; MEPEDS, 2008.

of the population studied and the type of provider records included in the study limit the generalizability of study results.

Risk Factors for Amblyopia and Strabismus

Amblyopia is typically a diagnosis of exclusion. When no other organic reason exists for observed symptoms, certain amblyogenic factors—the most common are strabismus, anisometropia, and deprivation (e.g., obstruction due to a cataract or drooping of the eyelid because of paralysis or a congenital condition)—suggest amblyopia (Flynn and Cassady, 1978; Hamm et al., 2014; Kemper et al., 2004). Studies in the United States have found that strabismus and significant refractive error (e.g., ansiometropia) are risk factors for unilateral amblyopia, whereas bilateral astigmatism and bilateral hyperopia increase the risk of developing bilateral amblyopia (Pascual et al., 2014; Tarczy-Hornoch et al., 2013).

Risk factors for strabismus identified through MEPEDS and BPEDS and other studies include maternal smoking throughout pregnancy, prematurity, and hereditary factors (Cotter et al., 2011; Maconachie et al., 2013; Torp-Pedersen et al., 2010). However, a more recent study of risk factors for strabismus in young children in Singapore, found no associations between strabismus or amblyopia and prematurity, maternal age, or maternal smoking (Chia et al., 2013). Other risk factors for strabismus in children include cerebral palsy, Noonan syndrome, Prader-Willi syndrome, and other neurological disorders (Cotter et al., 2011; Shah and Patel, 2015). Childhood hyperopia is also a well-established risk factor for certain types of strabismus (Cotter et al., 2011; von Noorden and Campos, 2002).

Adult-onset strabismus is generally linked to another condition, such as traumatic eye injury, thyroid eye disease, tumors, stroke, surgical procedures, cranial nerve palsies, or other neurologic disease and residual childhood strabismus. Martinez-Thompson and colleagues (2014) found that adult-onset strabismus was more likely to result from a paralytic disorder in a geographically limited study of residents of Olmstead County, Minnesota.

Cataracts

A cataract is a treatable condition that occurs when the lens of the eye becomes cloudy or discolored due to a pathological clumping of proteins within the lens (NEI/NIH, 2010d). Cataracts can occur in one or both eyes. Symptoms may include cloudy or blurred vision, color fading, glare, poor night vision, double vision. Frequent prescription changes may also signal developing cataracts (NEI/NIH, 2009). Cataracts vary by type[18] and in severity—not all require immediate action or the same type of intervention, depending on the stage of development. Eventually, cataracts worsen until subsequent vision impairment interferes with day-to-day life. Surgical removal of the lens is the only cure for cataracts, but regular monitoring by an eye care professional and updating one's prescription glasses may be sufficient for early cataracts.

In adults, cataract is the most common ocular diagnosis after refractive error, and it accounts for the largest proportion of vision impairment in adults over age 40 (NEI/NIH, 2010d). At the turn of the past century, 20.5 million Americans were diagnosed with a cataract in at least one eye; that number is projected to hit more than 33.6 million in the over-40 age group by 2045 (Congdon et al., 2004b; Wittenborn and Rein, 2016). Cataracts are rare in children, although congenital cataracts may be present upon birth, in which case they are usually surgically removed upon diagnosis.

The burden of cataract increases dramatically with age for all races and ethnicities, and prevalence rates are higher for women than men (Congdon et al., 2004b; NEI/NIH, 2010d; Prevent Blindness, 2012a). Overall prevalence rates increased from 2.5 percent for people ages 40 to 49, to 19.4 percent for those ages 60 to 69, and 42.2 percent of individuals ages 70 to 79 (Prevent Blindness, 2012d). Studies consistently report higher prevalence rates and numbers of individuals with cataracts among older white populations. Figure 2-10 illustrates how cataract prevalence rates are similar

---

[18] Nuclear sclerotic cataract involves a clouding or yellowing of the center of the lens, which progresses to hardening of the lens. A cortical cataract occurs when areas of white cloudiness develop along the outer edges of the lens, progressively moving inward. Posterior subcapsular cataracts begin as a small, cloudy, or opaque area on the back of the lens.

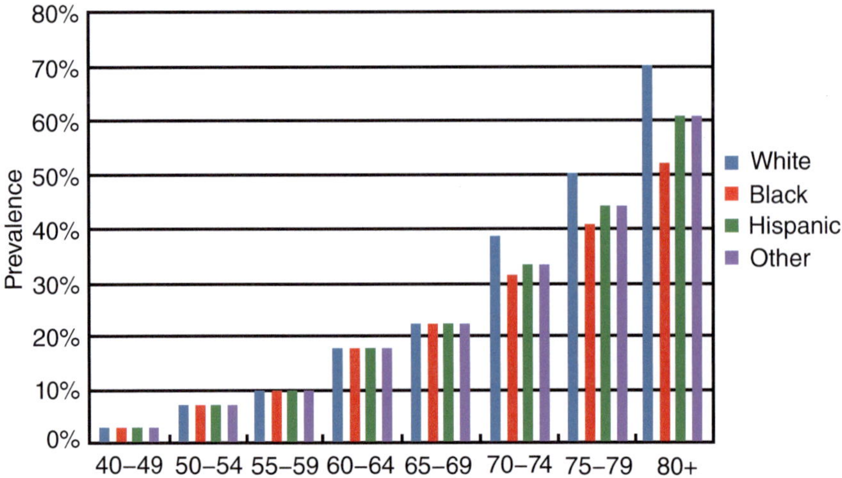

FIGURE 2-10 2010 U.S. prevalence rates for cataract by age and race.
SOURCE: NEI/NIH, 2010d.

across all racial and ethnic groups until age 70, after which the prevalence rates begin to increase faster for whites, followed by Hispanics, other races and ethnicities, and blacks.

Despite having lower prevalence rates of cataracts, minority populations are more likely to have vision impairment from untreated cataracts. For example, adult African American participants in the Baltimore Eye Survey were five times as likely as whites to have unoperated "senile" cataracts (Sommer et al., 1991; Zambelli-Weiner et al., 2012). The study also found that among one-third of African Americans under age 70 were blind because of unoperated cataracts (Sommer et al., 1991). A more recent study examined disparities in necessary cataract surgery for whites and African Americans ages 65 and older in the state of Florida. Shahbazi and colleagues (2015) found that African Americans were less likely than whites to have cataract surgery (cataract surgery rates were 7.9 percent for African American males, 6.2 percent for African American females, 12.1 percent for white males, and 10.5 percent for white females). In the Los Angeles Latino Eye Study population, 29.9 percent of Latino/Hispanic participants who needed cataract surgery had not undergone the procedure (Richter et al., 2009). NHANES data consistently show lower rates of cataract surgery among non-Hispanic blacks than among whites; cataract surgery rates for

Mexican Americans, on the other hand, are similar to whites, even after age- and sex-standardization of the data (Zhang et al., 2012).[19]

Common Risk Factors for Cataract

Although traumatic eye injury, eye surgery, and ultraviolet (UV) radiation exposure are all well-established risk factors for developing cataracts, the aging process is the primary cause of most cataracts (Glynn et al., 2009). The link between UV exposure and cataracts has been documented (McCarty and Taylor, 2002), but more research is emerging on the biochemical damage done by UV exposure, even to young human lenses (20 to 36 years), leading to formation of cataracts earlier in life (Linetsky et al., 2014; McCarty et al., 2001). The purported associations of cataracts with smoking, consumption of alcohol, and physical activity have been disputed, with studies arriving at contradictory or inconclusive results (Glynn et al., 2009; Tan et al., 2008; Ye et al., 2012). The confusion may be partly due to differences among nuclear, cortical, and posterior subcapsular cataracts, each of which possesses a unique set of risk factors (Chang et al., 2011; Mukesh et al., 2006; Williams, 2009). A meta-analysis by Ye and colleagues (2012b) concluded that there was an association of smoking with age-related cataract: current smokers are at greater risk than past smokers, and those who ever smoked are more at risk than those who never smoked. A recent prospective cohort study found a dose–response effect of smoking on the development of cataracts in men (Lindblad et al., 2014), complimenting an earlier study that had observed the same effect in women (Lindblad et al., 2005).

The association between obesity and cataracts has been reported in several epidemiological studies, although the findings are not consistent (Cheung and Wong, 2007; Hiller et al., 1998; Pan and Lin, 2014). Compared to nuclear cataract, cortical and posterior subcapsular cataracts (in particular) have been most consistently associated with obesity (Cheung and Wong, 2007; Pan and Lin, 2014). Obesity is associated with glucose intolerance, insulin resistance, diabetes, hyperlipidemia, and hypertension (Feingold and Grunfeld, 2000; George et al., 2015; Yu, 2014), which are all considered to be risk factors for cataract formation; however, the primary role of these factors in cataract formation is less clear (Cheung and Wong, 2007; Leske et al., 1999; Park and Lee, 2015; Yu et al., 2014). Increased

---

[19] According to NHANES III data, the rates of cataract surgery were 16.4 percent among African Americans, 19.3 percent among whites, and 20.4 percent among Mexican Americans; data from the NHANES 2005–2008 show the rates of cataract surgery were 13.5 percent among African Americans, 18.4 percent among whites, and 16.4 percent among Mexican Americans (Zhang et al., 2012).

physical activity, such as walking and biking, has been associated with a decreased risk of cataracts (Williams, 2009; Zheng Selin et al., 2015). Research also shows that heavy alcohol consumption is correlated with an increased cataract risk, although some studies have found that, after controlling for smoking status, the risk of heavy drinking is no higher than for moderate drinking (Gong et al., 2015; Kanthan et al., 2010). The literature does not clearly establish whether increasing dietary intake of specific vitamins or nutrients (e.g., supplementation with lutein or zeaxanthin) can reduce cataract formation (Chew et al., 2013). Other potential risk factors for cataracts, such as arthritis, the extended use of calcium channel blockers, thyroid hormone use, and corticosteroid use are in early stages of investigation. More research is needed to better understand the association and possible mechanism between weight (and associated chronic conditions), physical activity, diet, and cataract formation.

Eye Injuries and Damage to the Visual System

Injury to the visual system—including abrasions, chemical burns, lacerations, orbital wall fractures, and damage to the visual processing centers of the brain—are common. Each year, more than 2.5 million eye injuries occur in the United States, resulting in nearly 50,000 people permanently losing part or all of their vision (Owens and Mutter, 2011). Many eye injuries are preventable, especially in occupational and sports-related settings. In fact, a few studies have suggested that as much as 90 percent of sports-related eye injuries in particular populations can be prevented by wearing protective eyewear (Harrison and Telander, 2002; Mishra and Verma, 2012). Channa and colleagues (2016) analyzed nationally representative data from 2006 to 2011 and found that, among nearly 12 million eye-related emergency department visits, 13.7 percent were for corneal abrasions, 7.5 percent were related to a foreign body on the external eye, 2.8 percent were for contusion of the eye and orbital tissues, and 2.3 percent were related to lacerations of eyelids or skin near the eye. Among children and adolescents ages 0 to 5, 15.4 percent presented with corneal abrasions, contusions of the eye and orbital structures, laceration of the eyelid and the periocular area, open wounds of the ocular adnexa, and closed fractures of the orbital floor (Channa et al., 2016). Among children ages 6 to 12 and adolescents ages 13 to 18, 23.2 and 26.1 percent, respectively, visited the emergency department each year with eye injuries (Channa et al., 2016).[20]

---

[20] Figures derived from Table 2. Total percentage among patients ages 0–5: 1.9 percent + 6.1 percent + 4.4 percent + 2.9 percent + 0.1 percent = 15.4 percent. Total number among patients ages 0–5: 36,383 + 114,521 + 83,113 + 54,339 + 1,377 = 289,733. Total percentage among patients ages 6–12: 4.7 percent + 11.4 percent + 4.0 percent + 2.6 percent + 0.5 percent

Occupational Eye Injuries

About 2,000 work-related eye injuries caused by blunt, sharp, or chemical trauma require medical treatment daily in the United States, and one-third of them are treated in hospital emergency departments (CDC, 2007). This translates to approximately 250,000 emergency room visits each year. In 2012, more than 20,000 eye injuries in private industry required time off from work (BLS, 2012), and eye injuries in general "cost an estimated $300 million a year in lost productivity, medical treatment, and worker compensation" (Dang, 2015). Common causes of workplace eye injuries include flying objects (such as bits of metal, wood, or glass), tools, particles, chemicals, radiation, blood-borne pathogens, and other hazards.

Data from the 2002 National Health Interview Survey (NHIS) reveal an overall lifetime prevalence of 4.4 percent for work-related injuries among adults 18 years and older (Forrest and Cali, 2009). The study also found the highest prevalence rate of eye injury (6 percent) among people between the ages of 45 and 54, but work injuries occurred at every age of 18 and older (Forrest and Cali, 2009). Another study found that people ages 20 to 34 were at greatest risk for work-related eye injury visits to emergency departments (Xiang et al., 2005). Men have four to five times the number of workplace injuries than women (Forrest and Cali, 2009; Luo et al., 2012). For instance, data from the 2005–2007 Behavioral Risk Factor Surveillance System found that the lifetime prevalence of workplace eye injury was significantly higher for men (13.5 percent) than for women (2.6 percent), although socioeconomic status was only associated with lifetime risk for men (Luo et al., 2012).

Workplace eye injuries vary by type of industry and are more likely to affect populations engaged in certain occupations. The more risky occupations include those in precision production, transportation, farming, mining, and construction (Forrest and Cali, 2009). For example, construction workers experience the highest prevalence of eye injury (CDC, 2007). Health care workers, laboratory staff, janitorial workers, animal handlers, and other workers are also at risk for infectious diseases via eye exposure (e.g., touching the eye with contaminated fingers, infected blood splashes, or respiratory droplets) (CDC, 2007). A 2009 study found that workers who are more likely to have eye injuries have less than a high-school education, are non-Hispanic whites, are self-employed, and live in the Midwest region (Forrest and Cali, 2009). Relatedly, another study found that men with no more than a high school education (compared with having more than a high school

---

= 23.2 percent. Total number among patients ages 6–12: 44,702 + 108,067 + 37,956 + 24,777 + 4,588 = 220,090. Total percentage among patients ages 13–18: 5.5 percent + 12.4 percent + 3.8 percent + 2.6 percent + 1.8 percent = 26.1 percent. Total number among patients ages 13–18: 48,555 + 109,350 + 33,590 + 22,667 + 15,783 = 229,945.

education) and men with an annual household income less than $15,000 (compared with greater than $50,000) were more likely to experience a lifetime workplace eye injury, after adjusting for age, race and ethnicity, eye care insurance, health status, and risk-taking behaviors (Luo et al., 2012).

Sports-Related Injuries

Estimates suggest that between 40,000 and 600,000 documented sports-related eye injuries occur in the United States every year (Goldstein and Wee, 2011), and approximately 13,500 result in a permanent loss of sight (Mishra and Verma, 2012). The leading cause of blindness in children is eye injury (NEI/NIH, 2016a). High-risk, moderate-risk, low-risk, and eye-safe activities accounted for 55, 27, 16, and 3 percent, respectively, of 208,517 sports-related eye injuries treatment in emergency departments from 2001 to 2009 (Kim et al., 2011). High-risk sports include air rifle, paintball, racquet sports, lacrosse, hockey, and boxing (Mishra and Verma, 2012). Moderate-risk activities include badmitton, tennis, volleyball, football, and fishing; swimming, diving, skiing, wrestling, and bicycling are considered low risk (Mishra and Verma, 2012). Although data suggest that high- and moderate-risk eye injuries decreased from 2001 to 2005, Kim and colleagues (2011) found that rates began to increase between 2007 and 2009. Beyond the use of protective eye injury, protective sunwear can reduce the risk of damage to the eye from UV radiation.

Eye Issues Associated with Traumatic Brain Injury

Traumatic brain injury (TBI), including concussions, results from "a bump, blow, or jolt to the head or a penetrating head injury" that causes local or diffuse disruption of normal brain function (CDC, 2016a). The CDC states that in 2010 there were approximately 2.5 million emergency department visits related to TBI, and that from 2006 to 2010, major identifiable causes of TBI included falls (40.5 percent), motor vehicle crashes (14.3 percent), and assaults (10.7 percent) (CDC, 2016e). Patients with TBI may experience a range of visual symptoms and disorders, including problems with visual acuity, visual fields, oculomotor function, among others (Brahm et al., 2009; Cockerham et al., 2009; Goodrich et al., 2013; Magone et al., 2014; Rosner et al., 2016). A recent study of 100 adolescents ages 11 to 17 examined for concussion, a mild form of TBI, found that 69 percent had one or more of the following disorders: accommodative disorders (51 percent), convergence insufficiency (49 percent), and saccadic dysfunction (29 percent) (Master et al., 2016).

Vision impairment as a result of TBI during active military duty is becoming a growing problem. The U.S. Department of Defense reports that more than 347,000 service members have been diagnosed with TBI since 2000 (Defense and Veterans Brain Injury Center, 2016). Brahm and colleagues (2009) reported that, among combat-injured military personnel with TBI who were inpatients at a polytrauma rehabilitation center, the prevalence of vision impairment (20/100 or worse visual acuity) and visual field defects was 13 percent and 32.3 percent, respectively. An observational study of 103 patients at a Veterans Affairs polytrauma network site found that 76 and 75 percent of service members with polytrauma and TBI, respectively, reported visual symptoms (Stelmack et al., 2009). Goodrich and colleagues (2013) found that greater than 65 percent of combat-injured military personnel with blast-related and non-blast-related TBI report vision problems, such as difficulty reading and sensitivity to light. Similarly, a retrospective study of 31 patients found that long-term visual dysfunction, despite good distance acuity, is common even years after blast-induced mild traumatic brain injury (Magone et al., 2014).

Infections and Vision Impairment

The eye and vision health of children and adults can be compromised by infection, including eye infections, systemic infections that can potentially affect the development or function of the visual system, and nosocomial infections following eye surgery. For example, exposure to certain viruses and bacteria in utero can have lifelong effects on the developing visual system, especially in the absence of effective treatments or vaccinations. No single database tracks all potentially vision-threatening infections in the United States. Instead, data are usually available by specific infections, with varying availability of eye and vision health outcomes. This section covers some of the more common eye and systemic infections and is not intended to provide a comprehensive listing of all potential infectious agents. Nosocomial infections, such as endophthalmitis, are not covered here but are considered later in this chapter when discussing treatment.

Fetal and Neonatal Infections

During the first trimester of pregnancy, the visual system undergoes significant development. The recent outbreak of the Zika virus and its potential to affect the developing fetus has underscored the need to consider the effects of maternal infections on children's health, including development of the visual system (Valentine et al., 2016). Historically, several maternal infections have been associated with interference in normal ocular development when the fetus is exposed during the first trimester. Maternal infections known to be teratogens (i.e., agents that have the potential to cause birth defects) are referred to as the TORCH constellation.

TORCH refers to toxoplasmosis, other (syphilis, varicella-zoster, parvovirus B19), rubella, cytomegalovirus (CMV), and herpes infections (Stegmann and Carey, 2002). Other ocular teratogens include, but are not limited to, alcohol, opioids, benzodiazepines, cocaine, thalidomide, anticonvulsants, vitamin A, radiation, and diabetes mellitus (Tandon and Mulvhill, 2009).

Some sexually transmitted diseases, along with other viruses or bacteria, can be passed from a mother to a fetus, which can lead to vision-threatening conditions. Neonatal conjunctivitis, may cause red eyes, swollen eye lids, and discharge of pus. Usually a minor eye infection, in some cases conjunctivitis can lead to scarring, eye damage, or vision loss. The most common neonatal infection is chlamydia, which presents as a milder case of conjunctivitis and requires oral antibiotic treatment (CDC, 2015a, 2016b). Gonococcal conjunctivitis can destroy the corneal barrier and rapidly damage the eye; intravenous antibiotics are usually given as treatment (CDC, 2016b). Herpes simplex viral neonatal conjunctivitis presents as corneal epithelial involvement and periocular vesicles on the skin (CDC, 2016b). Many forms of neonatal conjunctivitis can be treated by eye drops or ointment (commonly required by state law), or oral and intravenous antibiotics.

Eye Infections in Children and Adults

Eye infections can be caused by many different organisms, including bacteria, viruses, amoeba, and fungi (CDC, 2015b). Viral and bacterial conjunctivitis are highly contagious and may result from a number of common agents, including adenovirus, rubella, measles, herpes, *Staphylococcus aureus*, *Streptococcus pneumoniae*, among others (CDC, 2016c). Data from the National Ambulatory Medical Care Survey indicated that Americans made more than 4 million visits to ambulatory physicians for bacterial conjunctivitis in 2005 (Smith and Waycaster, 2009). Approximately 70 percent of patients with acute conjunctivitis present to primary and urgent care providers, which accounts for 1 percent of all primary care office visits (Kaufman, 2011; Shields and Sloane, 1990). Adenoviruses account for 65 to 90 percent of cases of viral conjunctivitis (O'Brien et al., 2009).

Bacterial conjunctivitis is another common cause of acute conjunctivitis. In a series of patients presenting with acute conjunctivitis in an inner city hospital, conjunctival scrapings indicated that 36 percent of patients had viral conjunctivitis and 40 percent had bacterial conjunctivitis (Fitch et al., 1989). The most common bacteria noted in adults are staphylococcal species, *Streptococcus pneumoniae*, and *Haemophilus influenzae*, whereas in children, *Haemophilus influenzae* is more common (Azari and

Barney, 2013). Among children in particular, *Haemophilus influenzae* can lead to orbital cellulitis, which can progress to meningitis. Keratoconjunctivitis secondary to herpes simplex is an important contributor to ocular pathology. Most commonly due to herpes simplex Type I, this potentially recurring infection can lead, if not appropriately treated, to either significant corneal pathology requiring corneal transplantation or corneal perforation leading to loss of the eye. Varicella zoster and herpes zoster are also associated with eye infections (Wu and Ariyasu, 1999). Chlamydial conjunctivitis, associated with the most common sexually transmitted disease in the United States, accounts for 1.8 to 5.6 percent of all cases of acute conjunctivitis (adults and infants) (Azari and Barney, 2013; CDC, 2016c).

Many ocular infections are associated with the use of extended wear contact lenses. Each year in the United States, approximately 1 million eye infections related primarily to keratitis, a fungal infection of the cornea, and contact lens infections account for estimated direct costs of $175 million (Collier et al., 2014). In severe cases, infectious keratitis can progress to corneal ulceration, which may lead to blindness if left untreated. The incidence of fungal keratitis is not known. Health care providers are not required to report cases to public health authorities, although public health departments, the CDC, and the U.S. Food and Drug Administration (FDA) have been involved in multi-state outbreaks (CDC, 2015c). However, as many as 40.9 million U.S. adults wear contact lenses, and 99 percent of 4,269 contact-lens wearers surveyed reported at least one contact lens–related hygiene behavior associated with an increased risk for eye infection or inflammation (Cope et al., 2015). This presents an opportunity to focus on hygiene in other health promotion activities to reduce the occurrence and risk of contact lens–related infections.

Diabetic Retinopathy

Diabetic retinopathy can occur when chronically high blood sugar levels from diabetes cause abnormal blood vessels to grow along the surface of the retina and into the eye. These fragile vessels can leak fluid or blood, resulting in blurred or spotted vision (NEI/NIH, 2012b). Diabetic retinopathy can progress through four stages of increasing severity: mild, moderate, severe, and proliferative (NEI/NIH, 2012b). The early stages of diabetic retinopathy usually have no symptoms. In some cases, scar tissue may form and contract, causing retinal detachment and potentially permanent vision loss. Left unchecked, diabetic retinopathy can also lead to diabetic macular edema (DME), a buildup of fluid in the macula of the retina, which can cause blurred vision.

In 2012, 29 million people in the United States were living with diabetes, and an additional 86 million adults were considered prediabetic (CDC, 2016d). These numbers are expected to grow, with one study predicting that as many as one-third of U.S. adults diagnosed with diabetes by 2050 (Boyle et al., 2010). In 2012, an estimated 208,000 children under age 20 were diagnosed with diabetes (CDC, 2014).

As cases of diabetes continue to rise in the United States, diabetic retinopathy has become the leading cause of new cases of blindness among U.S. adults ages 20 to 74 (CDC, 2011a). According to one study using data from NHANES 2005–2008, among persons ages 40 and older with diabetes, 28.5 percent had diabetic retinopathy and 4.4 percent had severe nonproliferative diabetic retinopathy, proliferative diabetic retinopathy, or clinically significant macular edema (Zhang et al., 2010). From 2010 to 2050, diabetic retinopathy is conservatively expected to rise from 7.7 million to 14.6 million among Americans ages 40 and older (NEI/NIH, 2010e). Diabetic retinopathy has been diagnosed in adolescents and patients as young as age 5 (Forlenza and Stewart, 2012). Although prevention and control of the underlying diabetes or prediabetes is crucial, additional treatments are available to help hold retinopathy and edema in check and slow the progression of vision loss.

In general, minority populations are more likely to develop diabetic retinopathy that whites in the United States (Lanting et al., 2005; Spanakis and Golden, 2013; Varma et al., 2016). Figure 2-11 shows that, among adults ages 40 and older in 2010, the prevalence of diabetic retinopathy by race and ethnicity was highest among Hispanics (8.0 percent), followed by blacks (5.4 percent), whites (5.1 percent), and other minorities (4.7 percent) (NEI/NIH, 2010e). Numerous studies have found diabetic retinopathy to be more common in men, citing differences in vascular and circulatory factors (Nittala et al., 2014; Varma et al., 2007; Zetterberg, 2016), although a recent study found no correlation after adjusting for metabolic and socioeconomic risk factors (Wong et al., 2008). A more limited number of studies have focused on age, specifically, as an independent risk factor, although the duration of diabetes in younger people is likely to exceed that of older people, increasing their risk for diabetic retinopathy.

Common Risk Factors for Diabetic Retinopathy

By definition, individuals with diabetic retinopathy have diabetes. Hyperglycemia, hypertension, and dyslipidemia (an abnormal amount of lipids) are associated with increased risk of all forms of diabetic retinopathy and are also modifiable (Nittala et al., 2014; Varma et al., 2007; Yau et al., 2012). Numerous studies have identified an increased duration of diabetes and insulin use as risk factors for developing diabetic retinopathy (Bertelsen

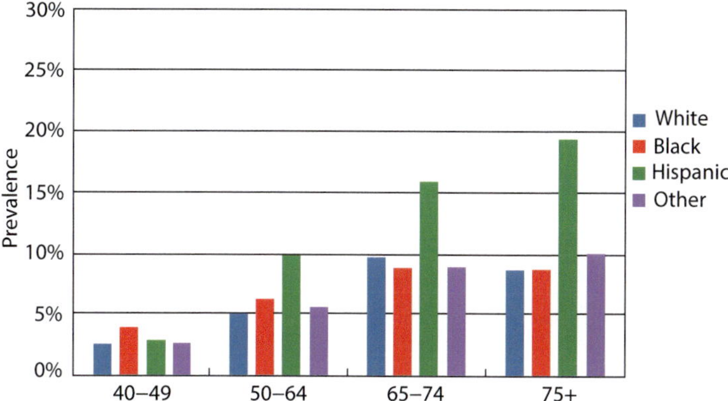

FIGURE 2-11 2010 U.S. age-specific prevalence rates for diabetic retinopathy by age and race/ethnicity.
SOURCE: NEI/NIH, 2010e.

et al., 2013; Fong et al., 2004; Jee et al., 2013; Lim et al., 2008; Nittala et al., 2014). An earlier population-based study in southern Wisconsin of 1,370 diabetic patients also found that more severe diabetic retinopathy was associated with longer duration of the disease, younger age at diagnosis, higher systolic blood pressure, insulin use, and small body mass, among other factors (Klein et al., 2008).

In addition to being an independent risk factor for type 2 diabetes, obesity is also associated with systemic diseases, including hyperlipidemia and hypertension (Cusick et al., 2003; Feingold and Grunfeld, 2000; George et al., 2015; Haslam and James, 2005; Stratton et al., 2001; Tapp et al., 2003). Other possible mechanisms related to obesity for diabetic retinopathy include increased vasoproliferative factors (e.g., vitreous vascular endothelial growth factor [VEGF]), increased oxidative stress associated with high leptin levels, platelet dysfunction, and increased blood viscosity, all of which are common conditions in obesity (Anfossi et al., 2009; Miyazawa-Hoshimoto et al., 2003; Solerte et al., 1997). Thus, efforts to reduce the rates of obesity, diabetes, or other chronic conditions associated with increased risk of diabetic retinopathy, especially in children, may help reduce the risk of associated vision impairment.

Glaucoma

Glaucoma is a chronic condition that includes a group of eye disorders characterized by deterioration in the optic nerve or specific changes in the visual field. In most types of glaucoma, fluid buildup in the anterior chamber of the eye causes increased intraocular pressure (IOP) that over time can damage the optic nerve, resulting in blindness. Glaucoma may occur in the absence of an increase in intraocular pressure. Initially individuals experience no pain and their vision remains normal. However, if glaucoma remains untreated, peripheral vision slowly deteriorates, and the vision field narrows progressively until it may seem as if a person is looking through a dark tunnel. Eventually, central vision disappears. In the United States, primary open-angle glaucoma (POAG) is the most common type of glaucoma. Unless otherwise noted, all discussions of glaucoma in this report refer to POAG.[21]

A 2010 estimate suggests that 2.7 million adults in the United States are affected by glaucoma, a number that is expected to rise to approximately 6.3 million individuals by 2050 (NEI/NIH, 2010i). Approximately 61 percent of glaucoma cases occur in women over age 40; in this age group, the prevalence rate of glaucoma in women and men is 2.2 percent and 1.6 percent, respectively (NEI/NIH, 2010i), although an earlier literature review found that men are more likely than women to have glaucoma after adjusting for age, race, year of publication, and study methods (Rudnicka et al., 2006). The prevalence of POAG increases with age and varies by race and ethnicity (Gordon et al., 2002; Varma et al., 2011). Prevalence is highest among African Americans (Gordon et al., 2002; Rudnicka et al., 2006), although Varma and colleagues (2011) found that Hispanics had comparable prevalence afer adjusting for age and gender. Figure 2-12 shows that the prevalence of glaucoma increases with age across all races and ethnicities, with the largest increases occurring for all racial and ethnic groups after age 80. Although overall prevalence rates are lower for the white population, white individuals still accounted for the majority of glaucoma cases (more than 66 percent) in 2010 (NEI/NIH, 2010i).

The severity of glaucoma and its effect on the eye is not uniform. One early study found that blindness from glaucoma was 6 to 8 times more common in African Americans than whites (Javitt et al., 1991). Another study found that visual impairment from glaucoma was 15 times more likely among African Americans than whites (Muñoz et al., 2000). A recent literature review concluded that older black populations tend "to present with more advanced disease at diagnosis" (Salowe et al., 2015,

---

[21] In POAG, fluid in the anterior chamber cannot exit through the open angle between the iris and cornea, resulting in increased IOP. Acute angle-closure glaucoma occurs when the open angle between the iris and cornea is blocked, preventing drainage of fluid in the anterior chamber and resulting in suddenly increased IOP. Normal-tension or low-tension glaucoma occurs when IOP is not elevated, but the optic nerve is still damaged. Other types of glaucoma include angle-closed glaucoma, low-tension or normal-tension glaucoma, secondary glaucoma, pigmentary glaucoma, exfoliation glaucoma, and congenital or infantile glaucoma; these are not discussed in this section.

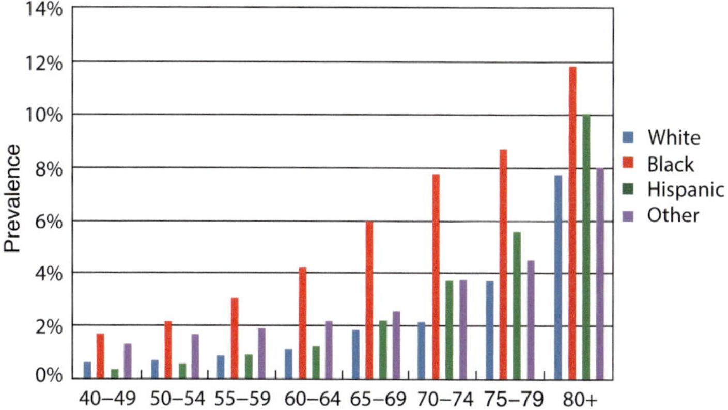

FIGURE 2-12 2010 U.S. prevalence rates for glaucoma by age and race/ethnicity. SOURCE: NEI/NIH, 2010h.

p. 3). Furthermore, race and ethnicity may interact with other risk factors to affect clinical presentation: white individuals diagnosed with glaucoma are more likely to be older yet also to have lower IOP (Fansi et al., 2009). Many studies have found that differences in surgical effectiveness vary by race and ethnicity (Taubenslag and Kammer, 2016; Wadwa and Higginbotham, 2005), although some studies have not and research is ongoing (Coleman et al., 2016a,b; Taubenslag and Kammer, 2016). More research is needed to understand the factors influencing glaucoma severity among different populations.

Common Risk Factors for Glaucoma

Certain physical and medical conditions are associated with increased risk of glaucoma. Physiological risk factors for developing glaucoma include an elevated IOP, greater cup to-disc ratio, and thin central corneal measurement (Coleman and Miglior, 2008; Gordon et al., 2002). Neovascular glaucoma can result from poorly controlled diabetes mellitus (Kersey and Broadway, 2006; Sayin et al., 2015; Watkinson and Seewoodhary, 2008). Increased risk of glaucoma has also been associated with eye surgeries, eye injuries, and the use of steroid drugs in some people (Bojikian et al., 2015; Worley and Grimmer-Somers, 2011). Available evidence suggests there may be an association between glaucoma and obesity, diabetes, or smoking, but the evidence is inconsistent (Cheung and Wong, 2007; Chiotoroiu et al., 2013; Edwards et al., 2008; Geloneck et al., 2015; Karadag et al., 2012; Oh et al., 2005; Ramdas et al., 2011; Wang et al., 2012; Yoshida et al., 2014;

Zhao et al., 2015). Other risk factors include family history and genetic predisposition (Gordon et al., 2002; Salowe et al., 2015).

Finally, some genes or genetic mutations may pose a risk for glaucoma: according to the National Eye Institute (NEI), 15 genes have been identified as associated with glaucoma (NEI/NIH, 2016b). Investigators in the population-based Rotterdam Study reported a lifetime risk of glaucoma of 22.4 percent in patients with relatives who had glaucoma, compared to 2.3 percent among controls (Wolfs et al., 1998). Researchers have also identified genetic loci that are associated with congenital, developmental, juvenile-onset primary open-angle glaucoma, and familial normal-tension glaucoma (Fingert, 2011).

Age-Related Macular Degeneration

AMD is a progressive, chronic condition that affects the retina, with most vision loss occurring in later stages of the disease (Lim et al., 2012). In neovascular, or "wet," AMD, damage to the macula is caused by fluid leaking from blood vessels that grow under the pigment epithelium in the retina. The extra fluid can cause the macula to bulge or lift up from its normal, flat position, thus distorting or destroying central vision. In geographical atrophy, or "dry," AMD, damage to the macula is caused by the breakdown of light-sensitive cells in the macula and accounts for 20 to 25 percent of legal blindness from AMD (Girmens et al., 2012). AMD is usually classified as early, intermediate, or advanced. Early and intermediate forms of AMD account for 90 percent of all cases, but the remaining 10 percent of cases cause 88 percent of all AMD-related blindness (Bourla and Young, 2006). Vision-related symptoms of AMD include blurred vision, dark areas or distortion in central field of vision, and a loss of central vision, which can be severe and rapid. Although AMD affects only older populations, certain drugs and other inherited diseases can cause other forms of macular degeneration in children and adolescents such as Stargardt's disease (DePaolis, 2014).

From 2000 to 2010, the number of U.S. adults ages 50 and older with AMD increased from 1.75 million to 2.07 million; by 2050 this number is expected to reach 5.44 million (NEI/NIH, 2010c). In 2004, when the Eye Diseases Prevalence Research Group first estimated the prevalence of AMD, it determined that 1.75 million U.S. adults ages 40 and older had "wet" AMD and another 7 million were at substantial risk of developing AMD (Friedman et al., 2004a).

Increasing age, white race, and female gender are associated with a higher risk of AMD. In the U.S. population ages 50 and older, women comprised 65 percent of the 2.1 million cases of late AMD in 2010 (NEI/NIH, 2010c). Figure 2-13 illustrates the dramatic rise in the prevalence rate

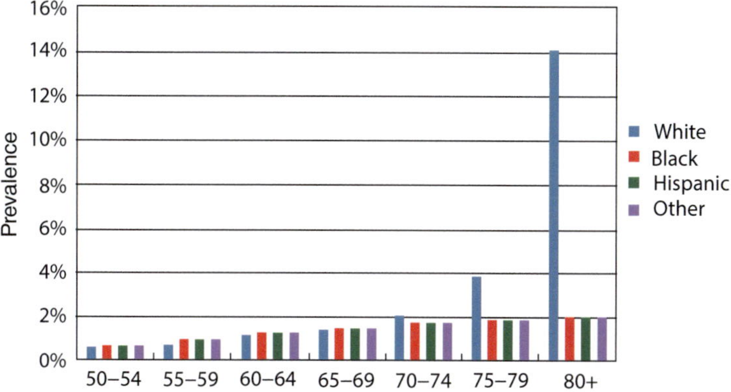

FIGURE 2-13 2010 U.S. age-specific prevalence rates for age-related macular degeneration by age and race/ethnicity.
SOURCE: NEI/NIH, 2010c.

of AMD after age 75 for the white population. The NEI reports an overall AMD prevalence rate of 2.5 percent for white persons and 0.9 percent for African American, Hispanic, and other minority populations ages 50 and older (NEI/NIH, 2010c). An earlier study found advanced AMD occurring in 11.9 percent and 16.4 percent of white men and white women ages 80 and older, respectively, compared with 1.56 percent and 2.44 percent among African American men and women in the same age group (Friedman et al., 2004b). A report from LALES found a prevalence rate for advanced AMD of 0 percent among Latinos ages 40 to 49 and 8.5 percent among those ages 80 and older (Varma et al., 2004b). Another study of any type of AMD in a 75- to 84-year-old group found prevalence varying from a low of 7.4 percent in African Americans to 15.8 percent in whites and Chinese (Klein et al., 2006). A 2004 study estimated that age-related macular degeneration accounted for approximately 54.4, 14.3, and 4.4 percent of blindness in white, Hispanic, and African American persons, respectively (Congdon, 2004a).

Common Risk Factors for AMD

A number of environmental, behavioral, genetic, and other physical conditions have been associated with the risk of AMD. By definition, increased age is the most significant risk factor for AMD, but race and ethnicity and family history are also correlated with increased prevalence (NEI/NIH, 2013). Multiple genes have been identified that appear to affect the risk of AMD development (Mousavi and Armstrong, 2013). One study found 10 different genetic loci associated with the progression of AMD from early to advanced stages of the disease (Seddon et al., 2015). In fact, recent studies have suggested that several of the genetic risk factors for AMD implicate a malfunctioning immune system (Mousavi and Armstrong, 2013; Nussblatt et al., 2014).

Smoking is one of the most consistently identified modifiable risk factors (Clemons et al., 2005; Shim et al., 2016). Less is known about the relationship between the risk of AMD and physical activity levels (Gopinath et al., 2014) or alcohol consumption (Adams et al., 2012; Chong et al., 2008). Two recent meta-analyses found a positive and inverse association between prevalent AMD and hyperopia and myopia, respectively (Lavanya et al., 2010; Pan et al., 2013). Pan and colleagues (2013) further found that no association existed between hyperopia or myopia and late AMD and called for further longitudinal research and study of the related pathophysiological mechanisms.

A few studies have found an association between obesity and AMD (AREDS Research Group, 2005; La Torre et al., 2013; Schaumberg et al., 2001). High body mass index, lens opacities, and use of some medications (i.e., antacids and thyroid hormones) are positively associated with advanced AMD, while arthritis has been associated with mild and moderate forms of AMD (Clemons et al., 2005). However, the underlying mechanisms for these associations are under investigation (Choi et al., 2013; Colak et al., 2012). Other proposed risk factors for AMD, such as hypertension and hyperlipidemia, are also associated with obesity (Cheung and Wong, 2014; Dasch et al., 2005; Feingold and Grunfeld, 2000; Hyman and Neborsky, 2002; Kyrou et al., 2000; Yu, 2014). Hypertension has been correlated with both advanced and intermediate AMD, but not early stages of the disease (AREDS Research Group, 2000). One study found synergistic effects among small groups of risk factors, such as obesity and alcohol, obesity and smoking, alcohol and high cholesterol, high cholesterol and smoking, and smoking and family history (La Torre et al., 2013).

The literature includes a number of studies examining the association between diet and the risk of AMD. Vitamins and minerals with antioxidant functions (e.g., vitamins C and E, carotenoids [lutein, zeaxanthin, β-carotene], and zinc) and compounds with anti-inflammatory properties (omega-3 fatty acids, docosahexaenoic acid) are associated with a lower risk of AMD (Rasmussen and Johnson, 2013). The association between vitamin D and A is controversial, with some studies finding a significant association between higher levels of blood 25-hydroxyvitamin D and an increased risk of AMD (Kim et al., 2014; Wu et al., 2014), and other studies finding no statistically significant association (Cougnard-Gregoire et al., 2015). One study documented a dose–response relationship between an increased prevalence of AMD and self-reported supplementary calcium consumption (more than 800 mg/d of supplementary calcium) (Kakigi et al., 2015).

Rarer and Inherited Eye Diseases

Although this chapter has focused on the conditions that affect the greatest number of persons in the United States, many other eye diseases can severely affect the eye and vision health of smaller numbers of individuals. Genetic studies have become a major focus of research programs, including those at the National Institutes of Health (NEI/NIH, 2012d). Researchers have found that about 5 percent of the human population carries genetic mutations that can cause inherited retinal diseases (Haddrill, 2016). In inherited retinal degenerations linked to recessive genes, gene therapy could possibly be used to replace a deficient gene and restore function. In other disease states, such as neovascular age-related macular degeneration or diabetic retinopathy, gene therapy has the potential to alter the production or function of existing cell proteins, such as vascular endothelial growth factor, which trigger conditions in the eye that can lead to vision loss (Campbell et al., 2016). Continued identification of molecular markers has also allowed researchers to identify individual classes of cells in the eye and may contribute to a better understanding of cell development and fate, which in turn has implications for future treatments for all who are at risk of vision impairment (NEI/NIH, 2012d; see, e.g., Chen et al., 2013). In addition to gene therapy, the use of embryonic or resident stem cells could lead to treatments that involve re-growing diseased cells or reprogramming existing cells within the eye to restore function. Some studies have identified resident stem cells that exist in the adult eye and that could potentially be activated to replace damaged or distressed cells within the eye (Mimeault and Batra, 2008, 2012; Ramsden et al., 2013).

CHARACTERIZING VISION IMPAIRMENT
FOR POPULATION HEALTH

Understanding the etiology of eye and vision health is important because it highlights which types of strategies are more likely to affect the greatest number of people over the longest time span. To this end, it can be helpful for public health professionals, clinicians, communities, and individuals to think about vision loss and impairment in terms of four categories:

1. Preventable (e.g., vision impairment that can potentially be prevented, such as that from untreated amblyopia and strabismus in children, acute eye injuries, infection, and diabetic retinopathy)

2. Modifiable (e.g., vision impairment from diseases and conditions for which available treatments can delay onset or slow the progression of vision loss, such as glaucoma or diabetic retinopathy)
3. Correctable (e.g., vision impairment from diseases and conditions for which available treatments can eliminate or correct for existing vision impairment, such as uncorrected refractive error and cataracts)
4. Uncorrectable (e.g., permanent vision impairment that cannot be improved through use of existing treatments, but whose impact on functionality, productivity, and independence can be lessened through access to vision rehabilitation services and reasonable accommodations)

Many diseases and conditions may fall into more than one category, based on the stage of a disease or condition or the severity of vision impairment. The examples provided below are meant to encourage discussions that meld public health and clinical approaches to eye and vision health and are not meant to be a comprehensive or exhaustive assessment of available treatments or their relative effectiveness. Subsequent chapters provide more in-depth discussion and specific examples of strategies to prevent, correct, and modify vision impairment.

Preventable Vision Impairment

As a general rule, prevention is the ultimate goal in a population health approach. In the case of eye and vision health, preventing injury, infection, and underlying chronic disease could have substantial effects on promoting eye and vision health before eye care is needed. Acute eye injuries may be preventable through better adherence to regulations and policies in workplace, school, and recreational settings that encourage the use of protective eyewear. Training employees to wear and properly don and doff personal protective equipment (such as eyewear), as required by the Occupational Safety and Health Administration (DOL, 2016), can prevent many eye injuries and reduce the impact on workers' health, finances, and productivity. Similarly, the American Academy of Ophthalmology, the American Academy of Pediatrics, the American Optometric Association, and Prevent Blindness all strongly recommend protective eyewear for all participants in sports for which there is a risk of eye injury (AAP, 2011; AOA, 2016). Preventing vision problems related to TBI will require more than using protective eyewear and may involve strategies to reduce concussions, falls, and motor vehicle accidents (CDC, 2016d; Master et al., 2016). Given the number of U.S. service members who experience TBI, it is also important to continue to follow the eye and vision health of active, reserve, and retired service members.

Preventing communicable diseases (including sexually transmitted diseases), ensuring adherence to vaccination schedules, and promoting proper hygiene can reduce the risk of vision-threatening infections. In general, prenatal screening and preventive treatment with antibiotics shortly after birth is the first line of defense against many sight-threatening infections in babies (CDC, 2016b). The risk of eye infections from contact lens can be reduced through proper hygiene (Cope et al., 2015). Noncompliance with recommended hygiene practices may account for the higher risk of corneal infiltrative and inflammatory events in the 15- to 25-year-old group (Chalmers et al., 2011). In the absence of new materials and modalities to reduce the risk of infection associated with contact lens wear, other health promotion activities to promote proper hygiene could help mitigate the risk of keratitis among contact lens wearers.

Efforts to stem the growth of non-vision-related chronic diseases can also directly and indirectly affect eye and vision health. Preventive treatment for nonproliferative diabetic retinopathy involves controlling diabetes through the maintenance of a healthy weight and the management of blood sugar, blood pressure, and blood cholesterol levels (NEI/NIH, 2012c). U.S. studies have found that tighter blood glucose control helps improve diabetic retinopathy and reduce the progression of diabetic retinopathy to the more proliferative and damaging form (ACCORDION, 2016; Klein et al., 2008). While progress has been made in improving other diabetes quality-of-care markers, improvements have not been made in access to annual dilated eye exams. According to data from the Dartmouth Atlas, 85 percent of diabetic Medicare enrollees achieved quality measures for hemoglobin A1c levels and lipid profiles in 2012, whereas only 67 percent had an eye exam (Dartmouth Atlas of Health Care, 2012).

Chronic disease can also increase the risk of complications for treatments of specific eye conditions, such as cataracts (Stein et al., 2011a). For example, among individuals with diabetes, cataract surgery can accelerate the development of diabetic retinopathy and increases the risk of macula edema (Hong et al., 2009; Pollreisz and Schmidt-Erfurth, 2010). Given that diabetes, the ultimate risk factor for developing diabetic retinopathy, is preventable, public health efforts to reduce diabetes prevalence and incidence would necessarily reduce the burden of diabetic retinopathy in the United States.

In addition to interventions that target specific forms of vision loss, the promotion of general social, environmental, and political determinants of health could also improve eye and vision health. For example, policies and interventions that promote healthy eating and reduce exposure to UV light could affect the prevalence of diabetic retinopathy, AMD, or cataracts.

Chapter 5 explores the link between multiple determinants of health and strategies to improve eye and vision health and prevent vision impairment in communities.

Modifiable and Correctable Vision Impairment

Early diagnosis and treatment can improve the trajectory of vision impairment by either slowing the progression of specific diseases or conditions or correcting the vision impairment itself. Many effective treatments exist to either modify or reverse vision loss in patients, but many of these diseases and conditions may present without symptoms in early stages. The issue is then promoting policies and conditions that enable populations most affected or at risk to access appropriate screenings, comprehensive eye examinations,[22] and follow-up treatments. These topics are discussed at length in Chapters 5, 6, 7, and 8.

Correctable Vision Impairment

Vision impairment associated with uncorrected refractive error can easily be avoided by correcting the refractive error with eyeglasses, contacts, or laser surgery (when appropriate), especially to correct hyperopia and myopia. Other advances in treating myopia include special glasses and contact lenses to alter eye growth "by focusing light from distant images across the entire field of view, rather than just at the centre [*sic*], as standard lenses do" (Dolgin, 2015, p. 278). Pharmacological treatments (e.g., anti-muscarinic medications and low-dose atropine) have been shown to slow the progression of myopia in children and adolescents (Chia et al., 2012; Walline et al., 2011), although corrective lenses may still be necessary.

The most common treatment for advanced cataracts is the removal of the opaque lens and implantation of an intra-ocular lens (IOL), and 90 percent of individuals who have their cataract lenses removed will experience improved vision (NEI/NIH, 2009). In the early stages of cataracts, the use of eyeglasses, better lighting, and magnifying glasses can help to reduce symptoms but they do not reverse or slow the progression of cataracts (NEI/NIH, 2009).

Early diagnosis and treatment of strabismus and amblyopia are essential to reducing the risk of long-term consequences. In children, the treatment of strabismus and amblyopia begins with the identification of the underlying causes or risk factors that lead to the development of the condition. For example, strabismus management varies based on the type of strabismus,

---

[22] For this report, the committee defines a comprehensive eye examination as a dilated eye examination that may include other tests.

the frequency and magnitude of the angle of turn, the age at which the eye turn presents, and other comorbidities. Available treatments for amblyopia and strabismus include observation, optical correction, prisms, botox injections, orthoptics or vision therapy, surgery, as well as other pharmaceutical interventions (Cotter and PEDIG, 2006; Cotter et al., 2012; Holmes et al., 2003; PEDIG, 2003; Repka et al., 2014; Scheiman et al., 2008). Although contemporary treatments can effectively improve visual acuity, there can be residual acuity deficits and even the risk of reoccurrence (Birch, 2013). There is ongoing research about when to correct, what treatments to use, and how much correction is appropriate for infants and young children with amblyopia and strabismus (Cotter et al., 2014; Jones-Jordan et al., 2014; PEDIG, 2012). Increased screening for vision loss in young children can help detect strabismus and amblyopia early when more promising treatment options are available.

Modifiable Vision Impairment

Comprehensive eye exams are important to ensure early detection and treatment of many eye diseases and conditions that cause modifiable vision impairment, such as diabetic retinopathy, glaucoma, and neovascular AMD (Sloan et al., 2014). For example, studies have found that the individuals most at risk for developing diabetic retinopathy are also those least likely to receive an exam to screen for the disease (Dumser et al., 2013; Lu et al., 2016; Nsiah-Kumi et al., 2009; Shi et al., 2014). Possible factors influencing access to high-quality care are described below and in Chapters 6 and 7.

Various surgical and pharmacological treatments are used to treat diabetic retinopathy, which are often used in combination to improve patient outcomes (Faghihi et al., 2008; Ferraz et al., 2015; Park et al., 2010). Intravitreal injections of anti-VEGFs and laser photocoagulation can slow the growth of abnormal blood vessels in patients with diabetic retinopathy or AMD (Evans et al., 2014; NEI/NIH, 2012b; Solomon et al., 2014). Along with photodynamic therapy, anti-VEGFs are also used for neovascular AMD to inhibit the growth of abnormal blood vessels in the retina. A vitrectomy, where the vitreous gel in the center of the eye is removed and replaced with a clear salt solution, can treat or prevent severe bleeding (NEI/NIH, 2012b; Wormald et al., 2007). Researchers are currently investigating long-acting drug delivery systems with the goal of decreasing the frequency of intraocular injections and improving long-term outcomes for neovascular AMD (Lim et al., 2012).

Common treatments for glaucoma include medications to lower intraocular pressure, incisional therapy (or surgery), laser trabeculoplasty, or aqueous shunts (Gedde et al., 2009; NEI/NIH, 2015; Ramulu et al., 2007; Weinreb et al., 2014). Recently, minimally invasive glaucoma surgeries have been introduced as surgical interventions to improve function and reduce various problems in glaucoma management, although several knowledge gaps persist (Richter and Coleman, 2016). High doses of vitamins C and E, lutein, zeaxanthin, and zinc have also been shown to slow the progression of intermediate AMD and late, advanced AMD that presents in a single eye (AREDS Research Group, 2001; AREDS 2 Research Group, 2013; Chew et al., 2014). Because many eye diseases and conditions that have modifiable vision impairment are chronic, repeated treatments may be necessary, which will require access to ongoing and coordinated eye care to maximize long-term benefits.

Uncorrectable Vision Impairment

Some diseases and conditions still do not have effective treatments. For example, there are no cures or treatments for some rarer diseases (e.g., AMD in children or adolescents related to Stargardt's disease) and dry AMD, although a recent study suggests that injections of a humanized anti-factor D antibody that targets VEGF could potentially stop the progression of dry AMD (Lim et al., 2012). Two other studies found that certain dietary supplements could slow dry AMD progression (Buschini et al., 2015; Schmidl et al., 2015). Additional efforts are under way to better understand potential pathophysiological pathways, which could lead to treatments (Querques et al., 2014). Public health strategies for uncorrectable vision impairment, including reasonable accommodations and access to rehabilitation services are discussed in Chapters 5 and 8. However, it is important to note that, when left untreated, modifiable vision impairment can progress to uncorrectable vision impairment (as with glaucoma, neovascular AMD, amblyopia, and diabetic retinopathy). Thus, early access to appropriate treatment can also be relevant to uncorrectable vision impairment.

Complications Following Treatment

Treatments to correct and modify vision impairment are effective, but complications can occur. Cataract surgery is relatively safe, but it does include some rare but potential risks such as bleeding, infection, and retinal detachment and success rates vary by treatment (Chen et al., 2015; Stein et al., 2011a). Potential complications of anti-VEGF therapy include retinal detachment, endophthalmitis, elevated blood pressure, and an increased risk of hypertension, stroke, and heart attack in patients with diabetic macular edema (Etminan et al., 2016; Osaadon et al., 2014). Injecting or implanting corticosteroids in the eye can suppress diabetic macular edema, but it can also cause increased eye pressure and glaucoma (NEI/NIH,

2012b). Laser photocoagulation to treat diabetic retinopathy can damage peripheral vision, as well as color and night vision (Arden and Ramsey, 2015), and the value of laser photocoagulation as a treatment of less severe forms of diabetic retinopathy is poorly understood (Royle et al., 2015). Risks associated with vitrectomy include retinal breaks and postoperative retinal detachment (Tan et al., 2011). Thus, it is important to minimize patient risk through prevention and early diagnosis, monitoring, and treatment in at-risk populations.

ESTIMATING THE PREVENTABLE BURDEN FROM REFRACTIVE ERROR AND CATARACTS

Uncorrected vision impairment is an important measure of eye and vision health in the United States because it represents the clearest opportunity to improve eye and vision health based on current knowledge and the relative effectiveness of specific treatments. When the committee began to analyze existing data to inform its deliberations, there were no national, peer-reviewed estimates of how much vision impairment could be eliminated or improved through changes in various policies and practices. To understand the magnitude of the undiagnosed and correctable visual impairment that currently exists in the United States, the committee commissioned an analysis to establish the preventable burden of vision impairment in the United States from five conditions (diabetic retinopathy, glaucoma, refractive error, cataracts, and age-related macular degeneration). The goal was to estimate the potential preventable burden attributable to five eye diseases or conditions when undiagnosed or untreated and to explore the potential costs and savings if all undiagnosed patients with eye disease were identified and treated using currently available medical technology. The results suggest that uncorrected refractive error and cataracts account for the vast majority of preventable and correctable vision impairment within the United States.

No single database exists that can support this type of analysis. Yet it is of fundamental importance to firmly establish the need for improved eye and vision health as a national health concern, as described in Chapter 4. Consequently, the estimates are based on a variety of sources, including population surveys and compilations of population-based studies, and reflect the best available data. The analysis required the authors to make assumptions about the status of eye and vision health in the United States. Numerous data gaps required several major assumptions related to undiagnosed prevalence, the costs associated with treating a specific disease or condition, and the costs savings that would accrue if the undiagnosed conditions were treated. In each case, the committee weighed the source and instructed the paper's authors to use the most conservative assumptions—that is, their assumptions minimized the potential benefits or maximized the potential costs of treatment. Although such practice is routine in the field of disease modeling, it does introduce bias or error due to differences in data source design. The full paper details the authors' methods, major assumptions, and findings including the preventable burden of each condition, the costs and savings associated with each, and the quality-adjusted life years (QALYs) saved.[23]

Most notably, for all causes except uncorrected refractive error, the committee relied on two data sources to calculate undiagnosed prevalence because of the limitations inherent to each data source. The first source, Vision Problems in the U.S. (VPUS), was used to estimate true prevalence, but it does not include diagnosis information.[24] VPUS prevalence rates were collected from population-based, epidemiological studies providing comprehensive eye examinations in set geographical areas, with eye diseases reported on the basis of age, race and ethnicity, and gender. The rates were multiplied by the 2010 census population estimates to provide national prevalence rates. To allocate prevalence by stage and to estimate the proportion of diagnosed cases, the committee relied on the second source—NHANES data. Undiagnosed cases were identified by subtracting the total number of identified cases in NHANES from overall prevalence using VPUS. In the case of uncorrected refractive error, visual acuity tests in NHANES data were used to identify the proportion of individuals with uncorrected refractive error. The proportion of severe uncorrected refractive error in working-age adults was derived from an overall estimate that included the elderly population, because of data limitations. Population-level prevalence, using U.S. Census projections, was then calculated using these data. This approach has been used in the published literature (Vitale et al., 2008). Vision impairment attributable to each condition was allocated according to the 2004 Eye Disease Prevalence Research Group rates for uncorrectable vision impairment (including blindness) among AMD, cataracts, diabetic retinopathy, glaucoma, and other.[25] The cost analysis assumes that all prevalent cases of visual impairment are treated in the first year and that incident cases are treated thereafter.

Although the authors used conservative estimates throughout their analysis, the committee only presents results related to cataracts and

---

[23] The Wittenborn and Rein commissioned paper includes a methodology section on pages 13–30. Chapter 4 describes NHANES, MEPS, and other surveys that include a vision component.

[24] These data are cited extensively by both the CDC and the NEI when characterizing the national prevalence of eye diseases and conditions (e.g., see https://nei.nih.gov/eyedata [accessed September 1, 2016]).

[25] These disease allocations are based on 2004 data, which are the most current, but they do not account for effective treatments introduced during the past 12 years.

uncorrected refractive error in this report because the analyses are most robust for these conditions. Thus, it would be possible to calculate a reasonably straightforward and accurate estimate of the preventable burden of uncorrected vision impairment in the United States and to assign potential expenditures and cost savings following treatment. Both conditions, in theory, are nearly 100 percent treatable, although appropriate treatment for cataracts varies by individual symptoms. The uncertainties and assumptions required to assign stages or severity—and, therefore, costs—for diabetic retinopathy, AMD, and glaucoma were substantial enough that the committee did not feel comfortable relying on these results to inform their deliberations or support recommendations.

The results presented in this report should be considered in the context of the limitations of this analysis and the underlying data, as well as with an understanding of how these results should be interpreted. In addition to the data limitations described above, this study also used a prevalence-based approach to estimate the current and future prevalent burden of eye disorders and vision loss. This approach is simpler than an incidence-based forecast analysis and does not require simulation of disease incidence and progression over time. However, a prevalence approach cannot account for any secular trends in disease epidemiology that would change the prevalence rates by age, race and ethnicity, and gender over time. In addition, because of the limited scope of this analysis as well as the fact that VPUS prevalence rates do not include confidence interval information, it was difficult to compare data from NHANES and VPUS. All parameters in the analysis model are static. The authors of the commissioned paper conducted a univariate sensitivity analysis of six major parameter categories, including disease and vision loss prevalence rates. These results are also included in the commissioned paper. These results, which are described in the paper, should only be used to demonstrate the potential magnitude of impact that could result from policies or demonstration programs aimed at evaluating the cost-effectiveness of early treatment and the improved quality of life related to uncorrected refractive error and cataracts, and these results warrant more extensive data collection and analysis, across all causes of vision impairment.

Uncorrected Refractive Error

Vitale and colleagues (2008) wrote that "because refractive error's impact on visual acuity can be mitigated relatively easily, it has sometimes been overlooked as an important cause of visual impairment" (p. 1117). Failure to address vision impairment in children can lead to developmental and social challenges that can have long-term, detrimental effects on educational, employment, health, and quality-of-life outcomes. Uncorrected or undercorrected refractive error is largely treatable, which should be a spur to action rather than a reason for inaction.

Although estimates of the size of the problem vary, all available statistics suggest that millions of people are needlessly affected by uncorrected refractive error in the United States. Wittenborn and Rein (2016) calculated that uncorrected (including undiagnosed) refractive error will affect an estimated 15.9 million people ages 12 and older in the United States in 2016. The CDC estimates that of the 14 million people ages 12 and older with a visual acuity of 20/50 or worse, 11 million (about 80 percent) could have their vision improved to 20/40 or better with appropriate refractive correction (CDC, 2015). Still Varma and colleagues (2016) estimate that in 2015 only 8.2 million people have vision impairment due to uncorrected refractive error based on their aggregation of data from six population-based studies. Smaller studies have found that 70 percent of all decreased visual acuity in non-Hispanic whites and Asian preschoolers (ages 30 to 72 months) and more than 90 percent of decreased visual acuity with an identifiable cause, is related to uncorrected refractive error or amblyopia resulting from refractive error (Tarczy-Hornoch et al., 2013). Similarly, the MEPEDS study found that the prevalence of poor visual acuity or amblyopia development due to uncorrected refractive error was 4.3 percent among African American and 5.3 percent among Hispanic preschoolers (ages 30 to 72 months) (MEPEDS, 2009).

Table 2-10 presents the prevalence of uncorrected refractive error in the United States by age, gender, and race and ethnicity, as calculated by Wittenborn and Rein (2016). For purposes of this analysis, the committee

TABLE 2-10 Prevalence of Uncorrected Refractive Error in the United States by Age, Gender, and Race/Ethnicity (in percent)

	White		Mexican American or Hispanic		Black		Other	
Age Group	Male	Female	Male	Female	Male	Female	Male	Female
12–17	0.06	0.06	0.14	0.15	0.12	0.15	0.09	0.16
18–29	0.04	0.05	0.12	0.10	0.09	0.10	0.10	0.08
30–39	0.04	0.04	0.04	0.11	0.12	0.10	0.11	0.03
40–49	0.04	0.04	0.08	0.05	0.10	0.08	0.07	0.06
50–59	0.03	0.01	0.04	0.08	0.02	0.05	0.05	0.02
60–69	0.03	0.04	0.04	0.07	0.03	0.03	0.10	0.06
70–79	0.04	0.05	0.11	0.11	0.08	0.07	0.04	0.07
80+	0.06	0.08	0.13	0.013	0.16	0.06	0.06	0.07

SOURCE: Adapted from Wittenborn and Rein, 2016, Table URE1, p. 31.

assumed 100 percent of these uncorrected or undercorrected refractive error cases are treatable with a vision examination, lenses, and frames at an average one-time cost of $397. Assuming annual refraction correction costs for each person as calculated in MEPS data (minimum of $36 for children ages 0 to 17 and maximum of $103 for individuals ages 40 to 64), net economic savings over the next 10 years would yield an average savings of more than $87.7 billion annually in direct and indirect costs, a remarkable 40-fold return for treatment of uncorrected refractive error.

Undercorrection of refractive error is also a concern. A 2014 study using NHANES data from 2005 to 2008 found that half of study participants ages 12 and older had correctable refractive error, but that 11.7 percent were inadequately corrected (defined as undercorrected or uncorrected) (Qiu et al., 2014). The study found significantly higher odds of inadequate correction of diagnosed refractive error for Mexican Americans and non-Hispanic black children than for non-Hispanic whites across all age groups, with the greatest disparity in the 12- to 19-year-old age group (Qiu et al., 2014).

Untreated Cataracts

Estimates from Wittenborn and Rein suggest that approximately 1.2 million Americans experience unnecessary vision impairment from cataracts, including approximately 157,000 cases of blindness.[26] To calculate the preventable burden, the committee assumed that 95 percent of all untreated cataracts cases were immediately treatable, at a one-time cost of $2,640 (persons ages 40 to 64) and $3,730 (persons over age 65). If all these individuals (prevalent cases) and all new (incident) cases were treated, about 300,000 QALYs would be saved, at an average net economic savings of more than $20 billion, including direct and indirect costs, over the next 10 years.

The committee was not able to find another national study estimating the preventable burden of cataracts, but other studies demonstrate the cost utility or cost-effectiveness of cataract surgery in the United States and other developed countries (Busbee et al., 2003; Sach et al., 2009). A 2013 study by Brown and colleagues examined the medical costs and associated financial return on investment and improvement in the quality of life for a 1-year cohort of patients who received cataract surgery (Brown et al., 2013). Results indicated that over a 13-year period, bilateral cataract surgery

---

[26] NHANES data found 51.92 percent of individuals with a self-reported history of cataract surgery; this estimate was applied to the VPUS prevalence populations under the assumption that the difference was the untreated population with cataracts.

conferred approximately 2.8 QALYs per patient, and the return on investment (ROI) was $123.4 billion (Medicare, $36.4 billion; Medicaid, $3.3 billion; other insurers, $9.6 billion; patients, $48.6 billion; and national productivity, $25.4 billion) (Brown et al., 2013). Moreover, another recent study found that cataract surgery was associated with decreased all-cause mortality for a national cohort of Medicare beneficiaries, although the study's authors identified a need for further studies to explore the causal mechanisms (Tseng et al., 2016). Studies such as these, in combination with committee estimates about the preventable burden of cataracts, suggest that it is not only possible but also practical to significantly reduce the burden of untreated vision impairment in the United States within a few years by implementing policies and programs that focus on the delivery of relatively inexpensive eyewear and treatments for these causes of vision loss.

Given the relative simplicity of treatment for refractive error and the effectiveness of surgery to correct many forms of cataracts, common sense suggests that eliminating these sources of correctable vision impairment should be achievable. Yet, the magnitude of vision impairment caused by uncorrected refractive error and cataracts suggest that barriers to access persist. Uncorrected refractive error and correctable cataracts should be a major component of any comprehensive population health approach to improving overall eye and vision health and health equity in the United States, especially among children.

KEY KNOWLEDGE AND RESEARCH GAPS

Despite the important contributions that existing literature has made to advance knowledge about eye and vision health in the United States, many key information gaps still remain. It is important to have accurate and timely estimates of the total number of individuals with vision impairment overall and with uncorrected vision impairment by disease and population characteristics because these measures provide the foundation from which to assess the need and possible impact of specific population health interventions. Future epidemiological research should attempt to better characterize disparities in terms of prevalence, incidence, and severity of disease. More research is needed to elucidate the causes and interactions that give rise to various forms and etiologies of vision loss in different populations. Box 2-1 provides a list of key knowledge and research gaps.

In efforts to advance knowledge about eye and vision health, it will be important for clinical, health care system, and social science researchers to work hand in hand with epidemiologists steeped in eye and vision health to track the impact of new knowledge on population health. As the NIH has stated in its overarching framework for guiding vision research, core principles must "use clinical, epidemiological, and statistical tools to

---

BOX 2-1
Key Knowledge and Research Gaps

- Total number of people affected by vision impairment (including uncorrected or untreated vision impairment) by age, sex, and race and ethnicity.
- Prospective studies to identify important risk and protective factors and their pathophysiologic pathways and modifiable mechanisms related to vision impairment, including specific etiologies, the impact of health care, and social determinants of health.
- Factors affecting utilization of available treatments for correctable and modifiable vision impairment.
- Tracking and comparing the safety and effectiveness of various prevention strategies and treatments to maximize the value and impact of eye and vision care, especially for certain patient groups.
- Treatment effectiveness, including combined treatments, among different populations.
- Systemic effects of treatment for vision impairment over the long term.
- Causes and potential treatments for rarer diseases and conditions, especially research that produces knowledge relevant to multiple types and causes of vision impairment.

---

identify populations at risk of blinding eye diseases and visual disorders, evaluate new therapeutics, and improve functional consequences of visual loss" (NEI/NIH, 2012d, p. 3). The committee stresses that efforts to expand knowledge about the epidemiology of vision impairment should balance the more common with rarer eye diseases and conditions in any population health approach to combat the immediate and long-term impacts of vision loss.

CONCLUSION

Several major themes emerge from this review of the scientific literature on the epidemiology of eye disease and vision impairment. First, the prevalence of vision impairment and many eye diseases increases with age, and can also vary with factors including race and ethnicity, gender, family history of eye disease, socioeconomic status, and geographic location. Second, some eye diseases can be corrected, cured, or prevented. Examples include refractive error, cataracts, and amblyopia. For many other eye diseases, interventions can only delay onset or slow the progression. Examples include diabetic retinopathy, AMD, and glaucoma. Third, some risk factors for eye disease are modifiable; these include UV exposure for cataracts, smoking for AMD, and elevated IOP for glaucoma.

Chapter 5 demonstrates how knowledge of these risk and protective factors can help shape public health interventions to ensure early diagnosis and follow-up care, prevent and control eye diseases and underlying comorbid conditions, and modify lifestyle behaviors both before and after eye disease occurs. This chapter has also identified several key knowledge and research gaps.

Using the best available data and methodological approaches to explore the epidemiology in the United States, it is clear that eye health and vision impairment constitute a major public health imperative—one which can be alleviated through a better understanding of populations affected, risk factors underlying specific disorders, and barriers to care that result in an unmet need for diagnosis and treatment. Assessing the prevalence and distribution of vision impairment across populations in the United States is critical to developing effective public health policy. The committee stresses that efforts to develop public health interventions should emphasize the more common diseases in any adopted population health approach to combat the immediate and long-term health-related effects of vision loss.

REFERENCES

AAP (American Academy of Pediatrics). 2011. AAP publications reaffirmed and retired. *Pediatrics* 128(3):e748 (referencing Committee on Sports Medicine & Fitness. 2004. Protective eyewear for young athletes. *Pediatrics* 113(3):619–622).

ACCORDION (Action to Control Cardiovascular Risk in Diabetes Follow-On Eye Study Group and the Action to Control Cardiovascular Risk in Diabetes Follow-On Study Group). 2016. Persistent effective of intensive glycemic control on retinopathy in type 2 diabetes in the Action to Control Cardiovascular Risk in Diabetes (ACCORD) Follow-On Study. *Diabetes Care* 39(7):1089–1100.

Adams, M. K., E. W. Chong, E. Williamson, K. Z. Aung, G. A. Makeyeva, G. G. Giles, D. R. English, J. Hopper, R. H. Guymer, P. N. Baird, L. D. Robman, and J. A. Simpson. 2012. 20/20—Alcohol and age-related macular degeneration: The Melbourne Collaborative Cohort Study. *American Journal of Epidemiology* 176(4):289–298.

Anfossi, G., I. Russo, and M. Trovati. 2009. Platelet dysfunction in central obesity. *Nutrition, Metabolism and Cardiovascular Diseases* 19(6):440–449.

AOA (American Optometric Association). 2016. School-aged vision: 6 to 18 years of age. http://www.aoa.org/patients-and-public/good-vision-throughout-life/childrens-vision/school-aged-vision-6-to-18-years-of-age?sso=y (accessed July 11, 2016).

AoA (U.S. Administration on Aging). 2014. Future growth. http://www.aoa.acl.gov/Aging_Statistics/Profile/2014/4.aspx (accessed April 8, 2016).

Arden, G. B., and D. J. Ramsey. 2015. Diabetic retinopathy and a novel treatment based on the biophysics of rod photoreceptors and dark adaptation. In H. Kolb, E. Fernandez, and R. Nelson (eds.), *Webvision: The organization of the retina and visual system*. Salt Lake City: University of Utah Health Sciences Center.

AREDS (Age-Related Eye Disease Study) Research Group. 2000. Risk factors associated with age-related macular degeneration: A case-control study in the age-related eye disease study: Age-Related Eye Disease Study report number 3. *Ophthalmology* 107(12):2224–2232.

———. 2001. A randomized, placebo-controlled, clinical trial of high-dose supplementation with vitamins C and E, beta carotene, and zinc for age-related macular degeneration and vision loss: AREDS report number 8. *Archives of Ophthalmology* 119(10):1417–1436.

———. 2005. Risk factors for the incidence of advanced age-related macular degeneration in the Age-Related Eye Disease Study (AREDS): AREDS report number 19. *Ophthalmology* 112(4):533–539, e531.

AREDS 2 Research Group. 2013. Lutein + zeaxanthin and omega-3 fatty acids for age-related macular degeneration: The Age-Related Eye Disease Study 2 (AREDS2) randomized clinical trial. *JAMA* 309(19):2005–2015.

Atkinson, J., O. Braddick, M. Nardini, and S. Anker. 2007. Infant hyperopia: Detection, distribution, changes and correlates—outcomes from the Cambridge infant screening programs. *Optometry & Vision Science* 84(2):84–96.

Azari, A. A., and N. P. Barney. 2013. Conjunctivitis: A systematic review of diagnosis and treatment. *JAMA* 310(16):1721–1730.

Barrett, B. T., A. Bradley, and T. R. Candy. 2013. The relationship between anisometropia and amblyopia. *Progress in Retinal and Eye Research* 36:120–158.

Bertelsen, G., T. Peto, H. Lindekleiv, H. Schirmer, M. D. Solbu, I. Toft, A. K. Sjølie, and I. Njølstad. 2013. Tromsø eye study: Prevalence and risk factors of diabetic retinopathy. *Acta Ophthalmologica* 91(8):716–721.

Birch, E. E. 2013. Amblyopia and binocular vision. *Progress in Retinal and Eye Research* 33:67–84.

BLS (Bureau of Labor Statistics). 2012. *Injuries, illnesses, and fatalities.* http://www.bls.gov/iif/oshwc/osh/case/ostb3594.pdf (accessed February 16, 2016).

Bojikan, K. D., A. L. Stein, M. A. Slaubaugh, and P. P. Chan. 2015. Incidence and risk factors for traumatic intraocular pressure elevation and traumatic glaucoma after open-globe injury. *Eye* 29:1579–1584.

Borchert, M. S., R. Varma, S. A. Cotter, K. Tarczy-Hornoch, R. McKean-Cowdin, J. H. Lin, G. Wen, S. P. Azen, M. Torres, J. M. Tielsch, D. S. Friedman, M. X. Repka, J. Katz, J. Ibironke, L. Giordano, and the Multi-Ethnic Pediartic Eye Disease Study and the Baltimore Pediatric Eye Disease Study groups. 2011. Risk factors for hyperopia and myopia in preschool children the Multi-Ethnic Pediatric Eye Disease and Baltimore Pediatric Eye Disease studies. *Ophthalmology* 118(10):1966–1973.

Bourla, D. H., and T. A. Young. 2006. Age-related macular degeneration: A practical approach to a challenging disease. *Journal of the American Geriatrics Society* 54(7):1130–1135.

Boyle, J. P., T. J. Thompson, E. W. Gregg, L. E. Barker, and D. F. Williamson. 2010. Projection of the year 2050 burden of diabetes in the U.S. adult population. Dynamic modeling of incidence, mortality, and prediabetes prevalence. *Population Health Metrics* 8(1):1.

Brahm, K. D., H. M. Wilgenburg, J. Kirby, S. Ingalla, C. Y. Chang, and G. L. Goodrich. 2009. Visual impairment and dysfunction in combat-injured service members with traumatic brain injury. *Optometry & Vision Sciences* 86(7):817–825.

Brown, G. C., M. M. Brown, A. Menezes, B. G. Busbee, H. B. Lieske, and P. A. Lieske. 2013. Cataract surgery cost utility revisited in 2012: A new economic paradigm. *Ophthalmology* 120(12):2367–2376.

Busbee, B. G., M. M. Brown, G. C. Brown, and S. Sharma. 2003. Cost-utility analysis of cataract surgery in the second eye. *Ophthalmology* 110(12):2310–2317.

Buschini, E., A. M. Fea, C. A. Lavia, M. Nassisi, G. Pignata, M. Zola, and F. M. Grignolo. 2015. Recent developments in the management of dry age-related macular degeneration. *Clinical Ophthalmology* 9:563–574.

Campbell, J. P., T. J. McFarland, and J. T. Stout. 2016. Ocular gene therapy. *Developments in Ophthalmology* 55:317–321.

CDC (Centers for Disease Control and Prevention). 2007. Eye safety tool box talk—instructor's guide. http://www.cdc.gov/niosh/topics/eye/toolbox-eye.html (accessed February 16, 2016).

———. 2009. The burden of vision loss. http://www.cdc.gov/visionhealth/basic_information/vision_loss_burden.htm (accessed March 24, 2016).

———. 2011a. National diabetes fact sheet: National estimates and general information on diabetes and prediabetes in the United States, 2011. Atlanta, GA: CDC. http://www.cdc.gov/diabetes/pubs/pdf/ndfs_2011.pdf (accessed September 2, 2016).

———. 2011b. The state of vision, aging, and public health in America. http://www.cdc.gov/visionhealth/pdf/vision_brief.pdf (accessed February 16, 2016).

———. 2014. *National diabetes statistics report: Estimates of diabetes and its burden in the United States, 2014.* Atlanta, GA: CDC.

———. 2015a. Chlamydia—CDC fact sheet (detailed). http://www.cdc.gov/std/chlamydia/stdfact-chlamydia-detailed.htm (accessed May 20, 2016).

———. 2015b. Definition of fungal eye infections. http://www.cdc.gov/fungal/diseases/fungal-eye-infections/definition.html (accessed August 19, 2016).

———. 2015c. Fungal eye infection statistics. http://www.cdc.gov/fungal/diseases/fungal-eye-infections/statistics.html (accessed August 19, 2016).

———. 2015d. National Health and Nutrition Examination Survey (NHANES). http://www.cdc.gov/visionhealth/data/systems/nhanes.htm (accessed August 19, 2016).

———. 2015e. Vision Health Initiative (VHI): National data. http://www.cdc.gov/vision-health/data/national.htm (accessed February 12, 2016).

———. 2016a. Basic information about traumatic brain injury and concussion. http://www.cdc.gov/traumaticbraininjury/basics.html (accessed February 16, 2016).

———. 2016b. Conjunctivitis (pink eye) in newborns. http://www.cdc.gov/conjunctivitis/newborns.html (accessed July 8, 2016).

———. 2016c. Conjunctivitis (pink eye). Causes. https://www.cdc.gov/conjunctivitis/about/causes.html (accessed July 8, 2016)

———. 2016d. Diabetes latest. http://www.cdc.gov/features/diabetesfactsheet (accessed June 16, 2016).

———. 2016e. Injury prevention & control: Traumatic brain injury & concussion—TBI: Get the facts. http://www.cdc.gov/traumaticbraininjury/get_the_facts.html (accessed June 4, 2016).

Chalmers, R. L., H. Wagner, G. L. Mitchell, D. Y. Lam, B. T. Kinoshita, M. E. Jansen, K. Richdale, L. Sorbara, and T. T. McMahon. 2011. Age and other risk factors for corneal infiltrative and inflammatory events in young soft contact lens wearers from the Contact Lens Assessment in Youth (CLAY) Study. *Investigative Ophthalmology & Visual Science* 52(9):6690–6696.

Chang, J. R., E. Koo, E. Agron, J. Hallak, T. Clemons, D. Azar, R. D. Sperduto, F. L. Ferris, 3rd, and E. Y. Chew. 2011. Risk factors associated with incident cataracts and cataract surgery in the Age-Related Eye Disease Study (AREDS): AREDS report number 32. *Ophthalmology* 118(11):2113–2119.

Channa, R., S. Zafar, J. K. Canner, R. Haring, E. B. Schneider, and D. S. Friedman. 2016. Epidemiology of eye-related emergency department visits. *JAMA Ophthalmology* 134(3):312–319.

Chen, X., W. Xiao, S. Ye, W. Chen, and Y. Liu. 2015. Efficacy and safety of femtosecond laser-assisted cataract surgery versus conventional phacoemulsification for cataract: A meta-analysis of randomized controlled trials. *Scientific Reports* 5:13123.

Chen, Y. K. Huang, M. N. Nakatsu, S. X. Deng, and G. Fan. 2013. Identification of novel molecular markers thorugh transcriptomic analysis in human fetal and adult corneal endothelial cells. *Human Molecular Genetics* 22(7):1271–1279.

Cheung, C., and T. Wong. 2014. Is age-related macular degeneration a manifestation of systemic disease? New prospects for early intervention and treatment. *Journal of Internal Medicine* 276(2):140–153.

Cheung, N., and T. Y. Wong. 2007. Obesity and eye diseases. *Survey of Ophthalmology* 52(2):180–195.

Chew, E. Y., J. P. SanGiovanni, F. L. Ferris, W. T. Wong, E. Agron, T. E. Clemons, R. Sperduto, R. Danis, S. R. Chandra, and B. A. Blodi. 2013. Lutein/zeaxanthin for the treatment of age-related cataract: AREDS2 randomized trial report number 4. *JAMA Ophthalmology* 131(7):843–850.

Chew, E. Y., T. E. Clemons, S. B. Bressler, M. J. Elman, R. P. Danis, A. Domalpally, J. S. Heier, J. E. Kim, and R. Garfinkel. 2014. Randomized trial of a home monitoring system for early detection of choroidal neovascularization Home Monitoring of the Eye (HOME) study. *Ophthalmology* 121(2):535–544.

Chia, A., W. H. Chua, Y. B. Cheung, W. L. Wong, A. Lingham, A. Fong, and D. Tan. 2012. Atropine for the treatment of childhood myopia: Safety and efficacy of 0.5%, 0.1%, and 0.01% doses (atropine for the treatment of myopia 2). *Ophthalmology* 119(2):347–354.

Chia, A., X. Lin, M. Dirani, G. Gazzard, D. Ramamurthy, B.-L. Quah, B. Chang, Y. Ling, S.-W. Leo, and T.-Y. Wong. 2013. Risk factors for strabismus and amblyopia in young Singapore Chinese children. *Ophthalmic Epidemiology* 20(3):138–147.

Chiotoroiu, S. M., D. Pop de Popa, G. I. Stefaniu, F. A. Secureanu, and V. L. Purcarea. 2013. The importance of alcohol abuse and smoking in the evolution of glaucoma disease. *Journal of Medicine and Life* 6(2):226–229.

Choi, J. A., J.-U. Hwang, Y. H. Yoon, and J.-Y. Koh. 2013. Methallothionein-3 contributes to vascular endothelial growth factor induction in a mouse model of choroidal neovascularization. *Metallomics* 5(10):1387–1396.

Chong, E. W., A. J. Kreis, T. Y. Wong, J. A. Simpson, and R. H. Guymer. 2008. Alcohol consumption and the risk of age-related macular degeneration: A systematic review and meta-analysis. *American Journal of Ophthalmology* 145(4):707–715.

Chou, C. F., C. E. Sherrod, X. Zhang, L. E. Barker, K. M. Bullard, J. E. Crews, and J. B. Saaddine. 2014. Barriers to eye care among people aged 40 years and older with diagnosed diabetes, 2006–2010. *Diabetes Care* 37(1):180–188.

Clemons, T. E., R. C. Milton, R. Klein, J. M. Seddon, F. L. Ferris 3rd, Age-Related Eye Disease Study Research Group. 2005. Risk factors for the incidence of advanced age-related macular degeneration in the Age-Related Eye Disease Study (AREDS): AREDS report number 19. *Ophthalmology* 112(4):533–539.

Cockerham, G. C., G. L. Goodrich, E. D. Weichel, J. C. Orcutt, J. F. Rizzo, K. S. Bower, and R. A. Schuchard. 2009. Eye and visual function in traumatic brain injury. *Journal of Rehabilitation Research & Development* 46(6):811–818.

Colak, E., N. Majkic-Singh, L. Zoric, A. Radosavljevic, and N. Kosanovic-Jakovic. 2012. The role of CRP and inflammation in the pathogenesis of age-related macular degeneration. *Biochemia Medica* 22(1):39–48.

Coleman, A. L., and S. Miglior. 2008. Risk factors for glaucoma onset and progression. *Survey of Ophthalmology* 53(6):S3–S10.

Coleman, A. L., F. Yu, E. Keeler, and C. M. Mangione. 2006. Treatment of uncorrected refractive error improves vision-specific quality of life. *Journal of American Geriatrics Society* 54(6):883–890.

Coleman, A. L., F. C. Lum, P. Velentgas, Z. Su, R. E. Gliklich, and RiGOR Study Group. 2016a. Impact of treatment strategies for open angle glaucoma on intraocular pressure: The RiGOR Study. *Journal of Comparative Effectiveness Research* 5(1):87–98.

Coleman, A. L., F. C. Lum, P. Velentgas, Z. Su, R. E. Gliklich, and RiGOR Study Group. 2016b. RiGOR: A prospective observational study comparing the effectiveness of treatment strategies for open-angle glaucoma. *Journal of Comparative Effectiveness Research* 5(1):65–78.

Collier, S. A., M. P. Gronostaj, A. K. MacGurn, J. R. Cope, K. L. Awsumb, J. S. Yoder, and M. J. Beach. 2014. Estimated burden of keratitis—United States, 2010. *Morbidity and Mortality Weekly Report* 63(45):1027–1030.

Congdon, N., B. O'Colmain, C. C. Klaver, R. Klein, B. Munoz, D. S. Friedman, J. Kempen, H. R. Taylor, and P. Mitchell. 2004a. Causes and prevalence of visual impairment among adults in the United States. *Archives of Ophthalmology* 122(4):477–485.

Congdon, N., J. R. Vingerling, B. E. Klein, S. West, D. S. Friedman, J. Kempen, B. O'Colmain, S. Y. Wu, and H. R. Taylor. 2004b. Prevalence of cataract and pseudophakia/aphakia among adults in the United States. *Archives of Ophthalmology* 122(4):487–494.

Cope, J. R., S. A. Collier, M. M. Rao, R. Chalmers, G. L. Mitchell, K. Richdale, H. Wagner, B. T. Kinoshita, D. Y. Lam, and L. Sorbara. 2015. Contact lens wearer demographics and risk behaviors for contact lens-related eye infections—United States, 2014. *Morbidity and Mortality Weekly Report* 64:865–870.

Cotch, M. F., R. J. Klein, K. M. Brett, and A. Ryskulova. 2005 Visual impairment and use of eye-care services and protective eyewear among children—United States, 2002. *Morbidity and Mortality Weekly* 54(17):425–429.

Cotter, S. A., and PEDIG (Pediatric Eye Disease Investigator Group). 2006. Treatment of anisometropic amblyopia in children with refractive correction. *Ophthalmology* 113(6):895–903.

Cotter, S. A., R. Varma, K. Tarczy-Hornoch, R. McKean-Cowdin, J. Lin, G. Wen, J. Wei, M. Borchert, S. P. Azen, M. Torres, J. M. Tielsch, D. S. Friedman, M. X. Repka, J. Katz, J. Ibironke, L. Giordano, and the Joint Writing Committee for the Multi-Ethnic Pediatric Eye Disease Study and the Baltimore Pediatric Eye Disease Study Groups. 2011. Risk factors associated with childhood strabismus: The Multi-Ethnic Pediatric Eye Disease and Baltimore Pediatric Eye Disease studies. *Ophthalmology* 118(11):2251–2261.

Cotter, S. A., N. C. Foster, J. M. Holmes, B. M. Melia, D. K. Wallace, M. X. Repka, S. M. Tamkins, R. T. Kraker, R. W. Beck, D. L. Hoover, E. R. Crouch, 3rd, A. M. Miller, C. L. Morse, and D. W. Suh. 2012. Optical treatment of strabismic and combined strabismic-anisometropic amblyopia. *Ophthalmology* 119(1):150–158.

Cotter, S. A., B. G. Mohney, D. L. Chandler, J. M. Holmes, M. X. Repka, M. Melia, D. K. Wallace, R. W. Beck, E. E. Birch, R. T. Kraker, S. M. Tamkins, A. M. Miller, N. A. Sala, and S. R. Glaser. 2014. A randomized trial comparing part-time patching with observation for children 3 to 10 years of age with intermittent exotropia. *Ophthalmology* 121(12):2299–2310.

Cougnard-Gregoire, A., B. M. Merle, J. F. Korobelnik, M. B. Rougier, M. N. Delyfer, C. Feart, M. Le Goff, J. F. Dartigues, P. Barberger-Gateau, and C. Delcourt. 2015. Vitamin D deficiency in community-dwelling elderly is not associated with age-related macular degeneration. *Journal of Nutrition* 145(8):1865–1872.

Cumberland, P. M., J. S. Rahi, for the UK Biobank Eye and Vision Consortium. 2016. Visual function, social position, and health and life changes: The UK Biobank Study. *JAMA Ophthalmology* 134(9):959–966.

Cummings, S. R., M. C. Nevitt, W. S. Browner, K. Stone, K. M. Fox, K. E. Ensrud, J. Cauley, D. Black, and T. M. Vogt. 1995. Risk factors for hip fracture in white women. Study of Osteoporotic Fractures Research Group. *New England Journal of Medicine* 332(12):767–773.

Cusick, M., E. Y. Chew, C.-C. Chan, H. S. Kruth, R. P. Murphy, and F. L. Ferris. 2003. Histopathology and regression of retinal hard exudates in diabetic retinopathy after reduction of elevated serum lipid levels. *Ophthalmology* 110(11):2126–2133.

Dang, S. 2015. Eye injuries at work. http://www.aao.org/eye-health/tips-prevention/injuries-work (accessed February 16, 2016).

Dartmouth Atlas of Health Care. 2012. Percent of diabetic Medicare enrollees receiving appropriate management, by race and type of screening. http://www.dartmouthatlas.org/data/table.aspx?ind=160 (accessed May 18, 2016).

Dasch, B., A. Fuhs, T. Behrens, A. Meister, J. Wellmann, M. Fobker, D. Pauleikhoff, and H.-W. Hense. 2005. Inflammatory markers in age-related maculopathy: Cross-sectional analysis from the Muenster Aging and Retina Study. *Archives of Ophthalmology* 123(11):1501–1506.

Defense and Veterans Brain Injury Center. 2016. DoD worldwide numbers for TBI. http://dvbic.dcoe.mil/dod-worldwide-numbers-tbi (accessed August 14, 2016).

DePaolis, M. 2014. Macular degeneration—FAQs. http://www.allaboutvision.com/faq/amd.htm (accessed February 17, 2016).

Dirani, M., L. Tong, G. Gazzard, X. Zhang, A. Chia, T. L. Young, K. A. Rose, P. Mitchell, and S. M. Saw. 2009. Outdoor activity and myopia in Singapore teenage children. *British Journal of Ophthalmology* 93(8):997–1000.

DOL (U.S. Department of Labor). 2016. Updating OSHA standards based on national consensus standards: Eye and face protection. *Federal Register* 81:16085–16093.

Dolgin, E. 2015. The myopia boom. *Nature* 519(7543):276–278.

Dotan, G., B. Truong, M. Snitzer, et al. 2015. Outcomes of an inner-city vision outreach program: Give kids sight day. *JAMA Ophthalmology* 133(5):527–532.

Dumser, S. M., S. J. Ratcliffe, D. R. Langdon, K. M. Murphy, and T. H. Lipman. 2013. Racial disparities in screening for diabetic retinopathy in youth with type 1 diabetes. *Diabetes Research and Clinical Practice* 101(1):e3–e5.

Edwards, R., J. Thornton, R. Ajit, R. A. Harrison, and S. P. Kelly. 2008. Cigarette smoking and primary open angle glaucoma: A systematic review. *Journal of Glaucoma* 17(7):558–566.

Etminan, M., D. A. Maberley, D. W. Babiuk, and B. C. Carleton. 2016. Risk of myocardial infarction and stroke with single or repeated doses of intravitreal bevacizumab in age-related macular degeneration. *American Journal of Ophthalmology* 163:53–58.

Evans, J. R., M. Michelessi, and G. Virgili. 2014. Laser photocoagulation for proliferative diabetic retinopathy. *Cochrane Database of Systematic Reviews* 11:CD011234.

Faghihi, H., R. Roohipoor, S. Mohammadi, K. Hojat-Jalali, A. Mirshahi, A. Lashay, N. Piri, and S. Faghihi. 2008. Intravitreal bevacizumab versus combined bevacizumab-triamcinolone versus macular laser photocoagulation in diabetic macular edema. *European Journal of Ophthalmology* 18(6):941.

Fansi, A. A., D. G. Papamatheakis, and P. J. Harasymowycz. 2009. Racial variability of glaucoma risk factors between African Caribbeans and Caucasians in a Canadian urban screening population. *Canadian Journal of Ophthalmology* 44(5):576–581.

Feingold, K. R., and C. Grunfeld. 2000. Obesity and dyslipidemia. In *Endotext*, L. J. De Groot, P. Beck-Peccoz, G. Chrousos, K. Dungan, A. Grossman, J. M. Hershman, C. Koch, R. McLachlan, M. New, R. Rebar, F. Singer, A. Vinik and M. O. Weickert (eds.). South Dartmouth, MA: MDText.com, Inc.

Ferraz, D. A., L. M. Vasquez, R. C. Preti, A. Motta, R. Sophie, M. G. Bittencourt, Y. J. Sepah, M. L. Monteiro, Q. D. Nguyen, and W. Y. Takahashi. 2015. A randomized controlled trial of panretinal photocoagulation with and without intravitreal ranibizumab in treatment-naive eyes with non-high-risk proliferative diabetic retinopathy. *Retina* 35(2):280–287.

Fingert, J. H. 2011. Primary open-angle glaucoma genes. *Eye (London)* 25(5): 587–595.

Fitch, C. P., P. A. Rapoza, S. Owens, F. Murillo-Lopez, R. A. Johnson, T. C. Quinn, J. S. Pepose, and H. R. Taylor. 1989. Epidemiology and diagnosis of acute conjunctivitis at an inner-city hospital. *Ophthalmology* 96(8):1215–1220.

Flynn, J. T., and J. C. Cassady. 1978. Current trends in amblyopia therapy. *Ophthalmology* 85:429–459.

Fong, D. S., L. Aiello, T. W. Gardner, G. L. King, G. Blankenship, J. D. Cavallerano, F. L. Ferris, 3rd, and R. Klein. 2004. Retinopathy in diabetes. *Diabetes Care* 27 (Suppl 1):S84–S87.

Forlenza, G. P., and M. W. Stewart. 2012. Diabetic retinopathy in children. *Pediatric Endocrinology Reviews* 10(2):217–226.

Forrest, K. Y., and J. M. Cali. 2009. Epidemiology of lifetime work-related eye injuries in the U.S. population associated with one or more lost days of work. *Ophthalmic Epidemiology* 16(3):156–162.

Fozailoff, A., K. Tarczy-Hornoch, S. Cotter, G. Wen, J. Lin, M. Borchert, S. Azen, and R. Varma. 2011. Prevalence of astigmatism in 6- to 72-month-old African American and Hispanic children: The Multi-Ethnic Pediatric Eye Disease Study. *Ophthalmology* 118(2):284–293.

Friedman, D. S., B. J. O'Colmain, B. Munoz, S. C. Tomany, C. McCarty, P. T. de Jong, B. Nemesure, P. Mitchell, and J. Kempen. 2004a. Prevalence of age-related macular degeneration in the United States. *Archives of Ophthalmology* 122(4):564–572.

Friedman, D. S., R. C. Wolfs, B. J. O'Colmain, B. E. Klein, H. R. Taylor, S. West, M. C. Leske, P. Mitchell, N. Congdon, J. Kempen, and Eye Diseases Prevalence Research Group. 2004b. Prevalence of open-angle glaucoma among adults in the United States. *Archives of Ophthalmology* 122(4):532–538.

Friedman, D. S., M. X. Repka, J. Katz, L. Giordano, J. Ibironke, P. Hawse, and J. M. Tielsch. 2009. Prevalence of amblyopia and strabismus in white and African American children aged 6 through 71 months: The Baltimore Pediatric Eye Disease Study. *Ophthalmology* 116(11):2128–2134, e2121–e2122.

Ganz, M. L., Z. Xuan, and D. G. Hunter. 2006. Prevalence and correlates of children's diagnosed eye and vision conditions. *Ophthalmology* 113(12):2298–2306.

Gedde, S. J., J. C. Schiffman, W. J. Feuer, L. W. Herndon, J. D. Brandt, and D. L. Budenz. 2009. Three-year follow-up of the tube versus trabeculectomy study. *American Journal of Ophthalmology* 148(5):670–684.

Geloneck, M. M., E. L. Crowell, E. B. Wilson, B. E. Synder, A. Z. Chuang, L. A. Baker, N. P. Bell, and R. M. Feldman. 2015. Correlation between intraocular pressure and body mass index in the seated and supine positions. *Journal of Glaucoma* 24(2):130–134.

George, A. M., A. G. Jacob, and L. Fogelfeld. 2015. Lean diabetes mellitus: An emerging entity in the era of obesity. *World Journal of Diabetes* 6(4):613.

Giordano, L., D. S. Friedman, M. X. Repka, J. Katz, J. Ibironke, P. Hawes, and J. M. Tielsch. 2009. Prevalence of refractive error among preschool children in an urban population: The Baltimore Pediatric Eye Disease Study. *Ophthalmology* 116(4):739–746.

Girmens, J.-F., J.-A. Sahel, and K. Marazova. 2012. Dry age-related macular degeneration: A currently unmet clinical need. *Intractable & Rare Diseases Research* 1(3):103.

Glynn, R. J., B. Rosner, and W. G. Christen. 2009. Evaluation of risk factors for cataract types in a competing risks framework. *Ophthalmic Epidemiology* 16(2):98–106.

Goldstein, M. H., and D. Wee. 2011. Sports injuries: An ounce of prevention and a pound of cure. *Eye & Contact Lens* 37(3):160–163.

Gong, Y., K. Feng, N. Yan, Y. Xu, and C. W. Pan. 2015. Different amounts of alcohol consumption and cataract: A meta-analysis. *Optometry & Vision Science* 92(4):471–479.

Goodrich, G. L., H. M. Flyg, J. E. Kirby, C. Y. Chang, and G. L. Martinsen. 2013. Mechanisms of TBI and visual consequences in military and veteran populations. *Optometry & Vision Science* 90(2):105–112.

Gopinath, B., G. Liew, G. Burlutsky, and P. Mitchell. 2014. Physical activity and the 15-year incidence of age-related macular degeneration. *Investigative Ophthalmology & Visual Science* 55(12):7799–7803.

Gordon, M. O., J. A. Beiser, J. D. Brandt, D. K. Heuer, E. J. Higginbotham, C. A. Johnson, J. L. Keltner, J. P. Miller, R. K. Parrish, and M. R. Wilson. 2002. The Ocular Hypertension Treatment Study: Baseline factors that predict the onset of primary open-angle glaucoma. *Archives of Ophthalmology* 120(6):714–720.

Haddrill, M. 2016. Stargardt's disease (fundus flavimaculatus). http://www.allaboutvision. com/conditions/stargardts.htm (accessed May 20, 2016).

Hamm, L. M., J. Black, S. Dai, and B. Thompson. 2014. Global processing in amblyopia: A review. *Frontiers in Psychology* 5:1–21.

Harrison, A., and D. G. Telander. 2002. Eye injuries in the young athlete: A case-based approach. *Pediatric Annals* 31(1):33–40.

Haslam, D., and W. James. 2005. Obesity. *Lancet* 366:1197–1209.

Hatt, S. R., and L. Gnanaraj. 2013. Interventions for intermittent exotropia. *Cochrane Database of Systematic Reviews* 5:1–35. http://doi.org/10.1002/14651858.CD003737.pub3 (accessed September 3, 2016).

He, M., F. Xiang, Y. Zeng, et al. 2015. Effect of time spent outdoors at school on the development of myopia among children in China: A randomized clinical trial. *JAMA* 314(11):1142–1148.

Hellgren, K. M., K. Tornqvist, P. G. Jakobsson, P. Lundgren, B. Carlsson, K. Kallen, F. Serenius, A. Hellstrom, and G. Holmstrom. 2016. Ophthalmologic outcome of extremely preterm infants at 6.5 years of age: Extremely Preterm Infants in Sweden Study (EXPRESS). *JAMA Ophthalmology*.

Hiller, R., M. J. Podgor, R. D. Sperduto, L. Nowroozi, P. W. Wilson, R. B. D'Agostino, T. Colton, and T. F. E. S. Group. 1998. A longitudinal study of body mass index and lens opacities: The Framingham studies. *Ophthalmology* 105(7):1244–1250.

Ho, V. H., and I. R. Schwab. 2001. Social economic development in the prevention of global blindness. *British Journal of Ophthalmology* 85(6):653–657.

Holmes, J. M., R. T. Kraker, R. W. Beck, E. E. Birch, S. A. Cotter, D. F. Everett, R. W. Hertle, G. E. Quinn, M. X. Repka, M. M. Scheiman, and D. K. Wallace. 2003. A randomized trial of prescribed patching regimens for treatment of severe amblyopia in children. *Ophthalmology* 110(11):2075–2087.

Hong, T., P. Mitchell, T. de Loryn, E. Rochtchina, S. Cugati, and J. J. Wang. 2009. Development and progression of diabetic retinopathy 12 months after phacoemulsification cataract surgery. *Ophthalmology* 116(8):1510–1514.

Hyman, L., and R. Neborsky. 2002. Risk factors for age-related macular degeneration: An update. *Current Opinion Ophthalmology* 13(3):171–175.

IOM (Institute of Medicine). 2003. *Unequal treatment: Confronting racial and ethnic disparities in health care.* Washington, DC: The National Academies Press.

Ip, J. M., S. C. Huynh, D. Robaei, K. A. Rose, I. G. Morgan, W. Smith, A. Kifley, and P. Mitchell. 2007. Ethnic differences in the impact of parental myopia: Findings from a population-based study of 12-year-old Australian children. *Investigative Ophthalmology & Visual Science* 48(6):2520–2528.

Ip, J. M., S. M. Saw, K. A. Rose, I. G. Morgan, A. Kifley, J. J. Wang, and P. Mitchell. 2008. Role of near work in myopia: Findings in a sample of Australian school children. *Investigative Ophthalmology & Visual Science* 49(7):2903–2910.

Javitt, J. C., A. M. McBean, G. A. Nicholson, J. D. Babish, J. L. Warren, and H. Krakauer. 1991. Undertreatment of glaucoma among Black Americans. *New England Journal of Medicine* 325(20):1418–1422.

Jee, D., W. K. Lee, and S. Kang. 2013. Prevalence and risk factors for diabetic retinopathy: The Korea National Health and Nutrition Examination Survey, 2008–2011. *Investigative Ophthalmology & Visual Science* 54(10):6827–6833.

Jones-Jordan, L. A., L. T. Sinnott, R. E. Manny, S. A. Cotter, R. N. Kleinstein, D. O. Mutti, J. D. Twelker, and K. Zadnik. 2010. Early childhood refractive error and parental history of myopia as predictors of myopia. *Investigative Ophthalmology & Visual Science* 51(1):115–121.

Jones-Jordan, L. A., G. L. Mitchell, S. A. Cotter, R. N. Kleinstein, R. E. Manny, D. O. Mutti, J. D. Twelker, J. R. Sims, and K. Zadnik. 2011. Visual activity before and after the onset of juvenile myopia. *Investigative Ophthalmology & Visual Science* 52(3):1841–1850.

Jones-Jordan, L. A., L. T. Sinnott, N. D. Graham, S. A. Cotter, R. N. Kleinstein, R. E. Manny, D. O. Mutti, J. D. Twelker, and K. Zadnik. 2014. The contributions of near work and outdoor activity to the correlation between siblings in the Collaborative Longitudinal Evaluation of Ethnicity and Refractive Error (CLEERE) study. *Investigative Ophthalmology & Visual Science* 55(10):6333–6339.

Kakigi, C. L., K. Singh, S. Y. Wang, W. T. Enanoria, and S. C. Lin. 2015. Self-reported calcium supplementation and age-related macular degeneration. *JAMA Ophthalmology* 133(7):746–754.

Kanthan, G. L., P. Mitchell, G. Burlutsky, and J. J. Wang. 2010. Alcohol consumption and the long-term incidence of cataract and cataract surgery: The Blue Mountains Eye Study. *American Journal of Ophthalmology* 150(3):434–440, e431.

Karadag, R., Z. Arslanyilmaz, B. Aydin, and I. F. Hepsen. 2012. Effects of body mass index on intraocular pressure and ocular pulse amplitude. *International Journal of Ophthalmology* 5(5):605.

Kaufman, H. E. 2011. Adenovirus advances: New diagnostic and therapeutic options. *Current Opinion Ophthalmology* 22(4):290–293.

Kemper, A. R. Harris, T. A. Lieu, C. J. Homer, and B. L. Whitener. 2004. *Screening for vision impairment in children younger than age 5 years: A systematic evidence review for the U.S. Preventive Services Task Force.* No. 27. Rockville, MD: Agency for Healthcare Research and Quality.

Kersey, J. P., and D. C. Broadway. 2006. Corticosteroid-induced glaucoma: A review of the literature. *Eye* 20:407–416.

Kim, E. C., K. Han, and D. Jee. 2014. Inverse relationship between high blood 25-hydroxyvitamin D and late stage of age-related macular degeneration in a representative Korean population. *Investigative Ophthalmology & Visual Science* 55(8):4823–4831.

Kim, T., A. P. Nunes, M. J. Mello, and P. B. Greenberg. 2011. Incidence of sport-related eye injuries in the United States: 2001–2009. *Graefes Archive for Clinical and Experimental Ophthalmology* 249:1743–1744.

Kirtland, K. A., J. B. Saaddine, L. S. Geiss, T. J. Thompson, M. F. Cotch, and P. P. Lee. 2015. Geographic disparity of severe vision loss—United States, 2009–2013. *Morbidity and Mortality Weekly Report* 64(19):513–517.

Klein, B. E. K., R. Klein, K. E. Lee, and K. J. Cruickshanks. 1998. Performance-based and self-assessed measures of visual function as related to history of falls, hip fractures, and measured gait time: The Beaver Dam Eye Study. *Ophthalmology* 105(1):160–164.

Klein, R., B. E. K. Klein, M. D. Knudtson, T. Y. Wong, M. F. Cotch, K. Liu, G. Burke, M. F. Saad, and D. R. Jacobs, Jr. 2006. Prevalence of age-related macular degeneration in 4 racial/ethnic groups in the multi-ethnic study of atherosclerosis. *Ophthalmology* 113(3):373–380.

Klein, R., M. D. Knudtson, K. E. Lee, R. Gangnon, and B. E. K. Klein. 2008. The Wisconsin epidemiologic study of diabetic retinopathy xxii. The twenty-five-year progression of retinopathy in persons with type 1 diabetes. *Ophthalmology* 115(11):1859–1868.

Kleinstein, R. N., L. A. Jones, S. Hullett, et al. 2003. Refractive error and ethnicity in children. *Archives of Ophthalmology* 121(8):1141–1147.

Ko, F., S. Vitale, C. F. Chou, M. F. Cotch, J. Saaddine, and D. S. Friedman. 2012. Prevalence of nonrefractive visual impairment in US adults and associated risk factors, 1999–2002 and 2005–2008. *JAMA* 308(22):2361–2368.

Kodjebacheva, G., E. R. Brown, L. Estrada, F. Yu, and A. L. Coleman. 2011. Uncorrected refractive error among first-grade students of different racial/ethnic groups in Southern California: Results a year after school-mandated vision screening. *Journal of Public Health Management Practice* 17(6):499–505.

Kodjebacheva, G., F. Yu, and A. L. Coleman. 2016. Vision conditions among first-graders of different racial/ethnic groups a year after vision screening by school nurses in Southern California. *Journal of Nursing Education and Practice* 6(2):27–34.

Kovarik, J. J., A. W. Eller, L. A. Willard, J. Ding, J. M. Johnston, and E. L. Waxman. 2016. Prevalence of undiagnosed diabetic retinopathy among inpatients with diabetes: The Diabetic Retinopathy Inpatient Study (DRIPS). *BMJ Open Diabetes Research & Care* 4(1).

Kulp, M. T., E. Ciner, M. Maguire, B. Moore, J. Pentimonti, M. Pistilli, L. Cyert, T. R. Candy, G. Quinn, and G. S. Ying. 2016. Uncorrected hyperopia and preschool early literacy: Results of the Vision in Preschoolers–Hyperopia in Preschoolers (VIP-HIP) study. *Ophthalmology* 123(4):681–689.

Kyrou, I., H. S. Randeva, and M. O. Weickert. 2000. Clinical problems caused by obesity. In *Endotext*, L. J. De Groot, P. Beck-Peccoz, G. Chrousos, K. Dungan, A. Grossman, J. M. Hershman, C. Koch, R. McLachlan, M. New, R. Rebar, F. Singer, A. Vinik and M. O. Weickert (eds.). South Dartmouth, MA: MDText.com, Inc.

La Torre, G., E. Pacella, R. Saulle, G. Giraldi, F. Pacella, T. Lenzi, O. Mastrangelo, F. Mirra, G. Aloe, P. Turchetti, C. Brillante, G. De Paolis, A. Boccia, and R. Giustolisi. 2013. The synergistic effect of exposure to alcohol, tobacco smoke and other risk factors for age-related macular degeneration. *European Journal of Epidemiology* 28(5):445–446.

Lanting, L. C., I. M. Joung, J. P. Mackenbach, S. W. Lamberts, A. H. Bootsma. 2005. Ethnic differences in mortality, end-stage complications, and quality of care among diabetic patients: A review. *Diabetes Care* 28(9):2280–2288.

Lavanya, R., R. Kawasaki, W. T. Tay, G. C. Cheung, P. Mitchell, S. M. Saw, T. Aung, and T. Y. Wong. 2010. Hyperopic refractive error and shorter axial length are associated with age-related macular degeneration: The Singapore Malay Eye Study. *Investigative Ophthalmology & Visual Science* 51(12):6247–6252.

Leske, M. C., S.-Y. Wu, A. Hennis, A. M. Connell, L. Hyman, A. Schachat, and B. E. S. Group. 1999. Diabetes, hypertension, and central obesity as cataract risk factors in a black population: The Barbados Eye Study. *Ophthalmology* 106(1):35–41.

Li, Y., S. Xirasagar, C. Pumkam, M. Krishnaswamy, and C. L. Bennett. 2013. Vision insurance, eye care visits, and vision impairment among working-age adults in the United States. *JAMA Ophthalmology* 131(4):499–506.

Lim, A., J. Stewart, T. Y. Chui, M. Lin, K. Ray, T. Lietman, T. Porco, L. Jung, S. Seiff, and S. Lin. 2008. Prevalence and risk factors of diabetic retinopathy in a multi-racial underserved population. *Ophthalmic Epidemiology* 15(6):402–409.

Lim, L. S., P. Mitchell, J. M. Seddon, F. G. Holz, and T. Y. Wong. 2012. Age-related macular degeneration. *Lancet* 379(9827):1728–1738.

Lindblad, B. E., N. Håkansson, H. Svensson, B. Philipson, and A. Wolk. 2005. Intensity of smoking and smoking cessation in relation to risk of cataract extraction: A prospective study of women. *American Journal of Epidemiology* 162(1):73–79.

Lindblad, B. E., N. Håkansson, and A. Wolk. 2014. Smoking cessation and the risk of cataract: A prospective cohort study of cataract extraction among men. *JAMA Ophthalmology* 132(3):253–257.

Linetsky, M., C. T. Raghavan, K. Johar, X. Fan, V. M. Monnier, A. R. Vasavada, and R. H. Nagaraj. 2014. UVA light-excited kynurenines oxidize ascorbate and modify lens proteins through the formation of advanced glycation end products: Implications for human lens aging and cataract formation. *Journal of Biological Chemistry* 289(24):17111–17123.

Lu, B., N. Congdon, X. Liu, K. Choi, D. S. Lam, M. Zhang, M. Zheng, Z. Zhou, L. Li, X. Liu, A. Sharma, and Y. Song. 2009. Associations between near work, outdoor activity, and myopia among adolescent students in rural China: The Xichang Pediatric Refractive Error Study report no. 2. *Archives of Ophthalmology* 127(6):769–775.

Lu, Y., L. Serpas, P. Genter, C. Mehranbod, D. Campa, and E. Ipp. 2016. Disparities in diabetic retinopathy screening rates within minority populations: Differences in reported screening rates among African American and Hispanic patients. *Diabetes Care* 39(3):e31–e32.

Luo, H., G. L. Beckles, X. Fang, J. E. Crews, J. B. Saaddine, and X. Zhang. 2012. Socioeconomic status and lifetime risk for workplace eye injury reported by a U.S. population aged 50 years and over. *Ophthalmic Epidemiology* 19(2):103–110.

Maconachie, G. D., I. Gottlob, and R. J. McLean. 2013. Risk factors and genetics in common comitant strabismus: A systematic review of the literature. *JAMA Ophthalmology* 131(9):1179–1186.

Magone, M. T., E. Kwon, and S. Y. Shin. 2014. Chronic visual dysfunction after blast-induced mild traumatic brain injury. *Journal of Rehabilitation Research & Development* 51(1):71–80.

Martinez-Thompson, J. M., N. N. Diehl, J. M. Holmes, and B. G. Mohney. 2014. Incidence, types, and lifetime risk of adult-onset strabismus. *Ophthalmology* 121(4): 877–882.

Master, C. L., M. Scheiman, M. Gallaway, A. Goodman, R. L. Robinson, S. R. Master, and M. F. Grady. 2016. Vision diagnoses are common after concussion in adolescents. *Clinical Pediatrics (Philadelphia)* 55(3):260–267.

McCarty, C. A., and H. R. Taylor. 2002. A review of the epidemiologic evidence linking ultraviolet radiation and cataracts. *Developments in Ophthalmology* 35:21–31.

McCarty, C. A., M. B. Nanjan, and H. R. Taylor. 2001. Vision impairment predicts 5 year mortality. *British Journal of Ophthalmology* 85(3):322–326.

McKean-Cowdin, R., S. A. Cotter, K. Tarczy-Hornoch, G. Wen, J. Kim, M. Borchert, R. Varma, and the Multi-Ethnic Pediatric Eye Disease Study Group. 2013. Prevalence of amblyopia or strabismus in Asian and non-Hispanic white preschool children: Multi-Ethnic Pediatric Eye Disease Study. *Ophthalmology* 120(10):2117–2124.

MEPEDS (Multi-Ethnic Pediatric Eye Disease Study) Group. 2008. Prevalence of amblyopia and strabismus in African American and Hispanic children ages 6 to 72 months: The Multi-Ethnic Pediatric Eye Disease Study. *Ophthalmology* 115(7):1229–1236, e1221.

———. 2009. Prevalence and causes of visual impairment in African-American and Hispanic preschool children: The Multi-Ethnic Pediatric Eye Disease Study. *Ophthalmology* 116(10):1990–2000, e1991.

———. 2010. Prevalence of myopia and hyperopia in 6 to 72 months old African American and Hispanic children: The Multi-Ethnic Pediatric Eye Disease Study. *Ophthalmology* 117(1):140.

Mimeault, M., and S. K. Batra. 2008. Recent progress on tissue-resident adult stem cell biology and their therapeutic implications. *Stem Cell Reviews* 4(1). DOI:10.1007/s 12015-12008-19008-12012.

———. 2012. Great promise of tissue-resident adult stem/progenitor cells in transplantation and cancer therapies. *Advances in Experimental Medicine and Biology* 741:171–186.

Mishra, A., and A. K. Verma. 2012. Sports related ocular injuries. *Medical Journal of Armed Forces India* 68(3):260–266.

Miyazawa-Hoshimoto, S., K. Takahashi, H. Bujo, N. Hashimoto, and Y. Saito. 2003. Elevated serum vascular endothelial growth factor is associated with visceral fat accumulation in human obese subjects. *Diabetologia* 46(11):1483–1488.

Mousavi, M., and R. A. Armstrong. 2013. Genetic risk factors and age-rated macular degeneration. *Journal of Optometry* 6(4):176–184.

Mukesh, B. N., A. Le, P. N. Dimitrov, S. Ahmed, H. R. Taylor, and C. A. McCarty. 2006. Development of cataract and associated risk factors: The Visual Impairment Project. *Archives of Ophthalmology* 124(1):79–85.

Muñoz, B., S. K. West, G. S. Rubin, et al. 2000. Causes of blindness and visual impairment in a population of older Americans: The Salisbury Eye Evaluation Study. *Archives of Ophthalmology* 118(6):819–825.

NEI/NIH (National Eye Institute/National Institutes of Health). 2009. Facts about cataract. https://nei.nih.gov/health/cataract/cataract_facts (accessed April 7, 2016).

———. 2010a. 2010 U.S. age-specific prevalence rates for hyperopia by age, and race/ethnicity. https://nei.nih.gov/eyedata/hyperopia (accessed April 7, 2016).

———. 2010b. 2010 U.S. age-specific prevalence rates for myopia by age, and race/ethnicity. https://nei.nih.gov/eyedata/myopia (accessed May 20, 2016).

———. 2010c. Age-related macular degeneration (AMD). https://nei.nih.gov/eyedata/amd (accessed May 20, 2016).

———. 2010d. Cataracts. https://nei.nih.gov/eyedata/cataract (accessed April 20, 2016).

———. 2010e. Diabetic retinopathy defined. https://nei.nih.gov/eyedata/diabetic (accessed May 20, 2016).

———. 2010f. Facts about refractive errors. https://www.nei.nih.gov/health/errors (accessed February 16, 2016).

———. 2010g. Facts about astigmatism. https://nei.nih.gov/health/errors/astigmatism (accessed August 10, 2016).

———. 2010h. Glaucoma, open-angle. https://nei.nih.gov/eyedata/glaucoma (accessed September 3, 2016).

———. 2010i. Open-angle glaucoma defined tables. https://nei.nih.gov/eyedata/glaucoma/tables (accessed May 20, 2016).

———. 2010j. Prevalence of adult vision impairment and age-related eye diseases in America. https://nei.nih.gov/eyedata/adultvision_usa (accessed February 17, 2016).

———. 2012a. Drawing of the eye. https://www.flickr.com/photos/nationaleyeinstitute/7544457228 (accessed May 20, 2016).

———. 2012b. Facts about diabetic eye disease. https://www.nei.nih.gov/health/diabetic/retinopathy (accessed May 20, 2016).

———. 2012c. Facts about diabetic retinopathy. https://www.nei.nih.gov/health/diabetic/retinopathy (accessed May 20, 2016).

———. 2012d. *Vision research needs, gaps, and opportunities.* Bethesda, MD: NIH. https://nei.nih.gov/sites/default/files/nei-pdfs/VisionResearch2012.pdf (accessed May 20, 2016).

———. 2013. Facts about age-related macular degeneration. https://www.nei.nih.gov/health/maculardegen/armd_facts (accessed May 20, 2016).

———. 2015. Facts about glaucoma. https://nei.nih.gov/health/glaucoma/glaucoma_facts (accessed October 7, 2015).

———. 2016a. About sports eye injury and protective eyewear. https://nei.nih.gov/sports (accessed May 20, 2016).

———. 2016b. NEI news. https://nei.nih.gov (accessed May 20, 2016).

Nittala, M. G., P. A. Keane, K. Zhang, and S. R. Sadda. 2014. Risk factors for proliferative diabetic retinopathy in a Latino American population. *Retina* 34(8):1594–1599.

Nsiah-Kumi, P., S. R. Ortmeier, and A. E. Brown. 2009. Disparities in diabetic retinopathy screening and disease for racial and ethnic minority populations—A literature review. *Journal of National Medical Association* 101(5):430–437.

Nussenblatt, R. B., R. W. Lee, E. Chew, B. Liu, H. N. Sen, A. D. Dick, F. L. Ferris. 2014. *American Journal of Ophthalmology* 158(1):5–11.

O'Brien, T. P., B. H. Jeng, M. McDonald, and M. B. Raizman. 2009. Acute conjunctivitis: Truth and misconceptions. *Current Medical Research Opinion* 25(8):1953–1961.

O'Donoghue, L., V. V. Kapetanankis, J. F. McClelland, N. S. Logan, C. G. Owen, K. J. Saunders, and A. R. Rudnicka. 2015. Risk factors for childhood myopia: Findings from the NICER study. *Investigative Ophthalmology & Visual Science* 56(3):1524–1530.

Oh, S. W., S. Lee, C. Park, and D. J. Kim. 2005. Elevated intraocular pressure is associated with insulin resistance and metabolic syndrome. *Diabetes/Metabolism Research and Reviews* 21(5):434–440.

Orlansky, G., J. Wilmer, M. B. Taub, D. Rutner, E. Ciner, and J. Gryczynski. 2015. Astigmatism and early academic readiness in preschool children. *Optometry and Vision Science* 92(3):279–285.

Osaadon, P., X. J. Fagan, T. Lifshitz, and J. Levy. 2014. A review of anti-VEGF agents for proliferative diabetic retinopathy. *Eye* 28(5):510–520.

Owens, P. L., and R. Mutter. 2011. Emergency department visits related to eye injuries, 2008. http://www.hcup-us.ahrq.gov/reports/statbriefs/sb112.pdf (accessed June 17, 2016).

Owsley, C. 2011. Aging and vision. *Vision Research* 51(13):1610–1622.

Pan, C.-W., and Y. Lin. 2014. Overweight, obesity, and age-related cataract: A meta-analysis. *Optometry and Vision Science* 91(5):478–483.

Pan, C.-W., D. Ramamurthy, and S. M. Saw. 2012. Worldwide prevalence and risk factors for myopia. *Ophthalmic and Physiological Optics* 32(1):3–16.

Pan, C.-W., M. K. Ikram, C. Y. Cheung, H. W. Choi, C. M. Cheung, J. B. Jonas, S. M. Saw, T. Y. Wong. 2013. Refractive errors and age-related macular degeneration: A systematic review and meta-analysis. *Ophthalmology* 120(10):2058–2065.

Park, D. H., J. P. Shin, and S. Y. Kim. 2010. Comparison of clinical outcomes between 23-gauge and 20-gauge vitrectomy in patients with proliferative diabetic retinopathy. *Retina* 30(10):1662–1670.

Park, S., and E.-H. Lee. 2015. Association between metabolic syndrome and age-related cataract. *International Journal of Ophthalmology* 8(4):804.

Parssinen, O., M. Kauppinen, and A. Viljanen. 2014. The progression of myopia from its onset at age 8–12 to adulthood and the influence of heredity and external factors on myopic progression: A 23-year follow-up study. *Acta Ophthalmologica* 92(8):730–739.

Pascual, M., J. Huang, M. G. Maguire, M. T. Kulp, G. E. Quinn, E. Ciner, L. A. Cyert, D. Orel-Bixler, B. Moore, and G. S. Ying. 2014. Risk factors for amblyopia in the vision in preschoolers study. *Ophthalmology* 121(3):622–629, e621.

PEDIG (Pediatric Eye Disease Investigator Group). 2003. The course of moderate amblyopia treated with patching in children: Experience of the Amblyopia Treatment Study. *American Journal of Ophthalmology* 136(4):620–629.

———. 2006. A randomized trial to evaluate two hours of daily patching for amblyopia in children. *Ophthalmology* 113(6):904–912.

———. 2012. Optical treatment of strabismic and combined strabismic-anisometropic amblyopia. *Ophthalmology* 119(1):150–158.

Petrash, J. M. 2013. Aging and age-related diseases of the ocular lens and vitreous body. *Investigative Ophthalmology & Visual Science* 54(14):ORSF54–ORSF59.

Pollreisz, A., and U. Schmidt-Erfurth. 2010. Diabetic cataract—Pathogenesis, epidemiology and treatment. *Journal of Ophthalmology* 2010:608751.

Prevent Blindness. 2012a. Vision impairment prevalence by age. http://www.visionproblemsus.org/vision-impairment/vision-impairment-by-age.html (accessed February 12, 2016).

———. 2012b. Vision problems in the U.S. http://www.visionproblemsus.org (accessed June 5, 2016).

———. 2012c. Vision problems in the U.S.: Blindness. http://visionproblemsus.org/cgi-bin/vpus.cgi (accessed July 5, 2016).

———. 2012d. Vision problems in the U.S.: Hyperopia. http://www.visionproblemsus.org/refractive-error/hyperopia.html (accessed February 16, 2016).

———. 2012e. Vision problems in the U.S.: Methods and sources. http://www.visionproblemsus.org/introduction/methods-and-sources.html (accessed July 5, 2016).

———. 2012f. Vision problems in the U.S.: Myopia. http://www.visionproblemsus.org/refractive-error/myopia.html (accessed February 16, 2016).

———. 2012g. Vision problems in the U.S.: Refractive error. http://www.visionproblemsus.org/refractive-error.html (accessed July 5, 2016).

———. 2012h. Vision problems in the U.S.: Vision impairment. http://visionproblemsus.org/cgi-bin/vpus.cgi (accessed July 5, 2016).

Qiu, M., S. Y. Wang, K. Singh, and S. C. Lin. 2014. Racial disparities in uncorrected and undercorrected refractive error in the United States. *Investigative Ophthalmology & Visual Science* 55(10):6996–7005.

Querques, G., P. J. Rosenfeld, E. Cavallero, E. Borrelli, F. Corvi, L. Querques, F. M. Bandello, and M. A. Zarbin. 2014. Treatment of dry age-related macular degeneration. *Ophthalmic Research* 52(3):107–115.

Ramdas, W. D., R. C. Wolfs, A. Hofman, P. T. de Jong, J. R. Vingerling, and N. M. Jansonius. 2011. Lifestyle and risk of developing open-angle glaucoma: The Rotterdam Study. *Archives of Ophthalmology* 129(6):767–772.

Ramsden, C. M., M. B. Powner, A.-J. F. Carr, M. J. K. Smart, L. da Cruz, and P. J. Coffey. 2013. Stem cells in retinal regeneration: Past, present and future. *Development (Cambridge, England)* 140(12):2576–2585.

Ramulu, P. Y., K. J. Corcoran, S. L. Corcoran, and A. L. Robin. 2007. Utilization of various glaucoma surgeries and procedures in Medicare beneficiaries from 1995 to 2004. *Ophthalmology* 114(12):2265–2270.

Rasmussen, H. M., and E. J. Johnson. 2013. Nutrients for the aging eye. *Clinical Interventions in Aging* 8:741.

Repka, M. X., F. Yu, F. Lum, and A. L. Coleman. 2013. Strabismus among aged Medicare beneficiaries: Impact of health status and region. *Journal of the American Association for Pediatric Ophthalmology and Strabismus* 17(4):391–394.

Repka, M. X., R. T. Kraker, J. M. Holmes, A. I. Summers, S. R. Glaser, C. N. Barnhardt, and D. R. Tien, and the Pediatric Eye Disease Investigator Group. 2014. Atropine vs patching for treatment of moderate amblyopia: Follow-up at 15 years of age of a randomized clinical trial. *JAMA Ophthalmology* 132(7):799–805.

Richter, G. M., and A. L. Coleman. 2016. Minimally invasive glaucoma surgery: Current status and future prospects. *Clinical Ophthalmology* 10:189–206.

Richter, G. M., J. Chung, S. P. Azen, R. Varma, and G. Los Angeles Latino Eye Study. 2009. Prevalence of visually significant cataract and factors associated with unmet need for cataract surgery: Los Angeles Latino Eye Study. *Ophthalmology* 116(12):2327–2335.

Rose, K. A., I. G. Morgan, W. Smith, G. Burlutsky, P. Mitchell, and S. M. Saw. 2008. Myopia, lifestyle, and schooling in students of Chinese ethnicity in Singapore and Sydney. *Archives of Ophthalmology* 126(4):527–530.

Rosner, M. S., D. L. Feinberg, J. E. Doble, and A. J. Rosner. 2016. Treatment of vertical heterophoria ameliorates persistent post-concussive symptoms: A retrospective analysis utilizing a multi-faceted assessment battery. *Brain Injury* 30(3):311–317.

Roy, M. S. 2000. Diabetic retinopathy in African Americans with type 1 diabetes: The New Jersey 725: II. Risk factors. *Archives of Ophthalmology* 118(1):105–119.

Roy, M. S., and M. Affouf. 2006. Six-year progression of retinopathy and associated risk factors in African American patients with type 1 diabetes mellitus: The New Jersey 725. *Archives of Ophthalmology* 124(9):1297–1306.

Royle, P., H. Mistry, P. Auguste, D. Shyangdan, K. Freeman, N. Lois, and N. Waugh. 2015. Pan-retinal photocoagulation and other forms of laser treatment and drug therapies for non-proliferative diabetic retinopathy: Systematic review and economic evaluation. *Health Technology Assessment* 19(51):v–xxviii, 1–247.

Rudnicka, A. R., S. Mt-Isa, C. G. Owen, D. G. Cook, and D. Ashby. 2006. *Investigative Ophthalmology & Visual Science* 47(10):4251–4261.

Sach, T. H., A. J. E. Foss, R. M. Gregson, A. Zaman, F. Osborn, T. Masud, and R. H. Harwood. 2009. Second-eye cataract surgery in elderly women: A cost-utility analysis conducted alongside a randomized controlled trial. *Eye* 24(2):276–283.

Salowe, R. J. Salina, N. H. Farbman, A. Mohammed, J. Z. Warren, A. Rhodes, A. Brucker, M. Regina, E. Miller, P. S. Sankar, A. Lehman, and J. N. O'Brien. 2015. Primary open-angle glaucoma in individuals of African descent: A review of risk factors. *Journal of Clinical & Experimental Ophthalmology* 6(4):1–13.

Salt, A., and J. Sargent. 2014. Common visual problems in children with disability. *Archives of Disease in Childhood* 99(12):1163–1168.

Salvi, S. M., S. Akhtar, and Z. Currie. 2006. Ageing changes in the eye. *Postgraduate Medical Journal* 82(971):581–587.

Sayin, N., N. Kara, and G. Pekel. 2015. Ocular complications of diabetes mellitus. *World Journal of Diabetes* 6(1):92–108.

Schaumberg, D. A., W. G. Christen, S. E. Hankinson, and R. J. Glynn. 2001. Body mass index and the incidence of visually significant age-related maculopathy in men. *Archives of Ophthalmology* 119(9):1259–1264.

Scheiman, M. M., R. W. Hertle, R. T. Kraker, R. W. Beck, E. E. Birch, J. Felius, J. M. Holmes, J. Kundart, D. G. Morrison, M. X. Repka, and S. M. Tamkins. 2008. Patching vs atropine to treat amblyopia in children aged 7 to 12 years: A randomized trial. *Archives of Ophthalmology* 126(12):1634–1642.

Schmidl, D., G. Garhöfer, and L. Schmetterer. 2015. Nutritional supplements in age-related macular degeneration. *Acta Ophthalmologica* 93(2):105–121.

Seddon, J. M., R. E. Silver, M. Kwong, and B. Rosner. 2015. Risk prediction for progression of macular degeneration: 10 common and rare genetic variants, demographic, environmental, and macular covariates. *Investigative Ophthalmology & Visual Science* 56(4):2192–2202.

Shah, J., and S. Patel. 2015. Strabismus: Symptoms, pathophysiology, management, and precautions. *International Journal of Science and Research* 4(7):1510–1514.

Shahbazi, S., J. Studnicki, and C. W. Warner-Hillard. 2015. A cross-sectional retrospective analysis of the racial and geographic variations in cataract surgery. *PLoS ONE* 10(11):e0142459.

Sharma, A., and H. B. Hindman. 2014. Aging: A predisposition to dry eyes. *Journal of Ophthalmology* Article ID 781683:1–8.

Shi, Q., Y. Zhao, V. Fonseca, M. Krousel-Wood, and L. Shi. 2014. Racial disparity of eye examinations among the U.S. working-age population with diabetes: 2002–2009. *Diabetes Care* 37(5):1321–1328.

Shields, T., and P. D. Sloane. 1990. A comparison of eye problems in primary care and ophthalmology practices. *Family Medicine* 23(7):544–546.

Shim, S. H., S. G. Kim, J. H. Bae, H. G. Yu and S. J. Song. 2016. Risk factors for progression of early age-related macular degeneration in Koreans. *Ophthalmic Epidemiology* 23(2):80–87.

Shweikh, Y., F. Ko, M. P. Y. Chan, P. J. Patel, Z. Muthy, P. T. Khaw, J. Yip, N. Strouthidis, and P. J. Foster. 2015. Measures of socioeconomic status and self-reported glaucoma in the UK Biobank Cohort. *Eye* 29(10):1360–1367.

Sloan, F. A., A. P. Yashkin, Y. Chen. 2014. Gaps in receipt of regular eye examinations among medicare beneficiaries diagnosed with diabetes or chronic eye diseases. *Ophthalmology* 121(12):2452–2460.

Smith, A. F., and C. Waycaster. 2009. Estimate of the direct and indirect annual cost of bacterial conjunctivitis in the United States. *BMC Ophthalmology* 9(1):1.

Solerte, S., M. Fioravanti, N. Pezza, M. Locatelli, N. Schifino, N. Cerutti, S. Severgnini, M. Rondanelli, and E. Ferrari. 1997. Hyperviscosity and microproteinuria in central obesity: Relevance to cardiovascular risk. *International Journal of Obesity and Related Metabolic Disorders* 21(6):417–423.

Solomon, S. D., K. Lindsley, S. S. Vedula, M. G. Krzystolik, and B. S. Hawkins. 2014. Antivascular endothelial growth factor for neovascular age-related macular degeneration. *Cochrane Database of Systematic Reviews* 8:CD005139.

Sommer, A., J. M. Tielsch, J. Katz, H. A. Quigley, J. D. Gottsch, J. C. Javitt, J. F. Martone, R. M. Royall, K. A. Witt, and S. Ezrine. 1991. Racial differences in the cause-specific prevalence of blindness in East Baltimore. *New England Journal of Medicine* 325(20):1412–1417.

Spanakis, E. K., and S. H. Golden. 2013. Race/ethnic difference in diabetes and diabetes complications. *Current Diabetes Reports* 13(6):1–18.

Stegmann, B. J., and J. C. Carey. 2002. TORCH infections. Toxoplasmosis, other (syphilis, varicella-zoster, parvovirus B19), rubella, cytomegalovirus (CMV), and herpes infections. *Current Women's Health Report* 2(4):253–258.

Stein, J. D., D. S. Grossman, K. M. Mundy, A. Sugar, and F. A. Sloan. 2011a. Severe adverse events after cataract surgery among Medicare beneficiaries. *Ophthalmology* 118(9):1716–1723.

Stelmack, J. A., T. Frith, D. Van Koevering, S. Rinne, and T. R. Stelmack. 2009. Visual function in patients followed at a Veterans Affairs polytrauma network site: An electronic medical record review. *Optometry* 80(8):419–424.

Stratton, I., E. Kohner, S. Aldington, R. Turner, R. Holman, S. Manley, and D. Matthews. 2001. UKPDS 50: Risk factors for incidence and progression of retinopathy in type II diabetes over 6 years from diagnosis. *Diabetologia* 44(2):156–163.

Tan, H. S., M. Mura, S. Y. Lesnik Oberstein, and H. M. Bijl. 2011. Safety of vitrectomy for floaters. *American Journal of Ophthalmology* 151(6):995–998.

Tan, J. S., J. J. Wang, C. Younan, R. G. Cumming, E. Rochtchina, and P. Mitchell. 2008. Smoking and the long-term incidence of cataract: The Blue Mountains Eye Study. *Ophthalmic Epidemiology* 15(3):155–161.

Tandon, A., and A. Mulvihill. 2009. Ocular teratogens: Old acquaintances and new dangers. *Science* 23:1269–1274.

Tapp, R. J., J. E. Shaw, C. A. Harper, M. P. de Courten, B. Balkau, D. J. McCarty, H. R. Taylor, T. A. Welborn, and P. Z. Zimmet. 2003. The prevalence of and factors associated with diabetic retinopathy in the Australian population. *Diabetes Care* 26(6):1731–1737.

Tarczy-Hornoch, K., Y. Wang, S. Cotter, M. Borchert, S. Azen, R. Varma, and MEPEDS Group. 2007. ATS HOTV visual acuity test results in African-American and Hispanic children: The Multi-Ethnic Pediatric Eye Disease Study. *Investigative Ophthalmology & Visual Science* 48(13):4827–4827.

Tarczy-Hornoch, K., R. Varma, S. A. Cotter, R. McKean-Cowdin, J. H. Lin, M. S. Borchert, M. Torres, G. Wen, S. P. Azen, J. M. Tielsch, D. S. Friedman, M. X. Repka, J. Katz, L. Giordano, and J. Ibironke. 2010. Risk factors for astigmatism in preschool children: The Multi-Ethnic Pediatric Eye Disease and Baltimore Pediatric Eye Disease Studies. *Ophthalmology* 118(10):1974–1981.

Tarczy-Hornoch, K., S. A. Cotter, M. Borchert, R. McKean-Cowdin, J. Lin, G. Wen, J. Kim, and R. Varma. 2013. Prevalence and causes of visual impairment in Asian and non-Hispanic white preschool children: Multi-Ethnic Pediatric Eye Disease study. *Ophthalmology* 120(6):1220–1226.

Taubenslag, K. J., and J. A. Kammer. 2016. Outcomes disparities between black and white populations in the surgical management of glaucoma. *Seminars in Ophthalmology* 31(4):385–393,

Thompson, J. R., J. M. Gibson, and C. Jagger. 1989. The association between visual impairment and mortality in elderly people. *Age and Ageing* 18(2):83–88.

Tielsch, J. M., A. Sommer, J. Katz, H. Quigley, and S. Ezrine. 1991. Socioeconomic status and visual impairment among urban Americans: Baltimore Eye Survey Research Group. *Archives of Ophthalmology* 109(5):637–641.

Torp-Pedersen, T., H. A. Boyd, G. Poulsen, B. Haargaard, J. Wohlfahrt, J. M. Holmes, and M. Melbye. 2010. In-utero exposure to smoking, alcohol, coffee, and tea and risk of strabismus. *American Journal of Epidemiology* 171(8):868–875.

Tseng, V. L., F. Yu, F. Lum, and A. L. Coleman. 2016. Cataract surgery and mortality in the United States Medicare population. *Ophthalmology* 123(5):1019–1026.

U.S. Census Bureau. 2015. New Census Bureau report analyzes U.S. population projections. http://www.census.gov/newsroom/press-releases/2015/cb15-tps16.html (accessed August 1, 2016).

USPSTF (U.S. Preventive Services Task Force). 2011. Evidence summary: Other supporting document for visual impairment in children ages 1–5: Screening. http://www.uspreventiveservicestaskforce.org/Page/Document/evidence-summary5/visual-impairment-in-children-ages-1-5-screening (accessed August 28, 2016).

Valentine, G., L. Marquez, and M. Pammi. 2016. Zika virus-associated microencephaly and eye lesions in the newborn. *Journal of the Pediatric Infectious Disease Society* 5(3):323–328.

Varma, R., S. Fraser-Bell, S. Tan, R. Klein, and S. P. Azen. 2004a. Prevalence of age-related macular degeneration in Latinos: The Los Angeles Latino Eye Study. *Ophthalmology* 111(7):1288–1297.

Varma, R., M. Ying-Lai, R. Klein, and S. P. Azen. 2004b. Prevalence and risk indicators of visual impairment and blindness in Latinos: The Los Angeles Latino Eye Study. *Ophthalmology* 111(6):1132–1140.

Varma, R., M. Ying-Lai, B. A. Francis, B. B.-T. Nguyen, J. Deneen, M. R. Wilson, and S. P. Azen. 2004c. Prevalence of open-angle glaucoma and ocular hypertension in Latinos. *Ophthalmology* 111(8):1439–1448.

Varma, R., G. L. Macias, M. Torres, R. Klein, F. Y. Pena, S. P. Azen, Los Angeles Latino Eye Study Group. 2007. Biologic risk factors associated with diabetic retinopathy: The Los Angeles Latino Eye Study. *Ophthalmology* 114(7):1332–1340.

Varma, R., P. P. Lee, I. Goldberg, and S. Kotak. 2011. An assessment of the health and economic burdens of glaucoma. *American Journal of Ophthalmology* 152(4):515–522.

Varma, R., T. S. Vajaranant, B. Burkemper, S. Wu, M. Torres, C. Hsu, F. Choudhury, and R. McKean-Cowdin. 2016. Visual impairment and blindness in adults in the United States: Demographic and geographic variations from 2015 to 2050. *JAMA Ophthalmology.*

Vitale, S., L. Ellwein, M. F. Cotch, F. L. Ferris, and R. Sperduto. 2008. Prevalence of refractive error in the United States, 1999–2004. *Archives of Ophthalmology* 126(8):1111–1119.

Vohr, B. R., L. L. Wright, A. M. Dusick, L. Mele, J. Verter, J. J. Steichen, N. P. Simon, D. C. Wilson, S. Broyles, C. R. Bauer, V. Delaney-Black, K. A. Yolton, B. E. Fleisher, L.-A. Papile, and M. D. Kaplan. 2000. Neurodevelopmental and functional outcomes of extremely low birth weight infants in the National Institute of Child Health and Human Development neonatal research network, 1993–1994. *Pediatrics* 105(6):1216–1226.

von Noorden G. K., and E. C. Campos. 2002. *Binocular vision and ocular motility: Theory and management of strabismus.* 6. St. Louis, MO: Mosby. P. 548.

Wadwa, S. D., and E. J. Higginbotham. 2005. Ethnic differences in glaucoma: Prevalence, management, and outcome. *Current Opinion Ophthalmology* 16(2):1010–1016.

Walline, J. J., K. Lindsley, S. S. Vedula, S. A. Cotter, D. O. Mutti, and J. D. Twelker. 2011. Interventions to slow progression of myopia in children. *Cochrane Database of Systematic Reviews* (12):Cd004916.

Wang, D., Y. Huang, C. Huang, P. Wu, J. Lin, Y. Zheng, Y. Peng, Y. Liang, J.-H. Chen, and M. Zhang. 2012. Association analysis of cigarette smoking with onset of primary open-angle glaucoma and glaucoma-related biometric parameters. *BMC Ophthalmology* 12(1):59.

Watkinson, S., and R. Seewoodhary. 2008. Ocular complications associated with diabetes mellitus. *Nursing Standard* 22(27):51–57.

Weinreb, R. N., T. Aung, and F. A. Medeiros. 2014. The pathophysiology and treatment of glaucoma: A review. *JAMA* 311(18):1901–1911.

Wen, G., K. Tarczy-Hornoch, R. McKean-Cowdin, S. A. Cotter, M. Borchert, J. Lin, J. Kim, R. Varma, and the Multi-Ethnic Pediatric Eye Disease Study Group. 2013. Prevalence of myopia, hyperopia, and astigmatism in non-Hispanic white and Asian children. *Ophthalmology* 120(10):2109–2116.

West, S. K., B. Munoz, G. S. Rubin, O. D. Schein, K. Bandeen-Roche, S. Zeger, S. German, and L. P. Fried. 1997. Function and visual impairment in a population-based study of older adults: The SEE project. *Investigative Ophthalmology & Visual Science* 38(1):72–82.

Williams, P. T. 2009. Prospective epidemiological cohort study of reduced risk for incident cataract with vigorous physical activity and cardiorespiratory fitness during a 7-year follow-up. *Investigative Ophthalmology & Visual Science* 50(1):95–100.

Wittenborn, J., and D. Rein. 2016 (unpublished). *The potential costs and benefits of treatment for undiagnosed eye disorders.* Paper prepared for the Committee on Public Health Approaches to Reduce Vision Impairment and Promote Eye Health. http://www.national academies.org/hmd/~/media/Files/Report%20Files/2016/UndiagnosedEyeDisorders CommissionedPaper.pdf (accessed September 15, 2016).

Wittenborn, J. S., X. Zhang, C. W. Feagan, W. L. Crouse, S. Shrestha, A. R. Kemper, T. J. Hoerger, and J. B. Saaddine. 2013. The economic burden of vision loss and eye disorders among the United States population younger than 40 years. *Ophthalmology* 120(9):1728–1735.

Wolfs, R. C., C. C. Klaver, R. S. Ramrattan, C. M. van Duijn, A. Hofman, and P. T. de Jong. 1998. Genetic risk of primary open-angle glaucoma: Population-based familial aggregation study. *Archives of Ophthalmology* 116(12):1640–1645.

Wong, T. Y., N. Cheung, W. T. Tay, J. J. Wang, T. Aung, S. M. Saw, S. C. Lim, E. S. Tai, and P. Mitchel. 2008. Prevalence and risk factors for diabetic retinopathy: The Singapore Malay Eye Study. *Ophthalmology* 115(11):1869–1875.

Worley, A., and K. Grimmer-Somers. 2011. Risk factors for glaucoma: What do they really mean? *Australian Journal of Primary Health* 17(3):233–239.

Wormald, R., J. Evans, L. Smeeth, and K. Henshaw. 2007. Photodynamic therapy for neovascular age-related macular degeneration. *Cochrane Database of Systematic Reviews* (3):CD002030.

Wu, E. W., D. A. Schaumberg, and S. K. Park. 2014. Environmental cadmium and lead exposures and age-related macular degeneration in U.S. adults: The National Health and Nutrition Examination Survey, 2005 to 2008. *Environmental Research* 133:178–184.

Wu, W., and R. G. Ariyasu. 1999. Cornea and external disease. In *Clinical guide to comprehensive ophthalmology*, edited by D. A. Lee and E. J. Higginbotham. New York: Thieme Medical Publishers. Pp. 183–264.

Xiang, H., L. Stallones, G. Chen, and G. A. Smith. 2005. Work-related eye injuries treated in hospital emergency departments in the U.S. *American Journal of Industrial Medicine* 48(1):57–62.

Yau, J. W., S. L. Rogers, R. Kawasaki, E. L. Lamoureux, J. W. Kowalski, T. Bek, S. J. Chen, J. M. Dekker, A. Fletcher, J. Grauslund, S. Haffner, R. F. Hamman, M. K. Ikram, T. Kayama, B. E. Klein, R. Klein, S. Krishnaiah, K. Mayurasakorn, J. P. O'Hare, T. J. Orchard, M. Porta, M. Rema, M. S. Roy, T. Sharma, J. Shaw, H. Taylor, J. M. Tielsch, R. Varma, J. J. Wang, N. Wang, S. West, L. Xu, M. Yasuda, X. Zhang, P. Mitchell, and T. Y. Wong. 2012. Global prevalence and major risk factors of diabetic retinopathy. *Diabetes Care* 35(3):556–564.

Ye, J., J. He, C. Wang, H. Wu, X. Shi, H. Zhang, J. Xie, and S. Y. Lee. 2012. Smoking and risk of age-related cataract: A meta-analysis. *Investigative Ophthalmology & Visual Science* 53(7):3885–3895.

Yip, J. L., R. Luben, S. Hayat, A. P. Khawaja, D. C. Broadway, N. Wareham, K. T. Khaw, and P. J. Foster. 2014. Area deprivation, individual socioeconomic status and low vision in the EPIC-Norfolk Eye Study. *Journal of Epidemiology & Community Health* 68(3):204–210.

Yoshida, M., M. Ishikawa, K. Karita, A. Kokaze, M. Harada, S. Take, and H. Ohno. 2014. Association of blood pressure and body mass index with intraocular pressure in middle-aged and older Japanese residents: A cross-sectional and longitudinal study. *Acta Medica Okayama* 68(1):27–34.

Yu, C-H. 2015. Origins of adolescent obesity and hypertension. *Pediatrics and Neonatology* 56(5):285–286.

Yu, X., D. Lyu, X. Dong, J. He, and K. Yao. 2014. Hypertension and risk of cataract: A meta-analysis. *PLoS ONE* 9(12):e114012.

Zadnik, K. 1997. Myopia development in childhood. *Optometry and Vision Science* 74(8):603–608.

Zadnik, K., W. A. Satariano, D. O. Mutti, R. I. Sholtz, and A. J. Adams. 1994. The effect of parental history of myopia on children's eye size. *JAMA* 271(17):1323–1327.

Zadnik, K., L. T. Sinnott, S. A. Cotter, L. A. Jones-Jordan, R. N. Kleinstein, R. E. Manny, J. D. Twelker, D. O. Mutti, Collaborative Longitudinal Evaluation of Ethnicity and Refractive Error (SLEERE Study Group). 2015. Prediction of juvenile-onset myopia. *JAMA Ophthalmology* 133(6):683–689.

Zambelli-Weiner, A., J. E. Crews, and D. S. Friedman. 2012. Disparities in adult vision health in the United States. *American Journal of Ophthalmology* 154(6 Suppl):S23–S30, e21.

Zebardast, N., B. K. Swenor, S. W. van Landingham, R. W. Massof, B. Munoz, S. K. West, and P. Y. Ramulu. 2015. Comparing the impact of refractive and nonrefractive vision loss on functioning and disability: The Salisbury Eye Evaluation. *Ophthalmology* 122(6):1102–1110.

Zetterberg, M. 2016. Age-related eye disease and gender. *Maturitas* 83:19–26.

Zhang, X., J. B. Saaddine, C. Chou, et al. 2010. Prevalence of diabetic retinopathy in the United States, 2005–2008. *JAMA* 304(6):649–656.

———. 2012. Vision health disparities in the United States by race/ethnicity, education, and economic status: Findings from two nationally representative surveys. *American Journal of Ophthalmology* 154(6 Suppl):S53–S62, e51.

Zhao, D., J. Cho, M. H. Kim, D. S. Friedman, and E. Guallar. 2015. Diabetes, fasting glucose, and the risk of glaucoma: A meta-analysis. *Ophthalmology* 122(1):72–78.

Zheng Selin, J., N. Orsini, B. Ejdervik Lindblad, and A. Wolk. 2015. Long-term physical activity and risk of age-related cataract: A population-based prospective study of male and female cohorts. *Ophthalmology* 122(2):274–280.

3

The Impact of Vision Loss

Vision loss has a significant impact on the lives of those who experience it as well as on their families, their friends, and society. The complete loss or the deterioration of existing eyesight can feel frightening and overwhelming, leaving those affected to wonder about their ability to maintain their independence, pay for needed medical care, retain employment, and provide for themselves and their families. The health consequences associated with vision loss extend well beyond the eye and visual system. Vision loss can affect one's quality of life (QOL), independence, and mobility and has been linked to falls, injury, and worsened status in domains spanning mental health, cognition, social function, employment, and educational attainment. Although confounding factors likely contribute to some of the harms that have been associated with vision impairment, testimony from visually impaired persons speaks to the significant role that vision plays in health, vocation, and social well-being.

The economic impact of vision loss is also substantial. One national study commissioned by Prevent Blindness found that direct medical expenses, other direct expenses, loss of productivity, and other indirect costs for visual disorders across all age groups were approximately $139 billion in 2013 dollars (Wittenborn and Rein, 2013), with direct costs for the under-40 population reaching $14.5 billion dollars (Wittenborn et al., 2013). These costs affect not only national health care expenditures, but also related expenses and the resources of individuals and their families. For example, Köberlein and colleagues (2013) found that the time spent by caregivers increases substantially as vision decreases.

This chapter explores the impact of chronic vision loss in the United States—both in terms of its financial costs and its effects on QOL. The first two sections of the chapter details the consequences of vision impairment and the relationship between chronic vision impairment and other chronic conditions. The third section of this chapter provides an overview of the economic impact of vision loss on individuals, insurers, and society, including estimates of direct and indirect costs, and life years lost. The final section discusses the state of cost-effectiveness research for clinical eye and vision care.

CONSEQUENCES OF VISION IMPAIRMENT

Quality of Life

Vision impairment is associated with a reduced QOL, which is a "complex trait that encompasses *vision functioning*, symptoms, emotional well-being, social relationships, concerns, and convenience as they are affected by vision" (Lamoureux and Pesudovs, 2011, p. 195). Numerous studies have shown that vision impairment is often associated with various negative health outcomes and poor QOL (Chia et al., 2006; Langelaan et al., 2007). A recent study using Behavioral Risk Factor Surveillance System (BRFSS) data from 22 states examined unadjusted health-related QOL among individuals ages 40 to 64 years by visual impairment status and found that the percentage of individuals reporting life dissatisfaction, fair or poor reported health, physical and mental unhealthy days, and days of limited activity increased as the self-reported severity of vision impairment increased (Crews et al., 2016b) (see Table 3-1). An earlier study found similar results among people ages 65 and older (Crews et al., 2014). Based on a variety of measurement instruments, reduced QOL has been related to the severity of disease in glaucoma, cataract, age-related macular degeneration, and strabismus (Chai et al., 2009; Chatziralli et al., 2012; Cheng et al., 2015; Freedman et al., 2014; Hassell et al., 2006; Orta et al., 2015). Although greater emphasis is traditionally placed on the better-seeing eye's role in visual function, one study concluded that the worse-seeing eye contributes importantly to patients' estimates of vision-related QOL, particularly when the underlying eye disease affects peripheral vision (e.g., in the case of glaucoma) (Hirneiss, 2014).

A study by Rein and colleagues (2007) found that the QOL begins to slowly decline with the onset of vision loss, and then decreases more precipitously as measures of visual field defects increase. A systematic literature review of studies that reported QOL in patients with central vision loss or peripheral vision loss, and found that both types of vision loss were associated with similar degrees of detriment to QOL, although "different

TABLE 3-1 Unadjusted Health-Related Quality of Life Among Those Ages 40 to 60 by Visual Impairment Status in 22 States,[a] 2006 to 2010, United States

Health-Related Quality of Life Measure	n	Total % (95% CI)	No Difficulty Seeing % (95% CI)	Little Difficulty Seeing % (95% CI)	Moderate/Severe Difficulty Seeing % (95% CI)
Life dissatisfaction (yes)	6,915	5.8 (5.6–6.1)	3.7 (3.5–4.0)	6.0 (5.6–6.5)	13.3 (12.3–14.3)
Disability (yes)	27,991	24.8 (24.3–25.4)	19.3 (18.6–19.9)	27.4 (26.2–28.5)	41.2 (39.7–42.8)
Self-reported health (fair/poor)	19,182	17.1 (16.6–17.6)	12.4 (11.8–13.0)	17.8 (16.9–18.7)	33.0 (31.4–34.5)
14 to 30 physical unhealthy days	14,196	12.4 (12.0–12.8)	9.2 (8.7–9.7)	12.7 (12.0–13.5)	23.7 (22.4–25.1)
14 to 30 mental unhealthy days	12,386	11.0 (10.6–11.4)	7.7 (7.3–8.2)	11.7 (11.0–12.4)	21.7 (20.4–23.1)
14 to 30 activity limitation days	9,571	8.2 (7.9–8.6)	5.5 (5.2–5.9)	8.5 (7.9–9.1)	17.8 (16.6–19.1)

NOTES: [a] The 22 states using the BRFSS vision module at least once in the years 2006–2010 were Alabama, Arizona, Arkansas, Colorado, Connecticut, Florida, Georgia, Indiana, Iowa, Kansas, Maryland, Massachusetts, Missouri, Nebraska, New Mexico, New York, North Carolina, Ohio, Tennessee, Texas, West Virginia, and Wyoming.
CI = confidence interval.
SOURCE: Crews et al., 2016b.

domains were affected" which "might be a function of the pathology of diseases" (Evans et al., 2009, p. 433). A recent Korean study, using the EQ-5D instrument[1] examined QOL scores based on whether participants were visually impaired[2] and whether they had 1 of 14 chronic conditions. The authors found that QOL scores in persons with each of the 14 chronic conditions, excepting coronary artery disease, were lower among individuals with that condition alone than individuals who also had any co-existing

---

[1] The EQ-5D is a generic instrument used to measure health-related QOL. The tool rates the impact of disease on a scale of 0 to 1 with a lower score indicating greater effect of the health condition. The EQ-5D has five dimensions—mobility, self-care, usual activities, pain or discomfort, and anxiety or depression.

[2] The authors defined "mild visual impairment" as visual acuity between 20/32 and 20/63; "moderate visual impairment" as visual acuity between 20/80 and 20/60; and "severe visual impairment" as visual acuity worse than or equal to 20/200.

vision impairment (Park et al., 2015). The impact of vision impairment on people with chronic conditions is explored further later in this chapter.

Two studies indicated that the QOL impact of vision loss may be perceived differently by health care providers than by the patients themselves. One study administered time-trade-off utilities to Canadian medical students and patients for different levels of vision loss (anchors were death = 0 and perfect vision = 1.0); the study found that medical students tended to underestimate the impact of vision loss (Chaudry et al., 2015). In a similar study in China, utility values for mild glaucoma and severe glaucoma were obtained from glaucoma patients and ophthalmologists; the ophthalmologists' utility ratings for mild glaucoma were significantly higher than the patients', suggesting that physicians may underestimate the impact of mild glaucoma on QOL (Zhang et al., 2015).

Dependence

Loss of vision affects patients' ability to work or care for themselves (or others), and it affects numerous casual activities such as reading, socializing, and pursuing hobbies (Brown et al., 2014). Vision impairment makes it more difficult to perform the basic self-care activities of daily living such as eating and dressing as well as instrumental activities of daily living such as shopping, financial management, medication management, and driving (Brown et al., 2014; Haymes et al., 2002; Whitson et al., 2007, 2014). Most studies have found that vision loss has a greater impact on dependency in instrumental activities of daily living than in basic activities of daily living. The instrumental activities of daily living are critical to one's ability to function in modern society. In particular, the loss of near vision affects one's ability to perform a variety of tasks that involve reading (e.g., getting information from medication labels, balancing bank statements, or following recipes), recognizing faces and images (e.g., socializing, playing cards, using a smartphone), or manipulating small objects (e.g., sewing, replacing batteries). One cross-sectional study found that individuals with visual impairment, defined as a best-corrected binocular presenting visual acuity of 20/30 or worse, had greater disability across functional measures, such as task performance, walking speeds, and driving when compared to people with normal vision and even uncorrected refractive error[3] (Zebardast et al., 2015). Visual field deficits affect one's ability to perform tasks that require ambulation in challenging settings (e.g., moving along crowded city streets, negotiating stairwells) or the use of peripheral vision (e.g., driving).

---

[3] Uncorrected refractive error was defined as a binocular visual acuity of less than or equal to 20/30 that improved to greater than 20/30 with subjective refraction.

Due to the challenges that vision impairment imposes for independent living, older adults with vision impairment may be more likely to require long-term care. In the Australian Blue Mountains Eye Study, with each line of reduction in presenting visual acuity at baseline, there was a 7 percent increased risk of subsequent nursing home placement (Wang et al., 2003). For participants in the Beaver Dam Eye Study, the odds ratio for nursing home placement was 4.23 (95% confidence interval [CI] = 2.34, 7.64) for low best-corrected visual acuity in the better eye, 5.00 (95% CI = 2.28, 10.94) for poor near vision, and 2.40 (95% CI = 1.46, 3.92) for poor contrast sensitivity, after adjustment for age, sex, self-rated health, and arthritis (Klein et al., 2003).

For persons with vision loss who desire to be a part of the workforce, vision impairment often poses barriers to employment opportunities (O'Day, 1999). Unfortunately, employment statistics pertaining to Americans with vision loss are lacking because available nationally representative data sources, such as the U.S. Census, group persons with vision impairment with all people who have sensory impairments or with people with sensory or communication impairments (U.S. Census Bureau, 2014).

Mobility and Falls

In a person with intact eyesight, the primary sense used to navigate three-dimensional space is vision. Mobility is therefore greatly affected by vision loss, whether resulting from changes in visual acuity, visual fields, depth perception, or contrast sensitivity (Bibby et al., 2007; Lord and Dayhew, 2001; Marron and Bailey, 1982). In the Salisbury Eye Evaluation (SEE) project, vision impairment (defined by visual acuity or visual field deficit) was significantly associated with self-reported difficulty with walking or going up or down steps (Swenor et al., 2013). Also in the SEE project, visual field deficits—but not visual acuity or contrast sensitivity deficits—were predictive of a slower-than-usual gait speed while navigating an obstacle course (Patel et al., 2006). A study from the United Kingdom found that 46 percent of frail elderly individuals admitted for hip fracture in two hospital districts had visual impairment, most frequently untreated cataract (49 percent) and macular degeneration (21 percent), but also uncorrected refractive error (17 percent); the visually impaired hip fracture patients were less likely than those without vision impairment to be under an eye provider's care and more likely to live in areas of social deprivation (Cox et al., 2005). In the Low Vision Rehabilitation Outcomes Study, 16.3 percent of participants referred to vision rehabilitation at 28 U.S. centers indicated that one of their chief vision-related problems was mobility (Brown et al., 2014).

Multiple peer-reviewed studies have documented a relationship between vision impairment and falls (Crews et al., 2016a; Lord, 2006). A 2016 study by Crews and colleagues that used 2014 BRFSS data to analyze the state-specific annual prevalence of falls among persons aged 65 years or older found that 46.7 percent of persons with severe vision impairment (state prevalence range 30.8–59.1 percent) and 27.7 percent of older adults without such impairment (state prevalence range 20.4–32.4 percent) reported having fallen during the previous year (Crews et al., 2016a). The visual parameters that have been strongly and consistently associated with falls include poor contrast sensitivity, reduced depth perception, and visual field loss (de Boer et al., 2004; Ivers et al., 1998; Klein et al., 2003; Lord and Dayhew, 2001; Lord et al., 1991, 1994; Nevitt et al., 1989). A review of studies that reported the univariate relationship between visual deficits (defined variously) and falls found that the relative risk ratios across studies was 2.5 (CI = 1.6, 3.5) (Rubenstein and Josephson, 2002).

Evidence is limited or conflicting on the need for vision assessment and specific interventions to reduce falls among visually impaired populations. The U.S. Preventive Services Task Force determined that vision correction was among several potential interventions that "lack[ed] sufficient evidence for or against use in prevention of falls in community-dwelling older adults" (Moyer, 2012, p. 200; see also, Schneider et al., 2012). Unfortunately, the visual deficits most strongly linked to fall risk (contrast sensitivity, depth perception, and visual field deficits) are generally less amenable to remediation than visual acuity. Other factors such as weakness, other chronic conditions, and the use of medications are also associated with falls, suggesting that successful interventions to reduce falls in visually impaired populations will require a multi-pronged approach (Steinman et al., 2011). Evidence is needed to determine which training aspects, equipment, and environmental modifications are most effective at reducing falls and improving mobility. However, it is the committee's assessment that there remains a role for vision rehabilitation in mitigating fall risk associated with vision loss.

Fractures

Vision impairment has been shown to be associated with an increased risk of fractures in multiple studies. In the Framingham Eye Study, which included a subset of participants from the Framingham Study Cohort, those participants with visual acuity worse than 20/100 were more than twice as likely to have had hip fractures than participants with visual acuity of 20/25 or better (relative risk [RR] = 2.17; 95% CI = 1.24, 3.80) (Felson et al., 1989). In the EPIDOS Prospective Study, among a prospective cohort of 7,575 French women, those with visual acuity of 2/10 (using the decimal Snellen fraction, thus equivalent to 20/100) or worse had a RR of 4.3 (95%

CI = 3.1, 6.1) of hip fracture compared to those with visual acuity better than 7/10 (roughly equivalent to 20/30) (RR = 1.0) (Dargent-Molina et al., 1996). Various other aspects of visual impairment besides poor visual acuity have been shown to be associated with an increased fracture risk. In the Study of Osteoporotic Fractures, white women in the lowest quartile of depth perception measures were estimated to have a 40 percent increased risk of fractures compared with women in the other three quartiles (RR = 1.4; 95% CI = 1.0, 1.9), and the risk of fractures increased by 20 percent for each standard deviation decrease in low-frequency contrast sensitivity (RR = 1.2; 95% CI = 1.0, 1.5) (Cummings et al., 1995). Furthermore, in the same cohort, women with mild, moderate, or severe binocular visual field loss had an increased risk of hip fractures when compared with women without binocular visual field loss, and women with moderate or severe visual field loss had an increased risk of non-hip and non-spine fractures compared with women without binocular visual field loss (Coleman et al., 2009).

Studies have suggested that reversing vision impairment from cataract may be protective against fractures. A randomized controlled trial that evaluated expedited versus routinely scheduled cataract surgery in 306 women found that women with expedited cataract surgery had a 67 percent lower risk of fractures within 1 year after surgery than women with routinely scheduled surgery (RR = 0.33; 95% CI = 0.1, 1.0) (Harwood et al., 2005). A large study of more than 1.1 million men and women with cataract in the national U.S. Medicare database found that compared to patients with cataract who did not undergo surgery, patients with cataract surgery had a 16 percent lower risk of hip fracture (odds ratio [OR] = 0.84; 95% CI = 0.81, 0.87) and a 5 percent lower risk of any fracture (OR = 0.95; 95% CI = 0.93, 0.97). Furthermore, this protective association was modified by the effects of age and systemic disease burden, and the apparent protective relationship between surgery and fracture, based on having a high Charlson Comorbidity Index score, was even stronger among participants who were elderly or ill (Tseng et al., 2012).

The protective association between cataract surgery and fractures may extend beyond a reduction in fracture risk. In a recent study of the same large population of Medicare beneficiaries with cataract, those who had cataract surgery experienced 27 percent decreased risk in long-term mortality compared with those without cataract surgery (hazards ratio [HR] = 0.73; 95% CI = 0.72, 0.74) (Tseng et al., 2016). Similar to what was seen in the study of cataract surgery and fractures, the protective association between cataract surgery and mortality was modified by the effects of age and systemic disease burden, where patients who were elderly or who had a moderate burden of systemic disease experienced even stronger protective effects than the overall population. Although this study did not examine the mechanisms of the protective effect between cataract surgery and mortality and the study design does not permit conclusions about causation, the reduction in the risk of fractures and accidents was proposed as a contributing factor in the reduced risk of death. The protective association between cataract surgery and mortality in this study was supported by additional data from two earlier studies in the Blue Mountains region, west of Sydney, Australia, both of which demonstrated that patients with vision improvement after cataract surgery had decreased mortality risk compared with patients with vision impairment due to cataract who had not undergone surgery or those with persistent vision impairment after cataract surgery (Fong et al., 2013, 2014).

Subsequent Injury

People with vision loss are at higher risk for several types of injury. Of these, the link between vision loss and fall-related injuries has been most clearly documented. In a population-based cohort of Latinos in California, a greater risk of injurious falls was reported in those with both central vision impairment (OR = 2.76; 95% CI = 1.10, 7.02) and peripheral vision impairment (OR = 1.40; 95% CI = 0.94, 2.05) (Patino et al., 2010). A loss of visual field was associated with fall-related fractures, and a relationship between a recently acquired decline in visual acuity and falls with fracture was observed in the Blue Mountain Eye Study (Hong et al., 2014; Klein et al., 2003). Interestingly, both falls and falls with fracture were more likely in participants with a unilateral, rather than bilateral, visual acuity deficit, which is similar to the findings of an earlier study, suggesting that poor depth perception may be a contributor to falls (Felson et al., 1989). Indeed, poor depth perception has been associated with hip fracture in other epidemiological studies (Cummings et al., 1995). Poor contrast sensitivity is also associated with risk of fall-related fractures (de Boer et al., 2004).

In a prospective study of seniors between the ages of 75 and 80 years, lowered vision[4] at baseline was associated with an increased risk of injurious accidents requiring hospitalization over 10 years of follow-up (Kulmala et al., 2008). A visual acuity worse than 0.3 on the Landolt ring chart (roughly equivalent to 20/65) was not associated with a risk of injurious accidents, possibly because persons with more severe visual impairment restricted their activities, resulting in less opportunity for injury. However, in a separate study that used the National Health Interview Survey (NHIS)

---

[4] Visual acuity was assessed using the Landolt ring chart, which consists of 13 lines in which visual acuity is scored from 0.125 (worst), if the person can only see the first line, to 2.0 (best) if the person can correctly see the last line. Visual acuity between 0.3 and 0.5 in the better eye was defined as lowered vision, and vision better than 0.5 was defined as normal vision.

to follow more than 100,000 adults for up to 7 years, severe bilateral vision impairment was associated with a risk of death due to unintentional injury (HR = 7.4; 95% CI = 3.0, 17.8) (Lee et al., 2003).

Mental Health

Compared to people with normal vision, those with vision impairment are at a higher risk for depression, anxiety, and other psychological problems (Kempen et al., 2012). Among older adults with vision impairment, the rates of depression and anxiety are significantly higher than among both individuals of similar ages without vision impairment and those of similar ages suffering from other chronic conditions, such as asthma or chronic bronchitis, heart conditions, and hypertension (Kempen et al., 2012). Distress related to vision loss is more strongly correlated with depression than other key risk factors such as negative life events or poor health status (Rees et al., 2010). Among visually impaired individuals, those with depressive symptoms report more functional limitations. The reasons for the relationship between depression and poor visual function are unclear and may be bi-directional, but patient-level differences in eye disease and general medical condition did not account for the observed relationship (Rovner and Casten, 2002; Rovner et al., 2006). One randomized, controlled trial of an integrated mental health and vision rehabilitation program (compared with vision rehabilitation with non-directed supportive therapy) for patients with macular degeneration and subsyndromal depressive symptoms found significantly reduced rates of depression symptoms and better functional outcomes in the intervention group (Rovner et al., 2014). This work suggests that some of the functional and affective consequences of vision loss are remediable.

As discussed in Chapter 2, children with uncorrected refractive error are more likely to underperform on some metrics of academic performance (Kulp et al., 2016). Academic problems have been found to be negatively associated with anxiety, with the frequency increasing with age in both children and adolescents (Mazzone et al., 2007). Similarly, among adolescents, vision impairment is associated with an increased prevalence of psychopathological symptoms, including depression and anxiety (Garaigordobil and Bernarás, 2009). An analysis of data from NHIS did not show evidence for a direct relationship between vision impairment and death from suicide (HR = 1.50; 95% CI = 0.90, 2.49); however, the study did indicate an indirect effect of visual impairment on death from suicide due to poorer self-rated health (HR = 1.05; 95% CI = 1.02, 1.08) and the number of non-ocular health conditions (HR = 1.12; 95% CI = 1.01, 1.24). These results suggest that people with vision impairment may be at greater risk of suicide due to vision impairment's association with poor general health (Lam et al., 2008).

Cognition

Several studies have found that cognitive impairment is more prevalent and progresses more rapidly in older adults with vision impairment than in those without (Lin et al., 2004; Ong et al., 2013; Reyes-Ortiz et al., 2005; Rogers and Langa, 2010; Tay et al., 2006; Whitson et al., 2007). About 4 percent of community-dwelling persons over age 65 have both cognitive and vision impairments, making the co-occurrence of these problems more prevalent than such well-recognized conditions as Parkinson's disease and emphysema (Whitson et al., 2007). People with age-related macular degeneration (AMD) have higher rates of cognitive impairment than their peers, lower scores on cognitive tests, and a higher risk of incident dementia (Baker et al., 2009; Clemons et al., 2006; Klaver et al., 1999; Pham et al., 2006; Wong et al., 2002; Woo et al., 2012). Other studies suggest that, even without dementia, AMD patients still perform more poorly on tests of verbal fluency and memory (Clemons et al., 2006; Whitson et al., 2010, 2015; Wong et al., 2002). Research has failed to demonstrate a clear genetic link between AMD and dementia (Butler et al., 2015; Souied et al., 1998). These results suggest more research is needed to fully assess the reasons behind the link between vision and cognitive impairment in adults.

In children, uncorrectable vision impairment frequently occurs in the context of comorbid conditions, making it difficult to quantify the direct impact of visual impairment and blindness on cognitive skills, academic performance, and QOL. Many children who have been diagnosed with neurodevelopmental disorders (genetic or acquired) have been found to also have an associated vision problem that has led to visual impairment. Current research focuses on determining the prevalence of these eye health and vision disorders that occur with the underlying neurodevelopmental diagnosis (Salt and Sargent, 2014). For example, children with cerebral palsy have been found to have a higher prevalence of strabismus, visual impairment due to uncorrected refractive error, eye movement disorders, and visual perceptual deficits than normally sighted children of the same age (Lew et al., 2015; Salt and Sargent, 2014). A higher rate of vision impairment has also been documented for children with Down syndrome (Cregg et al., 2003). It is difficult to ascertain the influence of the vision loss on cognitive or academic function in diagnoses that are already associated with cognitive impairment. One study demonstrated that children diagnosed with toxoplasmosis who present with reduced vision perform more poorly than children diagnosed with toxoplasmosis without vision impairment on verbal and performance measure of intellectual ability (Roizen et al., 2006). A meta-analysis on children with cerebral palsy found that visual perceptual deficits were prevalent in those children but none of the studies had a control comparison group (Ego et al., 2015). These children often perform below the level expected for their chronological ages, yet they have neither been categorized as visually impaired, nor referred for services (Flanagan et al., 2003).

Although an association exists between vision impairment—as well as some specific eye disorders—and cognition, the mechanisms underlying this relationship are unclear. One possibility is that diseases of the eye have a negative effect on cognitive processes, either directly or indirectly. In people with vision impairment, the loss of cognitively stimulating activities, such as reading, may diminish other cognitive abilities (Lindenberger and Baltes, 1994). Additionally, the brain is known to change in response to decreased visual input, and these changes may affect regions or neuronal pathways that support cognitive processes (Liu et al., 2007, 2010; Pascual-Leone et al., 2005). A second possibility is the "common cause" theory, which holds that genetic, environmental, or medical risk factors cause disease in the brain and eye simultaneously (Klaver et al., 1999; Lindenberger and Baltes, 1994). Another possibility is that confounding factors, such as behavior and economic status, contribute to the observed relationship between vision impairment and cognitive impairment.

Hearing Impairment

The prevalence of co-existing impairment in vision and hearing, also referred to as dual sensory impairment (DSI), increases markedly with age. A range from 9 to 21 percent of adults over the age of 70 possess some degree of DSI (Saunders and Echt, 2007). In an Australian cohort, the prevalence of DSI was even higher, reported to be 26.8 percent in participants ages 80 and older (Schneider et al., 2012). In a cross-sectional study of a random sample of 446 older adults (mean age 79.9 years) from Marin County, California, eight measures of visual ability were associated with risk of hearing impairment (defined as moderate bilateral hearing loss, threshold >40 dB) (Schneck et al., 2012). However, the relationship between vision impairment and hearing impairment only achieved statistical significance for three measures of visual acuity in low contrast conditions. Additional research is needed to determine whether vision loss is an independent risk factor for hearing loss and, if so, what factors underlie this relationship.

Mortality

Several studies report associations between vision impairment and an increased risk for all-cause and injury-related mortality, as compared to controls with normal vision (Christ et al., 2014; Lam et al., 2008; Lee et al., 2002, 2003; Zheng et al., 2014). One possible cause of the greater mortality in visually impaired people may be their elevated risk of accidents and falls. In the longitudinal study by Christ and colleagues (2014), the relationship between worse visual acuity and mortality was mediated by disability in instrumental activities of daily living, which suggests that some deaths may result from an impaired ability for self-care and disease management.

The relationship between vision impairment and mortality is certainly confounded by medical conditions (e.g., diabetes, obesity, hypertension, autoimmune disorders), lifestyle factors (e.g., smoking, alcohol use), and socio-demographic factors (e.g., race, age, socioeconomic disadvantage). As detailed in the next section, the complicated interplay between eye health and other medical comorbidities is an important factor in monitoring and reducing the overall public health burden of vision loss.

MULTIPLE COMORBID CONDITIONS

The Office of the Assistant Secretary for Health defines chronic conditions as, "conditions that last a year or more and require ongoing medical attention and/or limit activities of daily living" (Goodman et al., 2013, p. 3). Chronic conditions are associated with an increased risk of "early mortality, poor functional status, unnecessary hospitalizations, adverse drug events, duplicative tests, and conflicting medical advice" (HHS, 2010, p. 2; see also, Hwang et al., 2001; Vogeli et al., 2007; Wolff et al., 2002). Expenditures related to chronic conditions are substantial, with an estimated 66 percent of total health care spending attributable to care for Americans with multiple chronic conditions (HHS, 2010). Approximately 14 percent of Medicare beneficiaries with six or more chronic conditions accounted for 46 percent of total Medicare spending in 2010, while the 32 percent of beneficiaries with one or fewer chronic conditions accounted for 7 percent of spending (CMS, 2012).

Irreversible vision impairment resulting from eye disease should be considered a chronic condition; it can amplify the adverse effects of other illnesses and injuries, and people with vision loss commonly live with multiple chronic conditions. As of 2012, 117 million people had at least one chronic condition, with one in four adults reporting two or more chronic health conditions (CDC, 2016). Data from the Medical Expenditure Panel Survey show that among Americans over age 65 with eye disease, four out of five also had at least one of the following conditions: hypertension, heart disease, diabetes, or arthritis (Anderson and Horvath, 2004). According to a 2008 NHIS, a substantial number of people with chronic diseases reported trouble seeing: 34.8 percent of those with chronic kidney disease, 30.9 percent of those with stroke, 23.8 percent of those with coronary heart disease, 23.6 percent of those with diabetes, 22.1 percent of those with arthritis, 19.7 percent of those with patients, and 19.4 percent of those with hypertension (Crews and Chou, 2012). Whether or not any causal relationship exists between vision impairment and non-ocular comorbidities, it is clear that any successful efforts to alleviate the burden of vision impairment and loss will need to take comorbidities into account.

Vision Loss Amplifies the Effects of Other Conditions

A study of individuals ages 65 and older found that patients with a visual impairment and any of several other illnesses or conditions were many times more likely to have difficulty performing basic physical and social tasks than individuals in the same age range without visual impairment and without the particular illness or condition (Crews et al., 2006). For example, elderly individuals with severe depression, visual impairment, or both were 10.0, 2.9, and 23.9 times more likely, respectively, to have moderate or severe limitations in their ability to socialize than people without either severe depression or visual impairment. Table 3-2 details the increased odds of encountering difficulty when undertaking these basic physical and social tasks among persons with visual impairment or a given comorbidity, or both. Whether or not comorbid vision impairment directly caused the excess disability (which cannot be inferred from descriptive

TABLE 3-2 Adjusted Odds Ratio for the Self-Reported Difficulty Performing Tasks Among U.S. Adults Ages 65 and Older with Vision Impairment and/or Other Condition or Disease

Disease or Condition Reference Group	Condition or Disease		Vision Impairment Only		Condition or Disease + Vision Impairment	
	Physical	Social	Physical	Social	Physical	Social
Diabetes	2.3	2.0	2.8	3.4	5.7	6.4
Heart problems	2.6	2.4	2.7	3.1	6.6	7.4
Hypertension	1.9	1.5	2.9	3.5	5.1	5.2
Stroke	3.9	4.2	2.7	3.2	9.5	11.5
Severe depression	7.9	10.0	2.5	2.9	19.5	23.9
Low back pain	2.4	1.9	2.9	3.2	5.9	5.7
Breathing problems	2.3	2.0	2.8	3.4	5.8	6.0
Hearing impairment	1.8	1.7	2.7	3.3	4.6	5.4
Joint symptoms	2.6	2.0	2.6	3.2	6.1	5.5

NOTES: All figures describe adjusted odds ratio of encountering moderate to severe limitations when performing either physical or social activities among persons with vision impairment or a comorbidity or both as compared to persons without a vision impairment or the relevant illness/condition. Physical activity refers to ability to walk 0.25 mile. Social activity refers to ability to socialize.
SOURCE: Adapted from Crews et al., 2006.

data), vision impairment may help identify high-risk individuals or individuals with unmet needs who could be targeted for services and interventions across a variety of other clinical specialties.

Both cognitive impairment and vision impairment are disabling in their own right, but the co-occurrence of the two has been associated with even higher rates of disability and low self-rated health (Whitson et al., 2007, 2012a). Dual sensory impairment (concurrent vision and hearing deficits) has been associated with a higher risk of cognitive decline, disability, depression, and mortality (Gopinath et al., 2013; Heine and Browning, 2014; Lee et al., 2007; Lin et al., 2004; Schneider et al., 2011). Evidence is inconclusive regarding whether the combined effects of vision impairment and other impairments (cognition or hearing) on outcomes are synergistic or merely additive (Schneider et al., 2011; Whitson et al., 2007).

Vision Loss Complicates the Management of Other Conditions

As reviewed above, vision loss creates significant challenges in daily life. The challenge of not being able to see well can affect various vision-reliant tasks that are frequently required for good chronic disease management, including self-care (e.g., foot checks in diabetics, preparing nutritious meals) and transportation (e.g., getting to and from clinic visits). In addition, vision loss may create difficulties in medication adherence and management (e.g., reading pill bottles, ordering refills) so that individuals who develop vision loss associated with chronic conditions, such as diabetes or glaucoma, are at a disadvantage in managing those chronic conditions. For example, vision loss makes it difficult to properly administer medications such as insulin or eye drops. Thus, affected individuals are at risk of entering a "vicious cycle" of worsening health.

Other Conditions Affect the Management of Eye Disease

Comorbidities also affect patients' ability to manage and cope with their vision impairment and eye health. One area of eye care where the impact of comorbid conditions has been studied is vision rehabilitation. Both cognitive impairment and depression have been associated with worse functional outcomes in vision rehabilitation (Rovner et al., 2002; Whitson et al., 2012b). A qualitative study of 98 older adults and their companions/ caregivers in an outpatient vision rehabilitation clinic identified five themes regarding the impact of comorbid medical conditions on the patients' experiences in vision rehabilitation (Whitson et al., 2011). Comorbidities had the following implications for the success of vision rehabilitation: (1) concurrent medical problems resulted in fluctuating health status with "good days and bad days" that were unrelated to eye disease, (2) comorbid conditions (e.g., hearing impairment, cognitive impairment) often amplified communication barriers between patients and providers, (3) participants and caregivers felt "overwhelmed" by competing health care demands, (4) comorbidities tended to delay progress in vision rehabilitation programs because of unexpected health events (e.g., falls, hospitalization, disease flares), and (5) some barriers imposed by comorbid conditions seemed to be reduced by the effective involvement of an informal companion[5] (Whitson et al., 2011). A second qualitative study focused on the impact of comorbid cognitive impairment in vision rehabilitation (Lawrence et al., 2009). This study interviewed 17 individuals with co-existing vision impairment and dementia, 17 family caregivers, and 18 vision or dementia health specialists involved in the patients' care (Lawrence et al., 2009). The study found that vision-related service providers felt ill equipped to manage dementia-related needs, while visual needs were accorded a low priority by those providing dementia services; a lack of collaboration between the two services led to an overcautious approach (Lawrence et al., 2009).

Comorbidities can also affect patients' ability to manage specific aspects of their eye care. In particular, the administration of eye drops can be challenging for patients with a limited range of motion in the neck, with arthritis or neuropathy involving the hands, or with cognitive impairments. The precise impact of these comorbidities on medication adherence and the proper administration of eye drops merits further research, but one multisite study that video-taped glaucoma patients self-administering a single drop reported that individuals with arthritis were significantly less likely to have the drop land in their eye (Sayner et al., 2015).

OVERVIEW OF EXPENDITURES

Few studies are available that examine the total costs associated with all eye disease and vision impairment on a national level. A 2013 analysis of the economic burden of vision loss and eye disorders that was commissioned by Prevent Blindness estimated prevalence and costs from National Health and Nutrition Examination Survey (NHANES) data, Medical Expenditure Panel Survey (MEPS) data, and data from the Survey of Income and Program Participation, the 2011 U.S. Census, and federal budgets (Wittenborn and Rein, 2013). This analysis estimated the direct and indirect costs attributable to vision loss and eye disease to be $138.9 billion in the United States in 2013 dollars and found that costs for individual states ranged from $250 million in Wyoming to more than $15.6 billion in California

---

[5] A friend or relative with whom the participant had at least weekly contact.

(Wittenborn and Rein, 2013).[6] The direct medical costs summed across all age groups attributable to, for example, diagnosed disorders, undiagnosed visual loss, and optometry[7] visits were $48.7 billion, $3.0 billion, and $2.8 billion, respectively (Wittenborn and Rein, 2013). The total direct and indirect costs for eye disorders and vision loss per payer were $47.4 billion for government entities, $22.1 billion for private insurers, and $71.7 billion for patients (Wittenborn and Rein, 2013).

Table 3-3 provides a breakdown of the comprehensive costs by age group for major categories of direct and indirect costs associated with eye care in the United States. Directs costs associated with diagnosed vision impairments along with indirect costs associated with productivity loss account for approximately 70 percent of the comprehensive costs across all age groups. Medical vision aids, which include eyeglasses and contact lenses, are the next largest expense category. Nursing home expenses account for an additional 30 percent of indirect costs but are attributable only to the over-65 population. These data suggest that interventions targeting the prevention and reduction of vision impairment have the potential to reduce overall costs. Although more data are needed for a comprehensive analysis of this assertion, shifting the burden of vision expenditures away from the possible downstream consequences of severe vision impairment toward items and services that promote the earlier diagnosis and treatment of vision-threatening diseases or conditions would extend the productivity and function of populations with vision impairment.

The costs of eye disorders and subsequent vision loss are shared by the government, private insurance, and individuals, including patients and families. According to a recent analysis, the $47.4 billion that the government spends annually on eye disorders and vision loss is mostly for direct medical costs and long-term care (Wittenborn and Rein, 2013). One systematic review examined the average annual expense per patient in a cohort of Medicare beneficiaries and found per-patient costs in 2011 dollars to range from $12,175 to $14,029 for moderate vision impairment, $13,154 to $16,321 for severe visual impairment, and $14,882 to $24,180 for blindness (Köberlein et al., 2013). In comparison, the authors cited a mean expense of $8,695 for patients with no vision loss as the control, indicating

---

[6] The state cost estimates were a function of the states' populations within each age group. State populations were identified for the age groups 0–17, 18–39, 40–64, and 65+ based on the 2011 U.S. Census data. The burden estimate was divided by age for each age group to derive per-person costs for each group, then multiplied by the state population costs for each age group. These estimates do not include state-specific unit cost or utilization estimates (Wittenborn and Rein, 2013).

[7] "These costs are measured separately from other medical costs in MEPS; they are not associated with diagnosis codes and are based on non-confirmed, self-reported expenditures" (Wittenborn and Rein, 2013, p. 2).

TABLE 3-3 Economic Burden of Eye Disorders and Vision Loss (in millions of dollars)

Age Group	Comprehensive Costs (in $ millions)				
	0–17	18–39	40–64	65+	All Ages
Direct costs					
Diagnosed disorders	$2,844	$5,067	$14,218	$26,640	$48,769
Medical vision aids	$1,480	$3,335	$6,222	$2,199	$13,236
Undiagnosed vision loss	$48	$474	$1,702	$798	$3,022
Aids/devices	$38	$77	$81	$553	$749
Educational/school screening	$651	$119	—	—	$769
Assistance programs	$25	$13	$23	$145	$207
Total direct costs	**$5,086**	**$9,086**	**$22,246**	**$30,335**	**$66,752**
Indirect costs					
Productivity loss	—	$12,978	$10,828	$24,622	$48,427
Informal care	$601	—	$187	$1,264	$2,052
Nursing home	—	—	—	$20,248	$20,248
Entitlement programs[a]	$0.50	$165	$279	$1,782	$2,226
Tax deductions[a]	—	$6	$11	$10	$28
Transfer deadweight loss	$47	$98	$538	$808	$1,490
Total indirect costs	**$648**	**$13,075**	**$11,553**	**$46,941**	**$72,217**
Total economic burden	**$5,734**	**$22,161**	**$33,799**	**$77,276**	**$138,970**
Loss of well-being measures					
Disability adjusted life years lost	6.92	26.35	33.38	216.48	283.13

[a] Transfer payment costs are not included in total.
SOURCE: Wittenborn and Rein, 2013.

that expenses for blind individuals can sometimes be more than double the control cost at the upper end of the range (Köberlein et al., 2013). The total of all these costs is substantial, considering that Medicare had 52.2 million beneficiaries in 2013 (CMS, 2014).

Private insurers covered approximately one-third of the total, or $22.1 billion (Wittenborn and Rein, 2013). As with public insurance, the majority of these costs ($20.8 billion) were related to direct medical costs and supplies (Wittenborn and Rein, 2013). Costs associated with diagnosed disorders were by far the most substantial costs for private insurers, at more than $17 billion. The relatively small amount spent for medical vision aids ($2.6 billion) reflects the limited available reimbursement coverage and accounts for the high spending burden for such aids by the individual payer ($9.7 billion) (Wittenborn and Rein, 2013). The rest of the costs are attributable to reimbursement for long-term care. The costs associated with diagnosed blindness and vision impairment averaged (across all payers) $6,680 per year (Wittenborn and Rein, 2013). By way of comparison, the annual costs for all different types of diagnosed medical disorders average $3,432 per person (Wittenborn and Rein, 2013). Despite the high costs associated with vision impairment and loss, the per-person costs for vision correction average only $81 per year (Wittenborn and Rein, 2013). One expert suggested that the cost to expand all required pediatric vision-related services under the Patient Protection and Affordable Care Act of 2010 to all beneficiaries covered by private insurance would range from $1 to $2 per member per month (Spahr, 2015).

Individuals paid for slightly more than half—$71.7 billion—of the total cost of eye disorders and vision loss, "largely due to productivity and informal care losses" (Wittenborn and Rein, 2013, p. 5). Of that $71.7 billion covered by individuals, direct costs accounted for approximately $15.5 billion primarily for medical vision aids ($9.7 billion), diagnosed disorders ($4.7 billion), aids and devices ($749 million), and undiagnosed vision impairment ($372 million) (Wittenborn and Rein, 2013). Indirect costs accounted for more than $56 billion of the individual costs. Those indirect costs were due to productivity losses caused by reduced workforce involvement and lower wages, the costs of informal care, and long-term care costs (Wittenborn and Rein, 2013). One national survey of working age adults found that 52 percent of them had less than $1,000 on hand to pay for out-of-pocket expenses associated with the diagnosis of an unexpected serious illness; 28 percent had less than $500 (Aflac, 2015).

Figure 3-1 indicates that the costs attributed to eye and vision health increase with age across all payers and that the over-65 population is responsible for the vast majority of expenses for all payers, except private insurance. This is not surprising given the individual costs attributable to specific age-related eye diseases and conditions and the prevalence of diabetes in older populations. For example, diabetic retinopathy cost the United States $493 million in 2004, with 60 percent of the direct medical costs incurred by 40 to 60 years olds (Rein et al., 2006). Similarly, in 2009, the estimated costs to Medicare from glaucoma reached $748 million (Quigley et al., 2013). Schmier and Levine (2013) estimated the total loss in gross domestic product related to AMD was almost $42 billion in 2012 dollars. The costs attributable to individual cases vary by the severity of the disease or condition. For example, the distribution of AMD-associated costs varies by disease stage, "with greater cost for diagnosis procedures with earlier AMD and more on caregiving and institutional care with wet AMD" (Schmier and Levine, 2013). One study found a four-fold increase in direct ophthalmology-related costs between asymptomatic ocular hypertension/earliest glaucoma ($623 per year) and end-stage glaucoma/blindness ($2,511 per year) (Varma et al., 2011). The authors suggested

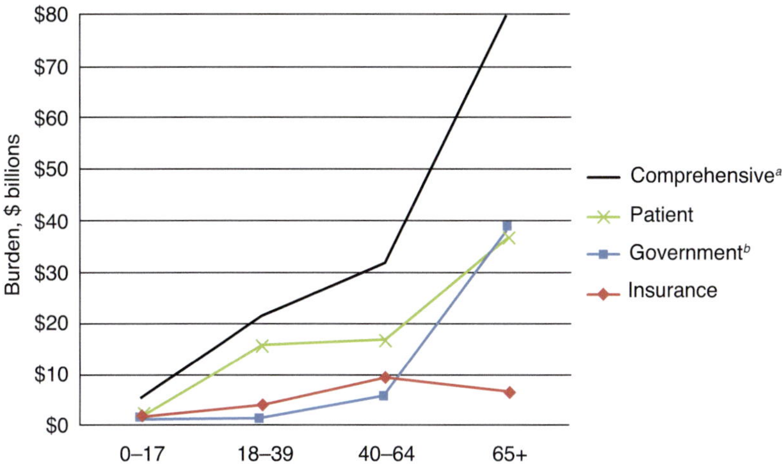

FIGURE 3-1 Costs by payer by age group for eye and vision health.
[a] "Comprehensive" is the cumulative sum of costs borne by the three payer categories: patient, government, and insurance providers.
[b] Government total includes transfer payment costs that are not included in "Comprehensive."
SOURCE: Wittenborn and Rein, 2013.

that "early identification and treatment of patients with glaucoma and those with ocular hypertension at high risk of developing vision loss may reduce the individual burden of disease on [health-related quality of life] and also may minimize personal and societal economic burdens" (p. 5).

In addition to incurring direct costs related to vision care, people with vision impairment tend to experience a lower QOL and decreased health status (as discussed in this chapter), and vision loss can complicate and exacerbate other comorbid conditions, driving up costs and worsening outcomes. For example, Bramley and colleagues (2008) demonstrated among Medicare beneficiaries with glaucoma that patients with any vision loss had 46.7 percent higher costs compared with patients without vision loss; the higher costs were the result of the increased risk for nursing home admission, depression, falls, accidents, and injury. These outcomes account for some of the most substantial health expenditures. As such, in order to secure population-level improvements in the field it will be critical to understand that the costs associated with vision impairment and eye disease are borne not only by individuals, but also by their caregivers, taxpayers, and employers. Without dedicated action, society as a whole will increasingly bear the burden of the direct costs from increasing yet avoidable Medicare spending and of the indirect costs from substantial lost productivity and a reduced labor force.

CONCLUSION

Vision impairment results in significant expenditures, both direct and indirect, and has the potential to affect almost every aspect of a person's life. Vision loss affects more than one's ability to see the world clearly. The consequences of vision impairment often negatively impact QOL, including the number of physical and mental unhealthy days and overall dissatisfaction with life. Individuals with vision impairment are also more likely to experience restrictions in their independence, mobility, and educational achievement, as well as an increased risk of falls, fractures, injuries, poor mental health, cognitive deficits, and social isolation.

Vision loss also amplifies the effects of other chronic conditions and is a chronic condition itself. People with a vision impairment and other illnesses or conditions are more likely to have difficulty performing tasks and reporting poor health. Vision loss can also complicate chronic disease management, including self-care, transportation to and from doctor's appointments, and the proper administration of medicine. Moreover, other conditions may affect the management of eye disease, including vision rehabilitation to improve the functionality and quality of life for those with vision impairments.

No studies are available on the total costs attributable to the promotion of eye and vision health and the economic impact of vision loss in the United States. However, the few studies available that have looked at overall direct and indirect costs found that national costs are in the billions each year and vary substantially by state. Total costs also vary by age and by payer, with substantial costs incurred by individuals, including costs of caring for family members with vision impairment. Population health approaches to improve eye and vision health will need to focus on the direct and indirect costs as objective measures of the impact of vision impairment but also as measures of equity among populations most likely to be affected by vision impairment.

REFERENCES

Aflac. 2015. National trends: 2015 fact sheet: Aflac workforces report. https://www.aflac.com/docs/awr/pdf/2015-detailed-findings/2015-national-fact-sheet.pdf (accessed April 7, 2016).

Anderson, G., and J. Horvath. 2004. The growing burden of chronic disease in America. *Public Health Reports* 119(3):263–270.

Baker, M. L., J. J. Wang, S. Rogers, R. Klein, L. H. Kuller, E. K. Larsen, and T. Y. Wong. 2009. Early age-related macular degeneration, cognitive function, and dementia: The Cardiovascular Health Study. *Archives of Ophthalmology* 127(5):667–673.

Bibby, S. A., E. R. Maslin, R. McIlraith, and G. P. Soong. 2007. Vision and self-reported mobility performance in patients with low vision. *Clinical and Experimental Optometry* 90(2):115–123.

Bramley, T., P. Peeples, J. G. Walt, M. Juhasz, and J. E. Hansen. 2008. Impact of vision loss on costs and outcomes in Medicare beneficiaries with glaucoma. *Archives of Ophthalmology* 126(6):849–856.

Brown, J. C., J. E. Goldstein, T. L. Chan, R. Massof, P. Ramulu, and Low Vision Research Network Study Group. 2014. Characterizing functional complaints in patients seeking outpatient low-vision services in the United States. *Ophthalmology* 121(8):1655–1662, e1651.

Butler, J. M., U. Sharif, M. Ali, M. McKibbin, J. P. Thompson, R. Gale, Y. C. Yang, C. Inglehearn, and L. Paraoan. 2015. A missense variant in CST3 exerts a recessive effect on susceptibility to age-related macular degeneration resembling its association with Alzheimer's disease. *Human Genetics* 134(7):705–715.

CDC (Centers for Disease Control and Prevention). 2016. Chronic disease overview. http://www.cdc.gov/chronicdisease/overview (accessed April 7, 2016).

Chai, Y., Y. Shao, S. Lin, K. Xiong, W. Chen, Y. Li, J. Yi, L. Zhang, G. Tan, and J. Tang. 2009. Vision-related quality of life and emotional impact in children with strabismus: A prospective study. *Journal of International Medical Research* 37(4):1108–1114.

Chatziralli, I. P., T. N. Sergentanis, V. G. Peponis, L. E. Papazisis, and M. M. Moschos. 2012. Risk factors for poor vision-related quality of life among cataract patients. Evaluation of baseline data. *Graefe's Archive for Clinical and Experimental Ophthalmology* 251(3):783–789.

Chaudry, I., G. C. Brown, and M. M. Brown. 2015. Medical student and patient perceptions of quality of life associated with vision loss. *Canadian Journal of Ophthalmology* 50(3):217–224.

Cheng, H.-C., C.-Y. Guo, M.-J. Chen, Y.-C. Ko, N. Huang, and C. J. L. Liu. 2015. Patient-reported vision-related quality of life differences between superior and inferior hemifield visual field defects in primary open-angle glaucoma. *JAMA Ophthalmology* 133(3):269–275.

Chia, E. M., P. Mitchell, E. Ojaimi, E. Rochtchina, and J. J. Wang. 2006. Assessment of vision-related quality of life in an older population subsample: The Blue Mountains Eye Study. *Ophthalmic Epidemiology* 13(6):371–377.

Christ, S. L., D. D. Zheng, B. K. Swenor, B. L. Lam, S. K. West, S. L. Tannenbaum, B. E. Munoz, and D. J. Lee. 2014. Longitudinal relationships among visual acuity, daily functional status, and mortality: The Salisbury Eye Evaluation study. *JAMA Ophthalmology* 132(12):1400–1406.

Clemons, T. E., M. W. Rankin, and W. L. McBee. 2006. Cognitive impairment in the Age-Related Eye Disease Study: AREDS report no. 16. *Archives of Ophthalmology* 124(4):537–543.

CMS (Centers for Medicare & Medicaid Services). 2012. *Chronic conditions among Medicare beneficiaries.* Baltimore, MD: CMS.

———. 2014. *Medicare enrollment—National trends 1966–2013.* Baltimore, MD: CMS. https://www.cms.gov/Research-Statistics-Data-and-Systems/Statistics-Trends-and-Reports/MedicareEnrpts/Downloads/SMI2013.pdf (accessed March 7, 2016).

Coleman, A. L., S. R. Cummings, K. E. Ensrud, F. Yu, P. Gutierrez, K. L. Stone, J. A. Cauley, K. L. Pedula, M. C. Hochberg, and C. M. Mangione. 2009. Visual field loss and risk of fractures in older women. *Journal of the American Geriatric Society* 57(10):1825–1832.

Cox, A., A. Blaikie, C. J. MacEwen, D. Jones, K. Thompson, D. Holding, T. Sharma, S. Miller, S. Dobson, and R. Sanders. 2005. Visual impairment in elderly patients with hip fracture: Causes and associations. *Eye (London)* 19(6):652–656.

Cregg, M., J. M. Woodhouse, R. E. Stewart, V. H. Pakeman, N. R. Bromham, H. L. Gunter, L. Trojanowska, M. Parker, and W. I. Fraser. 2003. Development of refractive error and strabismus in children with Down syndrome. *Investigative Ophthalmology & Visual Science* 44(3):1023–1030.

Crews, J., and C.-F. Chou. 2012. *Vision impairment and multiple chronic conditions: Findings from the 2002, 2008 National Health Interview Survey.* http://visionproblemsus.org/presentations/Crews.pdf (accessed April 7, 2016).

Crews, J. E., G. C. Jones, and J. H. Kim. 2006. Double jeopardy: The effects of comorbid conditions among older people with vision loss. *Journal of Visual Impairment and Blindness* 100:824.

Crews, J. E., C. F. Chou, X. Zhang, M. M. Zack, and J. B. Saaddine. 2014. Health-related quality of life among people aged ≥65 years with self-reported visual impairment: Findings from the 2006–2010 Behavioral Risk Factor Surveillance System. *Ophthalmic Epidemiology* 21(5):287–296.

Crews, J. E., C.-F. Chiu-Fung Chou, J. A. Stevens, and J. B. Saadine. 2016a. Falls among persons aged > 65 years with and without severe vision impairment—United States, 2014. *Morbidity and Mortality Weekly Report* 65(17):433–437.

Crews, J. E., C. F. Chou, M. M. Zack, X. Zhang, K. M. Bullard, A. R. Morse, and J. B. Saaddine. 2016b. The association of health-related quality of life with severity of visual impairment among people aged 40–64 years: Findings from the 2006–2010 Behavioral Risk Factor Surveillance System. *Ophthalmic Epidemiology* 23(3):145–153.

Cummings, S. R., M. C. Nevitt, W. S. Browner, K. Stone, K. M. Fox, K. E. Ensrud, J. Cauley, D. Black, and T. M. Vogt. 1995. Risk factors for hip fracture in white women. Study of Osteoporotic Fractures Research Group. *New England Journal of Medicine* 332(12): 767–773.

Dargent-Molina, P., F. Favier, H. Grandjean, C. Baudoin, A. Schott, E. Hausherr, P. Meunier, and G. Breart. 1996. Fall-related factors and risk of hip fracture: The EPIDOS prospective study. *Lancet* 348(9021):145–149.

de Boer, M. R., S. M. Pluijm, P. Lips, A. C. Moll, H. J. Volker-Dieben, D. J. Deeg, and G. H. van Rens. 2004. Different aspects of visual impairment as risk factors for falls and fractures in older men and women. *Journal of Bone and Mineral Research* 19(9):1539–1547.

Ego, A., K. Lidzba, P. Brovedani, V. Belmonti, S. Gonzalez-Monge, B. Boudia, A. Ritz, and C. Cans. 2015. Visual–perceptual impairment in children with cerebral palsy: A systematic review. *Developmental Medicine & Child Neurology* 57(s2):46–51.

Evans, K., S. K. Law, J. Walt, P. Buchholz, and J. Hansen. 2009. The quality of life impact of peripheral versus central vision loss with a focus on glaucoma versus age-related macular degeneration. *Clinical Ophthalmology* 3:433–445.

Felson, D. T., J. J. Anderson, M. T. Hannan, R. C. Milton, P. W. Wilson, and D. P. Kiel. 1989. Impaired vision and hip fracture: The Framingham Study. *Journal of the American Geriatric Society* 37(6):495–500.

Flanagan, N., A. Jackson, and A. Hill. 2003. Visual impairment in childhood: Insights from a community-based survey. *Child: Care, Health and Development* 29(6):493–499.

Fong, C. S.-U., P. Mitchell, E. Rochtchina, E. T. Teber, T. Hong, and J. J. Wang. 2013. Correction of visual impairment by cataract surgery and improved survival in older persons: The Blue Mountains Eye Study cohort. *Ophthalmology* 120(9):1720–1727.

Fong, C. S.-U., P. Mitchell, E. Rochtchina, T. De Loryn, A. G. Tan, and J. J. Wang. 2014. Visual impairment corrected via cataract surgery and 5-year survival in a prospective cohort. *American Journal of Ophthalmology* 157(1):163–170, e161.

Freedman, B. L., S. K. Jones, A. Lin, S. S. Stinnett, and K. W. Muir. 2014. Vision-related quality of life in children with glaucoma. *Journal of American Association for Pediatric Ophthalmology and Strabismus* 18(1):95–98.

Garaigordobil, M., and E. Bernarás. 2009. Self-concept, self-esteem, personality traits and psychopathological symptoms in adolescents with and without visual impairment. *Spanish Journal of Psychology* 12(01):149–160.

Goodman, R. A., S. F. Posner, E. S. Huang, A. K. Parekh, and H. K. Koh. 2013. Defining and measuring chronic conditions: Imperatives for research, policy, program, and practice. *Preventing Chronic Disease* 10:E66.

Gopinath, B., J. Schneider, C. M. McMahon, G. Burlutsky, S. R. Leeder, and P. Mitchell. 2013. Dual sensory impairment in older adults increases the risk of mortality: A population-based study. *PLoS ONE* 8(3):e55054.

Harwood, R. H., A. Foss, F. Osborn, R. Gregson, A. Zaman, and T. Masud. 2005. Falls and health status in elderly women following first eye cataract surgery: A randomised controlled trial. *British Journal of Ophthalmology* 89(1):53–59.

Hassell, J., E. Lamoureux, and J. Keeffe. 2006. Impact of age related macular degeneration on quality of life. *British Journal of Ophthalmology* 90(5):593–596.

Haymes, S. A., A. W. Johnston, and A. D. Heyes. 2002. Relationship between vision impairment and ability to perform activities of daily living. *Ophthalmic and Physiologic Optics* 22(2):79–91.

Heine, C., and C. J. Browning. 2014. Mental health and dual sensory loss in older adults: A systematic review. *Frontiers in Aging Neuroscience* 6:83.

HHS (U.S. Department of Health and Human Services). 2010. *Multiple chronic conditions— A strategic framework: Optimum health and quality of life for individuals with multiple chronic conditions.* Washington, DC: HHS.

Hirneiss, C. 2014. The impact of a better-seeing eye and a worse-seeing eye on vision-related quality of life. *Clinical Ophthalmology* 8:1703–1709.

Hong, T., P. Mitchell, G. Burlutsky, C. Samarawickrama, and J. J. Wang. 2014. Visual impairment and the incidence of falls and fractures among older people: Longitudinal findings from the Blue Mountains Eye Study. *Investigative Ophthalmology & Visual Science* 55(11):7589–7593.

Hwang, W., W. Weller, H. Ireys, and G. Anderson. 2001. Out-of-pocket medical spending for care of chronic conditions. *Health Affairs (Millwood)* 20(6):267–278.

Ivers, R. Q., R. G. Cumming, P. Mitchell, and K. Attebo. 1998. Visual impairment and falls in older adults: The Blue Mountains Eye Study. *Journal of the American Geriatric Society* 46(1):58–64.

Kempen, G. I., J. Ballemans, A. V. Ranchor, G. H. van Rens, and G. A. Zijlstra. 2012. The impact of low vision on activities of daily living, symptoms of depression, feelings of anxiety and social support in community-living older adults seeking vision rehabilitation services. *Quality of Life Research* 21(8):1405–1411.

Klaver, C. C., A. Ott, A. Hofman, J. J. Assink, M. M. Breteler, and P. T. de Jong. 1999. Is age-related maculopathy associated with Alzheimer's disease? The Rotterdam Study. *American Journal of Epidemiology* 150(9):963–968.

Klein, B. E., S. E. Moss, R. Klein, K. E. Lee, and K. J. Cruickshanks. 2003. Associations of visual function with physical outcomes and limitations 5 years later in an older population: The Beaver Dam Eye Study. *Ophthalmology* 110(4):644–650.

Köberlein, J., K. Beifus, C. Schaffert, and R. P. Finger. 2013. The economic burden of visual impairment and blindness: A systematic review. *British Medical Journal Open* 3(11):e003471.

Kulmala, J., P. Era, O. Parssinen, R. Sakari, S. Sipila, T. Rantanen, and E. Heikkinen. 2008. Lowered vision as a risk factor for injurious accidents in older people. *Aging Clinical and Experimental Research* 20(1):25–30.

Kulp, M. T., E. Ciner, M. Maguire, B. Moore, J. Pentimonti, M. Pistilli, L. Cyert, T. R. Candy, G. Quinn, and G.-S. Ying. 2016. Uncorrected hyperopia and preschool early literacy. *Ophthalmology* 123(4):681–689.

Lam, B. L., S. L. Christ, D. J. Lee, D. D. Zheng, and K. L. Arheart. 2008. Reported visual impairment and risk of suicide: The 1986–1996 National Health Interview Surveys. *Archives of Ophthalmology* 126(7):975–980.

Lamoureux, E., and K. Pesudovs. 2011. Vision-specific quality-of-life research: A need to improve the quality. *American Journal of Ophthalmology* 151(2):195–197, e192.

Langelaan, M., M. R. de Boer, R. M. van Nispen, B. Wouters, A. C. Moll, and G. H. van Rens. 2007. Impact of visual impairment on quality of life: A comparison with quality of life in the general population and with other chronic conditions. *Ophthalmic Epidemiology* 14(3):119–126.

Lawrence, V., J. Murray, D. Ffytche, and S. Banerjee. 2009. "Out of sight, out of mind": A qualitative study of visual impairment and dementia from three perspectives. *International Psychogeriatrics* 21(3):511–518.

Lee, D. J., O. Gomez-Marin, B. L. Lam, and D. D. Zheng. 2002. Visual acuity impairment and mortality in U.S. adults. *Archives of Ophthalmology* 120(11):1544–1550.

———. 2003. Visual impairment and unintentional injury mortality: The National Health Interview Survey 1986–1994. *American Journal of Ophthalmology* 136(6): 1152–1154.

Lee, D. J., O. Gomez-Marin, B. L. Lam, D. D. Zheng, K. L. Arheart, S. L. Christ, and A. J. Caban. 2007. Severity of concurrent visual and hearing impairment and mortality: The 1986–1994 National Health Interview Survey. *Journal of Aging Health* 19(3): 382–396.

Lew, H., H. S. Lee, J. Y. Lee, J. Song, K. Min, and M. Kim. 2015. Possible linkage between visual and motor development in children with cerebral palsy. *Pediatric Neurology* 52(3):338–343, e331.

Lin, M. Y., P. R. Gutierrez, K. L. Stone, K. Yaffe, K. E. Ensrud, H. A. Fink, C. A. Sarkisian, A. L. Coleman, and C. M. Mangione. 2004. Vision impairment and combined vision and hearing impairment predict cognitive and functional decline in older women. *Journal of the American Geriatric Society* 52(12):1996–2002.

Lindenberger, U., and P. B. Baltes. 1994. Sensory functioning and intelligence in old age: A strong connection. *Psychology and Aging* 9(3):339–355.

Liu, T., S. Cheung, R. Schuchard, C. Glielmi, X. Hu, S. He, and G. E. Legge. 2010. Incomplete cortical reorganization in macular degeneration. *Investigative Ophthalmology & Visual Science* 51(12):6826–6834.

Liu, Y., C. Yu, M. Liang, J. Li, L. Tian, Y. Zhou, W. Qin, K. Li, and T. Jiang. 2007. Whole brain functional connectivity in the early blind. *Brain* 130(Pt 8):2085–2096.

Lord, S. R. 2006. Visual risk factors for falls in older people. *Age and Ageing* 35(Suppl 2):ii42–ii45.

Lord, S. R., and J. Dayhew. 2001. Visual risk factors for falls in older people. *Journal of the American Geriatric Society* 49(5):508–515.

Lord, S. R., R. D. Clark, and I. W. Webster. 1991. Visual acuity and contrast sensitivity in relation to falls in an elderly population. *Age and Ageing* 20(3):175–181.

Lord, S. R., J. A. Ward, P. Williams, and K. J. Anstey. 1994. Physiological factors associated with falls in older community-dwelling women. *Journal of the American Geriatric Society* 42(10):1110–1117.

Marron, J. A., and I. L. Bailey. 1982. Visual factors and orientation-mobility performance. *American Journal of Optometry and Physiological Optics* 59(5):413–426.

Mazzone, L., F. Ducci, M. C. Scoto, E. Passaniti, V. G. D'Arrigo, and B. Vitiello. 2007. The role of anxiety symptoms in school performance in a community sample of children and adolescents. *BMC Public Health* 7(1):1–6.

Moyer, V. A. 2012. Prevention of falls in community-dwelling older adults: U.S. Preventive Services Task Force Recommendation statement. *Annals of Internal Medicine* 157(3):197–204.

Nevitt, M. C., S. R. Cummings, S. Kidd, and D. Black. 1989. Risk factors for recurrent nonsyncopal falls. A prospective study. *JAMA* 261(18):2663–2668.

O'Day, B. 1999. Employment barriers for people with visual impairments. *Journal of Visual Impairment and Blindness* 93(10):627–642.

Ong, S. Y., M. K. Ikram, B. A. Haaland, C. Y. Cheng, S. M. Saw, T. Y. Wong, and C. Y. Cheung. 2013. Myopia and cognitive dysfunction: The Singapore Malay Eye Study. *Investigative Ophthalmology & Visual Science* 54(1):799–803.

Orta, A. Ö., Z. K. Öztürker, S. Ö. Erkul, Ş. Bayraktar, and O. F. Yilmaz. 2015. The correlation between glaucomatous visual field loss and vision-related quality of life. *Journal of Glaucoma* 24(5):e121–e127.

Park, Y., J. A. Shin, S. W. Yang, H. W. Yim, H. S. Kim, Y.-H. Park, and Epidemiologic Survey Committee of the Korean Ophthalmologic Society. 2015. The relationship between visual impairment and health-related quality of life in Korean adults: The Korea National Health and Nutrition Examination Survey (2008–2012). *PLoS ONE* 10(7):e0132779.

Pascual-Leone, A., A. Amedi, F. Fregni, and L. B. Merabet. 2005. The plastic human brain cortex. *Annual Reviews of Neuroscience* 28:377–401.

Patel, I., K. A. Turano, A. T. Broman, K. Bandeen-Roche, B. Munoz, and S. K. West. 2006. Measures of visual function and percentage of preferred walking speed in older adults: The Salisbury Eye Evaluation project. *Investigative Ophthalmology & Visual Science* 47(1):65–71.

Patino, C. M., R. McKean-Cowdin, S. P. Azen, J. C. Allison, F. Choudhury, and R. Varma. 2010. Central and peripheral visual impairment and the risk of falls and falls with injury. *Ophthalmology* 117(2):199–206, e191.

Pham, T. Q., A. Kifley, P. Mitchell, and J. J. Wang. 2006. Relation of age-related macular degeneration and cognitive impairment in an older population. *Gerontology* 52(6):353–358.

Quigley, H. A., S. D. Cassard, E. W. Gower, P. Y. Ramulu, H. D. Jampel, and D. S. Friedman. 2013. The cost of glaucoma care provided to Medicare beneficiaries from 2002 to 2009. *Ophthalmology* 120(11):2249–2257.

Rees, G., H. W. Tee, M. Marella, E. Fenwick, M. Dirani, and E. L. Lamoureux. 2010. Vision-specific distress and depressive symptoms in people with vision impairment. *Investigative Ophthalmology & Visual Science* 51(6):2891–2896.

Rein, D. B., P. Zhang, K. E. Wirth, P. P. Lee, T. J. Hoerger, N. McCall, R. Klein, J. M. Tielsch, S. Vijan and J. Saaddine. 2006. The economic burden of major adult visual disorders in the United States. *Archives of Ophthalmology* 124(12):1754–1760.

Rein, D. B., K. E. Wirth, C. A. Johnson, and P. P. Lee. 2007. Estimating quality-adjusted life year losses associated with visual field deficits using methodological approaches. *Ophthalmic Epidemiology* 14(4):258–264.

Reyes-Ortiz, C. A., Y. F. Kuo, A. R. DiNuzzo, L. A. Ray, M. A. Raji, and K. S. Markides. 2005. Near vision impairment predicts cognitive decline: Data from the Hispanic Established Populations for Epidemiologic Studies of the Elderly. *Journal of the American Geriatric Society* 53(4):681–686.

Rogers, M. A., and K. M. Langa. 2010. Untreated poor vision: A contributing factor to late-life dementia. *American Journal of Epidemiology* 171(6):728–735.

Roizen, N., K. Kasza, T. Karrison, M. Mets, A. G. Noble, K. Boyer, C. Swisher, P. Meier, J. Remington, and J. Jalbrzikowski. 2006. Impact of visual impairment on measures of cognitive function for children with congenital toxoplasmosis: Implications for compensatory intervention strategies. *Pediatrics* 118(2):e379–e390.

Rovner, B. W., and R. J. Casten. 2002. Activity loss and depression in age-related macular degeneration. *American Journal of Geriatric Psychiatry* 10(3):305–310.

Rovner, B. W., R. J. Casten, and W. S. Tasman. 2002. Effect of depression on vision function in age-related macular degeneration. *Archives of Ophthalmology* 120(8):1041–1044.

Rovner, B. W., R. J. Casten, M. T. Hegel, and W. S. Tasman. 2006. Minimal depression and vision function in age-related macular degeneration. *Ophthalmology* 113(10):1743–1747.

Rovner, B. W., R. J. Casten, M. T. Hegel, R. W. Massof, B. E. Leiby, A. C. Ho, and W. S. Tasman. 2014. Low vision depression prevention trial in age-related macular degeneration. *Ophthalmology* 121(11):2204–2211.

Rubenstein, L. Z., and K. R. Josephson. 2002. The epidemiology of falls and syncope. *Clinical Geriatric Medicine* 18(2):141–158.

Salt, A., and J. Sargent. 2014. Common visual problems in children with disability. *Archives of Disease in Childhood* 99(12):1163–1168.

Saunders, G. H., and K. V. Echt. 2007. An overview of dual sensory impairment in older adults: Perspectives for rehabilitation. *Trends in Amplification* 11(4):243–258.

Sayner, R., D. M. Carpenter, A. L. Robin, S. J. Blalock, K. W. Muir, M. Vitko, M. E. Hartnett, S. D. Lawrence, A. L. Giangiacomo, G. Tudor, J. A. Goldsmith, and B. Sleath. 2015. How glaucoma patient characteristics, self-efficacy and patient-provider communication are associated with eye drop technique. *International Journal of Pharmaceutical Practice* 24(2):78–85.

Schmier, J. K., and J. A. Levine. 2013. Economic impact of progression of age-related macular degeneration. *Acta Ophthalmoligica* 93(2):105–121.

Schneck, M. E., L. A. Lott, G. Haegerstrom-Portnoy, and J. A. Brabyn. 2012. Association between hearing and vision impairments in older adults. *Ophthalmic and Physiological Optics* 32(1):45–52.

Schneider, J. M., B. Gopinath, C. M. McMahon, S. R. Leeder, P. Mitchell, and J. J. Wang. 2011. Dual sensory impairment in older age. *Journal of Aging and Health* 23(8):1309–1324.

Schneider, J., B. Gopinath, C. McMahon, E. Teber, S. R. Leeder, J. J. Wang, and P. Mitchell. 2012. Prevalence and 5-year incidence of dual sensory impairment in an older Australian population. *Annals of Epidemiology* 22(4):295–301.

Souied, E. H., P. Benlian, P. Amouyel, J. Feingold, J. P. Lagarde, A. Munnich, J. Kaplan, G. Coscas, and G. Soubrane. 1998. The epsilon 4 allele of the apolipoprotein E gene as a potential protective factor for exudative age-related macular degeneration. *American Journal of Ophthalmology* 125(3):353–359.

Spahr, J. 2015. *Presentation at second meeting on Public Health Approaches to Promote Eye Health and Reduce Vision Impairment.* Washington, DC.

Steinman, B., A. Nguyen, J. Pynoos, and N. Leland. 2011. Falls-prevention interventions for persons who are blind or visually impaired. *Insight: Research and Practice in Vision Impairment and Blindness* 4:83–91.

Swenor, B. K., B. Munoz, and S. K. West. 2013. Does visual impairment affect mobility over time? The Salisbury Eye Evaluation study. *Investigative Ophthalmology & Visual Science* 54(12):7683–7690.

Tay, T., J. J. Wang, A. Kifley, R. Lindley, P. Newall, and P. Mitchell. 2006. Sensory and cognitive association in older persons: Findings from an older Australian population. *Gerontology* 52(6):386–394.

Tseng, V. L., F. Yu, F. Lum, and A. L. Coleman. 2012. Risk of fractures following cataract surgery in Medicare beneficiaries. *JAMA* 308(5):493–501.

———. 2016. Cataract surgery and mortality in the United States Medicare population. *Ophthalmology*.

U.S. Census Bureau. 2014. American Community Survey (ACS). http://www.census.gov/people/ disability/methodology/acs.html (accessed June 7, 2016).

Varma, R., P. P. Lee, I. Goldberg, and S. Kotak. 2011. An assessment of the health and economic burdens of glaucoma. *American Journal of Ophthalmology* 152(4):515–522.

Vogeli, C., A. E. Shields, T. A. Lee, T. B. Gibson, W. D. Marder, K. B. Weiss, and D. Blumenthal. 2007. Multiple chronic conditions: Prevalence, health consequences, and implications for quality, care management, and costs. *Journal of General and Internal Medicine* 22(Suppl 3):391–395.

Wang, J. J., P. Mitchell, R. G. Cumming, W. Smith, and Blue Mountains Eye Study. 2003. Visual impairment and nursing home placement in older Australians: The Blue Mountains Eye Study. *Ophthalmic Epidemiology* 10(1):3–13.

Whitson, H. E., S. W. Cousins, B. M. Burchett, C. F. Hybels, C. F. Pieper, and H. J. Cohen. 2007. The combined effect of visual impairment and cognitive impairment on disability in older people. *Journal of the American Geriatric Society* 55(6):885–891.

Whitson, H. E., D. Ansah, D. Whitaker, G. Potter, S. W. Cousins, H. MacDonald, C. F. Pieper, L. Landerman, D. C. Steffens, and H. J. Cohen. 2010. Prevalence and patterns of comorbid cognitive impairment in low vision rehabilitation for macular disease. *Archives of Gerontology and Geriatrics* 50(2):209–212.

Whitson, H. E., K. Steinhauser, N. Ammarell, D. Whitaker, S. W. Cousins, D. Ansah, L. L. Sanders, and H. J. Cohen. 2011. Categorizing the effect of comorbidity: A qualitative study of individuals' experiences in a low-vision rehabilitation program. *Journal of the American Geriatric Society* 59(10):1802–1809.

Whitson, H. E., R. Malhotra, A. Chan, D. B. Matchar, and T. Ostbye. 2012a. Comorbid visual and cognitive impairment: Relationship with disability status and self-rated health among older Singaporeans. *Asia Pacific Journal of Public Health* 26(3):310–319.

Whitson, H. E., D. Whitaker, L. L. Sanders, G. G. Potter, S. W. Cousins, D. Ansah, E. McConnell, C. F. Pieper, L. Landerman, D. C. Steffens, and H. J. Cohen. 2012b. Memory deficit associated with worse functional trajectories in older adults in low-vision rehabilitation for macular disease. *Journal of the American Geriatric Society* 60(11):2087–2092.

Whitson, H. E., R. Malhotra, A. Chan, D. B. Matchar, and T. Ostbye. 2014. Comorbid visual and cognitive impairment: Relationship with disability status and self-rated health among older Singaporeans. *Asia Pacific Journal of Public Health* 26(3):310–319.

Wittenborn, J., and D. Rein. 2013. *Cost of vision problems: The economic burden of vision loss and eye disorders in the United States.* Chicago, IL: NORC at the University of Chicago.

———. 2016 (unpublished). *The potential costs and benefits of treatment for undiagnosed eye disorders.* Paper prepared for the Committee on Public Health Approaches to Reduce Vision Impairment and Promote Eye Health. http://www.nationalacademies.org/hmd/~/ media/Files/Report%20Files/2016/UndiagnosedEyeDisordersCommissionedPaper.pdf (accessed September 15, 2016).

Wolff, J. L., B. Starfield, and G. Anderson. 2002. Prevalence, expenditures, and complications of multiple chronic conditions in the elderly. *Archives of Internal Medicine* 162(20):2269–2276.

Wong, T. Y., R. Klein, F. J. Nieto, S. A. Moraes, T. H. Mosley, D. J. Couper, B. E. Klein, L. L. Boland, L. D. Hubbard, and A. R. Sharrett. 2002. Is early age-related maculopathy related to cognitive function? The Atherosclerosis Risk in Communities Study. *American Journal of Ophthalmology* 134(6):828–835.

Woo, S. J., K. H. Park, J. Ahn, J. Y. Choe, H. Jeong, J. W. Han, T. H. Kim, and K. W. Kim. 2012. Cognitive impairment in age-related macular degeneration and geographic atrophy. *Ophthalmology* 119:2094–2101.

Zebardast, N., B. K. Swenor, S. W. van Landingham, R. W. Massof, B. Munoz, S. K. West, and P. Y. Ramulu. 2015. Comparing the impact of refractive and nonrefractive vision loss on functioning and disability. *Ophthalmology* 122(6):1102–1110.

Zhang, S., Y. Liang, Y. Chen, D. C. Musch, C. Zhang, and N. Wang. 2015. Utility analysis of vision-related quality of life in patients with glaucoma and different perceptions from ophthalmologists. *Journal of Glaucoma* 24(7):508–514.

Zheng, D. D., S. L. Christ, B. L. Lam, S. L. Tannenbaum, C. L. Bokman, K. L. Arheart, L. A. McClure, C. A. Fernandez, and D. J. Lee. 2014. Visual acuity and increased mortality: The role of allostatic load and functional status. *Investigative Ophthalmology & Visual Science* 55(8):5144–5150.

4

Surveillance and Research

Surveillance is one of the cornerstones of public health, and it provides the basis for public health decision making (Lee et al., 2010). The World Health Organization defines surveillance as "the continuous, systematic collection, analysis and interpretation of health-related data," and notes that surveillance is critical for determining and monitoring the incidence and distribution of a health issue (WHO, 2016). Sound decisions about public policy and the prioritization of resources depend on having relevant and timely surveillance data. Surveillance of vision impairment and eye health is limited, however, and the lack of adequate surveillance has a substantial impact on public health efforts to address vision problems. The inability to detect and monitor prevalence and trends in the impact of vision impairment and blindness across the United States makes it difficult to characterize the burden of poor eye health among population groups and geographic locations and to then recommend specific effective interventions. A systematic and ongoing collection of relevant data about risk factors, the determinants of visual health, care practices and related health outcomes is needed to determine the nature and extent of the public health burden of eye disease and vision loss; to identify risk factors and at-risk populations; to discover disparities in access, care, and outcomes; and to tailor interventions to the needs of the public (West and Lee, 2012). This report has emphasized the need to prevent, correct, and slow the progression of eye disease; surveillance measures that focus only on an endpoint of vision impairment and blindness without regard to clinical measures that allow for identification of staging of diseases from early to advanced will miss opportunities to halt progression. A surveillance system for visual

163

health may also serve as a valuable source of data for etiologic studies (CDC, 2011a).

Research, which builds on surveillance, includes epidemiologic, behavioral, and laboratory research (Lee et al., 2010). Surveillance data can be used to suggest hypotheses that can be tested in research studies. Typically, such studies about eye health focus on the natural history of eye disease and vision loss, the risk and protective factors for eye disease and vision loss, and comorbidities. From a population health perspective, the role of the social determinants of eye health is important to understand. The relevant social determinants include socioeconomic, cultural, and environmental conditions, as well as social and community networks (Dahlgren and Whitehead, 1991).

Vision impairment and blindness are appropriate targets for surveillance and research because they adversely affect a large portion of the population, affect populations unequally, can be reduced by treatment and preventive efforts, and will become an increasing burden as the population ages (Saaddine et al., 2003). Eye health can be both an ultimate, or an intermediate outcome. It can be an endpoint that results from a malfunction or compromised physiological function of the eye or visual system. In other cases, reduced vision is an intermediate outcome that can signal the presence of underlying or co-existing diseases and conditions. Understanding the risk and protective factors (including treatment), the progression of eye diseases, related outcomes, and disparities associated with eye health for specific populations can, therefore, be used to reduce vision impairment and blindness more efficiently and to improve the overall management and treatment of diseases and conditions that affect population health. The determination of surveillance and research priorities should be similar to those used by Healthy People or Leading Health Indicators.

Surveillance and research on eye health and vision impairment can be used for a number of purposes, including

- Estimating the magnitude of the problem of vision impairment and the preventable burden;
- Understanding the natural history of eye disease from a population health perspective;
- Understanding how specific interventions halt the progression of disease from early to advanced stages;
- Understanding the relationship between risk factors and eye health outcomes;
- Documenting the existence of social determinants and policies affecting visual health;
- Evaluating prevention and control strategies;
- Detecting changes in health practice;

- Assessing the quality of eye care;
- Assessing the impact of occupational health and safety devices;
- Assessing the unmet need for timely care for specific disorders/conditions;
- Planning public health actions and the use of resources; and
- Identifying research needs.

This chapter identifies current surveillance and research methods, including surveys, population-based studies, patient information systems, and meta-analyses, and describes the strengths and limitations of each method. The chapter explores the challenges in obtaining data about eye diseases and vision impairment, and identifies opportunities to improve surveillance and research.

SURVEILLANCE

There is no current surveillance method that accurately and comprehensively measures the total burden of visual impairment and eye disease. Existing data collection methods and tools that are used to measure other health topics often ignore eye health, despite the available options for incorporating eye health measures into the data systems and tools that are used for other purposes. In addition, there is no single surveillance system that allows for the monitoring of prevalence and trends in eye health indicators within and between population groups. Vision health is a critical part of overall health, and the nation's health information system should be able to monitor its epidemiology and treatment patterns in order to improve public health practice.

Surveys

Numerous health-related surveys conducted by the federal government collect information about vision and eye health. (See a sampling of these surveys in Table 4-1.) Several state and regional surveys, such as the California Health Interview Survey, also include questions about eye exams and severe vision problems. These surveys use a variety of methods. For example, the Behavioral Risk Factor Surveillance System (BRFSS) employs a telephone-based survey (either by landline or cell phone), the National Ambulatory Medical Care Survey (NAMCS) uses information collected by clinicians during patient visits, and the National Health and Nutrition Examination Survey (NHANES) consists of both in-person interviews and physical examinations. Although the vision-related questions vary among surveys, most collect relatively little information about vision and eye health as part of the core instruments. The BRFSS, which collects state-level

TABLE 4-1 Select U.S. Department of Health and Human Services Nationwide Population and Organizational Surveys with Vision Components

Survey	Description
Behavioral Risk Factor Surveillance System (BRFSS)	A cross-sectional telephone-based survey that collects information on health conditions and risk factors (Mokdad, 2009). The sample includes about 430,000 adults, and the collected data include demographic variables on race, sex, age, income categories, education level, and the number of children in the household (Mokdad, 2009). Data are continuously collected and released annually.
Medical Expenditure Panel Survey (MEPS)	Annual surveys for families, individuals, medical providers, and employers that are divided into household and insurance components. The surveys collect data on the frequency and usage of specific health services, the costs, how services are paid for, and the characteristics (scope, cost, breadth) of health insurance coverage (AHRQ, 2009).
Medicare Claims Beneficiary Survey (MCBS)	A survey of a representative sample of Medicare beneficiaries that collects data to determine expenditures and the sources of payment, identify types of coverage, and trace the health outcomes and impacts of Medicare program changes (CMS, 2016b).
Monitoring the Future Study (MTF)	An annual survey of 50,000 8th, 10th, and 12th graders that collects data on the behaviors, attitudes, and values of students. A subset of the sample is sent follow-up questionnaires post-graduation (Monitoring the Future, 2016).
National Ambulatory Medical Care Survey (NAMCS)	An annual survey that collects information about the use of ambulatory medical services in the United States based on the results from office-based physicians, who provide data on symptoms, diagnoses, medications, patient demographics, diagnostic procedures, and planned future treatment (CDC, 2015a).
National Health and Nutrition Examination Survey (NHANES)	A program of studies conducted every 2 years among 5,000 individuals that includes an interview of demographic, socioeconomic, dietary, and health-related questions; an examination that consists of medical, dental, and physiological measurements; and laboratory tests (CDC, 2015c).
National Health Interview Survey (NHIS)	An annual survey that collects data from about 75,000 to 100,000 individuals of all ages. Surveys include a set of basic health and demographic items, and one or more sets of questions on current health matters from the noninstitutionalized civilian population (CDC Foundation, 2015).
National Hospital Ambulatory Medical Care Survey (NHAMCS)	Data are collected from hospital emergency, outpatient departments and ambulatory surgical centers during a randomly assigned 4-week reporting period. Staff are instructed on the completion of a patient record form that collects demographic data, complaints, source of payment, diagnoses, procedures, providers seen, cause of the injury, and characteristics of the facility (CDC, 2015a).

TABLE 4-1 Continued

Survey	Description
National Hospital Care Survey (NHCS)	A survey that describes patterns of hospital-based care delivery integrated with the NHAMCS, allowing episodes of care to be linked between different settings. Hospital-level characteristics, electronic health data, and abstracted clinical information are collected in this survey (CDC, 2015d).
National Hospital Discharge Survey (NHDS)	Annual collection of data through survey forms or from purchased computerized data files from 1965 to 2010, which was replaced with the NHCS in 2011. The surveys collected information on the characteristics of patients discharged from nonfederal, short-stay hospitals. These data included personal characteristics, the source of payment, admission and discharge dates, medical diagnoses, and procedures (CDC, 2015b).
National Notifiable Disease Surveillance System (NNDSS)	A national surveillance system used by public health officials to monitor, control, and prevent the transmission and occurrence of nationally notifiable communicable and noncommunicable diseases. This information is collected from providers, laboratories, and hospitals (CDC, 2015f).
National Profile of Local Health Departments (NPLHD)	A Web-based survey of local health departments (LHDs) in the United States (with the exception of Rhode Island and Hawaii). It is periodically conducted by the National Association of County and City Health Officials, and it collects information about LHDs' organization, responsibilities, workforce, funding, jurisdictional information, and core competencies (NACCHO, 2014).
National Survey of Children with Special Health Care Needs (NS-CSHCN)	A national survey of a sample size of about 40,000 children that explores the extent to which identified children with special health care needs have medical homes, adequate health insurance, access to needed services, and adequate care coordination. The survey includes questions regarding a child's need for eyeglasses or vision care and whether the need was met (CAHMI, 2016b).
National Survey of Children's Health (NSCH)	The survey examines the physical and emotional health of about 100,000 children ages 0 to 17 years throughout the United States. Special emphasis is placed on factors that may relate to well-being of children, including medical homes, family interactions, parental health, school and after-school experiences, and safe neighborhoods. In 2011, survey administration included two questions to ascertain whether a child had been screened or examined. The survey is sponsored by the Maternal and Child Health Bureau of the Health Resources and Services Administration. In 2017, this survey will be integrated with the National Survey of Children with Special Health Care Needs (CAHMI, 2016a).
National Vital Statistics System-Mortality (NVSS-M)	A source of geographic, demographic, and cause-of-death information collected through the collaboration of inter-government agencies. The data are collected from registration systems legally responsible for the processing of vital life events, with software available to automate the coding of medical information on the death certificate (CDC, 2016c).

continued

TABLE 4-1 Continued

Survey	Description
National Worksite Health Promotion Survey (NWHPS)	A nationally representative, cross-sectional telephone survey of employee health promotion programs, categorized by organization size and industry. Its key measures include worksite size, industry, how long the promotion program has been maintained internally, and barriers to offering a health promotion program. It has been conducted four times in 1985, 1992, 1999, and 2004 (Linnan et al., 2008).
Survey of Income and Program Participation (SIPP)	A series of national panels surveying from 14,000 to 52,000 interviewed households, with each panel lasting 2.5 to 4.0 years, the most recent having begun in February 2014. The panels collect data related to types of income, labor force participation, social program participation and eligibility, and general demographic characteristics in order to estimate coverage and outcomes of government programs (U.S. Census Bureau, 2016).

data and samples about 400,000 people annually, asked one vision question in the 2014 core questionnaire: "Are you blind or do you have serious difficulty seeing, even when wearing glasses?" An optional diabetes module that has questions about eye exams and whether diabetes has affected the respondent's eyes, and an optional vision module that was used from 2005 to 2010 asked about difficulty seeing, the receipt of eye exams, and diagnosed eye diseases. The National Health Interview Survey (NHIS) collects nationally representative data on nearly 100,000 respondents, using questions similar to BRFSS. A vision supplement was administered in 2002 and 2008. NHANES, which collects data on a representative sample of about 5,000 participants, is the only national survey that includes an objective, clinical measure of vision impairment (visual acuity of 20/50 or worse in the better-seeing eye) (Vitale et al., 2006). In addition, the NHANES examination has at times included components designed to measure the presence of eye diseases and conditions. For example, the 2005–2006 examination utilized two ophthalmological components in addition to vision measurements. Frequency doubling technology was used to test for visual field loss from diseases such as glaucoma, while the retinal imaging exam tested for retinal conditions such as diabetic retinopathy and age-related macular degeneration (AMD) (CDC, 2015e). However, NHANES has not conducted eye examinations or asked eye-related questions since 2008 (CDC, 2015e). In addition to information about vision and eye disease, these surveys collect demographic information and data about comorbidities and health risk factors.

These surveillance systems and the data collection instruments they use are powerful tools for measuring the prevalence of vision impairment and eye disease, along with the associated risk factors and outcomes. Because surveys use representative and often large samples, the results can be generalized to the noninstitutionalized population. Because the surveys are usually conducted annually, the resulting data can be used to document trends over time. However, there are limitations to these data: the metrics vary among surveys, most surveys rely on self-reported data, data on vision and eye disease are collected and reported relatively infrequently, and few surveys can provide information at a local level. Because of these limitations, a survey that produces vision-related data that is timely, representative, and standardized remains an unmet goal in advancing eye health.

The following methodological issues constitute the key challenges in constructing a national surveillance strategy. First, the metrics used to assess vision impairment and eye disease vary among surveys. There are no standardized survey questions to measure vision or eye health, and, as a result, estimates of vision impairment and prevalence of eye diseases vary significantly. Surveys may use objective clinical measures (NHANES) or self-reported assessments (BRFSS, NHIS). Surveys may ask a general question such as "Do you have serious difficulty seeing?" (BRFSS core questionnaire), or may use specific scenarios to assess distance and near vision acuity, such as whether the respondent has difficulty reading the print in a newspaper or recognizing a friend across the street (BRFSS vision module). Publications that use these data to define visual impairment may use any of these metrics or a combination of them. The eye conditions that are studied in these surveys are generally limited to AMD, diabetic retinopathy, cataracts, and glaucoma, even though there are other common and disabling conditions (Wittenborn and Rein, 2016).

Because the survey questions, definitions, and measurements differ across surveys, it is challenging to compare visual impairment and eye disease estimates across surveillance systems. As a result, simple questions such as "How many people are blind?" are difficult to answer, and the estimates vary widely (Wittenborn and Rein, 2016). In addition to the issue of the standardization of questions to measure eye-related conditions, NHANES, BRFSS, and NHIS pose demographic and comorbidity-related questions in ways that may prompt different answers from the same individual (Zambelli-Weiner et al., 2012).

Second, most surveys rely on self-reported answers to a small number of questions. While these types of less resource-intensive surveys yield a large, representative sample size, self-reported information can be unreliable, especially because vision impairment is difficult to assess via survey questions. For example, the BRFSS vision module provides five options for reporting the degree of difficulty in reading a newspaper or seeing a friend across the street: no difficulty, a little difficulty, moderate difficulty, extreme difficulty, and unable to do. It may not be easy for respondents to choose an answer from a spectrum of responses, and evidence suggests that individuals are not good at assessing their own vision (Wittenborn and Rein, 2016). The data gleaned from these survey responses provide an estimate of the prevalence of visual impairment, but the estimate is likely not as precise as would be an estimate obtained from a surveillance tool that uses clinical examinations to measure visual impairment.

Third, the frequency of data collection and reporting makes some surveys less suitable for recognizing trends or evaluating changes due to interventions. For example, NHANES data are collected annually but datasets and estimates are released only every 2 years in staggered amounts to accommodate the volume of data (CDC, 2015g). NAMCS and the National Hospital Ambulatory Medical Care Survey (NHAMCS) disseminate reports 24 months after data have been collected. Vision-specific data are not routinely or frequently collected. For example, NHIS had a vision supplement only in 2002 and 2008, NHANES has not consistently collected vision data since 2008, and the BRFSS vision module was discontinued after 2010.

Patient Data

Electronic Health Records

An enormous potential for surveillance exists in electronic health records (EHRs) from clinical providers. These records provide the most detailed health care data available, including examination and testing outcomes, diagnoses, procedures conducted, and services utilized (Rein, 2015). Public health programs in particular have the opportunity to benefit greatly from this newly available electronic health information, which has the potential to become a crucial component of surveillance. Public health practitioners need to leverage this electronic revolution by being innovative in their use of new and existing electronic data sources. For health departments, the use of EHR systems may be the next frontier in chronic disease surveillance (Maylahn, 2013). However, while EHRs present a huge opportunity to understand local conditions, access to these databases is often limited and can be proprietary. Local health department staff may not be able to make use of the data or may not have staff who can spend time analyzing the data.

The American Academy of Ophthalmology launched an ophthalmology electronic clinical registry, IRIS™ (Intelligent Research in Sight), in 2014. The IRIS registry collects uniform data, both clinical and patient-reported information, that can be analyzed to inform clinical decision making. IRIS captures data from 80 percent of U.S. ophthalmology practices

(Parke, 2015). As of January 2016, the IRIS registry represented data from 14 million unique patients (Parke et al., 2016).

Similarly, the American Optometric Association's Measures and Outcomes Registry for Eyecare (MORE), a clinical data registry launched in 2015, integrated EHR data from multiple systems to facilitate reporting for Centers for Medicare & Medicaid Services' (CMS's) Physician Quality Reporting System, and created an evidence base for future clinical decisions and research directions (AOA, 2015).

CMS has approved both IRIS and MORE as Qualified Clinical Data Registries, making substantial data available not only for quality reporting and CMS initiatives such as the EHR incentive program or the Value-based Payment Modifier program, but also for research utility through tracking outcomes and comparing clinical practice data (CMS, 2016a). However, Rein has cautioned that differences may exist between the clinical practices represented in the database and other populations of interest (i.e., populations without access to treatment) (Rein, 2015). In addition to IRIS and MORE, there are other commercial and not-for-profit sources of EHR data available, such as Epic Systems, though few of the data are related to vision or eye health (Rein, 2015).

Administrative Claims

Administrative claims from private insurers, Medicare, or Medicaid are a source of surveillance data about vision and eye-related health status and care utilization. Claims data rely on billing codes that indicate whether a service or procedure was performed or whether a patient received a diagnosis. These data are limited by the lack of detail inherent in billing codes and the possibility of human error in coding (Rein, 2015). Diagnostic codes may be too broad or too narrow, leading to under- or over-reporting of eye conditions (Elliott et al., 2012). However, administrative claims have many advantages versus other data sources. Data may be available over time for the same patient, provided that he or she remains enrolled in the same insurance plan (Rein, 2015). Large care providers, such as CMS or the U.S. Department of Veterans Affairs, have data that are representative of the subpopulations they serve (Elliott, 2012). Data from private insurers are not necessarily representative of the general population, but there are a few sources of data that include many patients. These include the MarketScan™ research databases, which are commercial products offering fully integrated patient-level data from more than 170 million patients, and claims from Vision Service Plan (VSP) vision and eye care insurance, which include acuity readings and cover 77 million patients (Truven Health Analytics, 2016; VSP, 2016).

Medicare data in particular have utility for surveillance. Medicare covers nearly all of the over-65 population. Medicare claims provide longitudinal data, because people generally stay enrolled in Medicare from age 65 on. The large amount of data available in Medicare claims allows for examination of lower-incidence conditions (Elliott et al., 2012). Medicare data have been used for a number of studies, including an analysis of 9 years of data to estimate how many beneficiaries with diabetes and chronic eye diseases receive annual eye exams (Lee et al., 2003).

Patient information from EHRs or administrative claims as a source of surveillance data has an advantage over data from surveys or research studies because it is real-world data collected in real time: it captures diagnostic information, how care is actually being provided, and the outcomes of that care (Elliott et al., 2012). However, these data are only collected when patients present themselves for care and therefore do not include information about the people who cannot or will not use clinical care. In addition, no one source of patient data covers the entirety of eye care. Services may be provided by optometrists, ophthalmologists, or general practitioners, and vision care is often paid for out of pocket or with separate vision insurance (Wittenborn and Rein, 2016). This division among multiple health and payment systems means that in order to get the full picture of eye care, patient data will have to be gathered from multiple sources.

Challenges

Although there is considerable quantitative and qualitative information about vision impairment and eye health available from myriad sources—surveys, EHRs, and administrative claims—each of these sources has its limitations. There is no existing surveillance system that systematically collects data to track prevalence, the incidence of new cases, and disparities in vision health in order to identify the causes of these disparities, to determine the stage of eye disease progression, and to develop and "monitor public health initiatives, programs, and policies aimed at reducing the burden of visual impairment and eye disease and eliminating existing disparities" (CDC, 2011a, p. 8). The lack of a comprehensive system is a major impediment to identifying and addressing the challenges and opportunities for public health action.

Vision and eye health surveillance is constrained by a number of overarching challenges. There are problems with data quality and collection, including a lack of standardized definitions to allow comparisons. Some populations—including groups that may be most at risk—are not captured by current surveillance methods. Technical and organizational challenges impede the integration of data sources and surveillance systems. Finally, there is a lack of sustained support for surveillance activities at the federal level, and very limited support at state and local levels.

Scope and Quality of Data

Vision surveillance suffers from the limited scope of data that are available at the national, state, and local levels. National and state surveys and patient data systems collect some information about the presence of eye disease and vision impairment, but they fail to measure many other factors linked to visual impairment or eye disease. None of the surveillance methods discussed above measures the total burden of vision impairment and blindness, which includes the extent of visual acuity loss; the presence and stage of specific eye disease, comorbidities, and health-risk behaviors; social or physical limitations imposed by low vision; quality of life (QOL) measures; and the existence of barriers to accessing health care and rehabilitation services. Most surveillance focuses primarily on prevalence and incidence, and instruments do not usually measure factors such as access to care, barriers to the use of care, health literacy, or access to assistance, all of which may greatly affect the health and QOL of a person with visual impairment or eye disease (Wittenborn and Rein, 2016).

The lack of standardized measures of vision impairment, eye health, and related health indicators also impairs the collection and analysis of surveillance data. No gold standard method of measuring vision impairment or the presence of eye disease has been developed or evaluated (Crews, 2015). Furthermore, current evaluation methods fall short of providing a comprehensive understanding of the impact of vision impairment and blindness. For example, the most commonly used instrument to assess vision-related QOL in the eye health literature is the National Eye Institute Visual Function Questionnaire (VFQ-25), although many other measurement approaches and instruments are in use (Heintz et al., 2012; Hirneiss, 2014; Mangione et al., 2001). Psychometric flaws have been noted concerning the VFQ-25 in its original structure, and other versions have been developed (Kowalski et al., 2012; Pesudovs et al., 2010). While generic QOL instruments capture some aspects of vision-related QOL, scales that only include items related to visual acuity or central vision are unlikely to capture the QOL impact of visual field deficits.

Consequently, surveys do not use the same metrics, and the ones that they use are not necessarily correlated with the clinical definitions coded in EHR and claims data. Standardized measures are difficult to implement in part because vision loss is not an all-or-nothing concept. The loss of sight occurs across a continuum, with varying degrees of impairment and functionality. Vision may be assessed with any number of measures, including acuity, contrast sensitivity, visual field, or night vision (Wittenborn and

Rein, 2016). There is no consensus on how vision impairment should be defined, so it is measured in different ways in different surveillance instruments (Wittenborn and Rein, 2016). Likewise, eye conditions can vary from minor to fatal and can be short-lived or chronic; this complexity makes it difficult to identify which conditions to include in surveillance and how. Because visual impairment and eye disease are often undiagnosed, a surveillance instrument that relies on self-reported diagnosis to identify people with eye disease may underestimate prevalence (Wittenborn and Rein, 2016). One population-based study analyzing the agreement between self-reported data and medical record for prevalence of eye disease and eye care utilization suggested national estimates tended to underestimate rates of eye disease and overestimate eye care utilization (MacLennan et al., 2013).

Limited Local Data

Although national surveillance collects information about vision impairment and eye health, there are limited data available at the local level, where interventions and policy decisions are often developed and implemented. The BRFSS provides state estimates, but the data are not broken down further by county or municipality, while other national surveys such as NHIS and NHANES provide only national or regional estimates (IOM, 2011). Increasingly, states and local communities are investing resources for data collection at the county level or in local jurisdictions. This trend has accelerated with the new requirements in the Patient Protection and Affordable Care Act of 2010 that tax-exempt hospitals must conduct an assessment of the health needs of their catchment areas and begin to address them (Rosenbaum and Margulies, 2011). This requirement builds on current best practices of hospitals and hospital systems, which include the strategic investment of resources and the building of community partnerships, including local groups and leaders in public health, with the goal of improving overall community health. Every 3 years, hospitals must conduct community health needs assessments (CHNAs). These coincide with assessments done by local health departments and others in the community. The goals of these assessments are to "identify existing health care resources and prioritize community health needs" (Stoto, 2013, p. 4). Each hospital also must develop an implementation strategy to meet the needs identified by its CHNA and a set of performance measures to track progress (Stoto, 2013). These actions must be reported to the Internal Revenue Service using Schedule H of Form 990 as an obligation for tax exemption. At the same time, the Public Health Accreditation Board established prerequisites of national accreditation for local health departments, including having completed a community health assessment, community health improvement plan, and an agency-wide strategic plan within the past 5 years (CDC, 2016d; PHAB, 2016; Riley et al., 2012). Data about the risk factors for eye disease and vision loss could be collected as part of these assessments, but eye-related issues must compete against the constellation of other public health problems present in communities.

One opportunity to improve the availability of local data involves combining data from community surveys with data from state and local surveillance systems to characterize patterns of risk, health outcomes, and relevant determinants. An example is the public health surveillance of cancer, in which data about cancer risk factors can be supplemented with information from cancer registries. Using geographic information system methods, data from different sources can be linked to help guide local cancer screening and treatment programs targeting high-risk or underserved communities (Birkhead and Maylahn, 2010). For vision surveillance, survey estimates of vision indicators can be augmented with clinical information about eye disease to produce a more complete picture of the eye health in a local community.

Availability of Data

Because public health surveillance is motivated by the public's concerns about a health issue, its impact on various groups, and what can be done to address it, surveillance data need to be made available, analyzed, and disseminated in a timely manner. However, as discussed above, some surveys collect and disseminate data infrequently. Furthermore, data on eye and vision health are often inaccessible to those who are not subject-matter experts, and it may be difficult for a policy maker or member of the public to easily find accurate estimates of vision impairment or eye disease (Wittenborn and Rein, 2016).

Populations Not Captured

The surveillance of visual impairment and eye disease, whether conducted by surveys or patient information databases, inevitably fails to include or represent some groups of people. For example, surveillance that relies on patient data, as found in EHRs or administrative claims, excludes people who are outside of the traditional clinical health system and who may be uninsured, underserved, or part of at-risk populations. People who cannot speak English may be underrepresented in surveys. While most national surveys that are conducted via interviews accommodate non-English speakers through the use of translators or bilingual interviewers, many of these services are restricted to the Spanish language or are only available in areas containing large numbers of non-English speaking respondents (Islam et al.,

2010). Low-resource communities—including rural, homeless, and undocumented populations—may be excluded from surveys and studies because they are difficult to contact. For example, the BRFSS, because it collects data by telephone, necessarily samples only those people who have access to a telephone. There are myriad ways in which surveillance methods fail to capture some populations; new or improved surveillance instruments should be designed to mitigate this as much as possible.

Lack of Integration Between Clinical and Public Health Data

Data from surveys and other population-based surveillance conducted by federal, state, and local public health agencies can contribute relevant information about eye health, especially for the country as a whole. Likewise, there is an abundance of data collected during patient health care visits that can be accessed from EHRs or administrative claims. Integrating these surveillance systems would allow for a more comprehensive picture of visual health. However, major constraints prevent this information from being aggregated or shared to create richer and more useful data. For example, there are technical constraints, including software incompatibility and lack of interoperability of datasets. Commercial and legal constraints affect data sharing and availability. Perhaps most importantly, coordination and collaboration among surveillance actors are limited. As a result, the nation lacks standard metrics for measuring vision impairment and eye health, there are limited sources for baseline data that can be used in surveillance and research, and significant hurdles stand in the way of integration or sharing between surveillance systems. Data that could be used to improve public health practice and clinical care are instead fragmented and siloed (CDC, 2011a).

Modest Funding Support

Vision and eye health surveillance efforts have received only modest attention and support from federal agencies. Several federal programs focus on eye health, including the National Eye Institute (NEI) and the National Eye Health Education Program (NEHEP) at the National Institutes of Health (NIH), and the Vision Health Initiative (VHI), which is housed in the Division of Diabetes Translation at the Centers for Disease Control and Prevention (CDC). These programs tend to emphasize research and education rather than surveillance activities. More recently, the NIH has begun to focus more heavily on genomics and personalized medicine than on population-level health. While these NIH research priorities are valuable in generating new knowledge, they may not offer the same potential impact as population-wide interventions and more traditional public health approaches to disease, which include the monitoring and tracking of diseases to identify populations at risk and how interventions affect subgroups.

Over the past several years, funding for eye-related activities at the NIH and the CDC has remained fairly constant or has dropped slightly. The NEI funding,[1] representing about 2 percent of all NIH funding, has remained around $700 million since 2010 (NIH, 2015). At the CDC, since 2010 the annual budget for the VHI has declined in both total amount and as a percentage of the overall CDC budget. The proportion of the VHI budget allocated to glaucoma-specific activities has remained relatively constant—at 86 percent—since 2011 (CDC, 2011b, 2012, 2013, 2014, 2016b). Funding and staffing for community surveillance activities is limited as well. Funding for local health departments has been cut on the federal, state, and local levels in recent years, and as a result, thousands of public health jobs have been eliminated (NACCHO, 2015).

However, integrating vision and eye components into the Multi-Ethnic Study of Atherosclerosis (MESA) was a way to "conduct surveillance by leveraging a relatively small investment of funds to build on an extensive existing study infrastructure" (Cotch, 2016, p. E1). MESA was originally designed as a multicenter community-based study on cardiovascular disease, risk factors, and outcomes in four different ethnic and racial groups (MESA, 2016a). Retinal photography and a refraction assessment were added to the study, and the inclusion of these components introduced access to the data collected from the rest of the study on comorbid conditions, genetic profiles, behaviors, and multiple health outcomes, with the potential of providing a broader, comprehensive picture of health (Cotch, 2016; MESA, 2016b). Research from the initiative included a study that published prevalence rates of AMD by age, gender, and four racial and ethnic groups using objective, clinical measures as the means to collect data (Klein et al., 2006).

RESEARCH

Surveillance is used to collect essential data on the prevalence of vision impairment and eye disease, the presence of risk factors, and details about the populations affected. Research builds on this data but is distinct in that it may include additional data on the causes and risk factors associated with vision impairment and eye disease, such as socioeconomic status, the presence of comorbidities, and access to eye care, and it may be used to

---

[1] Funding reported is the actual amount from the Congressional Appropriations, prior to obligations for HIV research and transfer costs.

identify correlations or causation between these factors and disease. Surveillance can lead to the identification of research gaps and helps justify the resources for research (Lee et al., 2012). As discussed earlier in this report, there is an urgent need for more research on vision health, including basic, clinical, applied, and translational research. Particularly important for the health of the population will be research that elucidates the effectiveness of population health interventions in preventing and reducing eye disease by addressing the underlying social determinants of health and primary and secondary prevention. Research can be performed by collecting original data, or through an analysis of existing data.

Types of Research

Analysis of Surveillance Data

Surveillance data, such as data from surveys, can be used to answer research questions by combining data from studies that compare vision and eye disease to other factors such as socioeconomic status, race and ethnicity, or geographic area. For example, Chou and colleagues (2012) used several years of BRFSS data in order to assess the prevalence of annual eye care among diabetic adults who were visually impaired, analyzed by state, race and ethnicity, education, and annual income. Participants were defined as "visually impaired" if they indicated that they had moderate or severe difficulty reading print or recognizing a friend across the street. Zhang and colleagues (2012) combined data from NHANES and NHIS in order to explore disparities in vision health by race and ethnicity, education, and economic status. Kirtland and colleagues (2015) analyzed American Community Survey data to describe the geographic pattern of severe vision loss and to assess its association with poverty level. These types of analyses allow researchers to stretch the utility of survey data by combining and comparing data across years and surveys. However, the ability to conduct meta-analyses is constrained because of the limitations of surveys discussed above: metrics that vary from survey to survey, reliance on self-reported data, and infrequent data collection and reporting.

Population-Based Community Studies

Population-based community studies are the "backbone of eye disease epidemiological knowledge" (Wittenborn and Rein, 2016). This type of research collects detailed information about a specific population. The population can be defined in a variety of ways—for example, by geographic area (e.g., Framingham Heart Study or Baltimore Eye Survey), ethnic group (e.g., Chinese American Eye Study), or occupation (e.g., Nurses' Health

Study)—and the population may be studied either in its entirety or by a representative sample. Population-based community studies can be either ongoing and long-term, or one-time assessments of a population.

Ongoing population-based community studies can provide valuable insight into the life course of a disease and the relationship of risk factors to disease outcomes. These prospective cohort studies collect a wide variety of data over a period of time from the same population. One of the longest-running eye studies is the Beaver Dam Eye Study, which began in 1988 with baseline examinations of nearly all of the 43- to 84-year-old residents of Beaver Dam, Wisconsin (about 5,000 initial participants) (Beaver Dam Eye Study, 2014). Researchers conducted follow-up examinations every 5 years on all cohort members (more than 1,900 in each follow-up period), resulting in more than 300 publications of the study findings. The study observed the natural history of several eye diseases, tracked the decline in vision as participants aged, and measured the relationship between eye conditions and long-term exposures such as blood pressure levels (Beaver Dam Eye Study, 2014). The Rotterdam Study in the Netherlands, another population-based community cohort study, has been collecting information on thousands of residents of Rotterdam since 1990 and is focused on cardiovascular, neurological, endocrine, and ophthalmological diseases (Hofman et al., 2007).

In addition to these long-term community studies, researchers also conduct one-time assessments of specific populations. For example, the Chinese American Eye Study sought to understand the prevalence of visual impairment and eye disease in Chinese Americans living in Monterey Park, California. Each of the 4,570 participants completed a questionnaire about health- and eye-related behaviors, risk factors, and their QOL, and underwent a clinical examination (Varma et al., 2013).

The main limitation to population-based community studies is the potential for differences between the study population and the general population and thus a lack of generalizability (IOM, 2011). Because the population studied is usually a specific group of people, rather than a representative sample of the general population, data about prevalence or risk factors may not be applicable to people outside the group. Moreover, respondents may differ from nonrespondents even in the population studied. However, these types of studies also have significant benefits. The data are usually based on examinations rather than on self-reporting, so prevalence and incidence numbers may be more accurate (Wittenborn and Rein, 2016). Using a prospective cohort allows researchers to draw correlations between disease outcomes and behavioral or environmental factors, while minimizing selection and recall bias (Kukull and Ganguli, 2012). In addition, in those cases when the participation of the cohort is ongoing, researchers can return to the cohort repeatedly for clinical examinations, biomarker measurements, or new areas of investigation. This study method can be optimal for collecting information about a minority group. For example, because the Chinese American Eye Study selected its participants from the U.S. city with the highest percentage of Chinese Americans, it was less time- and resource-intensive than drawing a representative sample of Chinese Americans from across the United States. While the results may not be generalizable to the entire U.S. population, the information may be used to estimate prevalence and health issues in the U.S. Chinese American population using census data (Rein, 2015).

Meta-Analysis of Population-Based Studies

The meta-analysis of population-based studies can provide insight into links between vision and eye health and other factors. The findings of individual population-based studies may not be applicable to the general population; however, if the results can be replicated across multiple studies, the validity and generalizability are strengthened (Kukull and Ganguli, 2012). In order to replicate findings, the studies must use the same standardized measurements and outcomes so that the data can be compared. The Beaver Dam Eye Study developed an imaging system and a standardized scale for the severity of certain eye conditions that were subsequently used in several other population-based community studies. As a result, it has been possible to compare data among these multiple studies and draw more robust conclusions from the findings. For example, the Beaver Dam Eye Study found an association between smoking and the development of cataract and AMD. Two other ongoing studies using the same system and scale—the Blue Mountains Eye Study in Australia and the Rotterdam Study in the Netherlands—found the same correlation, despite differences in the populations (The Board of Regents of the University of Wisconsin System, 2014). Similarly, a collaborative study between the Multi-Ethnic Pediatric Eye Disease Study and the Baltimore Pediatric Eye Disease Study used the same protocol and measurements to collect information on vision impairment from more than 10,000 children. The population studied lived in Los Angeles or Baltimore and included large percentages of minority children (44 percent African American and 32 percent Hispanic) (NEI/NIH, 2011). By using the same protocol on a large, diverse study population, researchers increased the generalizability of the results.

Vision Problems in the U.S. (VPUS), a project of Prevent Blindness America, is a meta-analysis of 12 population-based studies, including the 3 discussed above. VPUS uses the data from these studies, along with census data, to develop age-, race-, and sex-specific prevalence estimates on both the national and state levels (VPUS, 2012). The VPUS online database allows users to customize a research inquiry; for example, a user could compare glaucoma rates in black females between three different states, or look at vision impairment by age in California. VPUS has estimates for four eye conditions (AMD, cataract, diabetic retinopathy, and glaucoma) and four categories of vision (vision impairment, blindness, hyperopia, and myopia). While VPUS provides valuable, easy-to-understand information about vision and eye disease, there are several limitations to the data. The studies on which VPUS relies may not be representative of the current U.S. population—all of the study populations were from small geographic areas and were not probabilistically sampled, 5 of the 12 studies are international, and some of the data are up to 30 years old (Wittenborn and Rein, 2016). Furthermore, the scope of the VPUS data is limited, with data on only four eye disorders and no information on rates of under-diagnosis of eye conditions (Wittenborn and Rein, 2016).

Population Health Administrative Databases

Databases that link information from different sources at an individual level can be a useful tool for population-based research. Population health databases are used to track the health of a population of interest based on agreed-upon metrics. Although these databases rarely include measures specific to eye health, they may contain measures that are risk factors for poor eye health. For example, America's Health Rankings includes indicators on diabetes, high blood pressure, and smoking, all of which may affect eye health. These types of databases, which also include Healthy People 2020, Community Health Status Indicators, and data collected by the Trust for America's Health, can be linked to eye-specific databases in order to answer research questions about relationships between eye health and environmental, behavioral, or other risk factors.

Challenges

Although there are many potential avenues for conducting eye-related population health research, there are several challenges. First, there is no existing research database that includes comprehensive information about visual impairment and eye health, as well as comorbidities, QOL, and other issues that are affected by and affect eye health. The major population health databases do not include information about eye health, and eye-specific databases usually do not include general health information. As discussed above, VPUS is a valuable source of research data, but it is limited by the scope of the data. While it is possible to triangulate data between databases, a truly comprehensive database would allow for more in-depth, accurate research.

Second, there is limited coordination or integration among the research efforts of federal government agencies and private players. The federal government supports basic, clinical, applied, and translational research on vision and eye health, but this support is spread across multiple agencies. Eye-related research is supported by agencies including the Health Resources and Services Administration (HRSA), CMS, and the U.S. Department of Veterans Affairs. The NIH's support is spread across several institutes and programs including the NEI, NEHEP, the National Institute of Diabetes and Digestive and Kidney Diseases, and the National Institute of Minority Health and Health Disparities. VHI at the CDC has made an effort to create a coordinated public health framework for blindness and vision impairment and has promoted the inclusion of eye-related measures in the BRFSS and the NHANES (CDC, 2016a). However, there is no entity responsible for coordinating eye-related research, and federal budget support for eye and vision research has been fairly constant or has fluctuated. In the private sector, several organizations support population health eye research, including Research to Prevent Blindness, the Association for Research in Vision and Ophthalmology (ARVO), and the National Alliance for Eye and Vision Research. These organizations provide funding to researchers to perform basic clinical, applied, and translational research about eye disease and vision impairment. However, there is no coordinating body or national agenda to help integrate and prioritize these activities, and thus each agency or organization operates independently. On the local level, public health departments suffer from low funding, a plethora of competing demands, and a lack of coordination and leadership.

OPPORTUNITIES

Surveillance System

The United States needs a well-designed surveillance system that continuously collects, analyzes, and reports on population data in a standardized, timely, and continuous manner that accurately represents the population of interest (Lee et al., 2012; West and Lee, 2012; Zambelli-Weiner et al., 2012). Building this system from the local jurisdiction up would help ensure that the work of local, state, and federal public health agencies is coordinated and focused, and that the insights derived from the system can be widely and effectively disseminated. Standardization of the definitions, data elements, and collection methods would allow for comparisons among datasets that could validate the surveillance measures, strengthen evidence, and expand findings. More timely dissemination of surveillance data would enable decision makers to deploy resources in an expedient manner to better address the needs of at-risk populations. Representative sampling is essential to the methodological rigor and accuracy of surveillance findings, and it allows public health professionals to design appropriate and targeted interventions.

Steps have been taken to begin the process of creating a Visual Health Surveillance System. The CDC awarded a grant to investigators at NORC at the University of Chicago to develop a system that will produce new estimates for important eye health risk factors and outcomes including the use of eye care, as well as standardized visual health indicators and other resources for researchers (Rein, 2015). There are other opportunities to move forward in developing a comprehensive surveillance system; (1) Current surveillance methods, particularly national surveys, can be expanded and enhanced in order to better measure the total burden of eye disease and visual impairment and their impact in communities. National surveys should include eye-related questions in the core questionnaire each year, and eye examinations should be reincorporated into routine surveillance; (2) Clinical and public health data can be combined in a more integrated approach, taking advantage of recent developments in methods of measurement and technology; and (3) Collaboration and coordination can be increased among the surveillance community so that data and other resources are used more efficiently.

In addition to expanding and enhancing current surveillance instruments, surveillance should include other variables that would likely be helpful in identifying and characterizing important risk and protective factors for poor eye health. For example, along with prevalence and incidence data, a surveillance instrument could collect information on the determinants of eye health, including social and environmental determinants, and the impacts of eye disease and vision impairment. Given the stagnation in NIH and CDC funding for eye-related activities, it is difficult to imagine that new surveillance activities specific only to eye health and vision impairment would be sufficiently comprehensive. However, population health databases that track these types of variables are available and could be used to supplement vision-specific surveillance activities.

Opportunities to integrate and harmonize clinical and public health data into surveillance systems should be actively explored. As discussed above, a necessary first step toward integration will be the standardization of surveillance methods and tools used to collect surveillance data. The data elements are often not consistent across measurement approaches and may not align with the diagnostic criteria used by clinicians. Without standardization, it may not be possible to completely integrate these sources. However, efforts could be made to harmonize the data by identifying similar data elements in each instrument and linking these elements across instruments in order to compare and analyze the data (Wittenborn and Rein, 2016). Existing, non-standardized data can also be combined and analyzed through statistical techniques such as small-area estimation

(Wittenborn and Rein, 2016). This technique combines data from multiple sources in order to produce robust estimates that could not be produced by any one data source (Wittenborn and Rein, 2016). However, this technique generally requires state and local data, which are currently lacking. These methods of integrating data across settings and populations would give researchers access to rich, real-world data that could be used to improve our understanding and approach to visual impairment and eye health.

To ensure that surveillance activities are aligned across agencies, methods, and geographic areas and to avoid duplicate efforts, more collaboration and coordination will be needed between and within the eye and vision health community, and among population health surveillance experts. Key players include the NIH, Research to Prevent Blindness, ARVO, HRSA, the Agency for Healthcare Research and Quality, the Association of State and Territorial Health Officials (especially chronic disease directors and epidemiologists), and the National Association of County and City Health Officials, and the CDC. These players could work together to identify key elements of a surveillance system, including which conditions to include, consistent definitions that are correlated with clinical diagnosis criteria, standardized measurements, and methods for integrating and analyzing the data (Wittenborn and Rein, 2016). Bringing together a wide range of stakeholders at every step of the development process will help to ensure buy-in and acceptance for the resulting surveillance system (Wittenborn and Rein, 2016).

National Research Agenda

A research consortium dedicated to eye and vision health will be essential to promote and coordinate the above areas for potential improvement to eye-related surveillance and research. A research consortium can develop a national research agenda, which can serve to align and coordinate efforts, and to ensure that the most important areas of inquiry in instrument development and research design are prioritized. The CDC took steps toward this end through the creation of a panel of 14 experts "to identify action steps and priorities to strengthen national and state surveillance systems to help assess and monitor disparities in eye health, vision loss, and access to eye care over time and respond to national, state, and local needs" (CDC, 2015h). While this panel was a step in the right direction, an ideal research consortium would have a larger presence and focus. Likewise, the Vision Research Consortium at the University of California, Irvine, is a laudable effort; however, its focus only on basic, clinical, and applied research and its limited geographic range makes it insufficiently inclusive to serve as a national research consortium (University of California, 2016). There are several examples of other research consortia that could act as models for a national vision and eye health consortium. For example, the Pediatric Eye Disease Investigator Group (PEDIG) is a collaborative network, funded by the NEI, that coordinates multi-center research focusing on pediatric eye disorders. PEDIG's work is coordinated by a network chair, an executive committee, a steering committee, and a data and safety monitoring committee (PEDIG, 2016). PEDIG has conducted multiple randomized controlled trials on such disorders as amblyopia, strabismus, myopia, and nasolacrimal duct obstruction, and is an example of ophthalmology and optometry working together. Another model consortium is the Resuscitation Outcomes Consortium (ROC). ROC is a public–private collaboration among the National Heart, Lung, and Blood Institute; the U.S. Army Medical Research and Materiel Command; the Canadian Institutes of Health Research; Defence Research and Development Canada; the American Heart Association; and the Heart and Stroke Foundation of Canada. ROC supports research on cardiopulmonary arrest and severe traumatic injury by providing the infrastructure necessary to conduct multiple clinical trials in order to quickly translate scientific advances into clinical outcomes (ROC, 2016). Although financial support for ongoing ROC activities remains tenuous, it provides an example of how the public and private sectors can coordinate research and direct funding to conduct research more efficiently on

---

BOX 4-1
Key Surveillance and Research Limitations

- The lack of a national survey that produces vision-related data that are timely, representative, and standardized constitutes a significant challenge toward developing a surveillance strategy.
- The absence of a surveillance strategy is an impediment to identifying and addressing challenges and opportunities for public health action.
- Patient data captured from EHRs or administrative claims will not include information about the people who cannot or will not utilize care. Furthermore, these data may not provide a full picture of the entirety of one's care, because of fragmentation of eye and vision providers and their respective payment systems.
- Federally funded programs tend to emphasize research and education rather than surveillance activities. While these are valuable endeavors, research on interventions and public health approaches to disease prevention and control offer potential for impact on a population level.
- The lack of a research database that includes information about visual impairment and eye health, comorbidities, QOL, general health information, and associated social determinants poses a barrier toward conducting more in-depth, comprehensive research.

areas that promise the most change. Other examples of research consortia include the Vision Health Research Council in Canada, the Chronic Lymphocytic Leukemia Research Consortium, and the Public Health Research Consortium in the United Kingdom (CRC, 2016; PHRC, 2016; Vision Health Research Council, 2002).

The development of a national research consortium and a national research agenda would help promote vision and eye health by coordinating and prioritizing research to address causes, consequences, and unmet needs of those affected. The consortium, which should include private and public stakeholders, could develop an agenda to drive epidemiologic, clinical, and applied research, as well as health services and population health research. To support inquiry into other research gaps identified throughout this report, this consortium would need to address key surveillance and research limitations, such as those listed in Box 4-1.

CONCLUSION

A systematic and ongoing collection of relevant data about risk factors, determinants of visual health, care practices, and related health outcomes associated with eye health and visual impairment is currently lacking. Currently information is drawn from an array of surveys, EHRs, and administrative claims data, but it is difficult to triangulate information from these sources because of inconsistencies in definitions, measures, and other problems inherent in data collection activities that are discordant or developed independently. To fully understand the nature and extent of the public health burden of eye disease and to better inform practitioners and policy makers about what is needed to improve eye health, a coherent surveillance system is needed.

REFERENCES

AHRQ (Agency for Healthcare Research and Quality). 2009. Survey background. http://meps.ahrq.gov/mepsweb/about_meps/survey_back.jsp (accessed March 25, 2016).

AOA (American Optometric Association). 2015. *AOA announces initial registry EHR vendors*. St. Louis, MO: AOA.

Beaver Dam Eye Study. 2014. The Beaver Dam Eye Study. http://www.bdeyestudy.org (accessed April 7, 2016).

Birkhead, G. S., and C. M. Maylahn. 2010. State and local public health surveillance in the United States. In *Principles and practices of public health surveillance*, edited by L. M. Lee, S. M. Teutsch, S. B. Thacker, and M. E. St. Louis. Oxford, UK: Oxford University Press. Pp. 381–398.

The Board of Regents of the University of Wisconsin System. 2014. About the Beaver Dam Eye Study. http://www.bdeyestudy.org (accessed April 1, 2016).

CAHMI (Child and Adolescent Health Measure Initiative). 2016a. The National Survey of Children's Health. http://childhealthdata.org/learn/NSCH (accessed April 22, 2016).

———. 2016b. National Survey of Children with Special Health Care Needs. http://www.childhealthdata.org/learn/NS-CSHCN (accessed April 22, 2016).

CDC (Centers for Disease Control and Prevention). 2011a. *Enhancing public health surveillance of visual impairment and eye health in the United States.* Atlanta, GA: CDC. https://www.cdc.gov/visionhealth/pdf/surveillance_background.pdf (accessed June 21, 2016).

———. 2011b. FY 2011 operating plans. http://www.cdc.gov/budget/documents/fy2011/fy-2011-operating-plan-table.pdf (accessed April 8, 2016).-

———. 2012. FY 2012 operating plans. http://www.cdc.gov/budget/documents/fy2012/fy-2012-cdc-operating-plan-summary.pdf (accessed April 8, 2016).

———. 2013. FY 2013 operating plans. http://www.cdc.gov/budget/documents/fy2013/fy-2013-operating-plan.pdf (accessed April 8, 2016).

———. 2014. FY 2014 operating plans. http://www.cdc.gov/budget/fy2014/operating-plans.html (accessed April 8, 2016).

———. 2015a. About the Ambulatory Health Care Surveys. http://www.cdc.gov/nchs/ahcd/about_ahcd.htm (accessed March 25, 2016).

———. 2015b. About the Hospital Care Surveys. http://www.cdc.gov/nchs/nhds/about_nhds.htm (accessed June 22, 2016).

———. 2015c. About the National Health and Nutrition Examination Survey. http://www.cdc.gov/nchs/nhanes/about_nhanes.htm (accessed March 25, 2016).

———. 2015d. Has your hospital been selected to take part in the National Hospital Care Survey? http://www.cdc.gov/nchs/nhcs/about_nhcs.htm (accessed April 21, 2016).

———. 2015e. National Health and Nutrition Examination Survey 1996–2016 survey content brochure. http://www.cdc.gov/nchs/data/nhanes/survey_content_99_16.pdf (accessed April 21, 2016).

———. 2015f. National Notifiable Disease Surveillance System (NNDSS). https://wwwn.cdc.gov/nndss (accessed March 29, 2016).

———. 2015g. NHANES data release and access policy. http://www.cdc.gov/nchs/data/nhanes/nhanes_release_policy.pdf (accessed June 22, 2016).

———. 2015h. Vision surveillance in the U.S. http://www.cdc.gov/visionhealth/surveillance/index.htm (accessed April 7, 2016).

———. 2016a. Data sources. http://www.cdc.gov/visionhealth/data/systems/index.html (accessed April 7, 2016).

———. 2016b. FY 2016 operating plans. http://www.cdc.gov/budget/documents/fy2016/fy-2016-cdc-operating-plan.pdf (accessed April 8, 2016).

———. 2016c. Mortality data. http://www.cdc.gov/nchs/deaths.htm (accessed March 29, 2016).

———. 2016d. National voluntary accreditation for public health departments. http://www.cdc.gov/stltpublichealth/Accreditation (accessed September 1, 2016).

CDC Foundation. 2015. What is public health. http://www.cdcfoundation.org/content/what-public-health (accessed October 7, 2015).

Chou, C. F., X. Zhang, J. E. Crews, L. E. Barker, P. P. Lee, and J. B. Saaddine. 2012. Impact of geographic density of eye care professionals on eye care among adults with diabetes. *Ophthalmic Epidemiology* 19(6):340–349.

CMS (Centers for Medicare & Medicaid Services). 2016a. *2016 physician quality reporting system qualified clinical data registries.* Baltimore, MD: CMS.

———. 2016b. Medicare current beneficiary survey (MCBS). https://www.cms.gov/Research-Statistics-Data-and-Systems/Research/MCBS/index.html?redirect=/mcbs (accessed March 25, 2016).

Cotch, M. F. 2016. Public health surveillance—the integral role of community-based studies. *JAMA Ophthalmology* 134(5):578–579.

CRC (Chronic Lymphocytic Leukemia Research Consortium). 2016. Welcome to the CLL research consortium. http://cll.ucsd.edu (accessed April 22, 2016).

Crews, J. E. 2015. The conundrum of vision surveillance. Presentation to the IOM Committee on Public Health Approaches to Reduce Vision Impairment and Promote Eye Health. Washington, DC, May 19, 2015. http://www.nationalacademies.org/hmd/~/media/Files/Activity%20Files/PublicHealth/Vision/Meeting%201/04%20Crews%20IOM%20Vision%20Briefing%20Crews.pdf (accessed September 1, 2016).

Dahlgren, G., and M. Whitehead. 1991. *Policies and strategies to promote social equity in health*. Stockholm: Institute for Future Studies. https://core.ac.uk/download/files/153/6472456.pdf (accessed June 21, 2016).

Elliott, A. F., A. Davidson, F. Lum, M. F. Chiang, J. B. Saaddine, X. Zhang, J. E. Crews, and C. F. Chou. 2012. Use of electronic health records and administrative data for public health surveillance of eye health and vision-related conditions in the United States. *American Journal of Ophthalmology* 154(6 Suppl):S63–S70.

Heintz, E., A. B. Wirehn, B. B. Peebo, U. Rosenqvist, and L. A. Levin. 2012. QALY weights for diabetic retinopathy—A comparison of health state valuations with HUI-3, EQ-5D, EQ-VAS, and TTO. *Value Health* 15(3):475–484.

Hirneiss, C. 2014. The impact of a better-seeing eye and a worse-seeing eye on vision-related quality of life. *Clinical Ophthalmology (Auckland, N.Z.)* 8:1703–1709.

Hofman, A., M. M. Breteler, C. M. van Duijn, G. P. Krestin, H. A. Pols, B. H. C. Stricker, H. Tiemeier, A. G. Uitterlinden, J. R. Vingerling, and J. C. Witteman. 2007. The Rotterdam Study: Objectives and design update. *European Journal of Epidemiology* 22(11): 819–829.

IOM (Institute of Medicine). 2011. *A nationwide framework for surveillance of cardiovascular and chronic lung diseases*. Washington, DC: The National Academies Press.

Islam, N. S., S. Khan, S. Kwon, D. Jang, M. Ro, and C. Trinh-Shevrin. 2010. Methodological issues in the collection, analysis, and reporting of granular data in Asian American populations: Historical challenges and potential solutions. *Journal of Health Care for the Poor and Underserved* 21(4):1354–1381.

Kirtland, K. A., J. B. Saaddine, L. S. Geiss, T. J. Thompson, M. F. Cotch, and P. P. Lee. 2015. Geographic disparity of severe vision loss—United States, 2009–2013. *Morbidity and Mortality Weekly Report* 64(19):513–517.

Klein, R., B. E. K. Klein, M. D. Knudtson, T. Y. Wong, M. F. Cotch, K. Liu, G. Burke, M. F. Saad, and D. R. Jacobs Jr. 2006. Prevalence of age-related macular degeneration in 4 racial/ethnic groups in the multi-ethnic study of atherosclerosis. *Ophthalmology* 113(3):373–380.

Kowalski, J. W., A. M. Rentz, J. G. Walt, A. Lloyd, J. Lee, T. A. Young, W. H. Chen, N. M. Bressler, P. Lee, J. E. Brazier, R. D. Hays, and D. A. Revicki. 2012. Rasch analysis in the development of a simplified version of the National Eye Institute visual-function questionnaire-25 for utility estimation. *Quality of Life Research* 21(2):323–334.

Kukull, W. A., and M. Ganguli. 2012. Generalizability: The trees, the forest, and the low-hanging fruit. *Neurology* 78(23):1886–1891.

Lee, L. M., S. M. Teutsch, S. B. Thacker, and M. E. S. Louis (eds.). 2010. *Principles and practice of public health surveillance*. 3rd ed. New York: Oxford University Press.

Lee, P. P., Z. W. Feldman, J. Ostermann, D. S. Brown, and F. A. Sloan. 2003. Longitudinal rates of annual eye examinations of persons with diabetes and chronic eye diseases. *Ophthalmology* 110(10):1952–1959.

Lee, P. P., S. K. West, S. S. Block, J. Clayton, M. F. Cotch, C. Flynn, L. S. Geiss, R. Klein, T. W. Olsen, C. Owsley, S. A. Primo, G. S. Rubin, A. Ryskulova, S. Sharma, D. S. Friedman, X. Zhang, J. E. Crews, and J. B. Saaddine. 2012. Surveillance of disparities in vision and eye health in the United States: An expert panel's opinions. *American Journal of Ophthalmology* 154(6 Suppl):S3–S7.

Linnan, L., M. Bowling, J. Childress, G. Lindsay, C. Blakey, S. Pronk, S. Wieker, and P. Royall. 2008. Results of the 2004 National Worksite Health Promotion Survey. *American Journal of Public Health* 98(8):1503–1509.

MacLennan, P. A., G. McGwin, K. Searcey, and C. Owsley. 2013. Medical record validation of self-reported eye diseases and eye care utilization among older adults. *Current Eye Research* 38(1):1–8.

Mangione, C. M., P. P. Lee, P. R. Gutierrez, K. Spritzer, S. Berry, R. D. Hays, and National Eye Institute Visual Function Questionnaire Field Test Investigators. 2001. Development of the 25-item National Eye Institute visual function questionnaire. *Archives of Ophthalmology* 119(7):1050–1058.

Maylahn, C. 2013. Health departments in a brave new world. *Preventing Chronic Disease* 10:E41.

MESA (Multi-Ethnic Study of Atherosclerosis). 2016a. About MESA. https://www.mesa-nhlbi. org/aboutMESA.aspx (accessed May 30, 2016).

———. 2016b. MESA classic components by exam. https://www.mesa-nhlbi.org/about MESAStudyTime.aspx (accessed May 30, 2016).

Mokdad, A. H. 2009. The Behavioral Risk Factors Surveillance System: Past, present, and future. *Annual Reviews of Public Health* 30:43–54.

Monitoring the Future. 2016. Monitoring the Future: A continuing study of American youth. http://www.monitoringthefuture.org (accessed March 25, 2016).

NACCHO (National Association of County and City Health Officials). 2014. *2013 national profile of local health departments.* Washington, DC: NACCHO. http://archived.naccho. org/topics/infrastructure/profile/resources/2010report/upload/2010_profile_main_report-web.pdf (accessed June 21, 2016).

———. 2015. The changing public health landscape. http://nacchoprofilestudy.org/wp-content/uploads/2015/04/2015-Forces-of-Change-Slidedoc-Final.pdf (accessed May 3, 2016).

NEI/NIH (National Eye Institute/National Institutes of Health). 2011. National Institutes of Health releases data from largest pediatric eye study. https://nei.nih.gov/news/statements/pediatric (accessed May 27, 2016).

NIH (National Institutes of Health). 2015. National Institutes of Health: History of congressional appropriations, fiscal years 2000–2016. https://officeofbudget.od.nih.gov/pdfs/FY16/Approp%20History%20by%20IC%20FY%202000%20-%20FY%202016.pdf (accessed April 22, 2016).

Parke, D. W. 2015. Ophthalmic innovation 2015: A view from AAO. Presention at Ophthalmology Innovation Summit. Las Vegas, NV, November 12, 2015. http://www. healio.com/ophthalmology/technology/news/online/%7Bf2b7a043-d40c-4075-9254-63cb9625869c%7D/iris-registry-advances-science-of-ophthalmology (accessed April 7, 2016)

Parke, D. W., F. Lum, and W. L. Rich. 2016. The IRIS® registry: Purpose and perspectives. *Der Ophthalmologe* 113(6):463–468.

PEDIG (Pediatric Eye Disease Investigator Group). 2016. Pediatric Eye Disease Investigator Group (PEDIG) organizational structure. http://publicfiles.jaeb.org/pedig/Misc/PEDIG_OrgStructure_4_1_16.pdf (accessed May 27, 2016).

Pesudovs, K., V. K. Gothwal, T. Wright, and E. L. Lamoureux. 2010. Remediating serious flaws in the National Eye Institute visual function questionnaire. *Journal of Cataract & Refractive Surgery* 36(5):718–732.

PHAB (Public Health Accreditation Board). 2016. Welcome to the Public Health Accreditation Board. http://www.phaboard.org (accessed April 7, 2016).

PHRC (Public Health Research Consortium). 2016. Public Health Research Consortium. http://phrc.lshtm.ac.uk (accessed April 22, 2016).

Rein, D. B. 2015. Status of visual health surveillance and opportunities for improvement. Presentation to the IOM Committee on Public Health Approaches to Reduce Vision Impairment and Promote Eye Health. Washington, DC, October 29, 2015.

Riley, W. J., K. Bender, and E. Lownik. 2012. Public health department accreditation implementation: Transforming public health department performance. *American Journal of Public Health* 102(2):237–242.

ROC (Resuscitation Outcomes Consortium). 2016. Resuscitation Outcomes Consortium. https://roc.uwctc.org/tiki/tiki-index.php?page=roc-public-home (accessed April 22, 2016).

Rosenbaum, S., and R. Margulies. 2011. Tax-exempt hospitals and the Patient Protection and Affordable Care Act: Implications for public health policy and practice. *Public Health Reports* 283–286.

Saaddine, J. B., K. Venkat Narayan, and F. Vinicor. 2003. Vision loss: A public health problem? *Ophthalmology* 110(2):253–254.

Stoto, M. A. 2013. Population health in the Affordable Care Act era. Washington, DC: Academy Health. http://community-wealth.org/sites/clone.community-wealth.org/files/downloads/paper-stoto.pdf (accessed September 1, 2016).

Truven Health Analytics. 2016. Marketscan research databases. http://truvenhealth.com/your-healthcare-focus/analytic-research/marketscan-research-databases (accessed April 22, 2016).

University of California. 2016. Vision Research Consortium. http://www.ghei.uci.edu/consortium.asp (accessed April 7, 2016).

U.S. Census Bureau. 2016. Survey of income and program participation. https://www.census.gov/programs-surveys/sipp/about/sipp-introduction-history.html (accessed March 29, 2016).

Varma, R., C. Hsu, D. Wang, M. Torres, and S. P. Azen. 2013. The Chinese American Eye Study: Design and methods. *Ophthalmic Epidemiology* 20(6):335–347.

Vision Health Research Council. 2002. Vision is our most important sense. http://vhrc.net/ (accessed April 22, 2016).

Vitale, S., M. F. Cotch, R. Sperduto, and L. Ellwein. 2006. Costs of refractive correction of distance vision impairment in the United States, 1999–2002. *Ophthalmology* 113(12):2163–2170.

VPUS (Vision Problems in the U.S.). 2012. Methods and sources. http://www.visionproblemsus.org/introduction/methods-and-sources.html (accessed April 7, 2016).

VSP (Vision Service Plan). 2016. About VSP. https://vsp.com/about-vsp.html (accessed April 22, 2016).

West, S. K., and P. Lee. 2012. Vision surveillance in the United States: Has the time come? *American Journal of Ophthalmology* 154(6):S1–S2, e2.

WHO (World Health Organization). 2016. Public health surveillance. http://www.who.int/topics/public_health_surveillance/en (accessed April 4, 2016).

Wittenborn, J., and D. Rein. 2016 (unpublished). *The potential costs and benefits of treatment for undiagnosed eye disorders*. Paper prepared for the Committee on Public Health Approaches to Reduce Vision Impairment and Promote Eye Health. http://www.national academies.org/hmd/~/media/Files/Report%20Files/2016/UndiagnosedEyeDisorders CommissionedPaper.pdf (accessed September 15, 2016).

Zambelli-Weiner, A., J. E. Crews, and D. S. Friedman. 2012. Disparities in adult vision health in the United States. *American Journal of Ophthalmology* 154(6 Suppl):S23–S30, e21.

Zhang, X., M. F. Cotch, A. Ryskulova, S. A. Primo, P. Nair, C. F. Chou, L. S. Geiss, L. E. Barker, A. F. Elliott, J. E. Crews, and J. B. Saaddine. 2012. Vision health disparities in the United States by race/ethnicity, education, and economic status: Findings from two nationally representative surveys. *American Journal of Ophthalmology* 154(6):53–62.

5

The Role of Public Health and Partnerships to Promote Eye and Vision Health in Communities

Health has been defined as "a state of complete physical, mental, and social well-being and not merely the absence of disease or infirmity" (WHO, 1948). A population health approach involves multiple actors who work separately and cooperatively "on the interrelated conditions and factors that influence the health of populations over the life course, . . . systematic variations in their patterns of occurrence, and . . . the resulting knowledge to develop and implement policies and actions to improve the health and well-being of those populations" (Kindig and Stoddart, 2003, p. 380). Health is affected by multiple determinants, including

- innate individual traits (e.g., age, sex, race, genetics);
- individual behaviors;
- social, family, and community networks;
- living and working conditions (e.g., psychosocial factors, employment status and occupational factors, socioeconomic status, health care services); and
- broad social, economic, cultural, health, and environmental conditions and policies at the global, national, state, and local levels (e.g., economic inequality, urbanization, mobility, cultural values) (IOM, 2003).

Greater understanding of the determinants of health supports engaging the entire community in efforts to improve population health—hence the emergence of the concept of health in all policies (see, e.g., Wernham and Teutsch, 2015). Eye and vision health is no different. Although there are

191

specific system-related considerations that affect eye and vision outcomes, including the access to and quality of a complex health system (see Chapters 6 and 7), there are also societal-level factors that influence whether certain practices, policies, and conditions are available to reduce the risk of vision loss and decrease related health inequities. Good eye and vision health can reduce health disparities, but promoting optimal conditions for eye and vision health can also positively influence many other social ills, including poverty, other health inequities, increasing health care costs, and avoidable mortality and morbidity (Christ et al., 2014; Rahi et al., 2009; Rein, 2013).

The role of governmental public health is to ensure "the conditions in which people can be healthy" (IOM, 1988, p. 16). In contrast to medical care, which focuses on treating individual patients, the governmental public health departments (PHDs)[1] concentrate on the risks to the population's health and on improving health equity. As described in Chapter 1 when discussing the committee's approach to its statement of task, the committee distilled the fundamental aspects of governmental public health work into three core public health functions: assessment, policy development, and assurance. These functions include 10 essential public health services: (1) monitoring health; (2) diagnosing and investigating; (3) informing, educating, and empowering; (4) mobilizing community partnerships; (5) developing policies; (6) enforcing laws; (7) linking to and providing care; (8) assuring a competent workforce; (9) evaluating; and (10) conducting research (CDC, 2014b). To this end, governmental PHDs provide a wide range of services to protect (preventing diseases, chronic conditions, and injuries), promote (educating and changing behavior), monitor (carrying out surveillance), and improve the population's health.

The responsibility for improving population health, however, has never been the sole province of the governmental PHDs. Governmental PHDs work with and through other stakeholders, including other government agencies, the clinical care system, employers and businesses, media, nonprofit organizations, the education sector, and the community (IOM, 2003, 2011c) (see Figure 5-1). Within these categories are stakeholders such as religious organizations, sports organizations, clinical and public health associations, community living centers, nursing homes, assisted living facilities, and others. Successful health promotion in eye and vision health will require innovative partnerships engaged in a variety of activities that advance different objectives within population health. A key role for the governmental PHDs is to act as a convener of the different stakeholders who then develop and implement action plans that may complement national initiatives and that reflect a community's needs and goals.

----

[1] Governmental PHDs in this chapter encompasses federal, state, and local public health agencies.

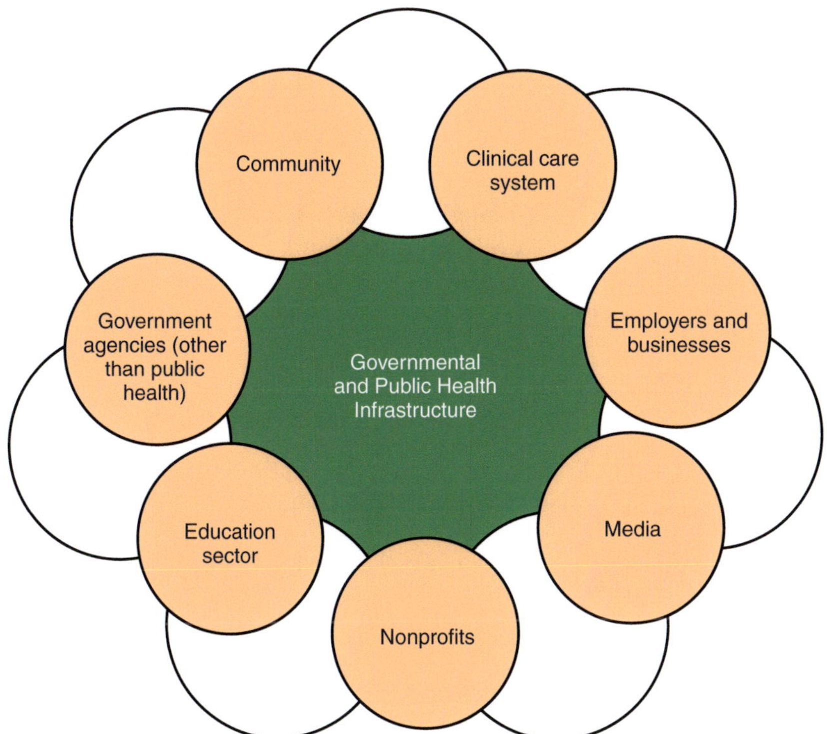

FIGURE 5-1 The population health system.
NOTES: This figure includes an additional circle for nonprofit organizations, which are also an important partner to advance population health objectives. The term "public health infrastructure" refers to the array of public entities charged with keeping the public healthy (e.g., agencies, laboratories, and partners) and to their operational capacity (IOM, 2003).
SOURCE: Adapted from IOM, 2011b.

The central issue we address in this chapter is the governmental PHD's capacity to improve and promote eye and vision health and how partnerships between actors in the population health system can enhance this capacity. Programs to address the risk factors for vision loss, such as diabetes, tobacco use, and injury are common. But public health strategies to promote vision health are rarely supported as a categorical focus or even as part of chronic disease programs in state and local health departments (LHDs) because of resource limitations and competing priorities. Although eye and vision health is not a current public health priority, this chapter demonstrates the ways in which the governmental PHDs, working in conjunction with the private sector, can transform eye and vision health into a public health imperative.

This chapter begins with a general overview of the governmental PHDs. In subsequent sections, we elaborate on the key governmental PHD functions as applied to eye and vision health. The second section introduces strategies for building capacities. The third section considers a variety of opportunities for governmental PHDs and other community stakeholders to incorporate eye and vision health into public health platforms. The final section concludes with a discussion of accountability, which includes priority setting and the evaluation of impact within governmental PHDs.

OVERVIEW OF THE GOVERNMENTAL PUBLIC HEALTH SYSTEM

Advancing eye and vision health as a population health priority will require more than simply asking governmental public health agencies and departments to place greater emphasis on the issue. Governmental public health professionals are responsible for a wide range of federal, state, and local activities and programs that are faced with dwindling resources and, simultaneously, increasing demand. Different levels of emphasis, resources, and staffing are required at each locus of government. In the absence of either increased funding overall or increased support for expanding programmatic focus, it will be difficult to rely on governmental PHDs to continue to provide current support or expand their footprints related to eye and vision health independently from other stakeholders.

This section provides an overview of the general responsibilities, structure, and current capacity constraints of federal, state, and local public health agencies to better understand the roles they could play to improve eye and vision health. In particular, it is important to understand the resource limitations of these systems as well as to recognize the heterogeneity among state and local PHDs because these factors underscore the need to embrace diverse partnerships and a wide range of strategies and programmatic emphases in order to adequately address the pressing public health needs related to eye and vision health and to vision impairment.

Federal Agencies and Organizations

Public health officials can use an array of legal and public health interventions to promote the population's health, such as issuing and then enforcing regulations. At the federal level, there are numerous agencies, institutes, and centers whose work affects eye health and the impact of vision impairment on populations (see Appendix D). Current federal activities influence eye and vision health and the response to vision impairment through various mechanisms, including (1) programs and funding that directly target the promotion of eye and vision health and are aimed at slowing the progression of vision impairment within defined populations; (2) tracking possible outcomes of poor eye and vision health, including activities to promote functionality following vision impairment; (3) promoting health more generally by addressing the underlying determinants of health that can also affect the risk of vision impairment; (4) establishing and enforcing policies related to the safety and functionality of occupational settings and built environments (i.e., the physical environment constructed by human activity), discrimination, and disability; (5) conducting research to advance scientific, medical, and public health knowledge; and (6) facilitating the delivery of services to promote access to the broader population.

The U.S. Department of Health and Human Services (HHS) supports a number of federal programs and institutes, such as the Centers for Disease Control and Prevention's (CDC's) Vision Health Initiative and the National Institutes of Health's National Eye Institute (NEI) and National Eye Health Education Program (NEHEP), both of which focus on vision loss and the funding of various activities targeting at-risk populations (CDC, 2015a; NEI/NIH, 2015b). The Health Resources and Services Administraion (HRSA) funds grants and innovative projects to support its programmatic activities and delivers educational material on eye and vision health (HRSA, n.d.). Various federal and private grants are used to support HHS's Healthy People 2020 objectives, which include eight goals that specifically address eye and vision conditions and emphasize early detection, timely treatment, and rehabilitation (ODPHP, 2016e).[2] For eye health and safety, the Occupational Safety and Health Administration (OSHA) within the U.S. Department of Labor sets workplace safety standards. For example, employers must ensure that employees use appropriate eye or face protection when exposed to eye or face hazards. Other federal agencies involved with vision and eye health include the U.S. Department of Agriculture, the U.S. Department of Defense, the U.S. Department of Veterans Affairs, the U.S. Environmental Protection Agency, and the U.S. Food and Drug Administration, among others (see Appendix D).

Despite these activities, eye and vision health are insufficiently represented as a programmatic focus in federal government programs overall,

---

[2] These goals include (1) increase the proportion of preschool children ages 5 years and under who receive vision screening, (2) reduce blindness and visual impairment in children and adolescents aged 17 years, (3) reduce occupational eye injuries, (4) increase the proportion of adults who have a comprehensive eye examination including dilation, within the past 2 years, (5) reduce visual impairment, (6) increase the use of personal protective eyewear in recreational activities and hazardous situations around the home, (7) increase vision rehabilitation, and (8) (developmental) increase the proportion of federally qualified health centers that provide comprehensive vision health services (ODPHP, 2016e).

and existing programs lack coordination within and across federal agencies and institutes. Support for more traditional public health activities has also been waning, which has affected the support available for grants that may target eye and vision health. For example, during fiscal year 2015, Iowa was the only state that used funds from a Preventive Health and Health Services federal block grant for any vision-related programming (CDC, 2015f). The funding for this grant program was eliminated in fiscal year 2016.

As described later in this chapter, chronic vision impairment is notably absent from government lists of priority chronic diseases, which means that eye and vision health are passively excluded from many federal programs and initiatives aimed at reducing the burden of chronic disease. Moreover, as described in Chapter 4, vision and eye health surveillance efforts have received only modest attention and support from federal agencies. Eye-related activities are not specifically listed as an area for funding or as an emphasis in the federal budget, unlike, for instance, oral health, and funding for the NEI has remained relatively stagnant over the past 5 years (NEI/NIH, 2016).

The Organization of State Health Departments

State health departments could provide substantial contributions to national eye and vision health efforts. First, their involvement in the planning process helps in the development of feasible action plans and ensures that the appropriate high-risk populations are targeted. Second, state health departments provide an important link between federal and community programs into incorporating eye and vision health strategies that are consistent with local needs and resources. State health departments offer grant opportunities that can be used to support specific eye and vision activities in LHDs or as part of a more comprehensive strategy in partnership with other groups. Third, as described more fully below, state health departments are expected to ensure that needed programs, regulations, and practices are monitored and improved.

The organizational model adopted for the state health department within each state offers insight into the roles they may play in relation to statewide and local public health services and priorities. There are four primary organizational models: a decentralized or home rule arrangement, under which local public health agencies operate independently of the state and report to local government; a centralized model in which there are no local public health agencies, though the state agency may have regional offices; a shared authority model; and a mixed authority model. In shared or mixed models, LHDs are generally responsible to both the state public health agency and to local government, but the details vary from state to state (NACCHO, 1998; Novick et al., 2005). As of 2012, 27 states had decentralized governance, 14 states and the District of Columbia have centralized (or state) governance, and 10 had shared or mixed (state and local) governance (ASTHO, 2012).

In most states, public health is a component of a broader health department, which might be combined with other functions, such as Medicaid, mental health, substance abuse, environmental health, and human services programs (ASTHO, 2014). Moreover, public health responsibilities at the state level generally reside in multiple agencies. For instance, most states have a separate environmental agency. All states have public health codes that provide the agencies with the authority to conduct public health activities and permit them to promulgate regulations and take action. These codes are based on the police powers that the states have as sovereign governments under the U.S. Constitution, to safeguard their populations' health, safety, and welfare (Lopez and Frieden, 2007). States may delegate this power to local governments, especially for public health activities. Surveillance and required disease reporting are exercises of state police powers.

Boards of Health provide additional oversight of governmental public health activities. The Institute of Medicine's (IOM's) report *For the Public's Health: Revitalizing Law and Policy to Meet New Challenges* (2011b, p. 30) sums up the responsibilities that boards of health at different levels of governance have across the country:

> Boards of health are [one] historical mechanism for public health governance at the state and local level, but their roles have evolved over time, and some have dismantled entirely (Nicola, 2005). Eighty percent of local public health agencies have an associated local board of health (NACCHO, 2009a), and 23 states have a state board of health (Hughes et al., 2011). Some local boards are advisory, and others play a role in governance and policymaking. Their functions may include adopting public health regulations, setting and imposing fees, approving the agency budget, hiring or firing the top agency administrator, and requesting a public health levy (Beitsch et al., 2010; Leahy and Fallon, 2005). State boards play varying roles as well, including agency oversight, appointing the health officer, a quasi-legislative function (i.e., adopting/rejecting rules) and a quasi-judicial function (i.e., enforcing rules) (Hughes et al., 2011).

The Organization of Local Health Departments

Except in states that use a centralized model, LHDs have broad authority to take actions necessary to protect and promote the public's health. LHDs can use the full range of legal and policy initiatives as provided under the state's and local public health code to achieve these objectives. For instance, LHDs can directly and indirectly use their regulatory authority to require an industry to make certain changes to their products, and they have the authority to require individuals to operate within certain limits (e.g., using seatbelts). LHDs may also use their bully pulpit to motivate shifts in how private-sector entities operate with regard to its products, often working with industry to develop voluntary standards instead of governmental regulation (see, e.g., Mello et al., 2008). In the case of eye and vision health, for example, businesses could voluntarily adopt initiatives to improve worker safety (i.e., requiring and paying for safety glasses and monitoring their use).

For the most part, public health activities are conducted at the local level through approximately 2,800 regional or LHDs (Salinsky, 2010). Many LHDs are small agencies with limited resources and capabilities in certain areas, such as legal and policy analysis. Sixty-four percent of LHDs serve populations of 50,000 or less, often in rural areas (Salinsky, 2010). Some LHDs are regional (combining several smaller counties into one LHD), but most are countywide, stand-alone agencies (Salinsky, 2010). Because LHD workforces are not standardized across the United States, general statements about the nature of positions and tasks performed are difficult to make at a national level. Not surprisingly, smaller LHDs are likely to have fewer resources and less capacity to meet their obligations than larger departments (usually located in metropolitan areas) (Mays et al., 2006). Health departments are also dealing with an aging workforce and the imminent retirements of key staff (Hearne et al., 2015). From 2008 to 2010, the LHD workforce declined by 19 percent (NACCHO, 2011).

LHD capabilities and human resources are important in the context of eye and vision health because numerous LHDs are already struggling to provide their mandated services, which currently have higher priority than eye and vision health. Information regarding the distribution and trends of optometrists or ophthalmologists in LHDs is limited. A 2000 report from HRSA, which remains the most current and comprehensive report of the U.S. public health workforce, identified only five federal and four LHD public health optometrists (Gebbie, 2000). Nonetheless, many LHDs employ professionals such as physicians, behavioral health specialists, health educators, nurses, nutritionists, and epidemiologists (NACCHO, 2009b) whose educational background and training could make them valuable allies in promoting eye and vision health. Similarly, policy development and policy analysis capabilities are crucial elements lacking in many smaller health departments. This poses additional barriers to changing or adapting a programmatic emphasis within communities to include eye and vision health.

BUILDING CAPACITY AND STRATEGIES TO PROMOTE EYE AND VISION HEALTH

A fundamental challenge confronting state and local public health agencies is the availability of dedicated funding and staff resources to identify and respond to eye and vision health needs and to sustain a focus on efforts to improve vision health over time. Providing the full range of expected public health services requires significant capacity (i.e., financial resources, adequate staffing, and an adequately trained staff) that even large health departments struggle to meet. Unabated public demand for services and new legislative mandates exacerbate an already challenging environment. PHDs currently face "declining public investment, sustained attacks from opponents (including affected industries and anti-government political groups), limited political power, and competitors encroaching on its responsibilities" (Jacobson et al., 2015, p. S318). Moreover, flexibility in how state and local governments use federal grant funds varies (e.g., block grants provide broad parameters for spending decisions, whereas state and local governments generally do not have as much latitude for categorical focus grants) (CBO, 2013).

The result for this situation is that other more traditional public health activities, such as surveillance, health promotion, and policy development (including tracking underlying social and environmental conditions as well as eye and vision health) do not receive adequate attention or the necessary resources to address the growing need (Brooks et al., 2009; Honoré and Schlechte, 2007; Jacobson et al., 2015). Some studies suggest that a large, disproportionate percentage of public health funds is dedicated to linking and assuring access to health care services, to the detriment of agencies' ability to adequately attend to other essential services (Brooks et al., 2009; Honoré and Schlechte, 2007). Programmatic emphasis may be narrowed and may reflect national public health priority lists, which do not typically include eye and vision health. For example, in its 2015 *Prevention Status Reports*, the CDC identified 10 top priority public health problems: motor vehicle injuries, obesity and nutrition, food safety, alcohol-related harms, health care–acquired infections, heart disease and stroke, HIV, prescription drug overdose, teen pregnancy, and tobacco use (CDC, 2015e). In the absence of federal directives and programs to advance eye and vision health, state and local PHDs are hard pressed to incorporate reduction of vision impairment as a categorical programmatic focus. Nor is eye and vision health well integrated into related programs, such as chronic disease and health education programs, although the risk of vision impairment is associated with a number of current public health issues, such as smoking rates. This opportunity is discussed later in this chapter.

An assessment of state-level activities for preventing eye disease and blindness found that the efforts of vision health stakeholders were generally uncoordinated and recommended the mobilization of partnerships to improve collaboration among public- and private-sector organizations (NACDD, 2004).

Public–Private Partnerships to Build Capacity

One response to the capacity constraints is for governmental PHDs to develop robust public–private partnerships, understood as arrangements in which public agencies formally or informally partner with private or non-profit entities to provide or improve public services (The National Council for Public-Private Partnerships, 2016; Nishtar, 2004). Such partnerships can improve population health by advancing public health strategies and policies, improving public health education and advocacy, fostering trust and collaboration among sectors and stakeholders, and improving access to health care (Nishtar, 2004). For example, community and religious organizations involved with health promotion campaigns can increase knowledge about and awareness of disease, encourage screening, and help reduce risky behaviors (DeHaven et al., 2004). These partnerships have the potential to fill gaps in expertise and provide services that would not otherwise be supported through government hiring. They also may allow health departments to focus on meeting other core and essential services.

Eye and vision health can become an important component of public–private collaborations with effective leadership and sustained commitment and funding to track meaningful measures of eye and vision health as a population health outcome and risk factor for other social determinants of health. For example, health departments can serve as navigators between medical care and the community (e.g., arranging transportation, working with providers to use community health workers in coordinating eye health in the community). For example, the National Association of Chronic Disease Directors, with input from the CDC and Prevent Blindness America, recommended that states designate an integration specialist to take responsibility for coordinating vision services within the state department of health and among external actors and that they form a community-based coalition of actors led by a public health coordinator to provide basic vision services (PBA/NACDD, 2005). Similarly, a well-functioning medical care system can expand access to appropriate eye and vision care services, allowing public health agencies to focus on preventive policies and action and assurance. A well-functioning medical care system could hire navigators within their own organization or through contractual relationships with governmental public health systems or nonprofit organizations to assure coordinated eye and vision care and population-wide improvements in, and reduction in inequalities associated with, eye and vision health. This includes linking people to needed care, assessing care quality, and promoting community support, policies, and environmental conditions that maximize health (IOM, 2003). Likewise, health care providers can collaborate with health departments to identify and refer individuals previously undiagnosed and to work with diagnosed individuals to secure needed services. The best collaborations should build on the unique strengths of partners to create a systemic effect that is greater than any single partner can produce.

At the same time, partnerships have limitations and may incur risks. The obligations of government to provide public services may conflict with the profit motives of for-profit private businesses or the political, economic, and social agendas of nonprofit organizations. Particular risks include the degradation of social safety nets, inappropriate reorientation of governmental health policy, fragmentation of health care systems, undesirable power imbalances among partner organizations, and unsustainable program operations (Nishtar, 2004). Most importantly, the failure to carefully select private-sector partners or to adequately delineate the partnership terms can erode traditional public-sector values such as accountability, transparency, responsibility, and quality (Reynaers, 2014).

Regionalization and Cross-Jurisdictional Sharing

Public health capacity can be expanded by consolidating smaller LHDs into a larger agency (also called regionalization) or at least by the cross-jurisdictional sharing of staff and services, two strategies that have been used most prominently in the context of emergency preparedness (Koh et al., 2008). Among others, Koh et al. (2008) and Stoto and Morse (2008) have argued that the benefits of regionalization and cross-jurisdictional sharing include improving LHD capacity, making more efficient use of funds, achieving economies of scale, and optimizing coordination—for example, in managing problems that are not bounded by municipal borders.

Consolidation offers several potential opportunities to elevate eye and vision health on the public health agenda. First, anything that expands staff capacity will enable an LHD to develop new initiatives or broaden current activities. As discussed below in the section Public Health Interventions to Promote Eye and Vision Health, the committee identified numerous opportunities for LHDs to improve eye and vision health if they have adequate staff and resources. Second, consolidation increases the number of people in the service area who might have vision impairment, making it more likely to detect changes in eye and vision health in response to specific interventions and initiatives. Third, consolidation improves the likelihood that LHDs will be active participants in the community health needs assessment process (discussed later in this chapter), which could then support public–private collaborations to improve eye and vision health. Finally, for smaller LHDs, "combining resources and operations, sharing different types of capacities (e.g., legal guidance and policy analysis), and specialized positions (e.g., epidemiologists) could help smaller agencies meet [accreditation] standards (Konkle, 2009; Libbey and Miyahara, 2011; Mays et al., 2006)" (IOM, 2011b, p. 43). This can generate new opportunities to discuss the insertion of eye and vision health metrics into public health debates related to health care quality and access. However, this approach could also lead to a loss of local identity and responsiveness, particularly those related to local needs and priorities.

OPPORTUNITIES TO INCORPORATE EYE AND VISION HEALTH: THE PUBLIC HEALTH AGENDA

A public health agenda represents informed decisions and prioritizations about specific health threats based on the nature of those threats and the ability to influence the occurrence or impact on the overall health and well-being of populations. The agenda should represent thoughtful consideration within a community about what health threats command attention, the availability and application of resources across health and non-health sector domains to successfully address these priorities, agreed upon metrics to measure impact and correct course where applicable, and the appropriate community oversight to hold stakeholders accountable for short- and long-term successes and failures.

Establishing public health priorities requires an informed public. Simply put, "public health depends on laypeople's ability to understand the health-related choices that they and their societies face" (Fischhoff et al., 2009, p. 940). To make such decisions wisely, individuals need to understand the risks and the benefits associated with alternative courses of action (Fischhoff et al., 1993). Health promotion and education are important components of any governmental PHDs population health approach to reducing the eye and vision health burden on society. Health promotion is "the process of enabling people to increase control over, and to improve, their health. It moves beyond a focus on individual behavior towards a wide range of social and environmental interventions" (WHO, n.d.b.). Therefore, health promotion activities include not only the communication of information to encourage changes in individual behaviors, but also larger policies and practices intended to promote social, economic, and structural environments that are more conducive to health. The related concept of health education includes strategies to promote optimal eye health, prevent vision impairment, and provide people with the skills and ability they need to manage vision impairment and rehabilitation, if necessary. This includes interventions to promote public awareness, change behaviors, and build community environments that promote eye health. Another goal of health education is also to give people the skills they need (e.g., health literacy) and the wherewithal to use them (e.g., an equitable health system). Strategies to promote and protect vision and eye health that are available to governmental PHDs include

- Altering the informational environment (e.g., promoting eye and vision health);
- Altering the built/physical environment (e.g., removing barriers to mobility);
- Directly regulating and monitoring (e.g., requiring eye protections and reporting for sports-related activities and safer work environments);
- Self-regulating (e.g., promoting voluntary employer initiatives to provide accommodations for vision-impaired employees);
- Developing robust state-level surveillance strategies (e.g., incorporating eye health into community health needs assessments and health impact assessments) to collect and analyze data regarding eye health status;
- Monitoring access to vision care services;
- Assuring access to clinical services, especially for undiagnosed and low-income populations at risk of eye disease;
- Incorporating vision care as a strategic planning priority and in conducting health impact assessments;
- Incorporating vision care as an integral component of "health in all policies" programs; and
- Facilitating community engagement in order to promote eye health and obtain community collaboration in implementing policies and programs.

The remainder of this chapter explores some of these strategies in more detail, including efforts to improve public awareness and education, expand access to vision care services and appropriate follow-up care, develop policies to encourage eye healthy environments, promote eye and vision health as part of formal population health programs, and enhance accountability for activities (or lack thereof) related to eye and vision health.

Improving Public Awareness and Education

Understanding that a problem exists and what can be done to ameliorate that problem is the first step to combating any public health threat. Although rarely adequate by themselves, public awareness campaigns can be an effective way to improve knowledge about key messages related to health within populations (Bray et al., 2015; Oto et al., 2011) and are one essential part of an effective population health strategy. In fact, the CDC has stated that public health strategies, which include efforts "to enhance awareness, to promote education, and to increase access to successful prevention, treatment, and rehabilitation services among populations at risk for poor vision outcomes[,] can improve vision health in the United States and globally" (Zambelli-Weiner et al., 2012, p. S23).

Knowledge About the Major Causes of Vision Loss

It is important to understand what the different causes of vision loss are because the types and scopes of applicable interventions vary based on the etiology of vision impairment. According to a recent online poll to examine the importance of eye and vision health among the U.S. population, 88 percent of the 2,044 respondents surveyed identified good vision as vital to maintaining overall health, and 47 percent rated losing their vision compared to loss of limb, memory, hearing, or speech as "potentially having the greatest effect on their day-to-day life" (Scott et al., 2016, p. E3). This same poll found that blindness ranked either first or second among African Americans, Asians, Hispanics, and whites as the worse disease or ailment.[3] Yet a lack of awareness around vision and eye health issues is "a major public health concern," especially for linking patients into care and attempting to make population-level changes in behavior and health practice (Bailey et al., 2006; Zhang et al., 2012).

Unfortunately, the peer-reviewed literature contains remarkably little comprehensive data from the past decade about eye and vision health knowledge and the impact of public awareness and health promotion in the United States nationally. In 2005 the NEI and the Lions Club International Foundation (LCIF) conducted a telephone survey of more than 3,000 English- and Spanish-speaking adults in the United States about public knowledge, attitudes, and practices related to eye health and disease. The study found that public awareness of glaucoma, age-related macular degeneration (AMD), diabetic eye disease, and low vision varied substantially by disease[4] (see Figure 5-2). While the majority of people who were aware of glaucoma (90 percent) or diabetic eye disease (51 percent) knew that

---

[3] Asians, Hispanics, and whites ranked blindness behind cancer and Alzheimer's disease, respectively (Scott et al., 2016).

[4] Low vision was defined as a visual impairment not correctable by standard eyeglasses, contact lenses, medication, or refractive surgery that interferes with the ability to perform everyday activities (NEI/LCIF, 2008).

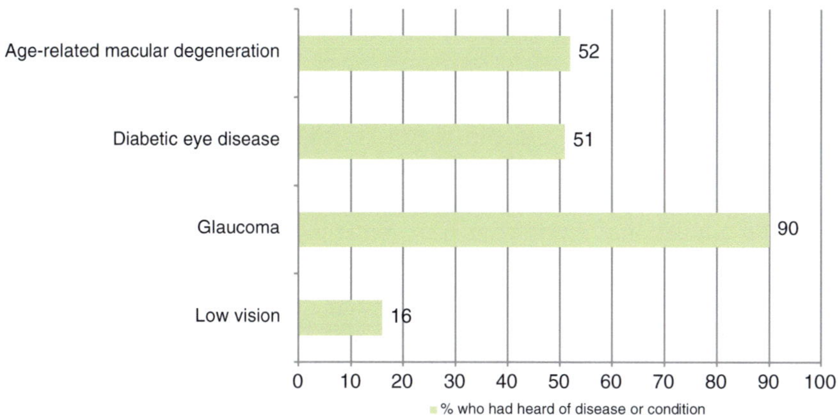

FIGURE 5-2 Percentage of adults ages 18 and older who are aware of four common eye-related diseases or conditions.
SOURCE: NEI/LCIF, 2008.

these conditions could be treated, the vast majority of these individuals did not know that glaucoma (92 percent) or diabetic retinopathy (89 percent) could present clinically with no early warning signs (NEI/LCIF, 2008). The most current, national data on vision loss awareness indicate that public knowledge about specific eye diseases and available treatment varies substantially.

Some improvements in knowledge over time have been observed. From 1991 to 2005, for instance, the percentage of adults who had heard of diabetic eye disease increased from 39 percent to 51 percent. The percentage of adults who had heard of glaucoma remained high (91 compared to 90 percent) during the same 14-year period (NEI/LCIF, 2008). The survey has not been updated since 2005, so there are no more recent statistics on public awareness of the major causes of eye disease. However, in its Five-Year Agenda for 2012–2017, NEHEP stated that "trends in the public's knowledge, attitude, and practices will be examined through updates of the Knowledge, Attitude, and Practices (KAP) Survey" (NEHEP, 2011, p. 22). The committee supports this endeavor and encourages federal support for updating data on the public's perception of and familiarity with eye health behaviors, risk factors, the relationship between eye and vision health and other measures of health, and available interventions, including the use of protective lenses, the utilization of health care, and the detection of uncorrected and correctable refractive error.

Awareness of Relevant Risk Factors for Vision Loss and Impairment

Knowing that a health threat exists is not the same as knowing what to do to avert that threat. Various factors are associated with an individual's level of knowledge about eye and vision health. The NEI-LCIF KAP survey analyzed data by age, household income, and educational attainment. Although the findings varied by condition, individuals with higher income levels and educational attainment were generally found to have a greater awareness of eye health (NEI/LCIF, 2008; see also Jaggernath et al., 2014). An awareness of eye health and disease has also been shown to be positively correlated with age (NEI/LCIF, 2008). Hispanic Americans are less likely to have knowledge of eye health and disease than Caucasians, African Americans, and Asian Americans (NEI/LCIF, 2008; Zhang et al., 2012). Studies outside of the United States found similar results. For example, a study in Canada about cataract, glaucoma, and macular degeneration found that both non-European ancestry and low educational attainment were associated with a poor knowledge of eye diseases, suggesting "that innovative education programs in primary and secondary schools and in non-English languages are needed to improve knowledge, attitudes, and practices" (Noertjojo et al., 2006, p. 617).

Not surprisingly, the evidence about public awareness is more robust when one examines risk factors that overlap with major public awareness initiatives. For example, two studies have analyzed the public's knowledge of smoking as a risk factor for AMD; these found, that 68 percent and 54 percent of the adults surveyed did not know that smoking was associated with specific types of vision impairment (AMD Alliance International, 2005; Caban-Martinez et al., 2011). A 2011 study investigating awareness of the relationship between smoking and vision impairment among smokers in the United States found that only 9.5 percent of smokers believed that smoking caused blindness, with those with a lower education level significantly more likely to doubt the association (Kennedy et al., 2011).

Even people who know that they have an eye disease or condition may not understand how that should affect their behavior. A primary reason that those who would benefit from an examination give for not seeing an eye care professional, even when they have an existing visual impairment and eye disease risk factors such as diabetes, is that "no need" exists (Bailey et al., 2006; Chou et al., 2014; McGwin et al., 2010; Varano et al., 2015). Substantial variation exists by state, and older populations are more likely to cite "no need" as a reason for not having their eyes examined (Chou et al., 2012, 2014). Patients are significantly more likely to receive annual eye examinations if they understand that examinations can detect eye disease (Sheppler et al., 2014). A 2008 American Optometric Association survey found that, although 81 percent of Americans use some form of vision correction, 32 percent were unaware that chronic and systemic diseases can be detected during an eye exam (AOA, 2008). A more recent survey found that, although African American participants with diabetes knew that they needed to have their eyes checked, they did not know why (NEHEP, 2014). A lack of awareness is also a barrier to accessing rehabilitation services among people who have uncorrectable impaired vision (Lam and Leat, 2015). The NEI-LCIF KAP survey revealed that only 31 percent of individuals with low vision had been told to see a low vision specialist (NEI/LCIF, 2008). These findings suggest that many eye care providers may not be providing sufficient education to their patients about low vision and the resources available to help them face the challenges associated with it—a topic that is explored further in Chapter 8.

In the absence of more robust data on public awareness about eye and vision health in general, it is reasonable to assume that members of the public know less about risk factors and appropriate actions to reduce the risk for specific eye diseases or conditions than about the existence of those diseases or conditions. The combination of a lack of awareness and the asymptomatic nature of much of early treatable disease leads to delayed diagnoses and treatment, which in turn leads to a greater risk of developing blindness (Alexander et al., 2008; Sloan et al., 2005). This suggests a need for additional public education activities and policies that encourage health care providers and public health practitioners to actively promote eye and vision health.

Efforts to Improve National Public Awareness of Eye and Vision Health

Enhancing public knowledge about a health threat is a fundamental first step in informing discussions that promote behavior change across multiple determinants of health and aligning health policies with general public health interests. Having reliable, consistent, evidence-based information that is available and accessible by a variety of stakeholders can help increase overall knowledge and lead individuals to behave in ways that promote good eye and vision health or seek appropriate care to slow progression of a vision-threatening disease or condition or to improve function when vision impairment is irreversible.

Public awareness campaigns—generally in combination with other public health strategies—have been used extensively and successfully in population health for decades. These campaigns often focus on behavior change that reduces the risk of poor health (e.g., smoking cessation, improved nutrition and exercise, increased cancer screenings) or the risk of injury (e.g., seatbelt use, reducing drunk driving and drug use, water safety). For example, campaigns targeting population tobacco use in adults have been identified as an important component in comprehensive tobacco control programs intended to affect knowledge, behaviors, and agenda setting (Bala et al., 2013; Chang et al., 2011; Durkin et al., 2012; Fosson et al., 2014; Hershey et al., 2005; Niederdeppe et al., 2004). Public education mass media campaigns in the United States and Australia have also been shown to be effective at reducing morbidity, mortality, and the economic costs due to skin cancer (Doran et al., 2016; Kyle et al., 2008; Shih et al., 2009). Public awareness campaigns also serve to raise the visibility of an issue among the national electorate, which can lead to changes in laws, regulations, and policies at the federal, state, and local levels that are intended to support and enforce individual behavior change (e.g., legislation to increase seatbelt use or increase the drinking age) or increase the resources and programmatic focus for specific diseases or conditions (e.g., breast cancer or HIV/AIDS).

Current national activities A number of national and state programs are designed to advance public awareness about eye issues. Many of these programs target particular threats to vision, especially among the most at-risk populations. For example, NEHEP partners with more than 60 professional, civic, and voluntary organizations and government agencies concerned with eye health in order to increase public awareness through culturally appropriate, health-literate, and evidence-based health information about the importance of early detection and timely treatment of eye disease and the use of vision rehabilitation services among health care professionals and the public (NEI/NIH, 2015b). Specifically, NEHEP includes five vision education programs focusing on (1) people living in Hispanic/ Latino communities, (2) people at risk for glaucoma, (3) diabetic eye disease, (4) age-related conditions, and (5) people living with low vision. NEHEP's printable cards, pamphlets, and infographics are geared toward use by a community health organizer. NEHEP partners with local governments to create culturally appropriate educational materials (NEHEP, 2011). The Lions Eye Health Program is a community-based education program that promotes healthy vision and raises awareness of the causes of preventable vision loss (Lions Club, 2016).

Various organizations design websites and related promotional materials to support national awareness months for specific eye diseases and conditions. For example, the NEI identifies January as Glaucoma Awareness Month (NEI/NIH, n.d.). Prevent Blindness has declared February to be National AMD and Low Vision Awareness Month and June to be Cataract Awareness Month (Prevent Blindness, 2016b). These types of activities provide valuable information about vision loss, but they fail to create a cohesive message that can advance eye and vision health as a larger public health priority among the general public.

Data on the impact of public awareness campaigns related to eye and vision health have largely been limited to data on exposure—e.g., the number of imprints, webpage views, or followers on social media websites—rather than on specific measures of health outcomes or on such determinants as attitudes and beliefs. There are no data to assess whether NEHEP activities have had an impact on health outcomes, behavioral change, or even general public awareness because the focus is not on behavior change and no funds are available to formally evaluate the program.[5,6] Moreover, there is no recent information about the number of Americans exposed to health education initiatives that are vision centric. In the future, large-scale public awareness campaigns will need to explicitly include resources to assess impact at different stages of the campaign.

Targeted education programs There are various smaller-scale, more conservative efforts to improve consumer education, and advocacy, professional, and patient organizations and other stakeholders can play an important role in their coordination. Smaller-scale health education initiatives have been shown to be effective at increasing the numbers of people receiving vision care and improving patient outcomes (Livingston et al., 1998). In the United States, for example, multiple health education interventions to promote screening for diabetic retinopathy have proven effective at increasing the rates of dilated fundus examinations (Jones et al., 2010; Walker et al., 2008; Weiss et al., 2015). After implementing a major vision health education campaign targeted to populations at higher risk for developing eye disease, Australia saw significant increases in the use of eye services and decreases in the prevalence of behaviors that are associated with increased risk to vision health (Müller et al., 2007). Similar findings emerged from a Norwegian study among diabetics (Sundling et al., 2008). A 2005 study of metal-ware factories in Italy found that the use of educational materials to prevent work-related eye injuries could be effective when it was coupled with increases in official inspections to promote compliance with workplace regulations (Mancini et al., 2005). More generally, health education has been shown to improve perceived security, quality of life, and functionality among patients with irreversible vision impairment (Dahlin Ivanoff et al., 2002; Eklund et al., 2004, 2005, 2008). Simple educational interventions

---

[5] It is important to note that NEHEP is not a behavioral change campaign per se and does not conduct general public outreach about eye health.

[6] Personal communication, N. Ammary-Risch, National Eye Health Education Program, 2016.

with patients can improve adherence to prescribed therapies and treatment schedules (Ellish et al., 2011; Weiss et al., 2015).

Examples of local public awareness campaigns include the Marshall B. Ketchum University's Children's Vision Initiative in California, the Day with the Doctor Intervention in Indiana, the Eye Exams in Putnam City Schools project in Oklahoma, the See to Read Vision Awareness Program in Tennessee, and the All The Kids project in Mississippi (AOA, 2014). Again, data on the impact of these types of programs vary and need to be linked to patient health outcomes, in addition to monitoring health care utilization rates.

The role of the media Mass and social media play a central role in shaping the lives and priorities of societies and individual communities. The media is an important public health tool for shaping public sentiment and political poignancy and their downstream effects on community attention and political priorities, respectively (Convissor et al., 1990; McCombs and Shaw, 1972). Furthermore, how the media portrays a particular health concern, such as visual impairment, may also be able to reduce the stigma or negative public perception related to that condition (e.g., IOM, 2012b; NASEM, 2016). For example, in the case of drug policy research, one study found that the media influences audiences by "setting the agenda and defining public interest; framing issues through selection and salience; indirectly shaping individual and community attitudes towards risk; and feeding into political debate and decision making" (Lancaster et al., 2011, p. 397). In its 2003 report *The Future of the Public's Health in the 21st Century*, the IOM cited media coverage of AIDS as a good example of how the media can enhance the visibility of important health topics among the general public (IOM, 2003). This knowledge can then serve as a catalyst to promote changes at the federal, state, local and community levels.

Little academic research exists on the role of the media in promoting eye and vision health in the United States. Some of the more common topics in the literature are various causes of eye injury (e.g., party foam–induced, work-related eye injuries, fireworks), although many of these studies call for additional awareness campaigns rather than evaluating the effectiveness of existing campaigns (Abulafia et al., 2013; Glazier et al., 2011; Korchak et al., 2012; Zohar et al., 2004). However, the Community Preventive Services Task Force has found strong evidence supporting the effectiveness of those health communication campaigns designed to influence behaviors "that use multiple channels, one of which must be mass media (e.g., television, radio, and billboards) but can also include small media, social media, and interpersonal communication, combined with the distribution of free or reduced-price health-related products" (ODPHP,

2010). The media's significance will continue to grow as more traditional news outlets (e.g., television, radio, and newspapers) are being replaced with ever-evolving communication technologies (e.g., smartphones, tablet computers) and social media outlets. The ubiquity of social media continues to expand opportunities to engage and educate the public about the importance of maintaining eye and vision health, and social media can serve as a valuable resource to connect visually impaired people to needed services and advocacy platforms. The effective use of social media platforms in health promotion intervention programs, in general, remains a fluid topic of discussion (Chou et al., 2009, 2013; Korda and Itani, 2013; Lefebvre and Bornkessel, 2013; Moorhead et al., 2013; Neiger et al., 2012). The use and efficacy of social media to educate the public and increase awareness concerning eye and vision health warrants additional research and consideration.

A national public awareness campaign to promote eye and vision health
Large-scale public awareness campaigns for eye and vision health will require substantial resources, which will necessitate a federal presence and collaboration with a variety of stakeholders in the public and private sectors. The most effective public awareness campaigns are usually large scale and multifaceted, involving a range of outreach activities, stakeholders and sponsors, educational materials, messaging, and media platforms. For example, to influence ultraviolet (UV) radiation-protective behaviors, a systematic review by the Community Preventive Services Task Force recommends "combinations of individual-directed strategies, mass media campaigns, and environmental and policy changes across multiple settings within a defined geographic area (city, state, province, or country)" (CPSTF, 2014).

Likewise, a comprehensive public awareness campaign for eye and vision health would need to be one component of a larger, long-term effort to change attitudes, knowledge, behavior, and practice across the lifespan. For example, the Partnership for a Healthier America and the Let's Move! initiative have raised the visibility of childhood obesity as a public health priority using a variety of media platforms to increase awareness (e.g., Chanel One News in schools, websites, mass marketing campaigns with industry, agreements with Sesame Street) (Spinweber and Honeysett, 2013). The media messaging is part of a larger effort to engage a wide range of public and private partners in diverse activities in order to catalyze large-scale changes in behaviors, interventions, and education around childhood obesity. Some of the other activities include increasing access to healthier, quality, affordable meals, maintaining and creating safe places for children to play, offering more opportunities for kids to get involved in active play, and educating parents on ways to increase healthy eating habits and active play (The White House, 2010).

Given the current and projected number of individuals with varying degrees and types of vision impairment in the United States (see Chapter 2), it will be necessary for advocacy organizations, government agencies, health care professionals, public health practitioners, researchers, and private industry to collaborate in order to amplify messaging from public health entities within and across the federal government, governmental PHDs, and population health systems. A large-scale public awareness campaign will need to be centered around concise and concrete goals and to consider a combination of individual-directed strategies, mass media campaigns, and environmental and policy changes across multiple settings within defined geographic areas (e.g., city, state, province, or country). Ascertaining the impact of specific campaigns and the elements most closely predictive of success will require careful evaluation. As with anti-smoking campaigns, the intensity and duration of mass vision health media campaigns may influence effectiveness, but the population characteristics, length of follow-up, and concurrent secular trends and events will also be important to monitor (Doyle et al., 2008). Necessary outcomes should include, but not be limited to

- changes in knowledge about high prevalence conditions, diseases, and events;
- risk and protective factors that account for multiple determinants of health;
- behavior changes (e.g., access to and use of eye health services, and adherence to risk reduction practices); and
- health outcomes, including more downstream effects from vision impairment.

Federal support for the infrastructure and engagement in public awareness campaigns, and large-scale public health initiatives, is "more likely when a field has a united front of advocates to communicate the urgency of a problem, why that problem should be addressed now, and how best to solve the problem" (IOM, 2015, p. 346). This will require the eye and vision field to establish a common platform from which to advance messages to improve eye and vision health that extend beyond the delivery of health care services. Moreover, because a lack of knowledge about vision loss and the possible prevention or treatment of subsequent vision impairment requires increased knowledge among vulnerable populations and practitioners, public awareness campaigns hold promise as a tactic to mitigate these deficits, when included as one component of a larger population health strategy. Assessing the impact of specific campaigns will require carefully designed evaluations, to not only provide some evidence of return on investment, but also provide the foundation from which to generate sustained support for ongoing efforts in future years.

EXPANDING ACCESS TO COMMUNITY-BASED VISION SCREENING SERVICES AND FOLLOW-UP CARE

Ensuring that at-risk populations are linked to appropriate clinical care is a public health function. Vision screening can be a critical connection between the clinical vision services system, the larger public health system, and the populations they serve. It is a means of strengthening clinical vision service actions in community settings and an opportunity for refocusing the clinical vision services system and its providers on the public health objectives of preventing and treating vision loss and approaches to accomplishing those objectives. In the absence of adequate resources to provide comprehensive eye examinations to every person in accordance with evidence-based guidelines, vision screenings may be performed by both optometrists and ophthalmologists, as well as by other properly trained individuals in order to expand entry into appropriate eye and vision care systems, as well as into the overarching health care system.

Vision screenings allow for the identification—but not diagnosis—of eye disease. In this report, unless otherwise stated, the term "vision screening" is used to refer to any of a set of general eye health assessments that can be used to identify potential problems with visual functioning or symptoms suggestive of an eye disease or condition. Screenings cannot diagnose the cause of vision problems, but they can be used to expand entry to the health care system and access to appropriate follow-up care for more vulnerable populations. Mobile screening and imaging units can improve access to vision care, promote follow-up care, optimize the capacity of a limited workforce, and promote multidisciplinary collaborations (Beynat et al., 2009; Boucher et al., 2008; Griffith et al., 2016; Hautala et al., 2009; Kodjebacheva et al., 2011). Vision screenings are generally less expensive and less time-consuming than comprehensive eye examinations, but there are also concerns about the sensitivity and specificity of vision screenings. These concerns and more technical aspects of screenings and comprehensive eye examinations are described in Chapter 7.

In the United States, emerging diagnostic technologies and innovative screening programs have extended the services of the vision care system to schools in remote and medically underserved areas. For example, photoscreening and remote autorefraction have been shown to be effective at screening schoolchildren for amblyopia and vision disorders in urban and rural Alaska (Arnold et al., 2008; Lang et al., 2007). Screening high-risk populations such as children for refractive error and amblyopia and then assuring access to proper treatment, including eye examinations for clinical diagnosis and corrective lenses, are key actions that can be advanced through a variety of population health partnerships and strategies.

Vision Screening for Children and Other At-Risk Populations

As in adults, refractive error is a major cause of preventable vision impairment in children and young adults (Tarczy-Hornoch et al., 2013; Vitale et al., 2008). For example, the Collaborative Longitudinal Evaluation of Ethnicity and Refractive Error Study evaluated more than 2,500 children ages 5 through 17 and found "overall, 9.2 percent of the children were myopic, 12.8 percent were hyperopic, and 28.4 were astigmatic," with pronounced differences between the four ethnic/racial groups studied (Kleinstein et al., 2003, p. 1141). Undiagnosed vision impairment in children can have substantial effects on social development and health, with the potential to negatively impact social, physical, educational, and professional activities (Davidson and Quinn, 2011; Kulp et al., 2016). Uncorrected refractive error can have significant effects on educational performance and is a risk factor for amblyopia (Tarczy-Hornoch et al., 2013). Glewwe and colleagues explore disparities in vision care utilization by low-income and minority children, noting that they "have a greater than average risk of under-diagnosis and under-treatment . . . [and] Title 1 students are two to three times more likely than non-Title 1 students to have undetected or untreated vision problems" (Glewwe et al., 2014, p. 1).

Mobile clinics and school-based vision screenings that are provided at no cost offer a means of addressing demonstrated financial, social, and political barriers to accessing eye care for children and other at-risk populations (Castanes, 2003). One school-based screening program in the United Kingdom achieved a screening acceptance rate of greater than 95 percent among 3,721 children; of the 11.14 percent of students referred who were for follow-up care, more than half had refractive errors correctable by eyeglasses (Toufeeq and Oram, 2014). In a screening program in North Carolina, school nurses evaluated 2,726 elementary school children during the 2009–2010 school year and identified 3 cases needing intervention out of every 100 evaluations (Kemper et al., 2012). Mobile clinics have been used to provide vision screenings for pre-kindergarten, kindergarten, and first-grade public school children, with one program performing more than 63,000 evaluations, representing 55 percent of the eligible population during a 12-year period (Griffith et al., 2016). Similarly, the University of California, Los Angeles (UCLA) Mobile Eye Clinic identified 906 out of 11,302 first-graders as having decreased visual acuity and found that eyeglasses would correct vision in 94.7 percent of those cases, although the investigation did not record rates of follow-up care after screening (Kodjebacheva et al., 2011).

Independent scholars have similarly recommended that policy makers implement vision programs that bring vision services to children, including screening, into classroom environments (Ethan and Basch, 2008). Head Start and Early Head Start programs are required, in collaboration with parents, to "obtain linguistically and age appropriate screenings to identify concerns regarding a child's developmental, sensory (*visual* and auditory), behavioral, motor, language, social, cognitive, perceptual, and emotional skills" within 45 calendar days of the child's entry into the program and facilitate implementation of follow-up plans and treatment.[7] The American Academy of Ophthalmology, the American Academy of Pediatric Ophthalmologists and Strabismus, and the American Academy of Pediatrics have recommended that vision screening be included in routine school-based vision checks because it can maximize the rate of early detection of amblyopia, strabismus, refractive error, and other eye conditions in children, among other benefits (AAO, 2013). Many states have imposed vision screening requirements for school-age children to help identify students in need of eye care (see, AAPOS, 2011, for a current list of state-by-state school screening requirements). Box 5-1 details the example of how the state of Michigan has promoted vision screening programs for children. However, specific requirements and screening practices vary among and even within states, with implications for the percentage of students with visual impairments that are identified as requiring eye care (AAPOS, 2011; Marshall et al., 2010). Some states—including Arizona, Hawaii, Idaho, New Hampshire, North Dakota, South Carolina, and South Dakota—have no pediatric vision screening policies at all, though the governments of New Hampshire and South Carolina do recommend screenings (AAPOS, 2011).

Promoting Follow-Up Care After Screenings

Screening programs cannot lead to reduced vision impairment if the process does not include a mechanism to assure appropriate follow-up care. One demonstration project that provided vision screening of preschool-age children at two primary care practices and two community-based centers achieved monocular visual acuity and stereopsis screening rates between 70 and 93 percent and 88 and 98 percent for 3- and 4-year-olds, respectively. However, the rates of follow-up varied widely—from 29 to 100 percent and from 41 to 100 percent for the 3- and 4-year-olds, respectively (Hartmann et al., 2006). A quality improvement project to enhance the rate of pediatric vision screenings at 13 clinics in North Carolina saw significant

---

[7] 45 C.F.R. 1304.20 (italic added).

BOX 5-1
Case Study on Michigan's Public Health
Vision Screening Program

Michigan's Public Health Hearing and Vision Screening Programs are the result of a 60-year collaboration between LHDs and the education system. The vision program includes an initial screening, retesting, and referral of children through a standardized program that tests visual acuity, eye muscle function, refractive error, and symptoms of other eye and vision problems (State of Michigan, 2016). Upon failing the initial screening, children are retested. If they fail the retest, they are referred for follow-up care. Approximately 1.1 million children are screened every year for both hearing and vision problems, with about 87,000 children referred for follow-up care (State of Michigan, 2016).

The program is supported through Michigan law, which states that vision testing or screening must be presented at the time of registration for kindergarten. Parents or guardians must present either a statement confirming receipt of screening from the U.S. Department of Health and Human Services Vision Screening or from a licensed provider (optometrist, ophthalmologist, or medical physician) stating an eye examination had occurred after the age of 3 but prior to school entry (MDHHS, 2016b). The state subsequently mandates vision screenings for children in first grade, third grade, fifth grade, seventh grade, and ninth grade, though there may be some variations in schedule depending on the local PHD (State of Michigan, 2016).

Screenings are facilitated by schools and LHDs. These screenings are available free of charge at the health department (MDHHS, 2016b; State of Michigan, 2016). These screenings are conducted by technicians employed by the PHD. The technicians undergo a 4-week training with practicum and maintain training through regular evaluation and mandatory attendance at a continuing education workshop every 2 years (State of Michigan, 2016). The program's website notes that this program "routinely identifies 10-15 percent of those screened as needing eye care" (MDHHS, 2016a).

improvements in the rate of screening among children ages 3 to 5 years over a 6-month period; vision distance testing increased from 92 to 97 percent, and stereopsis screening rates increased from 80 percent to 89 percent. Yet, follow-up rescreening for initially untestable children was infrequently documented, and referral rates for abnormal screens remained low at 48 percent (Kemper et al., 2011). Other studies have also found that the rates of appropriate referral and follow-up care can be sub-optimal (Hered and Wood, 2013).

Simple logic dictates that programs that provide eyeglasses following screenings or eye examinations will improve the sight of more people with correctable refractive error than screenings or examinations alone. A number of programs available through various philanthropic and charitable

BOX 5-2
Examples of Programs to Improve Eye Care in Communities

EyeCare America, the public service program of the Foundation of the American Academy of Ophthalmology, may provide a medical eye exam and up to 1 year of care at no cost for any disease condition during the initial exam for individuals who are ages 65 and older and who have not seen an EyeMD in 3 or more years. People who are found to be at increased risk for eye diseases and who have not had an eye exam in 12 months or more may also be eligible. Eyeglasses are not covered (AAO, 2016b).

InfantSEE® is a program developed in 2005 by the American Optometric Association and the Vision Care Institute of Johnson & Johnson Vision Care Inc. The program connects participating optometrists with families to provide children ages 6 to 12 months a comprehensive infant eye assessment as a no-cost public service (AOA, 2012).

The Lions Club OneSight program is a partnership between various nonprofit organizations that offers education, outreach, and free prescription eyeglasses to those who qualify. The program's Vision Vans are mobile units and vans that deliver new eyeglasses and free eye care to disadvantaged children. However this program was eliminated in 2015. The program also offers discounted eyeglasses vouchers. Once per year, a Lions Club partner, the Luxottica Retail stores (e.g., Sears Optical, LensCrafters, Pearle Vision, and Target Optical) offers free eyeglasses and eye exams to the needy and uninsured (OneSight, 2016).

New Eyes for the Needy provides vouchers to people who need to buy new prescription eyeglasses in the United States and distributes used eyeglasses to disadvantaged populations in developing countries. Voucher applications are available through the New Eyes website and must be submitted by a social service agency. The website provides a link to national programs that may provide free or low-cost eye examinations (New Eyes, n.d.).

The Philadelphia Eagles Eye Mobile visits a different school each day to deliver free eye examinations, prescription eyeglasses, and follow-up care from an ophthalmologist to under-insured and uninsured children in the Greater Philadelphia area (Phildelphia Eagles, 2016). Since its inception, the program has served more than 71,000 children and distributed more than 52,000 pairs of eyeglasses.

Sight for Students is a national gift certificate program founded in 1997 by Vision Service Plan (VSP) and part of VSP's larger Eyes of Hope initiative, which provides free eye exams and eyeglasses to low-income and uninsured children ages 19 and younger who qualify for the program (VSP, 2016). VSP partners with Boys & Girls Clubs of America, Communities in Schools, Lions Club International Foundation, the National Association of Community Health Centers, the National Association of School Nurses, the National Council of LaRaza, the National Head Start Association, and Prevent Blindness to deliver a free comprehensive exam

continued

BOX 5-2 Continued

and, if needed, corrective lenses if needed to more than 50,000 children each year (VSP, n.d.).

Vision To Learn, founded in 2012 in Los Angeles, provides children with free eye exams and free eyeglasses in California, Delaware, Hawaii, Iowa, and Virginia (Vision To Learn, 2016). Vision To Learn partners with other neighborhood youth and community organizations to conduct vision screenings. The Mobile Eye Clinic then visits each school or community site to conduct free eye examinations and fit children for free eyeglasses. Greater than 89 percent of children served by Vision To Learn live in poverty and 87 percent are minorities. Vision To Learn recently partnered with the Los Angeles Clippers, adding to the group's list of committed community advocates.

VISION USA is a program that provides free eye care from an optometrist to eligible low-income and uninsured people in 39 states and the District of Columbia. To apply you must work with a charitable organization, social worker, case worker, or community health agency to submit an application (AOA Foundation, 2016). Eyewear may be provided at no cost or for a small fee in some states.

---

organizations, professional organizations, and industry provide free eyecare screenings, examinations, and eyeglasses for children and other vulnerable populations to better ensure the detection of potential vision problems and improve eyesight. Box 5-2 provides some examples. Many of these programs are designed to link children and low-income individuals to available eye and vision services, including in some cases, provision of eyeglasses. Only a few recent peer-reviewed articles on population-level impact are available for these programs. A 2015 study on 689 students at 28 different schools served by the Philadelphia Eagles Eye Mobile found that false-positive rates of school nurse screening averaged 16.11 percent (range 0 to 44 percent), suggesting the need for better training to reduce false-positive screenings. The same study found that the use of prescribed glasses was 71 percent at 12 months, but only 53 percent of children followed through with their pediatric ophthalmology referral (Alvi et al., 2015).

Recently, Vision To Learn partnered with Johns Hopkins University, the Baltimore City Health Department, and the Baltimore City Public School System to launch a citywide initiative, Vision for Baltimore, which will provide vision screenings and free eyeglasses for pre-kindergarteners to eighth-graders in all 50 Baltimore City public schools (Naron and Mendes,

2016). The Baltimore City Health Department will administer initial screenings, with the support of the Anne E. Casey Foundation, the Abell Foundation, and Vision To Learn, the latter of which has mobile eye clinics for onsite services. Warby Parker, a New York City–based online eyewear retailer, has agreed to provide eyeglasses (Naron and Mendes, 2016). Staff from the School of Education and the Wilmer Eye Institute will work with the schools to train school staff and maximize the use of prescribed eyeglasses. A formal evaluation of the program's impact is planned. Results documenting the impact on student achievement and eyewear compliance have been submitted for publication (Naron and Mendes, 2016). A similar initiative exists in New York City, where the Community Schools Initiative will expand its vision screening program to all 130 Community Schools (including elementary, middle, and high schools) through a partnership with Warby Parker to provide free eyeglasses to every student in need (City of New York, 2016). Evaluations of the impacts of these programs will be essential to establishing better evidentiary support for investment in similar programs. As indicated by even the short list of activities provided in Box 5-2, a wide range of partners is already committed to improving the eye and vision health of the nation. It will be important to follow the impact of these programs and evaluate critical success and failure factors when considering whether similar initiatives will work in other communities and on larger scales. Policy makers could collaborate with PHDs, school administrators, and other stakeholders on a national effort to standardize state requirements for vision screening in schools.

Medicaid and the Children's Health Insurance Program are public health programs that can also provide eye and vision care coverage for certain low-income and disabled people and families (Kaiser Family Foundation, 2013; Medicaid, 2016b). All plans that cover children and adolescents must provide basic eye care services as an essential health benefit (Healthcare.gov, 2016). Optional eye and vision benefits under Medicaid are determined by individual states and so vary from state to state, but they may include the provision of eyeglasses and optometric, diagnostic, screening, preventive, and rehabilitative services, as well as prescription drugs, dental care, physical and occupational therapy, and podiatric services, among others (Medicaid, 2016a). Efforts to expand the benefits of these programs are considered in Chapter 6.

ENCOURAGING ENVIRONMENTS THAT SUPPORT EYE HEALTH AND VISUAL FUNCTION: POLICY DEVELOPMENT AND ENFORCEMENT

Health departments can play an important role in influencing the built environment, i.e., the physical environment constructed by human activity, although "exact [legal] mechanisms vary by state and locality" (see, e.g., Perdue et al., 2003, p. 1392). The built environment includes all the physical parts of where we live, including homes, buildings, worksites, transportation systems, civic infrastructure, and public places (Dannenberg et al., 2011). State and LHDs have the legal authority and capacity to work across sectors to improve the environmental conditions that impede eye and vision health; these environmental conditions include both the built and social determinants of eye and vision health. Two of the more obvious issues related to the built environment are accessibility and injury prevention, although building design regulations may now explicitly address vision-related conditions, such as eyestrain. Accessibility barriers can range from poorly designed pavement to inadequate pedestrian crossings. Poorly designed physical spaces (such as difficult-to-navigate subway platforms and poorly lighted building interiors) can cause injuries to people with low vision (Imrie and Kumar, 1998). These are important elements to consider when developing a comprehensive population health approach to address eye and vision health. Indeed, based on a variety of factors, health departments may take a leading role in recommending changes to the built environment. Arguably, for example, Frieden's (2010) Health Impact Pyramid places greater reliance on changing the environment (the context in the pyramid) than on medical care as the basis for health department interventions at the population level.

Ensuring Equal Access to Facilities and Services

The Americans with Disabilities Act (ADA) of 1990 (42 U.S.C. 12181),[8] including changes by the ADA Amendments Act of 2008,[9] prohibits discrimination on the basis of disability by state and local governments, places of public accommodation (e.g., hotels, shopping centers, pharmacies, doctor's offices, hospitals, libraries, private schools, health spas), commercial facilities, and private entities. The Rehabilitation Act of 1973 provides similar protections in relation to programs operated or funded by the federal government, as well as requiring equal employment opportunity within the federal government.[10] The ADA's definition of disability includes "blindness" (defined as meaning having less than 20/200 visual acuity even with corrective lenses or a visual field that is 20 degrees or less, regardless of acuity).[11] People with "low vision" (eyesight that is better than 20/200 or a visual field that is greater than 20 degrees but that includes a significant

---

[8] P.L. 101-336, enacted July 26, 1990.
[9] P.L. 110-325, enacted January 1, 2009.
[10] P.L. 93-112, enacted September 26, 1973.
[11] Social Security Act § 216(i)(1)(B).

vision impairment that substantially limits the ability to see well under different circumstances) may also require accommodations.

Entities subject to regulations must

> follow accessibility standards when constructing or altering facilities; remove architectural or structural communication barriers in existing facilities where it is readily achievable to do so; make reasonable modifications in policies and procedures (e.g., allow person to be accompanied by service animal or guide dog, even if a hotel has a "no pets" policy); eliminate discriminatory eligibility criteria (e.g., allow a guest to use alternative state ID to substitute for driver's license at check-in); and provide auxiliary aids and services leading to effective communication if it is not an undue burden and does not fundamentally alter the nature of the goods or services provided (e.g., provide alternate format materials such as Braille, large print, and audio tape when a guest cannot read standard print materials due to a disability). (DOJ, n.d.)

The facilities and services covered by the ADA includes, but are not limited to, transportation services; academic, medical, and recreational facilities; and government programs, activities, and services. For example, mass transit systems should design their facilities and equipment to be accessible to disabled individuals (AFB, 2016a). Airlines could offer additional services such as pre-boarding, a guided tour of the aircraft, and providing menus and evacuation information in Braille (SATH, 2013). Similarly, libraries, museums, shopping malls, community health clinics, courthouses, and city sidewalks should all be accessible to individuals with disabilities, including those who are legally blind. The ADA also requires that regulated entities promote effective communication with people who have disabilities that can affect different communication capabilities (DOJ, 2015). The U.S. Department of Justice has offered guidance on the types of services and practices that can be considered to better accommodate people with vision impairment under the ADA (see Box 5-3).

The Equal Employment Opportunity Commission, the agency responsible for enforcing the ADA, has also issued regulations regarding vision needs under the ADA Amendments Act of 2008. The statute, at 42 U.S.C. 12102(4)(c)(ii), states, inter alia, that mitigating measures include low-vision devices (excluding ordinary eyeglasses or contact lenses), the use of assistive technology, and reasonable accommodations or auxiliary aids or services. With regard to eyeglasses, the regulations state,

> The ameliorative effects of the mitigating measures of ordinary eyeglasses or contact lenses shall be considered in determining whether an impairment substantially limits a major life activity. The term "ordinary eyeglasses or contact lenses" means lenses that are intended to fully correct visual acuity

or eliminate refractive error; and the term "low-vision devices" means devices that magnify, enhance, or otherwise augment a visual image.

Likewise, adaptive behaviors to compensate for low vision (such as side-to-side movement for someone with monocular vision) are included. Problems associated with the affordability of eyeglasses are discussed in Chapter 6.

Ensuring and enforcing equal access under the ADA will require collaboration among federal, state, and local governments, architects and engineers, city planners, disability rights advocates, and others.

BOX 5-3
Examples of Services and Practices That May
Assist People with Vision Impairment Under
the Americans with Disabilities Act

- **Architectural Barriers** "Remove architectural barriers in existing facilities . . . where such removal is readily achievable, i.e., easily accomplishable and able to be carried out without much difficulty or expense."[a]
- **Guiding Techniques** Offer assistance to guests in navigating the facility, including finding and orienting to their rooms and other facilities, emphasizing safety information (e.g., nearest emergency exit).[b]
- **Verbalizing Directions** Be cognizant of how you provide directions, refraining from using gestures and other non-verbal cues.
- **New Construction and Alteration Requirements** Comply with minimum requirements of the ADA Standards for Accessible Design (Standards), as applicable.[a]
- **Signs** Include signs with:
  - Raised and Braille letters or numbers;
  - Appropriate character proportion and height;
  - Mounting location;
  - Color contrast; and
  - Non-glare surface.[b]
- **Elevators** Add Brailled or raised markings on elevator control buttons.[a]
- **Lighting** Provide ample lighting to promote visual function.[b]
- **Service Animals** Permit the use of a service animal.[a]
- **Auxiliary Aids and Services** Provide a "qualified" interpreter on-site or via video remote interpreting services; notetakers; transcription services; qualified readers; information in large print, Braille, or electronically for use with a wide variety of technologies including screen reader software, magnification software, and optical readers; or "other effective methods of making visually delivered materials available to individuals who are blind or have low vision."[a]

SOURCES: [a] 28 CFR § 36.101 et seq.; [b] DOJ, 2001.

Coordinating these actions to derive maximum value and efficiency from individual efforts is the difficult but necessary task of stakeholders in all sectors. Governmental PHDs can help facilitate these efforts by convening and working with local employers, regulators, and low-vision community advocates to create a long-term strategy to continue to improve ADA compliance.

Building Design and the Consideration of Light Sources

Appropriate architectural design can promote and maintain good eye and vision health as well as the functionality of individuals with vision impairment, especially in home-like settings. According to the Low Vision Design Committee of the National Institute of Building Sciences (NIBS), "while treatment of low vision and other visual disorders are medical issues, assuring optimal access to the built environment for persons with visual impairments is a design issue" (NIBS, 2015, p. 5). The NIBS committee recently published guidelines to help those planning and designing building sites to create building access, interior spaces with appropriate visual cues, and lighting design that optimizes the functioning of people with chronic visual impairments. For example, the implementation and manipulation of lighting design is an effective means to compensate for aging eyes and diminished abilities (Gordon, 2003; Krusen, 2010). Low-level lighting can contribute to falls (Paul and Liu, 2012). Creating office spaces and public open spaces with appropriate visual cues can help individuals with visual impairment navigate these spaces. Using high contrast colors can help make signing, light switches, or stairs more visible, and the use of matte paint can reduce glare. Tactile flooring and variations in ceiling height can reflect sound in ways that create cues for the visually impaired (Anderson, 2014). Using uniform lighting in hallways and stairwells can eliminate confusing shadows that may mimic changes in elevation (AFB, 2016b). Currently, it is not known whether these guidelines are widely observed (Sawyer and Kaup, 2014).

As the population ages and more people experience the vision loss typically associated with the aging process, it will become increasingly important to ensure that retirement communities, assisted living and nursing facilities, and general rehabilitation facilities are designed or furnished to enhance visual function in order to reduce the potential negative downstream consequences of vision impairment. Similar considerations are useful in individual homes and should be incorporated into public awareness campaigns targeting older populations.

Maintaining Eye Health: Going Green and Eyestrain

Eyestrain is a common condition that occurs when eyes become tired from continuous use, but it usually does not have serious or long-term consequences. In some cases, eyestrain can be suggestive of an underlying eye condition (e.g., accommodation insufficiency or convergence insufficiency) necessitating treatment (Chase et al., 2009). The causes of eyestrain may include reading without resting one's eyes if underlying factors are present; driving long distances and performing other activities involving extended focus; being exposed to bright light or glare; working with insufficient light; having an underlying eye problem such as dry eyes, uncorrected refractive error, eye teaming disorder, or accommodative or binocular vision disorders; being stressed or fatigued; and exposure to conditions that may contribute to dry eyes (Barnhardt et al., 2012; Gowrisankaran and Sheedy, 2015). The phenomenon of computer vision syndrome, which is "a group of visual symptoms experienced in relation to the use of computers," is relatively new and is associated with reduced productivity at work and reduced quality of life (Ranasinghe et al., 2016). Visual symptoms may include eyestrain, eye fatigue, headaches, ocular discomfort, dry eye, photophobia, diplopia, and blurred vision (Rosenfield, 2011; Sheedy et al., 2003).

Appropriate architectural design can help reduce eyestrain. Proper lighting, anti-glare filters, the ergonomic positioning of computer monitors, physical breaks away from screens, lubricating eye drops, and special computer glasses all may help improve visual comfort (Blehm et al., 2005). In recent decades, there have been efforts to promote the concept of "green buildings," which are meant to ensure the healthiest possible environment while representing the most efficient and least disruptive use of land, water, energy, and resources (EPA, 2015). Many of these new buildings reduce energy consumption by incorporating large windows or exteriors, allowing daylight to reach more space (EPA, 2015). Daylighting, "the practice of placing windows or other openings and reflective surfaces so that during the day natural light provides effective internal lighting," creates new challenges related to eye comfort (Spellman and Bieber, 2012, p. 256). Existing guiding principles for new construction require that facilities achieve a minimum daylight factor while providing appropriate lighting controls and glare control to minimize eyestrain (GSA, 2014). Such lighting controls can include building maintenance to keep windows free from glare, installing screen-type shading devices that are automatically controlled according to the seasons and the time, veiling reflections on monitors to reduce visual display terminal glare, and providing artificial lighting (Hwang and Kim, 2011). These controls protect occupants' eyes and also contribute to improved psychological health and productivity (Hwang and Kim, 2011). The committee believes that policies encouraging these practices are advisable and can encourage a broader range of stakeholders, including architects and human resource professionals, to think about their roles in promoting eye and vision health. As the use of computers and digital electronic devices for both vocational and non-vocational activities continues to expand in terms of the length of time as well as of the type of digital electronic screen available, it will become increasingly important to monitor how this environmental exposure affects eye health and development, especially in younger populations.

Improving Eye Injury Protection

Occupational and sports-related eye injuries occur frequently. Goldstein and Wee (2011) estimate that approximately 40,000 to 600,000 sports-related eye injuries alone occur annually. Many instances of eye injury can be avoided by using protective eyewear. The CDC, professional societies, and others recommend wearing eye protection during specific high-risk activities to reduce the risk of occupational eye injury and the associated potential for vision loss (AAO, 2016a; CDC, 2013a; OSHA, 2003; Prevent Blindness, 2016a). To reduce eye injuries, OSHA requires employers to use three eye safety strategies, as appropriate, in workplaces. These include (1) using engineering controls (i.e., the best strategy) such as machine guards that prevent the escape of particles or welding curtains for arc flash protection; (2) using administrative controls such as making certain that areas designated as "off limits" are visited only by those assigned to work there; and (3) providing for and enforcing the use of proper protective eyewear (CDC, 2013b). Employers must ensure that eye and face protection, which meets specified safety standards, is provided whenever necessary to protect workers from occupational hazards, and that all workers required to wear eye and face protection receive proper training and, when appropriate, fittings (OSHA, 2009, 2016).

Unfortunately, factors such as uncomfortable fit, the lack of available protection, and the lack of a culture of workplace safety may contribute to poor adherence rates (Lombardi et al., 2009). To improve compliance among workers, state agencies have produced simple materials for posting or distribution that seek to educate employees about the risks of injury and the benefits of eye protection (CDPH, 2008; TDI, 2007). The National Institute for Occupational Safety and Health and eye health safety and advocacy organizations have produced similar materials, available online, and OSHA has made an e-tool available to assist employers and employees with understanding the requirements for eye protection in their specific industries or occupations (CDC, 2013b; CPWR, 2014; OSHA, 2016; Prevent Blindness, 2016c). There are also concerns about certain under-regulated (and culturally distinct) agricultural worker communities, but more research is needed to demonstrate the effectiveness of community-based participatory models of education on the state-level enforcement of federal OSHA standards (Earle-Richardson et al., 2014; Tovar-Aguilar et al., 2014; Verma et al., 2011).

Nationally representative surveys have found that the rates of appropriate use of recreational eye protection in adults and children are low (approximately 30 percent and 15 percent, respectively) (Forrest et al., 2008; Matter et al., 2007). Estimates suggest that more than 90 percent of sports-related eye injuries could be prevented by using appropriate eye protection (Prevent Blindness, 2016c). The American Academy of Ophthalmology, the American Academy of Pediatrics, the American Association for Pediatric Ophthalmology and Strabismus, and the American Public Health Association, and the American Academy of Optometry all recommend protective eyewear for children in sports that pose a risk of eye injury (AAP, 2011; AOA, 2016). Appendix F shows examples of recommended eye protection for different sports (NEI/NIH, 2015a). Ordinary prescription glasses, contact lenses, and sunglasses do not protect against eye injuries (CDC, 2013b). In fact, regular eye glasses do not mitigate the risk of more serious injury and may shatter on impact (Goldstein and Wee, 2011).

The committee considers the use of protective eyewear in recreational and hazardous environments (e.g., home settings or around hazardous materials) to be amenable to change through policy implementation and education campaigns. Interventions targeted at multiple, engaged stakeholders can result in players more likely to change their behavior as a result (Eime et al., 2004, 2005). A 2009 systematic review (looking at both occupational and recreational eye protection) concluded that current research "[does] not provide reliable evidence that educational interventions are effective in preventing eye injuries," primarily due to the low quality of existing research and significant variation in study design (Shah et al., 2009, p. 11). However, Healthy People 2020 recommends such campaigns that could be combined with relevant policies and the provision of protective eyewear—to increase the use of protective eyewear in sports (CPSTF, 2010; ODPHP, 2016e). Surveillance systems monitor injuries, but more is needed to ensure compliance with occupational safety standards and to have more widespread adoption of protective eyewear in high-risk sports. Public awareness accompanied by policies, monitoring, and the provision of appropriate protective gear is essential so that athletes, parents, coaches, trainers, referees, and health care providers can help decrease morbidity from eye injuries (CDC, 2012; Goldstein and Wee, 2011; NEI/NIH, 2015a,b). Most importantly, school and organized sports programs can establish policies that promote and enforce the use of protective devices in particularly high-risk activities. Governmental PHDs can work with local communities to help develop and adopt regulations and policies that support the use of protective eyewear in both workplace and sports settings. Future research in this area should focus on the factors affecting policy adoption and compliance with established policies.

Promote Infection Control and Immunization

Poor hygiene, infrequent replacement of contact lens storage cases, and overnight contact lens wear are avoidable risk factors for microbial keratitis, contact lens–related inflammation, and other ophthalmic complications affecting eye health (Collier et al., 2014; Keay et al., 2007; Radford et al., 2009; Stapleton et al., 2008, 2012; Szczotka-Flynn et al., 2010). The CDC issued recommendations for keeping eyes healthy in contact lens wearers, but a recent review of the literature on past and recent trends found that the incidence of serious contact lens–related eye infections (e.g., microbial keratitis), which can lead to vision impairment, is rising (CDC, 2015g; Yildiz et al., 2012). This suggests that the public may not be adhering to published recommendations for various reasons.

The primary obstacle to eliminating contact lens–related infection and associated vision loss is not a lack of clarity on best practices, but rather improving patient education, awareness, and adherence. The CDC reported in 2015 that 99 percent of surveyed contact lens wearers engage in at least one risk behavior (including sleeping in their contact lenses, swimming or showering with them, rinsing/storing them in water, and failure to follow replacement schedules) (Cope et al., 2015). The impact of increased health promotion or education activities (e.g., at each eye care professional follow-up appointments) on contact lens–related infections and associated vision loss, while potentially helpful, remains ambiguous (Donshik et al., 2007; Kuzman et al., 2014; Robertson and Cavanagh, 2011). The degree to which industry-wide solutions (e.g., improved contact lens materials or case design) could ameliorate case-related infection rates is unclear (Wu et al., 2015b).

Beyond infections stemming from improper use and maintenance of prescription contact lenses, infectious keratitis, corneal abrasions, and other types of eye damage have also been documented as results of wearing decorative contact lenses (Steinemann et al., 2005). These lenses are classified by the U.S. Food and Drug Administration (FDA) as "medical devices" and should be obtained only with a prescription (FDA, 2006). Nonetheless, one study found that approximately 54 percent of patients attained these lenses from an unlicensed optical shop without a prescription (Singh et al., 2012). A previous study found similar results, with 51 percent of the patients surveyed reporting they obtained their decorative lenses from an unlicensed provider (Steinemann et al., 2005). The same study found that none of the patients had ever worn contact lenses, predisposing them to unhygienic lens handling techniques. The FDA and the CDC provide information directed at consumers, eye care professionals, and the industry regarding the policies, regulations, and health risks associated with unlicensed decorative contact lenses (FDA, 2006). The American Academy of Ophthalmology has also published articles in multiple languages warning against the purchase of such lenses (AAO, 2015). Large-scale public awareness campaigns may include messages related to the threat to eye health from non-prescription decorative lenses. Moreover, working with industry and the FDA, governmental PHDs can assist in enforcing laws intended to stop the sale and purchase of such lenses.

Infection control and immunization have had great success in stemming the transmission of infectious agents that can have a profound effect on sight (Rao, 2015). For example, interventions to prevent transmission in pre- and peri-natal circumstances and to maintain high immunization rates have helped eliminate rubella (ODPHP, 2016b). Shingles affects approximately one third of the population and is associated with conjunctivitis, keratitis, uveitis, and optic neuritis (Opstelten and Zaal, 2005). Improving the vaccination rates for the herpes zoster virus may help reduce related vision loss. Similarly, sexually transmitted disease (STD) programs should take into account the effect that a particular disease can have on sight.

Governmental PHDs are traditionally on the frontline for many issues related to infection control and prevention and can serve as a logical and informed point of contact for providers, industry, and consumer groups to help organize responses and emphasize the threat to eye and vision health when applicable. Similarly, there is an opportunity for eye care professionals and other health care providers to help one another reiterate the role that eye and vision health can play in improving overall health through broader public health initiatives.

Promotion of Eye and Vision Health as a Programmatic Focus: Provision of Technical Expertise and Resources

Federal agencies charged with a wide range of responsibilities in the promotion of public health are uniquely situated to provide the needed resources and expertise that will allow state and LHDs to incorporate eye and vision health as a programmatic focus. The Vision Health Initiative (VHI) is a multilevel collaboration between the CDC's Division of Diabetes Translation and state and national partners, designed to promote vision health and quality of life for all populations, throughout all life stages, by preventing and controlling eye disease, eye injury, and vision loss resulting in disability. VHI has the unique role of collaborating with state and national partners to strengthen science and develop interventions to improve eye health, reduce vision loss and blindness, and promote the health of people with vision loss (CDC, 2015a). In addition to its leadership role in VHI, the CDC also

- Provides technical assistance to national, state, and local organizations oriented to preserving, protecting, and enhancing vision;
- Offers scientific bases for collaboration among provider groups, financing systems, and policy makers so that health care systems can respond effectively to vision and eye health as a major public health concern;
- Aids in translating science into programs, services, and policies and in coordinating service activities with partners in the public, private, and voluntary sectors; and
- Addresses issues related to the cost of vision loss, vision disability, eye disease, and quality of life (CDC, 2015a).

VHI provides a number of examples of how federal support and involvement in eye and vision health can translate into information and practices at the state level (see Box 5-4). Many of these examples are specific to eye and vision health, including specific eye diseases, but the supported partnerships have also been extended to chronic conditions more broadly. For example, in 2003, the CDC entered into a partnership with Prevent Blindness America to build capacity in states to address vision and eye health, which led to the active engagement of the National Association of Chronic Disease Directors, an organization that represents the leaders of state health department chronic disease programs (NACDD, n.d.).

In 2016, the CDC implemented a vision grant program in partnership with state-based chronic disease programs and other clinical and non-clinical stakeholders "to engage in strategic initiatives or activities designed to improve vision and eye health" (NACDD, 2016, p. 1). The current grant program will award three states an average of $25,000 toward the development of activities that (1) "achieve the overall goal of advancing vision loss and eye health as public health priorities"; (2) "implement a vision and eye health intervention that focuses on [characterizing the burden of eye disease or vision loss, promote systems change, or implement interventions related to eye and vision health]"; and . . . (3) "focus on sustainability . . . beyond the initial funding period" (NACDD, 2016, p. 4). This is an important step in the right direction, but more extensive resources will be needed to allow each state the opportunity to invest resources in the eye and vision health of its population.

Similarly, the NEI provides funding opportunities and resources that have helped to increase understanding about eye and vision health problems. The NEI reports awarding approximately 1,600 research grants and training awards related to vision research, in addition to laboratory and

---

BOX 5-4
Examples of Vision Health Initiative Activities and Support to Expand Resources and Capacity for State and Local Health Departments and Other Essential Stakeholders

- From 2005 to 2011, VHI implemented a nine-question vision module as part of the Behavioral Risk Factor Surveillance System (BRFSS) to provide state-level data. Beginning in 2013, VHI reported state data using the BRFSS core question on severe vision loss and blindness, which are available on the website for end users to download and share with their programs.
- From 2005 to 2008, VHI supplemented the National Health and Nutrition Examination Survey adding an eye exam that included fundus photography and visual field testing.
- In 2015, VHI funded a research project to develop, test, and implement a vision and eye health surveillance system using existing surveys, as well as administrative and electronic data sources. The findings will be disseminated and shared with researchers, epidemiologists, decision makers, providers, and other end users for implementation and evaluation of programs aimed at improving the vision and eye health of the nation.
- VHI funded the Innovative Network for Sight Research, a collaborative vision research network of investigators at Johns Hopkins University, University of Alabama at Birmingham, University of Miami, and Wills Eye Institute that assesses and evaluates system-level and individual-level factors that affect access to and the quality of eye care. Site-specific and network studies will investigate barriers to and enablers of the delivery of efficacious and cost-effective eye care that prevents vision loss and promotes eye health.
- From 2005 to 2011, VHI provided support to Prevent Blindness to address three compelling problems: preschool and school vision health, integrating vision care into federally qualified health centers, and building capacity within states to integrate vision across state public health initiatives.
- In 2012, VHI supported two projects to determine whether large numbers of people with suspected glaucoma could be detected through aggressive outreach in communities where high-risk populations, including older people, African Americans, and Hispanics, reside.

SOURCE: Excerpts adapted from a document prepared and shared by the CDC at the request of the committee: Personal communication, J. Saaddine, Centers for Disease Control and Prevention, January 21, 2016.

---

patient-oriented research at its own facilities, and it supports NEHEP, as described earlier in this chapter (NEI/NIH, 2015c). A review of the major advances reported by the NEI on its website suggests a heavy focus on the development and evaluation of effective treatments for specific eye diseases and conditions. Moreover, a review of the NEI's pioneering new advances to prevent and treat vision loss indicates that much research focused on stem cell research, gene therapy, the genetics of complex diseases, and the regeneration of the retina and connections to the brain (NEI/NIH, 2015c). Again, this is valuable information, but this programmatic emphasis needs to balance the need for novel scientific discoveries against the need for research that focuses on diseases and conditions that affect a larger proportion of the public. Regardless, clinical advances should be evaluated in terms of their clinical effectiveness as well as improved population health.

Despite the CDC's and the National Institutes of Health's (NIH's) current commitment to improving the population's eye and vision health, doing so is not a prominent line item in either's budget (see Chapter 4). Furthermore, no part of the federal government has the statutory responsibility to ensure an adequately funded population health vision care agenda. At the state and local levels, vision care remains subordinate to other public health mandates and competing priorities. In short, to elevate eye and vision health as a population health issue, more coordination is needed within the federal government to expand the number and scope of opportunities to enhance state and local capacities.

Integration of Eye and Vision Health into Other Health Initiatives and Programs

The link between chronic diseases and the various determinants of health has been of interest to public health professionals for several decades (Ford et al., 2013). The risk of vision loss may be a direct consequence of an uncontrolled chronic disease, such as diabetes. Conversely, vision loss may put an individual at greater risk for poor health by affecting that person's ability to engage in health-promoting activities such as physical activity, by affecting treatment adherence (e.g., taking medications), or by increasing the risk of falls or injuries (see Chapter 3). High priority public health problems, such as population smoking rates, can be a direct risk factor for vision loss. The obvious overlap between eye and vision health and other aspects of health priorities provides a unique opportunity to improve surveillance and research that can reduce vision impairment and improve health equity. In fact, the CDC has suggested that public service announcements that tie chronic vision impairment to specific unhealthy behaviors (e.g., smoking) and other chronic conditions (e.g., diabetes) may improve public awareness of eye disease (CDC, 2015d).

The following subsections provide examples of existing programs that could be integrated with eye and vision health. These do not represent the full spectrum of programs that are available and amenable to these efforts. Rather they are intended to provide helpful illustrations that public health officials and other stakeholders can use to interpret their own programmatic work in the context of eye and vision health.

Anti-Tobacco and Smoking Cessation Programs

In 2014, the Surgeon General released a 50-year follow-up report about the health consequences of smoking, which highlighted new evidence about the causal relationship between cigarette smoking and AMD, as well as possible links to other smoking-related ocular morbidities, such as diabetic retinopathy or dry eye (U.S. Surgeon General, 2014). Several studies have linked smoking to various common and severe eye diseases, such as cataract, glaucoma, AMD, and inflammation (Chakravarthy et al., 2010; DeAngelis et al., 2007; Delcourt et al., 2011; Edwards et al., 2008; Evans et al., 2005; Galor and Lee, 2011; Khan et al., 2006; Klein et al., 2010; Lechanteur et al., 2015; Lindblad et al., 2014; Thornton et al., 2005; Zhang et al., 2011). Smoking may have a more pronounced impact on the vision health of some patients, such as older adults, genetically at-risk populations, and those with certain chronic health conditions and behaviors, than on others (Coleman et al., 2010; Liang et al., 2014; Schaumberg et al., 2007; Schmidt et al., 2006; Wu et al., 2015a). Even non-smokers exposed to secondhand smoke have an increased risk of AMD (Khan et al., 2006). Smoking may also decrease the effectiveness of AMD treatments (Lee et al., 2013a), and studies have found that the risk of AMD is higher among current smokers than among former smokers.

Smoking cessation programs have been implemented in community and clinical settings, targeted to both specific populations and diverse communities, and have employed varying methods and technologies using multiple types of care providers (Asvat et al., 2014; Chen et al., 2012; Gao et al., 2013; Kim et al., 2015; Lee et al., 2013b; Lin et al., 2013; Mussener et al., 2016; Omana-Cepeda et al., 2016; Papadakis et al., 2013; Sarna et al., 2014; Simpson and Nonnemaker, 2013; Stanczyk et al., 2014). These programs have been moderately successful at decreasing the prevalence of smoking among targeted populations, and programs that are effective at reducing smoking in the general population may also accomplish the same outcomes in patients with AMD. A meta-analysis of observational studies concluded that the beneficial impact of smoking cessation increased over time (Cong et al., 2008; Myers et al., 2014; Neuner et al., 2009).

Vision loss has already been incorporated into some public health activities related to smoking. The Vision Integration and Preservation Program, a collaboration between the New York State Department of Health and Prevent Blindness Tri-State, integrated vision health "preservation strategies into existing programs and functions within [the] state health department to promote public health strategies among community-based organizations and vision partners" (VHIPP, 2012, p. 2). The program produced vision health education resources on sports-related eye injuries and the impact of smoking, diabetes, and diet on vision health (Prevent Blindness, 2012).

Three programs were evaluated in terms of their efforts to integrate vision into existing program, and the results showed that sustained programming was feasible when vision fit into the existing deliverables and that it could be achieved with minimal effort and "very good" or "excellent" value (VHIPP, 2012). The New York State Department of Health also developed a "Smoking Causes Blindness" awareness campaign based on ads that had previously proved successful in increasing rates of smoking cessation in Australia (Asfar et al., 2015). The $2.5 million campaign ran on the radio and television and appeared on internet ads from December 2009 to February 2010 (NYSDOH, 2009). A 9 percent increase in calls to the state tobacco quit line was attributed to this public campaign, but rates to the call line decreased after the campaign's end (Asfar et al., 2015). Despite such successes, questions remain about the effectiveness of smoking cessation programs, especially in the context of specific eye diseases, such as cataracts (Lindblad et al., 2005, 2014; Weintraub et al., 2002).

Incorporating eye and vision health into anti-smoking initiatives may have other benefits, which may affect ongoing and future collaborations between eye care professionals and other health care providers. A recent survey found that optometrists and ophthalmologists may not routinely advise patients to quit smoking (Caban-Martinez et al., 2011). Asfar and colleagues suggested that eye care professionals can "integrate smoking cessation treatment in the standard care of patients' management" and can "serve as powerful public advocates against tobacco use, thereby significantly enhancing public awareness about the link between smoking and eye disease" and reducing vision loss in the long term (Asfar et al., 2015, p. 1120). This highlights a new role for eye care professionals in combating other high-priority health problems in at-risk populations, although more research is needed on systems-level strategies that include tobacco control in eye care settings (Asfar et al., 2015; Loo et al., 2009).

Skin Cancer and UV Exposure

UV radiation, both from natural sunlight and from artificial UV rays, can damage both the surface tissues (i.e., cornea) and the internal structures (i.e., lens and retina) of the eye (Behar-Cohen et al., 2014; Sliney, 2001). Because most UV radiation comes from the sun, outdoor behavior can significantly influence the risk of subsequent and cumulative eye damage. Multiple studies have documented an increased risk of UV-caused damage to the eyes among pilots (Chorley et al., 2011, 2015, 2016). Sun shields, hats, and contact lenses can provide some protection again UV damage, but sunglasses (and even non-tinted plastic spectacles) worn close to the head can reduce most UV back reflection and transmission (Citek, 2008; Krutmann et al., 2014). The back reflection of radiation from lenses to the eye is also a concern, and antireflective coatings can considerably increase UV radiation back reflection (Citek, 2008). Better assessment and comparison of the UV-protective properties of lenses in actual use is needed (Behar-Cohen et al., 2014).

Recommendations for reducing the risk of skin cancer often focus on avoiding UV exposure to eyes and surrounding areas by wearing sunglasses (Glanz et al., 2002). For example, in Australia, "SunSmart" policies encourage school children to wear hats, especially broad-brimmed hats, during outdoor activities to reduce the risk of cancer from the sun, which can also benefit eye health (Gies et al., 2006). Similar policies in the United States encourage use of hats and sunwear in schools and in specific occupations (especially for workers who are often outside, such as migrant workers), although concerns about dress codes for reasons unrelated to eye health can present barriers (Hammond et al., 2009; Wright et al., 2007). Longitudinal studies that are designed to track the incidence of skin cancer (including on the skin around the eyes) in relation to UV exposure and the use of protective equipment could include eye health as another related health outcome.

Obesity and Physical Activity

A number of eye diseases and conditions may have risk factors that are associated, directly or indirectly, with obesity and exercise levels. For example, diabetic retinopathy may result from diabetes, and type 2 diabetes can be a consequence of obesity. Thus, understanding the risk factors for developing diabetes may also provide data relevant to the risk of developing diabetic retinopathy.

Increased exercise, including outdoor activity, is encouraged to reduce childhood and adult obesity (IOM, 2011a; U.S. Surgeon General, 2016). Outdoor activity has also been inversely associated with the likelihood of myopia in school children (Guo et al., 2013; Parssinen et al., 2014; Rose et al., 2008), although the exact mechanism is unknown. Recent increases in myopia among Chinese students (almost 82 percent of 16- to 18-year-olds were diagnosed with myopia) have highlighted the need for more information about the duration and characteristics of near-work activity and the risk of myopia in school children (Dolgin, 2015; Guggenheim et al., 2012). Another recent Chinese study found that watching television and playing on the computer, among other factors, was associated with increased prevalence of myopia (Zhou et al., 2016). The degree to which screen time exposure alone affects the development or progression of refractive error remains unknown. Screen time and other sedentary activities are already tracked as a contributor to the obesity epidemic in the United States (Boone et al., 2007; Council on Communications and Media, 2011; Rey-Lopez et al., 2008). Including measures of eye and vision health (such as myopia) in studies on obesity and physical activity, especially those tracking physiological metrics, could provide valuable information about shared risk factors and related physiological mechanisms, maximizing efficiencies, resources, and overall impact on health. Furthermore, incorporating dilated eye examinations could provide another mechanism by which to identify other comorbid conditions (e.g., diabetes, multiple sclerosis) (CDC, 2016b; Frohman et al., 2008).

The committee concluded that governmental PHDs and other stakeholders should consider including eye and vision health measures and metrics into existing programs to better understand the risk and protective factors for vision impairment and the relationship that exists between eye and vision health and other chronic diseases. The committee recognized that incorporating other measures and metrics into existing programs will increase the scope and expense of such trials and studies. However, establishing partnerships between the eye and vision research communities and the cancer research communities, to the extent that they do not sufficiently exist within specific areas, could help improve efficiency and increase the impact of limited resources, requiring less horse trading to advance both eye and vision health and other governmental PHD duties.

Vision Impairment as a Chronic Condition

The designation of a health condition as a chronic condition is important because HHS

> administers a large number of federal programs directed toward preventing and managing chronic conditions, including, for example, financing health care services (Centers for Medicare & Medicaid Services); delivering care and services to persons with chronic conditions (Administration on Aging, Health Resources and Services Administration, and Indian Health Service); conducting basic, interventional, and systems research (Agency for Healthcare Research and Quality, National Institutes of Health); implementing programs to prevent and manage chronic disease (Centers for Disease Control and Prevention, and Substance Abuse and Mental Health Services Administration); promoting the economic and social well-being of families, children, individuals, and communities (Administration for Children and Families); and overseeing development of safe and effective drug therapies (Food and Drug Administration). (HHS, 2010a, p. 4)

HHS has released a framework on multiple chronic conditions, with one of the overarching goals being to "foster health care and public health system changes to improve the health of individuals with multiple chronic conditions" (HHS, 2010a, p. 6). Under this framework, HHS encourages payment reform and incentives to reduce and avoid health outcomes that negatively affect both the individual and the health care system, such as hospital readmissions. The framework also promotes preventive interventions to mitigate the progression and exacerbation of existing chronic conditions (HHS, 2010a).

Chronic vision impairment qualifies as a general chronic condition under the Assistant Secretary of Health's definition. In Chapter 1, the committee defined chronic vision impairment as "a vision impairment that is present and must be managed over the lifespan to maintain the activities of daily living." An analysis of legally blind adults included in National Health Interview Survey data found that 46 percent of blind adults reported a limited ability to perform personal care activities, and 52 percent reported problems with at least one instrumental activity of daily living[12] (Zuckerman, 2004). Vision-threatening eye diseases and conditions (such as glaucoma, AMD, and diabetic retinopathy) cannot be cured, but permanent damage to the eye can be mitigated or their progression slowed through continuous medical management. In the case of refractive error, prescriptions must be monitored with some frequency (usually less so in mid-life), and new eyeglasses must be acquired if needed. Without these services and items, vision impairment can affect the performance of daily activities or even, in the case of amblyopia and strabismus in children, lead to permanent vision impairment. Even in the case of cataract, the progression and monitoring of the condition may occur over many years before surgery is necessary. Following surgery, examinations may be necessary to check for complications or to monitor the development of other eye conditions for which cataract surgery is a known risk factor.

The Centers for Medicare & Medicaid Services (CMS) have identified certain eye diseases and conditions as chronic conditions. Cataracts and glaucoma comprise the "eye disease" category. Medicare/Medicaid beneficiaries with cataracts and glaucoma equaled, respectively, 15.4 percent and 8.6 percent of all enrollees in 2008 (CMS, 2014). A CMS analysis grouped clinical and chronic conditions into categorical condition groups (CCGs), of which glaucoma and cataracts comprised the aggregate CCG "Eye Disease." The total expenditure for possessing two CCGs at the per-member/per-month rate of $1,628 totaled more than $1.47 billion in 2008 (CMS, 2014). Analysis of comorbidity CCG pairs among enrollees with a diagnosed condition in the "Eye Disease" CCG found co-occurring CCG diagnoses in lung disease (26 percent), anemia (39 percent), mental health conditions (39 percent), diabetes (43 percent), musculoskeletal disorders (48 percent), and heart conditions (86 percent) (CMS, 2014).

---

[12] Instrumental activities of daily living defined here as using telephones, shopping, preparing meals, managing money, and doing housework.

Nonetheless, vision impairment is generally excluded as a categorical focus for multiple chronic condition improvement. In 2013, Goodman and colleagues published an article that outlined a conceptual model for "improving understanding of and standardizing approaches to defining, identifying, and using information about chronic conditions in the United States" (Goodman et al., 2013, p. 1). As part of this exercise, the article included an appendix of 20 conditions[13] that were chronic, prevalent, and "potentially amenable to public health or clinical interventions or both," as well as being identifiable through *International Classification of Diseases* (ICD) codes (Goodman et al., 2013, p. 1). When this definition was applied to sources from CMS, the Agency for Healthcare Research and Quality, and the Robert Wood Johnson Foundation (RWJF) to identify a "manageable number" of conditions, eye disease was overlooked despite its prevalence across the lifespan as well as the fact that it was addressed as a chronic condition in both the RWJF and CMS sources (Anderson, 2010; CMS, 2016). The article itself does note that "visual impairment" is a chronic condition stemming from permanent or long-standing anatomical problems. Although this article serves as an example of how to approach the identification and prioritization of chronic conditions for various clinical and public health initiatives, it was not meant to dictate a formal list of the conditions to be included in these initiatives and programs—although it has been interpreted as such in many cases (Bayliss et al., 2014).

Although the visibility of other chronic conditions certainly does and should affect the prioritization of eye disease and vision impairment, chronic vision impairment also affects the prevalence and health outcomes associated with other chronic conditions (see Chapter 2). To the extent that data and evidence-based guidelines are available to assess the impact of, and care processes for, vision impairment as a chronic condition, vision impairment should be considered for inclusion in any framework targeting multiple chronic conditions. Some existing programs designed to combat the costs and negative outcomes of comorbid conditions should, given the high-prevalence of co-occurring diagnoses, incorporate eye and vision health This is already being studied in the United Kingdom, with eye care services being reciprocally incorporated into depression treatment and screening for hearing loss (Court et al., 2014). It is important for government agencies to consider reevaluating the status of eye and vision health.

---

[13] These conditions include hypertension, congestive heart failure, coronary artery disease, cardiac arrhythmias, hyperlipidemia, stroke, arthritis, asthma, autism spectrum disorder, cancer, chronic kidney disease, chronic obstructive pulmonary disease, dementia, depression, diabetes, hepatitis, human immunodeficiency virus, osteoporosis, schizophrenia, and substance abuse disorders (Goodman et al., 2013, p. 1).

Upstream Determinants of Health

An elevated risk of vision impairment is often associated with other inequities associated with broader social, economic, and political conditions that either passively permit or inadvertently contribute to unhealthy conditions affecting a population, especially those already at-risk for poor health outcomes (see Chapters 1 and 2). The result is disparities in both the prevalence of vision-threatening eye diseases and conditions and also the severity of vision impairment among various race or ethnicity groups and genders and across geographic locations.

The World Health Organization's Commission on Social Determinants of Health called on national governments and organizations to achieve greater health equity by addressing important social determinants of health (WHO, n.d.a.). Healthy People 2020, which is led by the Office of Disease Prevention and Health Promotion in HHS,[14] has identified the creation of "social and physical environments that promote good health for all" as one of the four overarching goals for 2020 (ODPHP, 2016c). To this end, Healthy People 2020 includes measure such as "proportion of children ages 0 to 17 living with at least one parent," "employed year round, full time," "proportion of persons living in poverty," and "proportion of all households that spend more than 50 percent of income on housing" (ODPHP, 2016d). The sense of sight is critically important to an individual's communication, physical health, independence and mobility, social engagement, educational and employment opportunities, socioeconomic status, and performance of daily activities, such as reading, driving a car, and caring for family members (Alberti et al., 2014; Bowers et al., 2009; Bronstad et al., 2013; Davidson and Quinn, 2011; Rahi et al., 2009; Sengupta et al., 2015; Whitson and Lin, 2014; Whitson et al., 2007; Wood et al., 2012). Thus, part of the equation to maximize health equity will be to prevent vision loss and to adequately respond to the burden of vision impairment, including providing eyeglasses, treatments, and rehabilitation services.

Building Determinants of Health into Existing Programs

Intersectoral collaborative efforts to improve health and its determinants span various federal agencies. Some examples include First Lady Michelle Obama's Let's Move! campaign with its attention to the availability, accessibility, and promotion of nutrition; the Interagency Partnership for Sustainable Communities of the U.S. Department of Housing and Urban

---

[14] Other departments include the U.S. Department of Agriculture, U.S. Department of Education, U.S. Department of Housing and Urban Development, U.S. Department of Justice, U.S. Department of the Interior, U.S. Department of Transportation, U.S. Department of Veterans Affairs, and the U.S. Environmental Protection Agency.

Development, the U.S. Department of Transportation, and the U.S. Environmental Protection Agency; and the new RWJF's vision for a culture of health, which promotes healthy and safe environments, equal opportunity, and health care coverage as some of the elements necessary for people to lead healthier lives now and in the future (National Center for Appropriate Technology, 2014; RWJF, 2014; White House Task Force on Childhood Obesity, 2010). Other countries are also making strides in this area. For example, the Public Health Agency of Canada funded its national collaborating centers in 2005, which include a National Collaborating Centre for Determinants of Health, which focuses on advancing social determinants of health and health equity through public health practice and policy—engaging in many of the same broad categories of programmatic focus as the CDC's VHI.

The CDC is well positioned to incorporate into its programs many of these upstream determinants of eye and vision health, which may fall outside the scope of more traditional clinical, research, and public health endeavors to improve health. The CDC has several programs indirectly related to eye and vision health targeting social determinants of health, which could be used as templates to build eye- and vision-specific programs addressing social determinants. For example, the National Program to Eliminate Diabetes-Related Disparities in Vulnerable Populations provides funding to organizations to "help plan, develop, implement, and evaluate multi-sector community-based interventions to work on social, cultural, economic, and environmental issues that influence health disparities associated with diabetes" (CDC, 2016a). This is led by the Division of Diabetes Translation within the National Center for Chronic Disease Prevention and Health Promotion, and it calls attention to increased rates of mortality and "serious health complications, including heart disease, *blindness*, kidney failure, and lower-extremity amputation" (CDC, 2014a) [emphasis added]. The CDC also provides a toolbox to help partnerships develop initiatives that address the social determinants of health in communities (Ramirez et al., 2008). In the context of eye and vision health, VHI acknowledges primary prevention and how health is shaped by many factors (e.g., family, community, social network, cultural, beliefs, healthy literacy, economics and environment), but these factors are typically couched in terms of improving "the use, acceptance, and accessibility of quality vision care" rather than in terms of reducing the risk factors that contribute to poor health (CDC, 2007, p. 16). VHI is an example of a program that could be expanded to provide a more comprehensive focus on the upstream factors that affect eye and vision health.

More is needed to ensure that greater improvements in population eye health outcomes can be achieved by addressing both the social determinants of health and individual-level risk factors for vision impairment. Because social and environmental conditions contribute to almost all of the conditions that the CDC addresses, a more integrated focus may be needed across programs to address the upstream conditions of health. The committee encourages efforts to expand this focus on the broader determinants that affect all health conditions, with special attention placed on the role of eye and vision health as both an outcome and an intervening variable.

The Example of Health Literacy

Health literacy has been defined as the degree to which individuals have the capacity to obtain, process, and understand basic health information and the services needed to make appropriate health decisions (IOM, 2004, p. 2). Low health literacy is associated with less use of preventive services (e.g., mammograms, Pap smears, and flu shots), more use of health care services (i.e., emergency room visits and hospitalizations), higher health care costs, and a higher risk of death and poor treatment outcome (Al Sayah et al., 2015; Baker et al., 1997, 2002; Bennett et al., 1998; Cimasi et al., 2013; Glassman, 2013; Haun et al., 2015; McNaughton et al., 2015; Sentell et al., 2015). In glaucoma patients, several studies have shown that poor health literacy is associated with noncompliance to treatment, nonadherence to medications, worse disease understanding, greater disease progression, and poor visual outcomes (Freedman et al., 2012; Juzych et al., 2008; Muir et al., 2006, 2013). In addition, patients with poor health literacy have greater visual field loss on initial presentation than those with adequate health literacy (Juzych et al., 2008).

In 2003, both the IOM and the U.S. Surgeon General identified improving health literacy as critical to advancing the health of the nation (Carmona, 2003; IOM, 2003). In 2010, HHS introduced a National Action Plan to Improve Health Literacy, which highlights the need to develop and disseminate health and safety information, promote changes in the health care system to facilitate consumer decision making, incorporate appropriate curricula into educational settings, support local efforts to provide age-appropriate and culturally sensitive information, build partnerships to change policies, increase basic research and the evaluation of health literacy interventions, and increase the use of evidence-based practice (HHS, 2010b). The committee notes that the accompanying Health Literate Care Model does not specifically highlight any particular disease or condition, including eye and vision health (Koh et al., 2013). However, the proposed toolkit can be used by eye care professionals and public health practitioners together to design interventions that improve eye and vision health literacy, including raising awareness, communicating clearly, accounting for culture and other considerations, using health education materials effectively, and working with other health and literacy resources in the community. Available resources address health care organization, health information systems, self-management support, links to supportive systems, engagement of individuals as partners in care and improvement efforts, and activated patients and families (ODPHP, 2016a). These are useful resources for the eye and vision care community. Moreover, efforts to evaluate the impact of general health literacy initiatives should take into account the interdependent relationships that exist among vision, overall health, and other social determinants of health.

ENHANCING ACCOUNTABILITY

Accountability refers to "the principle that individuals, organizations and the community are responsible for their actions and may be required to explain them to others" (Benjamin et al., 2006, p. 78). A core governmental PHDs function is providing assurance that appropriate institutions are protecting the public's health, rather than a specific subset of the population (e.g., patients within a health care system). This is an essential accountability mechanism that only the governmental PHDs can provide for the population's eye and vision health. In any population health initiative, accountability is important because it forces partners and collaborators to measure and communicate a program's expectations and the magnitude of its impact to inform and influence the public and elected officials.

In 2011, the IOM released the report *For the Public's Health: The Role of Measurement in Action and Accountability*, which chronicled different types of measures and assessments for characterizing the public health system's impact and how decision makers can use these tools to inform policies and practices (IOM, 2011c). The report proposed that "assessing and measuring accountability at any level (local, state, or national) and holding organizations accountable require the following four foundational elements:

- An identified body with a clear charge to accomplish particular steps toward health goals.
- Ensuring that the body has the capacity to undertake the required activities.
- Measuring what is accomplished against the identified body's clear charge.
- The availability of tools to assess and improve effectiveness and quality (such as a feedback loop as part of a learning system, incentives, and technical assistance)." (IOM, 2011c, p. 113)

This will require a process for priority setting and for evaluating the impact of specific programs to maintain accountability to the public, partners, and policy makers.

Prioritizing Eye and Vision Health

Population health priorities should be driven by more than simple mortality rates and should account for the potential quality of adjusted life years, the economic impact of the particular problem across the lifespan, and the ability to prevent or eliminate a potential burden for a large proportion of the affected individuals. As discussed in Chapter 2, the burden of eye diseases and vision impairment affects individuals across the lifespan to varying degrees of severity. To begin to diminish this public health burden, state and LHDs can explicitly make eye and vision health a priority as part of their strategic planning and program implementation. To establish nationwide consistency, the CDC and other federal bodies would also need to prioritize eye and vision health within their official strategic plans. As noted earlier in the chapter, neither state nor LHDs will be able to give, or support, emphasis in the eye and vision health area without some consistent source of financial and staffing support. Thus, additional congressional funding specific to eye and vision health initiatives beyond current levels would also be necessary.

The CDC has recognized five definitional features of a public health problem: (1) the problem affects a large number of people; (2) the problem imposes large morbidity, quality-of-life, and cost burdens; (3) the severity of the problem is increasing and is predicted to continue increasing; (4) the public perceives the problem to be a threat; and (5) community- or public health-level interventions to the problem are feasible (CDC, 2009). As described in earlier chapters, eye and vision health meet this definition. There are many diseases, conditions, and injuries that meet this definition, however, so governmental PHDs and other community stakeholders must decide whether the promotion of eye and vision health is indeed a priority.

Priority setting helps balance the most pressing needs with the finite budget. A number of tools are available to help governmental PHDs and other population health stakeholders determine what will constitute health priorities within their communities. Box 5-5 describes the broad suggestions of the National Association of County and City Health Officials for prioritizing community health issues. For example, the Department of Public Health for the County of Los Angeles identifies four categories of criteria that could be used by decision makers: (1) a quantitative assessment of the magnitude of the issue, (2) a qualitative assessment of the importance of the issue, (3) the effectiveness of interventions, and (4) the feasibility of implementing interventions (Department of Public Health County of Los Angeles, 2010). For evaluating eye and vision disorders, these criteria may accurately depict the preventable and correctable burden that could potentially be alleviated through public health measures. Studies evaluating the use of these criteria for eye and vision health in the health department

---

BOX 5-5
Prioritizing Issues in a Community
Health Improvement Process

1. **Identifying Criteria:** Ensure community and stakeholder ownership of a diverse set of considered criteria for the priority selection process, which will increase the likelihood of action to improve health. Criteria considered should include, for example: size, seriousness, trends, equity, intervention, feasibility, value, consequences of inaction, and social determinants/root causes.
2. **Meaningful Engagement for the Issue Prioritization Process:** This will establish chosen priorities as those that reflect the experiences of those in the community. Ensure strategic and representative participation, strike appropriate balance between having a framework, while remaining flexible to participants, and plan for, recognize, and overcome barriers that impede the decision-making process.
3. **Utilize Tools in Issue Prioritization:** Several tools are available to support a strategic approach to decision making. These tools generally use some form of methodology to weigh criteria and processes when considering and assigning value to information. Some examples include the "Control and Influence" conceptual tool, a prioritization matrix, the Hanlon Method, and various voting techniques.

SOURCE: Adapted from NACCHO, 2016.

---

priority-setting processes would be particularly useful to serve as a model for implementation across the country.

In 2006 the National Association of Chronic Disease Directors with the support of the CDC's National Center for Chronic Disease Prevention and Health Promotion, convened a workshop on chronic disease program integration because of its growing interest in state public health agencies. Participants developed a list of eight principles for state health agencies to use as a guide for supporting chronic disease program integration initiatives. These principles can be instructive in the context of vision impairment:

1. Engage state health agency leadership,
2. Develop crosscutting epidemiology and surveillance programs,
3. Leverage the use of information technology,
4. Build state and local partnerships,
5. Develop integrated state plans,
6. Engage management and administration,
7. Implement integrated interventions, and
8. Evaluate integration activities. (Slonim et al., 2007)

The strategic alignment of resources includes combining programs or activities that currently focus on a particular topic, but it also includes the integration of new yet complementary topics into existing programs. This integration affords the opportunity to address upstream determinants of health that span health conditions beyond eye and vision health across the spectrum, yet are seldom the primary purview of any single program. When evaluating whether eye and vision health rises to the level of a "top priority" within a given community, the committee encourages governmental PHDs, policy makers, private industry, nonprofit organizations, the media, the public, and other stakeholders to carefully consider the scope of the problems associated with vision impairment, the availability of treatments to effectively and relatively easily correct or reverse vision impairment for millions of people, the lack of knowledge about relatively simple behaviors that can reduce the risk of vision loss, and the wide range of strategies available to ensure that eye and vision health are present within formal programmatic designs.

Strategies to Improve Accountability for Eye and Vision Health

Holding organizations accountable for specific eye and vision health outcomes will be difficult for several reasons. First, there are numerous problems related to basic surveillance of the prevalence and impact of vision impairment from an epidemiological perspective, as described in Chapter 4. Second, because vision impairment can both contribute to and result from other chronic conditions, it can be difficult to eliminate the effects of confounding variables and ascertain the effects of specific variables on eye and vision health metrics. Third, all health outcomes in a community naturally shift and change over time, regardless of whether a public health intervention has been implemented. Fourth, there is a lack of evidence-based research documenting the characteristics and long-term impact of known community-based interventions across representative populations. For example, the Healthy People 2020 website lists systematic reviews for interventions that are strongly supported in the literature to accomplish goals related to eye and vision health (ODPHP, 2016f). Only three resources are listed, and two of them apply to clinical services.[15] The community-based intervention pertains to health communication and social marketing

---

[15] The website discloses that "evidence-based resources ha[ve] been rated and classified according to a set of selection criteria based, in part, on publication status, publication type, and number of studies. This classification scheme does not necessarily consider all dimensions of quality, such as statistical significance, effect size (e.g., magnitude of effect), meaningfulness of effect, additional effect over control, and study design (e.g., sample size, power, internal validity, external validity, generalizability, potential biases, potential confounders)" (ODPHP, 2016f).

in general. The same problems are not as prevalent for clinical interventions in the context of eye and vision health. Fifth, because there is little research available about the effect of specific interventions, there is even less information about how and whether to scale those interventions to benefit different populations in different geographic locations. Sixth, because vision loss and impairment can be the cumulative effect of multiple exposures over the lifespan, it can take decades to determine whether a particular public health intervention has had an impact. Finally, there are other challenges associated with aligning the missions of diverse population-health partnerships, which may affect the outcomes most relevant to particular groups.

Despite these challenges, strategies are available to enhance accountability for population-health activities intended to advance eye and vision health. For instance, public health agencies and departments can support collaborative efforts by collecting, analyzing, and disseminating data related to the targeted public health problem. Public health agencies could track and report progress related to the 10 essential public health services (see Chapter 1), across a variety of actors. As discussed in Chapter 4, this may involve combining eye-specific databases and those that track other chronic conditions or health determinants. Vision impairment should be added to chronic disease surveillance systems. Government public health agencies "can also serve as managers or facilitators of incentives that both reward and serve as a tool for holding stakeholders accountable (i.e., driving other sectors to demonstrate accountability on contributions to health improvement) in some cases on behalf of the community in general or a community group" (IOM, 2011c, p. 123).

To improve the quality, effectiveness, and consistency of public health services, the IOM and other organizations have identified national accreditation as a mechanism by which to improve accountability (see, e.g., IOM, 2012c). The expansion of the Public Health Accreditation Board (PHAB) process for quality standards and measurement has the potential to assure accountability, improve public health service delivery, and offer a better understanding of which public health programs are working and which need to be improved (PHAB, n.d.). The committee recognizes that the national accreditation effort is not mature, continues to evolve, and must remain dynamic and responsive to a changing system. Moreover, as described above, although some states have maintained their own accreditation process, there are significant variations across states regarding the process. As the accreditation standards for required public health services and measures evolve, there may be an opportunity to mandate components related to vision impairment, such as the number of at-risk people who receive an eye examination, which could address disparities in access to care. In the absence of a specific vision components, there are also opportunities to incorporate eye and vision health metrics into health impact assessments and community health assessments and improvement plans, which are required elements for accreditation.

Health impact assessments Efforts to examine the ramifications of policy decisions on health outcomes are becoming possible through the use of tools, such as health-impact assessments, as part of the "health-in-all-policies" movement (CDC, 2015b; Koivusalo, 2010). The National Research Council defines a health impact assessment (HIA) as "a systematic process that uses an array of data sources and analytic methods and considers input from stakeholders to determine the potential effects of a proposed policy, plan, program, or project on the health of the population" (NRC, 2011, p. 5). As part of the requirements for public health accreditation, many state and LHDs conduct a systematic HIA on a regular basis. Through the HIA process, LHDs systematically collect and analyze data to identify the community's health needs, establish priorities for programs and investments, devise metrics for ongoing evaluation and quality assurance (PHAB, 2013), and monitor progress toward meeting health improvement objectives (i.e., developing and implementing a health improvement plan) (ASTHO, 2016; Rubin et al., 2015). Eye and vision health, however, is not commonly part of these assessments and plans (Shin and Finnegan, 2009) (see Chapter 4). PHBA could develop an eye and vision HIA module and offer appropriate guidance for data collection and analysis.

Community health assessments and planning A community health assessment and community health improvement plan are required for accreditation. Additionally, changes in the health care environment, particularly the Patient Protection and Affordable Care Act (ACA), offer specific opportunities for health departments to be significant actors and partners in vision and eye health. First, under the ACA, nonprofit hospitals and health systems must conduct a community health needs assessment (CHNA) in conjunction with the LHD in their catchment area at least once every 3 years and implement a community health improvement plan to address the identified priorities. The CHNA process is a convenient mechanism for identifying those with visual impairment who are likely to need educational accommodation, along with income and other social supports. Second, vision is an element of the Healthy People 2020 objectives. According to the Office of Disease Prevention and Health Promotion,

> The Healthy People 2020 Vision objectives focus on evidence-based interventions to preserve sight and prevent blindness. Objectives address screening and examinations for children and adults, early detection and timely treatment of eye diseases and conditions, injury prevention, and the use of vision rehabilitation services. (ODPHP, 2016e)

Third, the ACA created the National Prevention, Health Promotion, and Public Health Council with a process to set a national prevention strategy. The national prevention strategy could be a mechanism for promoting eye health, especially in the context of uncorrected refractive error.

Valuing community-based prevention Beyond current actionable items, there is also interest in establishing effective frameworks and models to assess the value of community-based prevention services and different types of partnerships. Although this area is still in the early stages, frameworks have been developed by the IOM and other organizations to guide communities, PHDs, and policy makers, among others, in thinking about quantifying the relationship between benefits and harms in terms of community health, well-being, and process and resource utilization (IOM, 2012a). Evaluating the impact of public–private partnerships will also be difficult. Partnerships vary in the scope, objectives, stakeholders involved, and the inclusion of multifaceted interventions to resolve complex health problems. As a result, improvements in public health outcomes cannot

---

BOX 5-6
Key Research Gaps

- Surveys on current public awareness about eye and vision health, including knowledge about the etiology and risk factors for specific eye diseases, conditions, and injuries; behavior to reduce the risk of vision loss; and the links between eye and vision health and overall health and wellness.
- Impact of school- and community-based screenings or eye examinations on eye and vision health, quality of life, and workplace or academic achievement, among other outcomes.
- Interventions to improve rates of appropriate follow-up care after an initial eye screening or examination.
- Impact of policies and strategies to improve the use of protective eyewear, reduce eye infections, and improve compliance with the Americans with Disabilities Act regulations.
- Impact of building design to promote visual function.
- Conditions that encourage the adoption of policies to improve the use of personal protective eyewear in professional, recreational, and personal settings, including factors influencing policy setting in school environments.
- Evaluation of programs that integrate eye and vision health into existing chronic disease programs, including the cost, design, and impact of these programs to promote broader adoption of these programs by governmental PHDs.
- Impact of partnerships between governmental PHDs and various community stakeholders to improve measures of eye and vision health.

always be reliably attributed to the actions of a partnership. In addition, partnership goals may be ambiguous or may shift over time, making it difficult to even define program success (Smith et al., 2009). Research into the effectiveness of public–private partnerships is generally limited, and many existing analyses conclude that further research is needed (Pedersen et al., 2015; Vrangbaek, 2008). Arthur Himmelman has suggested a matrix of strategies for working together, which includes networking, coordinating, cooperating, and collaborating, which may be good starting points from which to develop specific evaluation metrics (Himmelman, 2002). Population health research agendas would benefit from increased attention and support related to the systematic evaluation and valuation of the types of activities explored in this chapter. Evidence of their effectiveness would likely drive greater attention and provide more information on how best to target limited resources in order to best benefit population eye and vision health in various communities.

To better assist with the evaluation of the impact of specific interventions and programs and increase the accountability of specific governmental PHDs related to eye and vision health, it will be important to have additional information available to both establish a baseline for improvement and determine whether improvements in population eye and vision health have occurred. To this end, Box 5-6 provides a list of key research gaps that have been mentioned throughout this chapter.

CONCLUSION

Governmental PHDs are a critical lynchpin to advancing eye and vision health, but they are constrained by the current level of resources available and the overall emphasis of public health on communicable diseases and emergency preparedness. Governmental PHDs provide a range of services to promote population health, but capacity to provide these services is contingent on adequate and sustained resources (e.g., funding, personnel, and expertise) to meet increasing demands. It will be difficult to achieve better eye and vision health at a national level given current funding levels.

Because the role of governmental PHDs varies from the federal to the state and to the local level, and also by the specific organizational structure and resources of LHDs, advancing eye and vision health requires a broad range of activities that varies by jurisdiction based on available infrastructure, resource, and need. Short- and long-term population health strategies should address the broad determinants of health, including policies that influence individual behaviors, healthy environments, and social conditions, because of their potential impact on eye and vision health. Enhancing public awareness of the etiology, causes, and risk factors related to eye and vision health, as well as the behaviors that effectively reduce the risk of vision loss, is an important and essential first step to establishing eye and vision health as a public health priority. However, public awareness and education alone will not be sufficient. Eye and vision health promotion will require varied strategies to influence both individuals and to create social and physical environments that support those behaviors. This may include policies and regulations that encourage the use of protective eyewear in hazardous work environments and during some recreational activities; that expand access to essential eye and vision screenings, examinations, and treatments; and that encourage eye-friendly building design. It may also require governmental PHDs and other critical stakeholders to integrate eye and vision health as a complementary element within existing public health programs, especially those related to chronic diseases. Public health can facilitate the development of clinical care systems that assure the organized delivery of care to everyone in their jurisdiction (see Chapters 7 and 8).

Establishing a wide range of partnerships can help expand governmental PHDs capacity by either providing additional resources to expand services related to eye and vision health or by providing necessary clinical services in community environments, which could allow governmental PHDs to focus on other essential public health services in eye and vision health such as coordination of clinical care systems and community-based efforts. Partnerships should include a variety of stakeholders from the community, clinical care systems, employers and businesses, the media, nonprofit organizations, the education sector, and government agencies—including those that have already made substantial contributions to the field, as well as stakeholders for whom optimal eye and vision health may be a non-explicit but nevertheless mission-specific objective. These partnerships can complement existing federal, state, and local funding and activities and future efforts to integrate eye and vision health into public health messaging, research, policy and practice, as well as across agencies, departments, and institutes in order to maximize efficiencies and enhance public health capacities.

Improving the accountability of governmental PHDs and health care systems will be important to increasing the visibility of community eye and vision health. This will require formal responsibility to incorporate objectives related to eye and vision health into existing public health and health care initiatives, to measure the impact of specific interventions, and to evaluate the availability of resources necessary to scale effective interventions that benefit the most at-risk populations. Establishing eye and vision health as public health priorities will not be easy due to limitations in public health capacities, surveillance challenges, limited evidence-based research, among other challenges. However, the chronic nature of many vision impairments and their impact on other chronic diseases and health determinants require federal, state, and local governments and other diverse yet critical stakeholders to carefully and collaboratively consider the potential benefits and available opportunities to increase the prominence of eye and vision health among current population health priorities. Preventing disability and poor quality of life from preventable, modifiable, or correctable vision impairment is a health imperative in its own right. It is time to meet that challenge head on.

REFERENCES

AAO (American Academy of Ophthalmology). 2013. Vision screening for infants and children—2013. http://www.aao.org/clinical-statement/vision-screening-infants-children--2013 (accessed April 7, 2016).

———. 2015. Halloween warning from ophthalmologists: Over-the-counter contact lenses could contain dangerous chemicals. http://www.aao.org/newsroom/news-releases/detail/halloween-warning-from-ophthalmologists-over-count (accessed July 12, 2016).

———. 2016a. Eye injuries at work. http://www.aao.org/eye-health/tips-prevention/injuries-work (accessed April 6, 2016).

———. 2016b. Online referral center. https://secure.eyecareamerica.org/onlinematch/default.aspx?lang=en-US&refresh=1 (accessed July 11, 2016).

AAP (American Academy of Pediatrics). 2011. AAP publications reaffirmed and retired. *Pediatrics* 128(3):e748 (referencing Committee on Sports Medicine & Fitness. 2004. Protective eyewear for young athletes. *Pediatrics* 113(3):619–622).

AAPOS (American Association for Pediatric Ophthalmology and Strabismus). 2011. State-by-state vision screening requirements. http://www.aapos.org/resources/state_by_state_vision_screening_requirements/ (accessed April 7, 2016).

Abulafia, A., F. Segev, E. Platner, and G. J. Ben Simon. 2013. Party foam-induced eye injuries and the power of media intervention. *Cornea* 32(6):826–829.

AFB (American Foundation for the Blind). 2016a. Accessible mass transit. http://www.afb.org/info/living-with-vision-loss/getting-around/accessible-mass-transit/235 (accessed April 7, 2016).

———. 2016b. Creating a comfortable environment for people with low vision. http://www.afb.org/info/low-vision/living-with-low-vision/creating-a-comfortable-environment-for-people-with-low-vision/235 (accessed April 7, 2016).

Al Sayah, F., S. R. Majumdar, L. E. Egede, and J. A. Johnson. 2015. Associations between health literacy and health outcomes in a predominantly low-income African American population with type 2 diabetes. *Journal of Health Communication* 20(5):581–588.

Alberti, C. F., E. Peli, and A. R. Bowers. 2014. Driving with hemianopia: III. Detection of stationary and approaching pedestrians in a simulator. *Investigative Ophthalmology & Visual Science* 55(1):368–374.

Alexander, R. L., N. A. Miller, M. F. Cotch, and R. Janiszewski. 2008. Factors that influence the receipt of eye care. *American Journal of Health Behavior* 32(5):547–556.

Alvi, R. A., L. Justason, C. Liotta, S. Martinez-Helfman, K. Dennis, S. P. Croker, B. E. Leiby, and A. V. Levin. 2015. The Eagles Eye mobile: Assessing its ability to deliver eye care in a high-risk community. *Journal of Pediatric Ophthalmology and Strabismus* 52(2):98–105.

AMD (Age-related Macular Degeneration) Alliance International. 2005. *Awareness of age-related macular degeneration and associated risk factors.* Toronto, Ontario: AMD Alliance International.

Anderson, G. 2010. *Chronic care: Making the case for ongoing care.* Princeton, NJ: Robert Wood Johnson Foundation.

Anderson, L. 2014. How a San Francisco architect reframes design for the blind. http://www.curbed.com/2014/8/6/10064320/how-a-san-francisco-architect-reframed-design-for-the-blind (accessed April 6, 2016).

AOA (American Optometric Association). 2008. Third annual American Optometric Association American Eye-Q survey. http://texas.aoa.org/documents/2008-Eye-Q-Executive-Summary.pdf (accessed July 25, 2016).

———. 2012. Infantsee®. http://www.infantsee.org (accessed July 11, 2016).

———. 2014. 2014 HEHP projects. http://www.aoafoundation.org/hehp/hehp-projects/2014-hehp-projects (accessed February 4, 2016).

———. 2016. School-aged vision: 6 to 18 years of age. http://www.aoa.org/patients-and-public/good-vision-throughout-life/childrens-vision/school-aged-vision-6-to-18-years-of-age?sso=y (accessed July 11, 2016).

AOA Foundation. 2016. How the program operates. http://www.aoafoundation.org/vision-usa/how-the-program-operates (accessed July 11, 2016).

Arnold, R. W., L. Stark, R. Leman, K. K. Arnold, and M. D. Armitage. 2008. Tent photo-screening and patched HOTV visual acuity by school nurses: Validation of the ASD–ABCD protocol. (Anchorage School District–Alaska Blind Child Discovery Program). *Binocular Vision & Strabismus Quarterly* 23(2):83–94.

Asfar, T., B. L. Lam, and D. J. Lee. 2015. Smoking causes blindness: Time for eye care professionals to join the fight against tobacco. *Investigative Ophthalmology & Visual Science* 56(2):1120–1121.

ASTHO (Association of State and Territorial Health Officials). 2012. State and local health department governance classification system. http://www.astho.org/Research/Data-and-Analysis/State-and-Local-Governance-Classification-Tree (accessed July 7, 2016).

———. 2014. *ASTHO profile of state public health, volume three.* Arlington, VA: ASTHO.

———. 2016. Community health needs assessments. http://www.astho.org/Programs/Access/Community-Health-Needs-Assessments (accessed April 6, 2016).

Asvat, Y., D. Cao, J. J. Africk, A. Matthews, and A. King. 2014. Feasibility and effectiveness of a community-based smoking cessation intervention in a racially diverse, urban smoker cohort. *American Journal of Public Health* 104(Suppl 4):S620–S627.

Bailey, R. N., R. W. Indian, X. Zhang, L. S. Geiss, M. R. Duenas, and J. B. Saaddine. 2006. Visual impairment and eye care among older adults—Five states, 2005. *Morbidity and Mortality Weekly Report* 55(49):1321–1325.

Baker, D. W., R. M. Parker, M. V. Williams, W. S. Clark, and J. Nurss. 1997. The relationship of patient reading ability to self-reported health and use of health services. *American Journal of Public Health* 87(6):1027–1030.

Baker, D. W., J. A. Gazmararian, M. V. Williams, T. Scott, R. M. Parker, D. Green, J. Ren, and J. Peel. 2002. Functional health literacy and the risk of hospital admission among Medicare managed care enrollees. *American Journal of Public Health* 92(8):1278–1283.

Bala, M. M., L. Strzeszynski, R. Topor-Madry, and K. Cahill. 2013. Mass media interventions for smoking cessation in adults. *Cochrane Database of Systematic Reviews* 6:Cd004704.

Barnhardt, C., S. A. Cotter, G. L. Mitchell, M. Scheiman, M. T., Kulp, CITT Study Group. 2012. Symptoms in children with convergence insufficiency: Before and after treatment. *Optometry & Vision Science* 89(10):1512–1520.

Bayliss, E. A., D. E. Bonds, C. M. Boyd, M. M. Davis, B. Finke, M. H. Fox, R. E. Glasgow, R. A. Goodman, S. Heurtin-Roberts, S. Lachenmayr, C. Lind, E. A. Madigan, D. S. Meyers, S. Mintz, W. J. Nilsen, S. Okun, S. Ruiz, M. E. Salive, and K. C. Stange. 2014. Understanding the context of health for persons with multiple chronic conditions: Moving from what is the matter to what matters. *Annals of Family Medicine* 12(3):260–269.

Behar-Cohen, F., G. Baillet, T. de Ayguavives, P. O. Garcia, J. Krutmann, P. Pena-Garcia, C. Reme, and J. S. Wolffsohn. 2014. Ultraviolet damage to the eye revisited: Eye-sun protection factor (E-SPF (R)), a new ultraviolet protection label for eyewear. *Journal of Clinical Ophthalmology* 8:87–104.

Beitsch, L. M., C. Leep, G. Shah, R. G. Brooks, and R. M. Pestronk. 2010. Quality improvement in local health departments: Results of the NACCHO 2008 survey. *Journal of Public Health Management and Practice* 16(1):49–54.

Benjamin, G., M. Fallon, P. E. Jarris, and P. Libbey. 2006. *Final recommendations for a voluntary national accreditation program for state and local public health departments.* Alexandria, VA: Public Health Accreditation Board.

Bennett, C. L., M. R. Ferreira, T. C. Davis, J. Kaplan, M. Weinberger, T. Kuzel, M. A. Seday, and O. Sartor. 1998. Relation between literacy, race, and stage of presentation among low-income patients with prostate cancer. *Journal of Clinical Oncology* 16(9):3101–3104.

Beynat, J., A. Charles, K. Astruc, P. Metral, L. Chirpaz, A. M. Bron, and C. Creuzot-Garcher. 2009. Screening for diabetic retinopathy in a rural French population with a mobile non-mydriatic camera. *Diabetes & Metabolism* 35(1):49–56.

Blehm, C., S. Vishnu, A. Khattak, S. Mitra, and R. W. Yee. 2005. Computer vision syndrome: A review. *Survey of Ophthalmology* 50(3):253–262.

Boone, J. E., P. Gordon-Larsen, L. S. Adair, and B. M. Popkin. 2007. Screen time and physical activity during adolescence: Longitudinal effects on obesity in young adulthood. *The International Journal of Behavioral Nutrition and Physical Activity* 4:26.

Boucher, M. C., G. Desroches, R. Garcia-Salinas, A. Kherani, D. Maberley, S. Olivier, M. Oh, and F. Stockl. 2008. Teleophthalmology screening for diabetic retinopathy through mobile imaging units within Canada. *Canadian Journal of Ophthalmology* 43(6):658–668.

Bowers, A. R., A. J. Mandel, R. B. Goldstein, and E. Peli. 2009. Driving with hemianopia, I: Detection performance in a driving simulator. *Investigative Ophthalmology & Visual Science* 50(11):5137–5147.

Bray, J. E., L. Straney, B. Barger, and J. Finn. 2015. Effect of public awareness campaigns on calls to ambulance across Australia. *Stroke* 46(5):1377–1380.

Bronstad, P. M., A. R. Bowers, A. Albu, R. Goldstein, and E. Peli. 2013. Driving with central field loss I: Effect of central scotomas on responses to hazards. *JAMA Ophthalmology* 131(3):303–309.

Brooks, R. G., L. M. Beitsch, P. Street, and A. Chukmaitov. 2009. Aligning public health financing with essential public health service functions and national public health performance standards. *Journal of Public Health Management and Practice* 15(4): 299–306.

Caban-Martinez, A. J., E. P. Davila, B. L. Lam, S. R. Dubovy, K. E. McCollister, L. E. Fleming, D. D. Zheng, and D. J. Lee. 2011. Age-related macular degeneration and smoking cessation advice by eye care providers: A pilot study. *Preventing Chronic Disease* 8(6):A147.

Carmona, R. H. 2003. Health literacy: Key to improving American's health. http://www.surgeongeneral.gov/news/speeches/healthlit09192003.html (accessed April 6, 2016).

Castanes, M. S. 2003. Major review: The underutilization of vision screening (for amblyopia, optical anomalies and strabismus) among preschool age children. *Binocular Vision & Strabismus Quarterly* 18(4):217–232.

CBO (Congressional Budget Office). 2013. *Federal grants to state and local governments.* Washington, DC: CBO.

CDC (Centers for Disease Control and Prevention). 2007. *Improving the nation's vision health: A coordinated public health approach.* Atlanta, GA: CDC.

———. 2009. Why is vision loss a public health problem? http://www.cdc.gov/visionhealth/basic_information/vision_loss.htm (accessed October 7, 2015).

———. 2012. Eye health tips. http://www.cdc.gov/visionhealth/basic_information/eye_health_tips.htm (accessed September 17, 2015).

———. 2013a. Eye safety. http://www.cdc.gov/niosh/topics/eye/eyechecklist.html (accessed April 6, 2016).

———. 2013b. Eye safety tool box talk—Instructor's guide. http://www.cdc.gov/niosh/topics/eye/pdfs/instructor.pdf (accessed September 11, 2015).

———. 2014a. The National Program to Eliminate Diabetes-Related Disparities in Vulnerable Populations. http://www.cdc.gov/diabetes/prevention/pdf/vulnerablepopulationsfactsheet.pdf (accessed April 6, 2016).

———. 2014b. The public health system and the 10 essential public health services. http://www.cdc.gov/nphpsp/essentialservices.html (accessed March, 2016).

———. 2015a. About us. http://www.cdc.gov/visionhealth/about/index.htm (accessed April 6, 2016).

———. 2015b. Health in all policies. http://www.cdc.gov/policy/hiap/ (accessed April 6, 2016).

———. 2015c. NIOSH programs. http://www.cdc.gov/niosh/programs.html (accessed April 6, 2016).

———. 2015d. Powerful new "tips from former smokers" ads focus on living with vision loss and colorectal cancer. http://www.cdc.gov/media/releases/2015/p0326-tips.html (accessed June 13, 2016).

———. 2015e. *Prevention status reports*. Atlanta, GA: CDC.

———. 2015f. PHHS block grant. http://www.cdc.gov/phhsblockgrant/statehpprior.htm#i (accessed April 6, 2016).

———. 2015g. Protect your eyes. http://www.cdc.gov/contactlenses/protect-your-eyes.html (accessed April 6, 2016).

———. 2016a. CDC programs addressing social determinants of health. http://www.cdc.gov/socialdeterminants/cdcprograms/index.htm (accessed April 6, 2016).

———. 2016b. Keep an eye on vision health. http://www.cdc.gov/features/healthyvision (accessed July 12, 2016).

CDPH (Connecticut Department of Public Health). 2008. *Health alert! Keeping an eye on eye protection*. Hartford: CDPH.

Chakravarthy, U., T. Y. Wong, A. Fletcher, E. Piault, C. Evans, G. Zlateva, R. Buggage, A. Pleil, and P. Mitchell. 2010. Clinical risk factors for age-related macular degeneration: A systematic review and meta-analysis. *BMC Ophthalmology* 10:31.

Chang, F. C., C. H. Chung, Y. C. Chuang, T. W. Hu, P. T. Yu, K. Y. Chao, and M. L. Hsiao. 2011. Effect of media campaigns and smoke-free ordinance on public awareness and secondhand smoke exposure in Taiwan. *Journal of Health Communication* 16(4):343–358.

Chase, C., C. Tosha, E. Borsting, and W. H. Ridder, 3rd. 2009. Visual discomfort and objective measures of static accommodation. *Optometry & Vision Science* 86(7):883–889.

Chen, Y. F., J. Madan, N. Welton, I. Yahaya, P. Aveyard, L. Bauld, D. Wang, A. Fry-Smith, and M. R. Munafo. 2012. Effectiveness and cost effectiveness of computer and other electronic aids for smoking cessation: A systematic review and network meta-analysis. *Health Technology Assessment* 16(38).

Chorley, A. C., B. J. Evans, and M. J. Benwell. 2011. Civilian pilot exposure to ultraviolet and blue light and pilot use of sunglasses. *Aviation, Space, and Environmental Medicine* 82(9):895–900.

———. 2015. Solar eye protection practices of civilian aircrew. *Aerospace Medicine and Human Performance* 86(11):953–961.

Chorley, A. C., K. A. Baczynska, M. J. Benwell, B. J. Evans, M. P. Higlett, M. Khazova, and J. B. O'Hagan. 2016. Occupational ocular UV exposure in civilian aircrew. *Aerospace Medicine and Human Performance* 87(1):32–39.

Chou, C. F., L. E. Barker, J. E. Crews, S. A. Primo, X. Zhang, A. F. Elliott, K. McKeever Bullard, L. S. Geiss, and J. B. Saaddine. 2012. Disparities in eye care utilization among the United States adults with visual impairment: Findings from the Behavioral Risk Factor Surveillance System 2006–2009. *American Journal of Ophthalmology* 154 (6 Suppl):S45–S52, e41.

Chou, C. F., C. E. Sherrod, X. Zhang, L. E. Barker, K. M. Bullard, J. E. Crews, and J. B. Saaddine. 2014. Barriers to eye care among people aged 40 years and older with diagnosed diabetes, 2006–2010. *Diabetes Care* 37(1):180–188.

Chou, W.-Y. S., Y. M. Hunt, E. B. Beckjord, R. P. Moser, and B. W. Hesse. 2009. Social media use in the United States: Implications for health communication. *Journal of Medical Internet Research* 11(4):e48.

Chou, W.-Y. S., A. Prestin, C. Lyons, and K. Y. Wen. 2013. Web 2.0 for health promotion: Reviewing the current evidence. *American Journal of Public Health* 103(1):e9–e18.

Christ, S. L., D. D. Zheng, B. K. Swenor, B. L. Lam, S. K. West, S. L. Tannenbaum, B. E. Muñoz, and D. J. Lee. 2014. Longitudinal relationships among visual acuity, daily functional status, and mortality: The Salisbury Eye Evaluation Study. *JAMA Ophthalmology* 132(12):1400–1406.

Cimasi, R. J., A. R. Sharamitaro, and R. L. Seiler. 2013. The association between health literacy and preventable hospitalizations in Missouri: Implications in an era of reform. *Journal of Health Care Finance* 40(2):1–16.

Citek, K. 2008. Anti-reflective coatings reflect ultraviolet radiation. *Optometry* 79(3):143–148.

City of New York. 2016. Partnership with Warby Parker. http://www1.nyc.gov/site/communityschools/schools-and-partners/partnership-with-warby-parker.page (accessed July 11, 2016).

CMS (Centers for Medicare & Medicaid Services). 2014. *Physical and mental health condition prevalence and comorbidity among fee-for-service Medicare-Medicaid enrollees.* Washington, DC: CMS.

———. 2016. Condition categories. https://www.ccwdata.org/web/guest/condition-categories (accessed March 18, 2016).

Coleman, A. L., R. L. Seitzman, S. R. Cummings, F. Yu, J. A. Cauley, K. E. Ensrud, K. L. Stone, M. C. Hochberg, K. L. Pedula, E. Thomas, C. M. Mangione, and the Study of Osteoporotic Fractures Research Group. 2010. The association of smoking and alcohol use with age-related macular degeneration in the oldest old: The Study of Osteoporotic Fractures. *American Journal of Ophthalmology* 149(1):160–169.

Collier, S. A., M. P. Gronostaj, A. K. MacGurn, J. R. Cope, K. L. Awsumb, J. S. Yoder, and M. J. Beach. 2014. Estimated burden of keratitis—United States, 2010. *Morbidity and Mortality Weekly Report* 63(45):1027–1030.

Cong, R., B. Zhou, Q. Sun, H. Gu, N. Tang, and B. Wang. 2008. Smoking and the risk of age-related macular degeneration: A meta-analysis. *Annals of Epidemiology* 18(8):647–656.

Convissor, R. B., R. E. Vollinger, Jr., and P. Wilbur. 1990. Using national news events to stimulate local awareness of public policy issues. *Public Health Reports* 105(3):257–260.

Cope, J. R., S. A. Collier, M. M. Rao, R. Chalmers, G. L. Mitchell, K. Richdale, H. Wagner, B. T. Kinoshita, D. Y. Lam, L. Sorbara, A. Zimmerman, J. S. Yoder, and M. J. Beach. 2015. Contact lens wearer demographics and risk behaviors for contact lens–related eye infections—United States, 2014. *Morbidity and Mortality Weekly Report* 64(32):865–870.

Council on Communications and Media. 2011. Children, adolescents, obesity, and the media. *Pediatrics* 128(1):201–208.

Court, H., G. McLean, B. Guthrie, S. W. Mercer, and D. J. Smith. 2014. Visual impairment is associated with physical and mental comorbidities in older adults: A cross-sectional study. *BMC Medicine* 12:181.

CPSTF (Community Preventive Services Task Force). 2010. Health communication and social marketing: Health communication campaigns that include mass media and health-related product distribution. Guide to Community Preventive Services. http://www.thecommunity guide.org/healthcommunication/campaigns.html (accessed June 10, 2016).

———. 2014. Preventing skin cancer: Multicomponent community-wide interventions. Guide to Community Preventive Services. http://www.thecommunityguide.org/cancer/skin/community-wide/multicomponent.html (accessed June 1, 2016).

CPWR (Center for Protection of Workers' Rights). 2014. Eye protection. http://www.cpwr.com/sites/default/files/publications/CPWR_Eye_Protection_2.pdf (accessed April 6, 2016).

Dahlin Ivanoff, S., U. Sonn, and E. Svensson. 2002. A health education program for elderly persons with visual impairments and perceived security in the performance of daily occupations: A randomized study. *American Journal of Occupational Therapy* 56(3):322–330.

Dannenberg, A. L., H. Frumkin, and R. J. Jackson. 2011. *Making healthy places: Designing and building for health, well-being, and sustainability*. Washington, DC: Island Press.

Davidson, S., and G. E. Quinn. 2011. The impact of pediatric vision disorders in adulthood. *Pediatrics* 127(2):334–339.

DeAngelis, M. M., F. Ji, I. K. Kim, S. Adams, A. Capone, Jr., J. Ott, J. W. Miller, and T. P. Dryja. 2007. Cigarette smoking, CFH, APOE, ELOV14, and risk of neovascular age-related macular degeneration. *Archives of Ophthalmology* 125(1):49–54.

DeHaven, M. J., I. B. Hunter, L. Wilder, J. W. Walton, and J. Berry. 2004. Health programs in faith-based organizations: Are they effective? *American Journal of Public Health* 94(6):1030–1036.

Delcourt, C., M. N. Delyfer, M. B. Rougier, P. Amouyel, J. Colin, M. Le Goff, F. Malet, J. F. Dartigues, J. C. Lambert, and J. F. Korobelnik. 2011. Associations of complement factor H and smoking with early age-related macular degeneration: The alienor study. *Investigative Ophthalmology & Visual Science* 52(8):5955–5962.

Department of Public Health County of Los Angeles. 2010. Priority-setting in public health. Los Angeles, CA: Quality Improvement Division.

DOJ (U.S. Department of Justice). 2001. Americans with Disabilities Act: Guide for place of lodging: Serving guests who are blind or who have low vision. https://www.ada.gov/lodblind.htm (accessed August 14, 2016).

———. 2015. *ADA update: A primer for state and local governments*. Washington, DC: DOJ.

———. n.d. Americans with Disabilities Act: Guide for places of lodging: Serving guests who are blind or who have low vision. https://www.ada.gov/reachingout/lodblind(lesson2).html (accessed July 11, 2016).

Dolgin, E. 2015. The myopia boom. *Nature* 519(7543):276–278.

Donshik, P. C., W. H. Ehlers, L. D. Anderson, and J. K. Suchecki. 2007. Strategies to better engage, educate, and empower patient compliance and safe lens wear: Compliance: What we know, what we do not know, and what we need to know. *Eye & Contact Lens* 33 (6 Pt 2):430–433; discussion 434.

Doran, C. M., R. Ling, J. Byrnes, M. Crane, A. P. Shakeshaft, A. Searles, and D. Perez. 2016. Benefit cost analysis of three skin cancer public education mass-media campaigns implemented in New South Wales, Australia. *PLoS ONE* 11(1):e0147665.

Doyle, J., R. Armstrong, and E. Waters. 2008. Issues raised in systematic reviews of complex multisectoral and community based interventions. *Journal of Public Health (Oxford)* 30(2):213–215.

Durkin, S., E. Brennan, and M. Wakefield. 2012. Mass media campaigns to promote smoking cessation among adults: An integrative review. *Tobacco Control* 21(2):127–138.

Earle-Richardson, G., L. Wyckoff, M. Carrasquillo, M. Scribani, P. Jenkins, and J. May. 2014. Evaluation of a community-based participatory farmworker eye health intervention in the "black dirt" region of New York State. *American Journal of Industrial Medicine* 57(9):1053–1063.

Edwards, R., J. Thornton, R. Ajit, R. A. Harrison, and S. P. Kelly. 2008. Cigarette smoking and primary open angle glaucoma: A systematic review. *Journal of Glaucoma* 17(7):558–566.

Eime, R., N. Owen, and C. Finch. 2004. Protective eyewear promotion: Applying principles of behaviour change in the design of a squash injury prevention programme. *The American Journal of Sports Medicine* 34(10):629–638.

Eime, R., C. Finch, R. Wolfe, N. Owen, and C. McCarty. 2005. The effectiveness of a squash eyewear promotion strategy. *British Journal of Sports Medicine* 39(9):681–685.

Eklund, K., U. Sonn, and S. Dahlin Ivanoff. 2004. Long-term evaluation of a health education programme for elderly persons with visual impairment. A randomized study. *Disability and Rehabilitation* 26(7):401–409.

Eklund, K., U. Sonn, P. Nystedt, and S. Dahlin Ivanoff. 2005. A cost-effectiveness analysis of a health education programme for elderly persons with age-related macular degeneration: A longitudinal study. *Disability and Rehabilitation* 27(20):1203–1212.

Eklund, K., J. Sjöstrand, and S. Dahlin Ivanoff. 2008. A randomized controlled trial of a health-promotion programme and its effect on ADL dependence and self-reported health problems for the elderly visually impaired. *Scandinavian Journal of Occupational Therapy* 15(2):68–74.

Ellish, N. J., R. Royak-Schaler, and E. J. Higginbotham. 2011. Tailored and targeted interventions to encourage dilated fundus examinations in older African Americans. *Archives of Ophthalmology* 129(12):1592–1598.

EPA (U.S. Environmental Protection Agency). 2015. What is green infrastructure? https://www.epa.gov/green-infrastructure/what-green-infrastructure (accessed April 7, 2016).

Ethan, D., and C. E. Basch. 2008. Promoting healthy vision in students: Progress and challenges in policy, programs, and research. *Journal of School Health* 78(8):411–416.

Evans, J. R., A. E. Fletcher, and R. P. Wormald. 2005. 28,000 cases of age related macular degeneration causing visual loss in people aged 75 years and above in the United Kingdom may be attributable to smoking. *British Journal of Ophthalmology* 89(5):550–553.

FDA (U.S. Food and Drug Administration). 2006. Decorative, non-corrective contact lenses. http://www.fda.gov/MedicalDevices/DeviceRegulationandGuidance/GuidanceDocuments/ucm071572.htm (accessed April 6, 2016).

Fischhoff, B., A. Bostrom, and M. J. Quadrel. 1993. Risk perception and communication. *Annual Reviews of Public Health* 14:183–203.

Fischhoff, B., R. Detels, R. Beaglehole, M. Lansing, and M. Gulliford. 2009. Risk perception and communication. *Oxford Textbook of Public Health, Volume 2: The methods of public health* (Ed. 5):940–953.

Ford, E. S., J. B. Croft, S. F. Posner, R. A. Goodman, and W. H. Giles. 2013. Co-occurrence of leading lifestyle-related chronic conditions among adults in the United States, 2002–2009. *Preventing Chronic Disease* 10:E60.

Forrest, K. Y., J. M. Cali, and W. J. Cavill. 2008. Use of protective eyewear in U.S. adults: Results from the 2002 National Health Interview Survey. *Ophthalmic Epidemiology* 15(1):37–41.

Fosson, G. H., D. M. McCallum, and M. B. Conaway. 2014. Antismoking mass media campaigns and support for smoke-free environments, Mobile County, Alabama, 2011–2012. *Preventing Chronic Disease* 11:E150.

Freedman, R. B., S. K. Jones, A. Lin, A. L. Robin, and K. W. Muir. 2012. Influence of parental health literacy and dosing responsibility on pediatric glaucoma medication adherence. *Archives of Ophthalmology* 130(3):306–311.

Frieden, T. R. 2010. A framework for public health action: The health impact pyramid. *American Journal of Public Health* 100(4):590–595.

Frohman, E. M., J. G. Fujimoto, T. C. Frohman, P. A. Calabresi, G. Cutter, and L. J. Balcer. 2008. Optical coherence tomography: A window into the mechanisms of multiple sclerosis. Nature clinical practice. *Neurology* 4(12):664–675.

Galor, A., and D. J. Lee. 2011. Effects of smoking on ocular health. *Current Opinions in Ophthalmology* 22(6):477–482.

Gao, K., M. D. Wiederhold, L. Kong, and B. K. Wiederhold. 2013. Clinical experiment to assess effectiveness of virtual reality teen smoking cessation program. *Studies in Health Technology and Informatics* 191:58–62.

Gebbie, K. M. 2000. *The public health workforce: Enumeration 2000.* Washington, DC: Health Resources and Services Administration.

Gies, P., J. Javorniczky, C. Roy, and S. Henderson. 2006. Measurements of the UVR protection provided by hats used at school. *Photochemistry & Photobiology* 82(3): 750–754.

Glanz, K., M. Saraiya, and H. Wechsler. 2002. Guidelines for school programs to prevent skin cancer. *Morbidity and Mortality Weekly Report* 51(RR04):1–16.

Glassman, P. 2013. Health literacy. https://nnlm.gov/outreach/consumer/hlthlit.html (accessed April 6, 2016).

Glazier, R., M. Slade, and H. Mayer. 2011. The depiction of protective eyewear use in popular television programs. *Journal of Trauma and Acute Care Surgery* 70(4):965–969.

Glewwe, P., K. West, and J. Lee. 2014. *The impact of providing vision screening and free eyeglasses on academic outcomes: Evidence from a randomized trial in Title 1 elementary schools.* Minneapolis: University of Minnesota.

Goldstein, M. H., and D. Wee. 2011. Sports injuries: An ounce of prevention and a pound of cure. *Eye & Contact Lens* 37(3):160–163.

Goodman, R. A., S. F. Posner, E. S. Huang, A. K. Parekh, and H. K. Koh. 2013. Defining and measuring chronic conditions: Imperatives for research, policy, program, and practice. *Preventing Chronic Disease* 10:E66.

Gordon, G. 2003. *Interior lighting for designers.* New York: Wiley.

Gowrisankaran, S., and J. E. Sheedy. 2015. Computer vision syndrome: A review. *Work* 52(2):303–314.

Griffith, J. F., R. Wilson, H. C. Cimino, M. Patthoff, D. F. Martin, and E. I. Traboulsi. 2016. The use of a mobile van for school vision screening: Results of 63,841 evaluations. *American Journal of Ophthalmology* 163:108–114.e1.

GSA (U.S. General Services Administration). 2014. *Green building certification system.* Washington, DC: GSA.

Guggenheim, J. A., K. Northstone, G. McMahon, A. R. Ness, K. Deere, C. Mattocks, B. S. Pourcain, and C. Williams. 2012. Time outdoors and physical activity as predictors of incident myopia in childhood: A prospective cohort study. *Investigative Ophthalmology & Visual Science* 53(6):2856–2865.

Guo, Y., L. J. Liu, L. Xu, P. Tang, Y. Y. Lv, Y. Feng, M. Meng, and J. B. Jonas. 2013. Myopic shift and outdoor activity among primary school children: One-year follow-up study in Beijing. *PLoS One* 8(9):e75260.

Hammond, V., A. I. Reeder, and A. Gray. 2009. Patterns of real-time occupational ultraviolet radiation exposure among a sample of outdoor workers in New Zealand. *Public Health* 123(2):182–187.

Hartmann, E. E., G. E. Bradford, P. K. Chaplin, T. Johnson, A. R. Kemper, S. Kim, and W. Marsh-Tootle. 2006. Project universal preschool vision screening: A demonstration project. *Pediatrics* 117(2):e226–e237.

Haun, J. N., N. R. Patel, D. D. French, R. R. Campbell, D. D. Bradham, and W. A. Lapcevic. 2015. Association between health literacy and medical care costs in an integrated healthcare system: A regional population based study. *BMC Health Services Research* 15(1):1–11.

Hautala, N., P. Hyytinen, V. Saarela, P. Hagg, A. Kurikka, M. Runtti, and A. Tuulonen. 2009. A mobile eye unit for screening of diabetic retinopathy and follow-up of glaucoma in remote locations in northern Finland. *Acta Ophthalmologica* 87(8):912–913.

Healthcare.gov. 2016. Preventive health services. https://www.healthcare.gov/coverage/preventive-care-benefits (accessed May 18, 2016).

Hearne, S., B. C. Castrucci, J. P. Leider, E. K. Rhoades, P. Russo, and V. Bass. 2015. The future of urban health: Needs, barriers, opportunities, and policy advancement at large urban health departments. *Journal of Public Health Management and Practice* 21(Suppl 1):S4–S13.

Hered, R. W., and D. L. Wood. 2013. Preschool vision screening in primary care pediatric practice. *Public Health Reports* 128(3):189–197.

Hershey, J. C., J. Niederdeppe, W. D. Evans, J. Nonnemaker, S. Blahut, D. Holden, P. Messeri, and M. L. Haviland. 2005. The theory of "truth": How counterindustry campaigns affect smoking behavior among teens. *Health Psychology* 24(1):22–31.

HHS (U.S. Department of Health and Human Services). 2010a. *Multiple chronic conditions— A strategic framework: Optimum health and quality of life for individuals with multiple chronic conditions.* Washington, DC: HHS.

———. 2010b. *National action plan to improve health literacy.* Washington, DC: HHS.

Himmelman, A. 2002. *Collaboration for a change: Definitions, descision-making models, roles, and collaboration process guide.* Minneapolis, MN: Himmelman Consulting.

Honoré, P. A., and T. Schlechte. 2007. State public health agency expenditures: Categorizing and comparing to performance levels. *Journal of Public Health Management and Practice* 13(2):156–162.

HRSA (Health Resources and Services Administration). n.d. Vision screening. http://www.mchb.hrsa.gov/programs/visionscreening/index.html (accessed July 7, 2016).

Hughes, R., K. Ramdhanie, T. Wassermann, and C. Moscetti. 2011. State boards of health: Governance and politics. *The Journal of Law, Medicine & Ethics* 39:37–41.

Hwang, T., and J. T. Kim. 2011. Effects of indoor lighting on occupants' visual comfort and eye health in a green building. *Indoor and Built Environment* 20(1):75–90.

Imrie, R., and M. Kumar. 1998. Focusing on disability and access in the built environment. *Disability & Society* 13(3):357–374.

IOM (Institute of Medicine). 1988. *The future of public health.* Washington, DC: National Academy Press.

———. 2003. *The future of the public's health in the 21st century.* Washington, DC: The National Academies Press.

———. 2004. *Health literacy: A prescription to end confusion.* Washington, DC: The National Academies Press.

———. 2011a. *Early childhood obesity prevention policies.* Washington, DC: The National Academies Press.

———. 2011b. *For the public's health: Revitalizing law and policy to meet new challenges.* Washington, DC: The National Academies Press.

———. 2011c. *For the public's health: The role of measurement in action and accountability.* Washington, DC: The National Academies Press.

———. 2012a. *For the public's health: Investing in a healthier future.* Washington, DC: The National Academies Press.

———. 2012b. *An integrated framework for assessing the value of community-based prevention.* Washington, DC: The National Academies Press.

———. 2012. *Epilepsy across the spectrum: Promoting health and understanding.* Washington, DC: The National Academies Press.

———. 2015. *Strategies to improve cardiac arrest survival: A time to act.* Washington, DC: The National Academies Press.

Jacobson, P. D., J. Wasserman, H. W. Wu, and J. R. Lauer. 2015. Assessing enrepreneurship in governmental public health. *American Journal of Public Health* 105(S2):S318–S322.

Jaggernath, J., L. Verland, P. Ramson, V. Kovai, V. F. Chan, and K. S. Naidoo. 2014. Poverty and eye health. *Health* 6(14):1849–1860.

Jones, H. L., E. A. Walker, C. B. Schechter, and E. Blanco. 2010. Vision is precious: A successful behavioral intervention to increase the rate of screening for diabetic retinopathy for inner-city adults. *Diabetes Educator* 36(1):118–126.

Juzych, M. S., S. Randhawa, A. Shukairy, P. Kaushal, A. Gupta, and N. Shalauta. 2008. Functional health literacy in patients with glaucoma in urban settings. *Archives of Ophthalmology* 126(5):718–724.

Kaiser Family Foundation. 2013. *Medicaid: A primer.* Menlo Park, CA: The Henry J. Kaiser Family Foundation.

Keay, L., F. Stapleton, and O. Schein. 2007. Epidemiology of contact lens-related inflammation and microbial keratitis: A 20-year perspective. *Eye & Contact Lens* 33(6 Pt 2):346–353, discussion 362–363.

Kemper, A. R., A. Helfrich, J. Talbot, N. Patel, and J. E. Crews. 2011. Improving the rate of preschool vision screening: An interrupted time-series analysis. *Pediatrics* 128(5):e1279–e1284.

Kemper, A. R., A. Helfrich, J. Talbot, and N. Patel. 2012. Outcomes of an elementary school-based vision screening program in North Carolina. *Journal of School Nursing* 28(1):24–30.

Kennedy, R. D., M. M. Spafford, C. M. Parkinson, and G. T. Fong. 2011. Knowledge about the relationship between smoking and blindness in Canada, the United States, the United Kingdom, and Australia: Results from the International Tobacco Control Four-Country Project. *Optometry* 82(5):310–317.

Khan, J. C., D. A. Thurlby, H. Shahid, D. G. Clayton, J. R. Yates, M. Bradley, A. T. Moore, and A. C. Bird. 2006. Smoking and age related macular degeneration: The number of pack years of cigarette smoking is a major determinant of risk for both geographic atrophy and choroidal neovascularisation. *British Journal of Ophthalmology* 90(1):75–80.

Kim, S. S., S. H. Kim, H. Fang, S. Kwon, D. Shelley, and D. Ziedonis. 2015. A culturally adapted smoking cessation intervention for Korean Americans: A mediating effect of perceived family norm toward quitting. *Journal of Immigrant and Minority Health* 17(4):1120–1129.

Kindig, D., and G. Stoddart. 2003. What is population health? *American Journal of Public Health* 93(3):380–383.

Klein, R., K. J. Cruickshanks, S. D. Nash, E. M. Krantz, F. J. Nieto, G. H. Huang, J. S. Pankow, and B. E. K. Klein. 2010. The prevalence of age-related macular degeneration and associated risk factors: The Beaver Dam Offspring Study. *Archives of Ophthalmology* 128(6):750–758.

Kleinstein, R. N., L. A. Jones, S. Hullett, S. Kwon, R. J. Friedman, R. E. Manny, D. O. Mutti, J. A. Yu, K. Zudnik, and Collaborative Longitudinal Evaluation of Ethnicity and Refractive Error Study Group. 2003. Refractive error and ethnicity in children. *Archives of Ophthalmology* 121(8):1141–1147.

Kodjebacheva, G., E. R. Brown, L. Estrada, F. Yu, and A. L. Coleman. 2011. Uncorrected refractive error among first-grade students of different racial/ethnic groups in Southern California: Results a year after school-mandated vision screening. *Journal of Public Health Management and Practice* 17(6):499–505.

Koh, H. K., L. J. Elqura, C. M. Judge, and M. A. Stoto. 2008. Regionalization of local public health systems in the era of preparedness. *Annual Reviews of Public Health* 29:205–218.

Koh, H. K., C. Brach, L. M. Harris, and M. L. Parchman. 2013. A proposed "health literate care model" would constitute a systems approach to improving patients' engagement in care. *Health Affairs (Millwood)* 32(2):357–367.

Koivusalo, M. 2010. The state of health in all policies (HIAP) in the European Union: Potential and pitfalls. *Journal of Epidemiology and Community Health* 64(6):500–503.

Konkle, K. M. 2009. *Exploring shared services collaboration in Wisconsin local public health agencies: A review of the literature*. Madison: Institute for Wisconsin's Health Inc.

Korchak, M. E., R. U. Glazier, R. S. Slack, M. W. Plankey, and H. R. Mayer. 2012. Protective eyewear use as depicted in children's television programs. *Journal of Pediatric Ophthalmology and Strabismus* 50(2):118–123.

Korda, H., and Z. Itani. 2013. Harnessing social media for health promotion and behavior change. *Health Promotion Practice* 14(1):15–23.

Krusen, N. 2010. Home lighting: Understanding what, where and how much. *OT Practice* 15(19):8–9.

Krutmann, J., F. Behar-Cohen, G. Baillet, T. de Ayguavives, P. Ortega Garcia, P. Pena-Garcia, C. Reme, and J. Wolffsohn. 2014. Towards standardization of UV eye protection: What can be learned from photodermatology? *Photodermatology, Photoimmunology, & Photomedicine* 30(2–3):128–136.

Kulp, M. T., E. Ciner, M. Maguire, B. Moore, J. Pentimonti, M. Pistilli, L. Cyert, T. R. Candy, G. Quinn, G. S., Ying, for the VIP HIP Study Group. Uncorrected hyperopia and preschool early literacy: Results of the Vision in Preschoolers-Hyperopia in Preschoolers (VIP-HIP) Study. *Ophthalmology* 123(4):681–689.

Kuzman, T., M. B. Kutija, S. Masnec, S. Jandrokovic, D. Mrazovac, D. Jurisic, I. Skegro, M. Kalauz, and R. Kordic. 2014. Compliance among soft contact lens wearers. *Collegium Antropologicum* 38(4):1217–1221.

Kyle, J. W., J. K. Hammitt, H. W. Lim, A. C. Geller, L. H. Hall-Jordan, E. W. Maibach, E. C. De Fabo, and M. C. Wagner. 2008. Economic evaluation of the US Environmental Protection Agency's SunWise Program: Sun protection education for young children. *Pediatrics* 121(5):e1074–e1084.

Lam, N., and S. J. Leat. 2015. Reprint of: Barriers to accessing low-vision care: The patient's perspective. *Canadian Journal of Ophthalmology* 50(Suppl 1):S34–S39.

Lancaster, K., C. E. Hughes, B. Spicer, F. Matthew-Simmons, and P. Dillon. 2011. Illicit drugs and the media: Models of media effects for use in drug policy research. *Drug and Alcohol Review* 30(4):397–402.

Lang, D., R. Leman, A. W. Arnold, and R. W. Arnold. 2007. Validated portable pediatric vision screening in the Alaska bush. A VIPS-like study in the Koyukon. *Alaska Medicine* 49(1):2–15.

Leahy, E., and M. Fallon. 2005. Boards of health: Extinction or evolution? *Transformations in Public Health* 6(3):1–4.

Lechanteur, Y. T., P. L. van de Camp, D. Smailhodzic, J. P. van de Ven, G. H. Buitendijk, C. C. Klaver, J. M. Groenewoud, A. I. den Hollander, C. B. Hoyng, and B. J. Klevering. 2015. Association of smoking and CFH and ARMS2 risk variants with younger age at onset of neovascular age-related macular degeneration. *JAMA Ophthalmology* 133(5):533–541.

Lee, S., S. J. Song, and H. G. Yu. 2013a. Current smoking is associated with a poor visual acuity improvement after intravitreal ranibizumab therapy in patients with exudative age-related macular degeneration. *Journal of Korean Medical Science* 28(5):769–774.

Lee, S. M., J. Landry, P. M. Jones, O. Buhrmann, and P. Morley-Forster. 2013b. The effectiveness of a perioperative smoking cessation program: A randomized clinical trial. *Anesthesia & Analgesia* 117(3):605–613.

Lefebvre, R. C., and A. S. Bornkessel. 2013. Digital social networks and health. *Circulation* 127(17):1829–1836.

Liang, X. Y., L. J. Chen, T. K. Ng, J. Tuo, J. L. Gao, P. O. Tam, T. Y. Lai, C. C. Chan, and C. P. Pang. 2014. FPR1 interacts with CFH, HTRA1 and smoking in exudative age-related macular degeneration and polypoidal choroidal vasculopathy. *Eye (London)* 28(12):1502–1510.

Libbey, P., and B. Miyahara. 2011. *Cross-jurisdictional relationship in local public health: Preliminary summary of an environmental scan.* Princeton, NJ: Robert Wood Johnson Foundation.

Lin, P. R., Z. W. Zhao, K. K. Cheng, and T. H. Lam. 2013. The effect of physician's 30 s smoking cessation intervention for male medical outpatients: A pilot randomized controlled trial. *Journal of Public Health (Oxford)* 35(3):375–383.

Lindblad, B. E., N. Håkansson, H. Svensson, B. Philipson, and A. Wolk. 2005. Intensity of smoking and smoking cessation in relation to risk of cataract extraction: A prospective study of women. *American Journal of Epidemiology* 162(1):73–79.

Lindblad, B. E., N. Håkansson, and A. Wolk. 2014. Smoking cessation and the risk of cataract: A prospective cohort study of cataract extraction among men. *JAMA Ophthalmology* 132(3):253–257.

Lions Club. 2016. Lions eye health program. http://members.lionsclubs.org/EN/serve/sight/eye-health (accessed July 10, 2016).

Livingston, P. M., C. A. McCarty, and H. R. Taylor. 1998. Knowledge, attitudes, and self care practices associated with age related eye disease in Australia. *British Journal of Ophthalmology* 82(7):780–785.

Lombardi, D. A., S. K. Verma, M. J. Brennan, and M. J. Perry. 2009. Factors influencing worker use of personal protective eyewear. *Accident Analysis & Prevention* 41(4):755–762.

Loo, D. L., D. H. Ng, W. Tang, and K. G. Au Eong. 2009. Raising awareness of blindness as another smoking-related condition: A public health role for optometrists? *Clinical and Experimental Optometry* 92(1):42–44.

Lopez, W., and T. R. Frieden. 2007. Legal counsel to public health practitioners. In *Law in public health practice*, edited by R. A. Goodman, R. E. Hoffman, W. Lopez, G. W. Matthews, M. A. Rothstein and K. L. Foster. New York: Oxford University Press.

Mancini, G., A. Baldasseroni, G. Laffi, S. Curti, S. Mattioli, and F. S. Violante. 2005. Prevention of work related eye injuries: Long term assessment of the effectiveness of a multicomponent intervention among metal workers. *Occupational and Environmental Medicine* 62(12):830–835.

Marshall, E. C., R. E. Meetz, and L. L. Harmon. 2010. Through our children's eyes—The public health impact of the vision screening requirements for Indiana school children. *Optometry* 81(2):71–82.

Matter, K. C., S. A. Sinclair, and H. Xiang. 2007. Use of protective eyewear in U.S. children: Results from the National Health Interview Survey. *Ophthalmic Epidemiology* 14(1):37–43.

Mays, G. P., M. C. McHugh, K. Shim, N. Perry, D. Lenaway, P. K. Halverson, and R. Moonesinghe. 2006. Institutional and economic determinants of public health system performance. *American Journal of Public Health* 96(3):523–531.

McCombs, M., and D. Shaw. 1972. The agenda-setting function of mass media. *Public Opinion Quarterly* 36(2):176–187.

McGwin, G., R. Khoury, J. Cross, and C. Owsley. 2010. Vision impairment and eye care utilization among Americans 50 and older. *Current Eye Research* 35(6):451–458.

McNaughton, C. D., C. Cawthon, S. Kripalani, D. Liu, A. B. Storrow, and C. L. Roumie. 2015. Health literacy and mortality: A cohort study of patients hospitalized for acute heart failure. *Journal of the American Heart Association* 4(5).

MDHHS (Michigan Department of Health and Human Services). 2016a. Vision screening. http://www.michigan.gov/mdhhs/0,5885,7-339-73971_4911_4912_6238_76134---,00. html (accessed May 18, 2016).

————. 2016b. Vision screening and reporting for kindergarten. https://www.mcir.org/wp-content/uploads/2014/09/SS_Vision.pdf (accessed May 18, 2016).

Medicaid. 2016a. Benefits. https://www.medicaid.gov/medicaid-chip-program-information/by-topics/benefits/medicaid-benefits.html (accessed October 20, 2015).

————. 2016b. Eligibility. https://www.medicaid.gov/medicaid-chip-program-information/by-topics/eligibility/eligibility.html (accessed October 20, 2015).

Mello, M. M., J. Pomeranz, and P. Moran. 2008. The interplay of public health law and industry self-regulation: The case of sugar-sweetened bevarage sales in schools. *American Journal of Public Health* 98(4):595–604.

Moorhead, S. A., D. E. Hazlett, L. Harrison, J. K. Carroll, A. Irwin, and C. Hoving. 2013. A new dimension of health care: Systematic review of the uses, benefits, and limitations of social media for health communication. *Journal of Medical Internet Research* 15(4):e85.

Muir, K. W., C. Santiago-Turla, S. S. Stinnett, L. W. Herndon, R. R. Allingham, P. Challa, and P. P. Lee. 2006. Health literacy and adherence to glaucoma therapy. *American Journal of Ophthalmology* 142(2):223–226.

Muir, K. W., L. Christensen, and H. B. Bosworth. 2013. Health literacy and glaucoma. *Current Opinion in Ophthalmology* 24(2):119–124.

Müller, A., J. E. Keeffe, and H. R. Taylor. 2007. Changes in eye care utilization following an eye health promotion campaign. *Clinical & Experimental Ophthalmology* 35(4):305–309.

Mussener, U., M. Bendtsen, N. Karlsson, I. R. White, J. McCambridge, and P. Bendtsen. 2016. Effectiveness of short message service text-based smoking cessation intervention among university students: A randomized clinical trial. *JAMA Internal Medicine* 176(3):321–328.

Myers, C. E., B. E. K. Klein, R. Gangnon, T. A. Sivakumaran, S. K. Iyengar, and R. Klein. 2014. Cigarette smoking and the natural history of age-related macular degeneration: The Beaver Dam Eye Study. *Ophthalmology* 121(10):1949–1955.

NACCHO (National Association of County and City Health Officials). 1998. *NACCHO survey examines state/local health department relationships.* Washington, DC: NACCHO.

————. 2009a. *2008 national profile of local health departments.* Washington, DC: NACCHO.

————. 2009b. *The local health department workforce: Findings from the 2008 national profile of local health departments.* Washington, DC: NACCHO.

————. 2011. *Local health department job losses and program cuts: Findings from January 2011 survey and 2010 national profile study.* Washington, DC: NACCHO.

————. 2016. *Tip sheet: Prioritizing issues in a community health improvement process.* Washington, DC: NACCHO. http://archived.naccho.org/topics/infrastructure/CHAIP/upload/Final-Issue-Prioritization-Resource-Sheet.pdf (accessed August 15, 2015).

NACDD (National Association of Chronic Disease Directors). 2004. *Vision problems in the United States: Recommendations for a state public health response.* Chicago, IL: Prevent Blindness.

————. 2016. Vision and eye health initiative funding opportunity announcement (FOA #VIi2015a). http://c.ymcdn.com/sites/www.chronicdisease.org/resource/resmgr/Healthy_Aging/RFA_for_Vision_and_Eye_Healt.pdf (accessed November 29, 2016).

————. n.d. About NACDD. http://www.chronicdisease.org/?page=AboutUs (accessed April 5, 2016).

Naron, S., and M. Mendes. 2016. Baltimore City announces new citywide initiative to provide free universal vision screening and glasses to students. Baltimore, MD: City of Baltimore.

NASEM (The National Academies of Sciences, Engineering, and Medicine). 2016. *Hearing health care for adults: Priorities for improving access and affordability*. Washington, DC: The National Academies Press.

National Center for Appropriate Technology. 2014. Partnership for sustainable communities: Five years of learning from communities and coordinating federal investments. https://www.sustainablecommunities.gov/sites/sustainablecommunities.gov/files/docs/partnership-accomplishments-report-2014-reduced-size.pdf (accessed July 22, 2016).

The National Council for Public-Private Partnerships. 2016. 7 keys to success. http://www.ncppp.org/ppp-basics/7-keys (accessed April 6, 2016).

NEHEP (National Eye Health Education Program). 2011. National Eye Health Education Progam five-year agenda 2012–2017. Bethesda, MD: National Eye Institute.

———. 2014. Diabetes focus group findings. Bethesda, MD: National Eye Institute.

———. n.d. Glaucoma awareness month. https://nei.nih.gov/nehep/gam (accessed July 10, 2016).

NEI/LCIF (National Eye Institute/Lions Club International Foundation). 2008. 2005 survey of public knowledge, attitudes, and practices related to eye health and disease. https://nei.nih.gov/sites/default/files/nei-pdfs/2005KAPFinalRpt.pdf (accessed April 6, 2016).

NEI/NIH (National Eye Institute/National Institutes of Health). 2015a. Eye health tips. https://nei.nih.gov/healthyeyes/eyehealthtips (accessed April 6, 2016).

———. 2015b. Finding the right eye protection. https://nei.nih.gov/sports/findingprotection (accessed September 23, 2015).

———. 2015c. National Eye Health Education Program (NEHEP). https://nei.nih.gov/nehep/about (accessed June 12, 2016).

———. 2015d. NEI's research progress. https://nei.nih.gov/about/mission (accessed April 6, 2016).

———. 2016. Budget and Congress. https://nei.nih.gov/news/congress (accessed April 7, 2016).

Neiger, B. L., R. Thackeray, S. H. Burton, C. G. Giraud-Carrier, and M. C. Fagen. 2012. Evaluating social media's capacity to develop engaged audiences in health promotion settings: Use of Twitter metrics as a case study. *Health Promotion Practice* 14(2):157–162.

Neuner, B., A. Komm, J. Wellmann, M. Dietzel, D. Pauleikhoff, J. Walter, M. Busch, and H. W. Hense. 2009. Smoking history and the incidence of age-related macular degeneration—results from the Muenster Aging and Retina Study (MARS) cohort and systematic review and meta-analysis of observational longitudinal studies. *Addictive Behaviors* 34(11):938–947.

New Eyes. n.d. U.S. voucher program. http://www.new-eyes.org/us-voucher-program-1 (accessed July 11, 2016).

NIBS (National Institute of Building Sciences). 2015. *Design guidelines for the visual environment*. Washington, DC: NIBS.

Nicola, R. M. 2005. Boards of health give citizens a voice. *Transformations in Public Health* 5(3):2–7.

Niederdeppe, J., M. C. Farrelly, and M. L. Haviland. 2004. Confirming "truth": More evidence of a successful tobacco countermarketing campaign in Florida. *American Journal of Public Health* 94(2):255–257.

Nishtar, S. 2004. Public–private "partnerships" in health—A global call to action. *Health Research Policy and Systems* 2:5–5.

Noertjojo, K., D. Maberley, K. Bassett, and P. Courtright. 2006. Awareness of eye diseases and risk factors: Identifying needs for health education and promotion in Canada. *Canadian Journal of Ophthalmology* 41(5):617–623.

Novick, L. F., G. P. Mays, and G. Benjamin. 2005. *Public health administration: Principles for population-based management*. Burlington, MA: Jones and Bartlett.

NRC (National Research Council). 2011. *Improving health in the United States: The role of health impact assessment.* Washington, DC: The National Academies Press.

NYSDOH (New York State Department of Health). 2009. *Graphic ad campaign warns smokers of stroke and eye damage from cigarettes: TV, radio, internet ads promote free NYS quitline services to kick addiction.* Albany: NYSDOH.

ODPHP (Office of Disease Prevention and Health Promotion). 2010. Health communication and social marketing: Health communication campaigns that include mass media and health-related product distribution (community guide recommendation). https://www.healthypeople.gov/2020/tools-resources/evidence-based-resource/health-communication-and-social-marketing-health-0 (accessed April 6, 2016).

———. 2016a. Health literate care model. http://health.gov/communication/interactiveHLCM/resources.asp (accessed June 1, 2016).

———. 2016b. Immunization and infectious diseases. https://www.healthypeople.gov/2020/topics-objectives/topic/immunization-and-infectious-diseases/objectives (accessed April 6, 2016).

———. 2016c. Social determinants of health. https://www.healthypeople.gov/2020/topics-objectives/topic/social-determinants-of-health (accessed April 13, 2016).

———. 2016d. Social determinants of health: Objectives. https://www.healthypeople.gov/2020/topics-objectives/topic/social-determinants-of-health/objectives (accessed April 13, 2016).

———. 2016e. Vision. https://www.healthypeople.gov/2020/topics-objectives/topic/vision/objectives (accessed April 6, 2016).

———. 2016f. Vision interventions & resources. https://www.healthypeople.gov/2020/topics-objectives/topic/vision/ebrs (accessed April 6, 2016).

Omana-Cepeda, C., E. Jane-Salas, A. Estrugo-Devesa, E. Chimenos-Kustner, and J. Lopez-Lopez. 2016. Effectiveness of dentist's intervention in smoking cessation: A review. *Journal of Clinical and Experimental Dentistry* 8(1):e78–e83.

OneSight. 2016. FAQs. https://onesight.org/faqs (accessed July 11, 2016).

Opstelten, W., and M. J. W. Zaal. 2005. Managing ophthalmic herpes zoster in primary care. *British Medical Journal* 331(7509):147–151.

OSHA (Occupational Safety and Health Administration). 2003. Eye and face protection. https://www.osha.gov/Publications/osha3151.html#eyeandface (accessed April 6, 2016).

———. 2009. Regulations (Standards—29 CFR): Table of contents. https://www.osha.gov/pls/oshaweb/owadisp.show_document?p_table=STANDARDS&p_id=9778 (accessed April 6, 2016).

———. 2016. Eye and face protection eTool. https://www.osha.gov/SLTC/etools/eyeandface/employer/requirements.html (accessed April 6, 2016).

Oto, M. A., O. Ergene, L. Tokgozoglu, Z. Ongen, O. Kozan, M. Sahin, M. K. Erol, T. Tezel, and M. Ozkan. 2011. Impact of a mass media campaign to increase public awareness of hypertension. *Turk Kardiyoloji Dernegi Ars* 39(5):355–364.

Papadakis, S., P. W. McDonald, A. L. Pipe, S. T. Letherdale, R. D. Reid, and K. S. Brown. 2013. Effectiveness of telephone-based follow-up support delivered in combination with a multi-component smoking cessation intervention in family practice: A cluster-randomized trial. *Preventive Medicine* 56(6):390–397.

Parssinen, O., M. Kauppinen, and A. Viljanen. 2014. The progression of myopia from its onset at age 8–12 to adulthood and the influence of heredity and external factors on myopic progression: A 23-year follow-up study. *Acta Ophthalmologica* 92(8):730–739.

Paul, S., and Y. Liu. 2012. Inadequate light levels and their effect on falls and daily activities of community dwelling older adults: A review of literature. *New Zealand Journal of Occupational Therapy* 59(2):39–42.

PBA/NACDD (Prevent Blindness America/National Association of Chronic Disease Directors). 2005. *A plan for the development of state based vision preservation programs: Summary of a retreat on public health vision preservation.* Rensselaerville, NY: National Association of Chronic Disease Directors.

Pedersen, E. R., N. K. Eberhart, K. M. Williams, T. Tanielian, C. Epley, and D. M. Scharf. 2015. *Public–private partnerships for providing behavioral health care to veterans and their families: What do we know, what do we need to learn, and what do we need to do?* Santa Monica, CA: RAND Corporation.

Perdue, W. C., L. A. Stone, and L. O. Gostin. 2003. The built environment and its relationship to the public's health: The legal framework. *American Journal of Public Health* 93(9):1390–1394.

PHAB (Public Health Accreditation Board). 2013. Getting started. http://www.phaboard.org/accreditation-overview/getting-started (accessed April 11, 2016).

———. n.d. What is public health accreditation. http://www.phaboard.org/accreditation-overview/what-is-accreditation (accessed July 15, 2016).

Phildelphia Eagles. 2016. Eagles charitable foundation: Vision care. http://www.philadelphiaeagles.com/community/org-vision.html (accessed July 11, 2016).

Prevent Blindness. 2012. The vision connection: Integrating vision into state health programs. Chicago, IL: Prevent Blindness America.

———. 2016a. Eye safety at work. http://www.preventblindness.org/eye-safety-work (accessed April 6, 2016).

———. 2016b. Prevent Blindness eye health and safety observance calendar. http://www.preventblindness.org/prevent-blindness-eye-health-and-safety-observance-calendar (accessed July 10, 2016).

———. 2016c. Preventing eye injuries. http://www.preventblindness.org/preventing-eye-injuries (accessed April 6, 2016).

Radford, C. F., D. Minassian, J. K. Dart, F. Stapleton, and S. Verma. 2009. Risk factors for nonulcerative contact lens complications in an ophthalmic accident and emergency department: A case-control study. *Ophthalmology* 116(3):385–392.

Rahi, J. S., P. M. Cumberland, and C. S. Peckham. 2009. Visual function in working-age adults: Early life influences and associations with health and social outcomes. *Ophthalmology* 116(10):1866–1871.

Ramirez, L. B., E. Baker, and M. Metzler. 2008. *Promoting health equity: A resource to help communities address social determinants of health.* Atlanta, GA: CDC.

Ranasinghe, P., W. S. Wathurapatha, Y. S. Perera, D. A. Lamabadusuriya, S. Kulatunga, N. Jayawardana, and P. Katulanda. 2016. Computer vision syndrome among computer office workers in a developing country: An evaluation of prevalence and risk factors. *BMC Research Notes* 9(1):150.

Rao, G. 2015. The Barrie Jones lecture—Eye care for the neglected population: Challenges and solutions. *Eye* 29(1):30–45.

Rein, D. B. 2013. Vision problems are a leading source of modifiable health expenditures. *Investigative Ophthalmology & Visual Science* 54(14):ORSF18–ORSF22.

Rey-Lopez, J. P., G. Vicente-Rodriguez, M. Biosca, and L. A. Moreno. 2008. Sedentary behaviour and obesity development in children and adolescents. *Nutrition, Metabolism and Cardiovascular Diseases* 18(3):242–251.

Reynaers, A.-M. 2014. Public values in public–private partnerships. *Public Administration Review* 74(1):41–50.

Robertson, D. M., and H. D. Cavanagh. 2011. Non-compliance with contact lens wear and care practices: A comparative analysis. *Optometry & Vision Science* 88(12):1402–1408.

Rose, K. A., I. G. Morgan, J. Ip, A. Kifley, S. Huynh, W. Smith, and P. Mitchell. 2008. Outdoor activity reduces the prevalence of myopia in children. *Ophthalmology* 115(8):1279–1285.

Rosenfield, M. 2011. Computer vision syndrome: A review of ocular causes and potential treatments. *Ophthalmic and Physiologic Optics* 31(5):502–515.

Rubin, D. B., S. R. Singh, and G. J. Young. 2015. Tax-exempt hospitals and community benefit: New directions in policy and practice. *Annual Review of Public Health* 36(1):545–557.

RWJF (Robert Wood Johnson Foundation). 2014. *Building a culture of health*. Princeton, NJ: RWJF.

Salinsky, E. 2010. *Governmental public health: An overview of state and local public health agencies*. Washington, DC: National Health Policy Forum.

Sarna, L. P., S. A. Bialous, E. Kralikova, A. Kmetova, V. Felbrova, S. Kulovana, K. Mala, E. Roubickova, M. J. Wells, and J. K. Brook. 2014. Impact of a smoking cessation educational program on nurses' interventions. *Journal of Nursing Scholarship* 46(5):314–321.

SATH (Society for Accessible Travel & Hospitality). 2013. How to travel with a sight impairment or blindness. http://sath.org/how-to-travel-with-a-sight-impairment-or-blindness (accessed April 7, 2016).

Sawyer, J., and M. L. Kaup. 2014. Lighting, vision, and aging in place: The impact of living with low vision in independent living facilities. *Undergraduate Research Journal for the Human Sciences* 13.

Schaumberg, D. A., S. E. Hankinson, Q. Guo, E. Rimm, and D. J. Hunter. 2007. A prospective study of 2 major age-related macular degeneration susceptibility alleles and interactions with modifiable risk factors. *Archives of Ophthalmology* 125(1):55–62.

Schmidt, S., M. A. Hauser, W. K. Scott, E. A. Postel, A. Agarwal, P. Gallins, F. Wong, Y. S. Chen, K. Spencer, N. Schnetz-Boutaud, J. L. Haines, and M. A. Pericak-Vance. 2006. Cigarette smoking strongly modifies the association of LOC387715 and age-related macular degeneration. *American Journal of Human Genetics* 78(5):852–864.

Scott, A. W., N. M. Bressler, S. Ffolkes, J. S. Wittenborn, J. Jorkavsky. 2016. Public attitudes about eye and vision health. *JAMA Ophthalmology* 134(10):1111–1118.

Sengupta, S., A. M. Nguyen, S. W. van Landingham, S. D. Solomon, D. V. Do, L. Ferrucci, D. S. Friedman, and P. Y. Ramulu. 2015. Evaluation of real-world mobility in age-related macular degeneration. *BMC Ophthalmology* 15(1):1–11.

Sentell, T., K. L. Braun, J. Davis, and T. Davis. 2015. Health literacy and meeting breast and cervical cancer screening guidelines among Asians and Whites in California. *SpringerPlus* 4:432.

Shah, A., K. Blackhall, K. Ker, and D. Patel. 2009. Educational interventions for the prevention of eye injuries. *Cochrane Database of Systematic Reviews* (4):Cd006527.

Sheedy, J. E., J. N. Hayes, and J. Engle. 2003. Is all asthenopia the same? *Optometry & Vision Science* 80(11):732–739.

Sheppler, C. R., W. E. Lambert, S. K. Gardiner, T. M. Becker, and S. L. Mansberger. 2014. Predicting adherence to diabetic eye examinations: Development of the compliance with annual diabetic eye exams survey. *Ophthalmology* 121(6):1212–1219.

Shih, S. T., R. Carter, C. Sinclair, C. Mihalopoulos, and T. Vos. 2009. Economic evaluation of skin cancer prevention in Australia. *Preventive Medicine* 49(5):449–453.

Shin, P., and B. Finnegan. 2009. Assessing the need for on-site eye care professionals in community health centers. *George Washington University Center for Health Services Research and Policy* 1–23.

Simpson, S. A., and J. M. Nonnemaker. 2013. New York tobacco control program cessation assistance: Costs, benefits, and effectiveness. *International Journal of Environmental Research and Public Health* 10(3):1037–1047.

Singh, S., D. Satani, A. Patel, and R. Vhankade. 2012. Colored cosmetic contact lenses: An unsafe trend in the younger generation. *Cornea* 31(7):777–779.

Sliney, D. H. 2001. Photoprotection of the eye—UV radiation and sunglasses. *Journal of Photochemistry and Photobiology* B 64(2–3):166–175.

Sloan, F. A., G. Picone, D. S. Brown, and P. P. Lee. 2005. Longitudinal analysis of the relationship between regular eye examinations and changes in visual and functional status. *Journal of the American Geriatrics Society* 53(11):1867–1874.

Slonim, A. B., C. Callaghan, L. Daily, B. A. Leonard, F. C. Wheeler, C. W. Gollmar, and W. F. Young. 2007. Recommendations for integration of chronic disease programs: Are your programs linked? *Preventing Chronic Disease* 4(2):A34.

Smith, K. E., C. Bambra, K. E. Joyce, N. Perkins, D. J. Hunter, and E. A. Blenkinsopp. 2009. Partners in health? A systematic review of the impact of organizational partnerships on public health outcomes in England between 1997 and 2008. *Journal of Public Health* 31(2):210–221.

Spellman, F. R., and R. M. Bieber. 2012. *Environmental health and science desk reference.* Lanham, MD: Government Institutes.

Spinweber, E., and A. Honeysett. 2013. *Partnership for a healthier America and Channel One News to bring healthy messages into the classroom.* Washington, DC: Channel One News.

Stanczyk, N. E., E. S. Smit, D. N. Schulz, H. de Vries, C. Bolman, J. W. Muris, and S. M. Evers. 2014. An economic evaluation of a video- and text-based computer-tailored intervention for smoking cessation: A cost-effectiveness and cost-utility analysis of a randomized controlled trial. *PLoS ONE* 9(10):e110117.

Stapleton, F., L. Keay, K. Edwards, T. Naduvilath, J. K. Dart, G. Brian, and B. A. Holden. 2008. The incidence of contact lens–related microbial keratitis in australia. *Ophthalmology* 115(10):1655–1662.

Stapleton, F., K. Edwards, L. Keay, T. Naduvilath, J. K. Dart, G. Brian, and B. Holden. 2012. Risk factors for moderate and severe microbial keratitis in daily wear contact lens users. *Ophthalmology* 119(8):1516–1521.

State of Michigan. 2016. Michigan's public health hearing & vision screening programs: Information for healthcare providers. https://www.michigan.gov/documents/mdch/physicans_flyer_361187_7.pdf (accessed June 10, 2016).

Steinemann, T. L., M. Fletcher, A. E. Bonny, R. A. Harvey, D. Hamlin, P. Zloty, M. Besson, K. Walter, and M. Gagnon. 2005. Over-the-counter decorative contact lenses: Cosmetic or medical devices? A case series. *Eye & Contact Lens* 31(5):194–200.

Stoto, M. A., and L. Morse. 2008. Regionalization in local public health systems: Public health preparedness in the Washington Metropolitan area. *Public Health Reports* 123(4):461–473.

Sundling, V., P. Gulbrandsen, J. Jervell, and J. Straand. 2008. Care of vision and ocular health in diabetic members of a national diabetes organization: A cross-sectional study. *BMC Health Services Research* 8(1):1–8.

Szczotka-Flynn, L. B., E. Pearlman, and M. Ghannoum. 2010. Microbial contamination of contact lenses, lens care solutions, and their accessories: A literature review. *Eye & Contact Lens* 36(2):116–129.

Tarczy-Hornoch, K., S. A. Cotter, M. Borchert, R. McKean-Cowdin, J. Lin, G. Wen, J. Kim and R. Varma. 2013. Prevalence and causes of visual impairment in Asian and non-Hispanic white preschool children: Multi-Ethnic Pediatric Eye Disease Study. *Ophthalmology* 120(6):1220–1226.

TDI (Texas Department of Insurance). 2007. *Eye injury prevention factsheet.* Austin: TDI.

Thornton, J., R. Edwards, P. Mitchell, R. A. Harrison, I. Buchan, and S. P. Kelly. 2005. Smoking and age-related macular degeneration: A review of association. *Eye (London)* 19(9):935–944.

Toufeeq, A., and A. J. Oram. 2014. School-entry vision screening in the United Kingdom: Practical aspects and outcomes. *Ophthalmic Epidemiology* 21(4):210–216.

Tovar-Aguilar, J. A., P. F. Monaghan, C. A. Bryant, A. Esposito, M. Wade, O. Ruiz, and R. J. McDermott. 2014. Improving eye safety in citrus harvest crews through the acceptance of personal protective equipment, community-based participatory research, social marketing, and community health workers. *Journal of Agromedicine* 19(2):107–116.

U.S. Surgeon General. 2014. *The health consequences of smoking—50 years of progress: A report from the Surgeon General.* Rockville, MD: U.S. Department of Health and Human Services.

———. 2016. Active living. http://www.surgeongeneral.gov/priorities/prevention/strategy/active-living.html (accessed August 4, 2016).

Varano, M., N. Eter, S. Winyard, K. U. Wittrup-Jensen, R. Navarro, and J. Heraghty. 2015. Current barriers to treatment for wet age-related macular degeneration (WAMD): Findings from the WAMD patient and caregiver survey. *Journal of Clinical Ophthalmology* 9:2243–2250.

Verma, A., M. R. Schulz, S. A. Quandt, E. N. Robinson, J. G. Grzywacz, H. Chen, and T. A. Arcury. 2011. Eye health and safety among Latino farmworkers. *Journal of Agromedicine* 16(2):143–152.

VHIPP (Vision Health Integration and Preservation Program). 2012. *Centers for Disease Control & Prevention component 2a: Vision integration.* Albany, NY: VHIPP.

Vision To Learn. 2016. *Annual report 2015.* Los Angeles, CA: Vision To Learn.

Vitale, S., L. Ellwein, M. F. Cotch, F. L. Ferris, 3rd, and R. Sperduto. 2008. Prevalence of refractive error in the United States, 1999–2004. *Archives of Ophthalmology* 126(8):1111–1119.

Vrangbaek, K. 2008. Public–private partnerships in the health sector: The Danish experience. *Health Economics, Policy and Law* 3(02):141–163.

VSP (Vision Service Plan). 2016. Gift certificates. https://vspglobal.com/cms/vspglobal-outreach/gift-certificates.html (accessed July 11, 2016).

———. n.d. Become a partner. https://vspglobal.com/cms/vspglobal-outreach/giftcertificates-nationalpartner.html (accessed August 31, 2106).

Walker, E. A., C. B. Schechter, A. Caban, and C. E. Basch. 2008. Telephone intervention to promote diabetic retinopathy screening among the urban poor. *American Journal of Preventive Medicine* 34(3):185–191.

Weintraub, J. M., W. C. Willett, B. Rosner, G. A. Colditz, J. M. Seddon, and S. E. Hankinson. 2002. Smoking cessation and risk of cataract extraction among US women and men. *American Journal of Epidemiology* 155(1):72–79.

Weiss, D. M., R. J. Casten, B. E. Leiby, L. A. Hark, A. P. Murchison, D. Johnson, S. Stratford, J. Henderer, B. W. Rovner, and J. A. Haller. 2015. Effect of behavioral intervention on dilated fundus examination rates in older African American individuals with diabetes mellitus: A randomized clinical trial. *JAMA Ophthalmology* 133(9):1005–1012.

Wernham, A., and S. M. Teutsch. 2015. Health in all policies for big cities. *Journal of Public Health Management and Practice* 21(Suppl 1):S56–S65.

The White House. 2010. *First Lady Michelle Obama launches Let's Move: America's move to raise a healthier generation of kids.* Washington, DC: The White House, Office of the First Lady.

White House Task Force on Childhood Obesity. 2010. *Solving the problem of childhood obesity within a generation.* Washington, DC: The White House.

Whitson, H. E., and F. R. Lin. 2014. Hearing and vision care for older adults: Sensing a need to update Medicare policy. *JAMA* 312(17):1739–1740.

Whitson, H. E., S. W. Cousins, B. M. Burchett, C. F. Hybels, C. F. Pieper, and H. J. Cohen. 2007. The combined effect of visual impairment and cognitive impairment on disability in older people. *Journal of the American Geriatric Society* 55(6):885–891.

WHO (World Health Organization). 1948. Preamble to the Constitution of the World Health Organization as adopted by the International Health Conference, New York, 19–22 June, 1946; signed on 22 July 1946 by the representatives of 61 States. *Official Records of the World Health Organization* 2:100.

______. n.d.a. Commission on Social Determinants of Health, 2005–2008. http://www.who.int/social_determinants/thecommission/en (accessed August 14, 2016).

______. n.d.b. Health promotion. http://www.who.int/topics/health_promotion/en (accessed August 14, 2016).

Wittenborn, J., and D. Rein. 2016. *The potential costs and benefits of treatment for undiagnosed eye disorders*. Paper prepared for the Committee on Public Health Approaches to Reduce Vision Impairment and Promote Eye Health. http://www.nationalacademies.org/hmd/~/media/Files/Report%20Files/2016/UndiagnosedEyeDisordersCommissionedPaper.pdf (accessed September 15, 2016).

Wood, J. M., A. Chaparro, P. Lacherez, and L. Hickson. 2012. Useful field of view predicts driving in the presence of distracters. *Optometry & Vision Science* 89(4):373–381.

Wright, C. Y., A. I. Reeder, G. E. Bodeker, A. Gray, and B. Cox. 2007. Solar UVR exposure, concurrent activities and sun-protective practices among primary schoolchildren. *Photochemistry and Photobiology* 83(3):749–758.

Wu, Y., L. Tian, and Y. Huang. 2015a. Correlation between the interactions of ABCA4 polymorphisms and smoking with the susceptibility to age-related macular degeneration. *International Journal of Clinical and Experimental Pathology* 8(6):7403–7408.

Wu, Y. T., M. Willcox, H. Zhu, and F. Stapleton. 2015b. Contact lens hygiene compliance and lens case contamination: A review. *Contact Lens Anterior Eye* 38(5):307–316.

Yazar, S., A. W. Hewitt, L. J. Black, C. M. McKnight, J. A. Mountain, J. C. Sherwin, W. H. Oddy, M. T. Coroneo, R. M. Lucas, and D. A. Mackey. 2014. Myopia is associated with lower vitamin D status in young adults' myopia and vitamin D status. *Investigative Ophthalmology & Visual Science* 55(7):4552–4559.

Yildiz, E. H., S. Airiani, K. M. Hammersmith, C. J. Rapuano, P. R. Laibson, A. S. Virdi, T. Hongyok, and E. J. Cohen. 2012. Trends in contact lens–related corneal ulcers at a tertiary referral center. *Cornea* 31(10):1097–1102.

Zambelli-Weiner, A., J. E. Crews, and D. S. Friedman. 2012. Disparities in adult vision health in the United States. *American Journal of Ophthalmology* 154(6 Suppl):S23–S30, e21.

Zhang, X., J. Kahende, A. Z. Fan, L. Barker, T. J. Thompson, A. H. Mokdad, Y. Li, and J. B. Saaddine. 2011. Smoking and visual impairment among older adults with age-related eye diseases. *Preventing Chronic Disease* 8(4):A84.

Zhang, X., M. F. Cotch, A. Ryskulova, S. A. Primo, P. Nair, C.-F. Chou, L. S. Geiss, L. Barker, A. F. Elliott, J. E. Crews, and J. B. Saaddine. 2012. Vision health disparities in the United States by race/ethnicity, education, and economic status: Findings from two nationally representative surveys. *American Journal of Ophthalmology* 154(60): S53–S62, e51.

Zhou, J., Y. H. Ma, J. Ma, Z. Y. Zou, X. K. Meng, F. B. Tao, C. Y. Luo, J. Jing, D. H. Pan, J. Y. Luo, X. Zhang, H. Wang, and H. P. Zhao. 2016. Prevalence of myopia and influencing factors among primary and middle school students in 6 provinces of China. *Zhonghua Liu Xing Bing Xue Za Zhi* 37(1):29–34.

Zohar, Z., I. Waksman, J. Stolero, G. Volpin, E. Sacagiu, and A. Eytan. 2004. Injury from fireworks and firecrackers during holidays. *Harefuah* 143(10):698–701, 768.

Zuckerman, D. M. 2004. *Blind adults in America: Their lives and challenges*. Washington, DC: National Research Center for Women & Families.

6

Access to Clinical Vision Services: Workforce and Coverage

Vision impairment affects millions of people in the United States (Prevent Blindness, 2012), including approximately 6.4 million people who experience uncorrectable vision impairment and between 8.2 and 15.9 million people who have uncorrected refractive error (Varma et al., 2016; Wittenborn and Rein, 2016; Wittenborn et al., 2013). Different populations are higher risk for vision impairment from different types of conditions (see Chapter 2). For example, children are most commonly affected by amblyopia and strabismus, conditions that can lead to permanent vision loss without early intervention. Age-related diseases, such as glaucoma and cataract, are more prevalent in older population, but disease progression can be slowed with early and effective treatments. Diabetic retinopathy is a possible consequence of uncontrolled diabetes in almost any age group, but can be prevented if the underlying condition is controlled. For populations with uncorrectable vision impairment, access to rehabilitation services and appropriate accommodations can improve health and quality of life.

Although the etiologies of vision loss and the characteristics of affected populations differ, having access to appropriate care is a shared strategy to help mitigate the severity or impact of vision impairment. Combined with estimates of correctable and uncorrectable vision impairment, this prompts questions about broader conditions that may prevent access to existing eye and vision services. Access to health care services is influenced by numerous factors, such as income, distance from an eye care provider, wealth, and vision insurance coverage (Sloan et al., 2014; Zhang et al., 2008a). However, entry into the eye and vision care system is also affected by overaching social and policy barriers, including the availablity of trained eye and vision

271

care professionals (as well as primary care and public health practitioners familiar with eye and vision health) and payment policies that limit coverage for basic services and equipment, directly affecting populations who are most in need of assistance and likely to suffer from uncorrectable or uncorrected vision impairment.

This chapter focuses on two basic prerequisites to facilitate entry into the eye and vision care system: workforce adequacy and insurance coverage of eye and vision care services. Chapters 7 and 8 discuss strategies to improve care quality within the eye and vision care system and advance rehabilitation services and accessibility, respectively. The first section of this chapter explores the different types of providers, their distribution, and workforce diversity. The second section describes the status of insurance coverage for eye disease and vision impairment among both publicly subsidized and employment-based insurance providers and identifies policy options to expand coverage of specific eye and vision services. The final section highlights the importance of cost-effectiveness research to establish the value of specific policies and practices that can improve entry into the eye and vision care system for the most at-risk populations while maximizing health care resources and minimizing the downstream impacts of vision loss.

THE CLINICAL EYE AND VISION CARE WORKFORCE

A variety of professionals provide eye and vision services in the United States and have different education and training. This results in fragmentation between different professional groups, which is compounded by differing provider and patient preferences, the suboptimal use of electronic medical records and low levels of interoperability and confidentiality within the health care information technology infrastructure, and different state laws and regulations that govern practices and professions in the medical and optometric communities (AAO, 2011; Hall and Schulman, 2010). Understanding who to see for what services is important not only in terms of public messaging, but also in terms of effective collaboration with the general medical establishment to promote eye and vision health through appropriate referrals and care coordination, which are discussed in Chapter 7.

Defining Eye and Vision Care Providers

Ophthalmologists and optometrists are the two professional groups most commonly associated with eye and vision care. Ophthalmologists are physicians, having completed either allopathic (M.D.) or osteopathic (D.O.) medical education after a baccalaureate degree, followed by a mandatory internship and residency training. According to the American Academy of

Ophthalmology, approximately 40 percent of ophthalmologists complete fellowship subspecialty training (AAO, 2011). Optometrists, on the other hand, have completed a doctor of optometry (O.D.) degree after a baccalaureate degree and may have completed a post-graduate residency or fellowship training. The distinction between ophthalmologists and optometrists may drive health care decisions in the United States, including some payment policies, and may impose barriers or create opportunities affecting access to preventive and follow-up eye care.

In addition to ophthalmologists and optometrists, a variety of additional health care professionals (e.g., occupational therapists, orthoptists, opticians, ophthalmic technicians, ophthalmic medical assistants, ophthalmic medical technologists, and ophthalmic surgical assistants) and educational specialists (e.g., low-vision therapists, orientation and mobility specialists, and vision rehabilitation therapists) play intricate and necessary roles in supporting the eye and vision health of populations. Vision specialists, occupational therapists, mobility specialists, and blind-rehabilitation specialists provide an important care component that is explored in greater detail in Chapter 8. Ophthalmic medical assistants, ophthalmic medical technologists, and ophthalmic surgical assistants support ophthalmologists and optometrists in the provision of patient care. Primary care physicians, physician assistants, nurse practitioners, nursing staff, and other primary care providers aid in the early detection of vision problems and serve as an entry point into the eye and vision care system. Appendix F describes the educational requirements and professional responsibilities of many of these providers.

State regulations govern scope of practice for both medical doctors, such as ophthalmologists, and optometrists. None of the 50 states has any restrictions on medical and surgical practice for ophthalmologists, and all 50 states allow optometrists to "diagnose" diseases of the eye and vision system and to use diagnostic pharmaceutical agents to facilitate examination and therapeutic pharmaceutical agents to treat diseases or conditions of the eye and related structures (Cooper, 2012).[1] However, other aspects of eye and vision care for optometrists vary widely. For example, the legal authority to prescribe controlled narcotic substances, use injectables, or perform surgical and/or laser procedures varies state by state (Cooper, 2012). Kentucky and Oklahoma allow optometrists to perform all laser surgery procedures (with the exception of retina, laser in-situ keratomileusis, and cosmetic lid surgery in Oklahoma) (Webb, 2011). Other states, such as California and Colorado, explicitly prohibit optometrists from performing

---

[1] Massachusetts is currently the only state where optometrists do not possess the authority to treat glaucoma.

surgery.[2,3] Internal practice protocols and organizational barriers adopted by managed care organizations, as well as various other factors, may also affect the scope of practice (Soroka et al., 2000).

Although the committee was not constituted to define the appropriate scope of practice for each profession, the committee does find that differences in scope of practice can create confusion among members of the public and health care providers in general, hindering population health efforts to increase access to appropriate care. In addition, debates over scope of practice highlight tensions among eye and vision care providers, which can hamper efforts to create a unified advocacy platform from which to advance population eye and vision health.

Workforce Distribution and Projections

Healthy People 2020 identifies geographic location as a factor that affects an individual's ability to achieve good health and that contributes to health disparities (ODPHP, 2016). The distribution of different types of eye care providers varies among and within states, which affects the delivery of preventive services and effective treatments for many populations, especially those already at risk for poor health. Analyzing the current workforce distribution is important to maintaining or expanding adequate access to appropriate care through sufficiently trained eye care and health care professionals. As the U.S. population ages and the prevalence of age-related eye diseases and conditions increase accordingly (Varma et al., 2016; Wittenborn and Rein, 2016), it will be important to ensure adequate workforce supply to respond to growing demand and the need to control costs.

The availability of eye care professionals affects rates of care, especially for specific types of eye diseases and conditions. For example, access to ophthalmologists is associated with whether an individual obtains medically related eye care for diabetes, age-related macular degeneration (AMD), and glaucoma (Chou et al., 2012; Gibson, 2014; Sloan et al., 2004, 2014). Yet, recent studies have noted an absence of eye care professionals in a substantial percentage of counties with diabetic populations. Chou and colleagues (2012), using 2006 Behavioral Risk Factor Surveillance System (BRFSS) and 2007 Area Resource File (ARF) data, estimated that 10 percent of BRFSS respondents with diabetes lived in counties with neither an ophthalmologist nor an optometrist. Alabama has a high and growing prevalence of type 2 diabetes, but almost 15 percent of the counties in Alabama have neither an ophthalmologist nor an optometrist (MacLennan et al., 2014; The State of Obesity, 2016). Similarly, a survey of 597 primary care pediatricians

---

[2] S.B. 622 Optometry, 2015 Leg., Reg. Sess. (Cal. 2015).
[3] S.B. 11-094, 68th Gen. Assemb., Reg. Sess. (Colo. 2011).

found that 67.6 percent and 38.5 percent of those located in rural and non-rural areas, respectively, reported shortages of pediatric ophthalmologists (Pletcher et al., 2010).

The Current and Projected Eye and Vision Care Workforce

Given predicted increases in the prevalence of age-related eye diseases and conditions (see Chapter 2), it will be important to determine whether the eye and vision workforce supply and distribution is adequate to meet the rising demand. In 2013, the Association of American Medical Colleges (AAMC) reported 18,317 active ophthalmologists in the United States, with about 95 percent reporting their major activity as patient care rather than teaching or research (AAMC, 2014). From 2008 to 2013, there was a 2.6 percent increase in the number of active ophthalmologists and a 1.6 percent decrease in the number of first-year Accreditation Council for Graduate Medical Education residents and fellows (AAMC, 2014). A report released by the U.S. Department of Health and Human Services in 2008 projected that, based on patterns of graduates, specialty choice, and practice behavior, there would be more than 20,000 active ophthalmologists by 2015 (HHS, 2008). The report also calculated "baseline physician requirement projections"[4] from the number of ophthalmologists in 2000 and estimated that the need for ophthalmologists would grow by 28 percent by 2020 (HHS, 2008). This put ophthalmology third among all medical specialties, following closely behind estimated projected needs for cardiology (33 percent) and urology (30 percent) (HHS, 2008).

The Health Resources and Services Administration (HRSA) reports that, in 2013, an estimated 36,858 optometrists practices in the United States (HHS, 2013b).[5] The number of graduates from optometry degree programs increased by approximately 20 percent from 2007 to 2014, according to the Association of Schools and Colleges of Optometry's annual student data report (ASCO, 2009, 2015b). The number of new graduates per 100,000 in the population increased from 0.43 in 2007 to 0.49 in 2014 (ASCO, 2009, 2015b). The Bureau of Labor Statistics (BLS) (2015b) forecasts a faster-than-average growth over the next decade, with a projected 27 percent increase in the number of optometrists between 2014 and 2024.

The current distribution of different types of eye care providers varies among and within states, which can affect access to preventive services and

---

[4] "The baseline projections take into account the growth and aging of the population, but are calculated on the assumption that the United States will provide the same level of care in the future" that it provided in 2000 (HHS, 2008, p. 56).

[5] HRSA's U.S. Health Workforce Chartbook, which provides detailed data on workforce supply but not supply adequacy, does not include data on ophthalmologists because they are categorized more generally under "physicians and surgeons" (HHS, 2013b).

effective treatments for many populations, especially those already at risk for poor health (Gibson, 2014, 2015; Kilmer et al., 2010). Figures 6-1 and 6-2 show the approximate distribution of ophthalmologists and optometrists in the United States, respectively. A substantial number of U.S. counties have neither an ophthalmologist nor an optometrist. Using practitioner data from the ARF, Gibson reported that 24 percent of the 3,143 counties in the United States had neither type of practitioner in 2011 (Gibson, 2015). Furthermore, 60.7 percent of these counties fell into one of the two lowest quartiles on the number of both specialists per capita. The author noted that there may be opportunities to leverage the use of optometrists in the 24.1 percent of counties with high availability of optometrists, but insufficient numbers of ophthalmologists.

In analyzing the number of ophthalmologists and optometrists by county, the committee notes that Gibson and colleagues (2015) used population-weighted quartiles[6] that may lead to distortions in the presentation of the data. For example, in Alaska, the presence of one additional ophthalmologist or optometrist in one county of 1,000 residents could result in that county going from the lowest quartile to the highest quartile, which could be misleading. Another concern is that National Health and Nutrition Examination Survey (NHANES) data is not geographically representative of the entire country and could introduce selection bias that may affect the results. It is unclear if the ARF includes satellite offices that may be available in rural areas for ophthalmologists because there are not enough patients to support a full-time surgical practice. In addition, Gibson and co-authors did not take into account either the findings from the RAND group—that ophthalmologists are able to accommodate an approximately 30 percent greater patient load[7] than optometrists—or the numbers of family physicians, pediatricians, nurse practitioners, and physician assistants who can provide select eye care services, including medical treatment and/or the use of screening telemedicine services (Lee et al., 2007). For these reasons, the county-level availability estimates of optometrists and the ophthalmologists in the figures and manuscript may be misleading about the actual workforce availability and needs.

---

[6] "The definitions of population-weighted quartiles of the county-level number of ophthalmologists per 100,000 county residents are: low, ≤2.95; medium-low, >2.95 and ≤5.39; medium-high, >5.39 and ≤7.63; high, >7.63. The definitions of the population-weighted quartiles of the number of optometrists per 100,000 county residents are: low, ≤10.96; medium-low >10.96 and ≤14.09; medium-high >14.09 and ≤16.80; high, >16.80 (Gibson, 2015).

[7] Lee and colleagues (2007) calculated the surrogate work effort for optometrists, defined as average number of patients seen per week, compared to ophthalmologists and found an equivalence of 0.69.

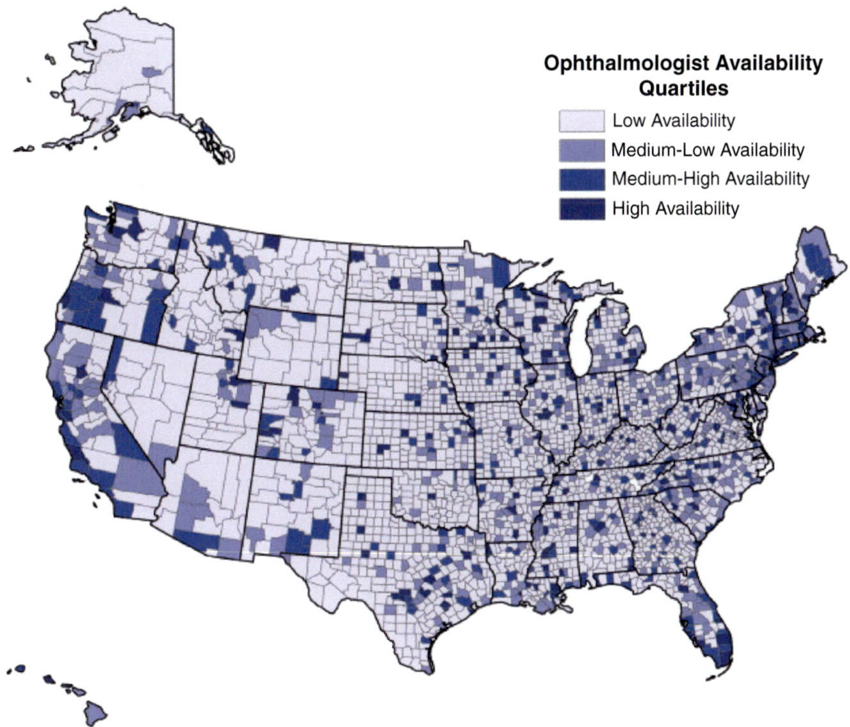

FIGURE 6-1 County-level availability of ophthalmologists in the United States. SOURCE: Gibson, 2015.

Challenges in Assessing Workforce Level

A number of challenges make it difficult to assess whether current workforce levels, distribution patterns, and projected trends will be sufficient to meet the growing demand for eye and vision care services as the U.S. population ages. Workforce projection studies produced by different advocacy groups vary substantially (see, e.g., AOA, 2013; Lee et al., 2007). Modeling projections make assumptions about the changing demographics of patient populations, the professional workforce, public health demand versus market demand, and the impact of new technologies and treatments on clinical practice, which can have substantial effects on projections (Higginbotham, 2012). For example, early projections from a RAND study found that whether ophthalmologists or optometrists were assumed to be primary eye care provider significantly affected whether models predicted an oversupply or no excess of ophthalmologists in the workforce (Lee et

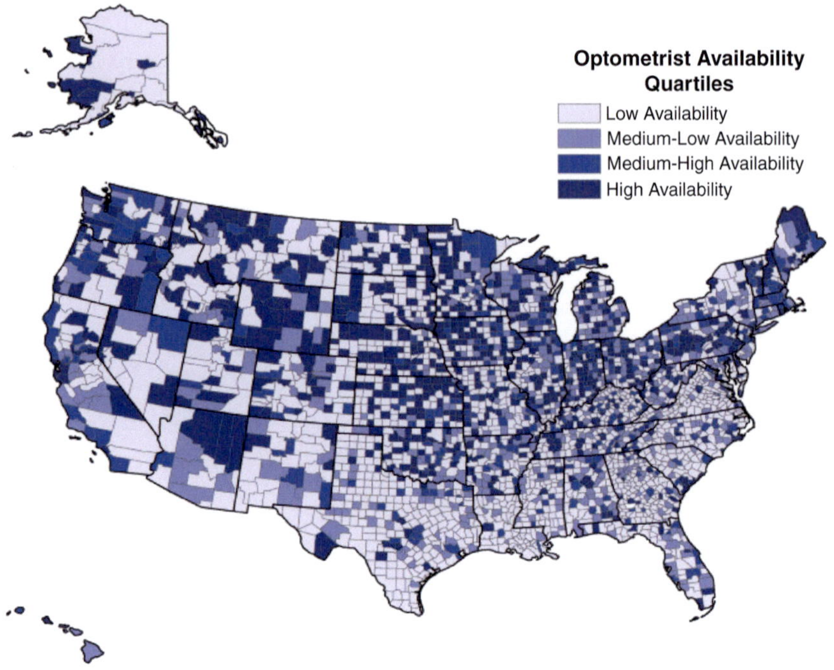

FIGURE 6-2 County-level availability of optometrists in the United States. SOURCE: Gibson, 2015.

al., 1995, 1998).[8] A more recent study by Lee and colleagues (2007) predicted that ophthalmology would face "substantial manpower challenges by 2020 or 2030" after accounting for changes in ophthalmic practice, new therapeutic opportunities, more recent data on the optometric work effort, U.S. population growth, and the growth of the ophthalmologist workforce. Another modeling study predicted that growth in the general, diabetic, and insured populations in the United States will lead to increased eye care

---

[8] Lee and colleagues (1998) describe an optometry-first model as one in which "all care that optometrists are legally entitled to provide, exclusive of laser or incisional surgery, are provided by optometrists preferentially" (p. 918). By contrast, in an ophthalmology-first model, "ophthalmologists provide all the care that they can provide before any care is allocated to optometrists" (p. 918). Oversupply occurs when total full-time equivalents (defined as "the total number of hours, per year, in which eye care services can be provided and is a function of the number of hours worked per day and the number of weeks worked per year") exceed the total need for eye care (Lee et al., 1995, pp. XIII–XV). The need for eye care services was defined as "the level of eye-related pathology in the population that requires monitoring or medical treatment."

demand and that demand will exceed the total supply of eye care by 2025, although the degree of excess was affected by the estimates of workforce capacity (Lewin Group, 2014).[9]

Changes in policy, payment practices, and referral patterns will also affect workforce patterns. For example, predictions must also account for the effect of the Patient Protection and Affordable Care Act (ACA) on demand for pediatric eye care services (see Chapter 7), renewed emphasis on population health, the emergence of the medical home, and the focus on team-based care (Higginbotham and Lippa, 2010). In the absence of trained eye care professionals or in response to evolving practice patterns, using public health practitioners and primary care providers to administer specific eye and vision care screenings or services will also affect demand.

More data could provide a more accurate, representative depiction of the workforce distribution for both optometrists and ophthalmologists. Research is also needed to fill existing knowledge gaps about workforce sufficiency, the likely impacts to care access and quality, and which workforce policies are best suited to addressing workforce capacity concerns.

Workforce Diversity

Diversity in the eye and vision care workforce is important to address some of the inequities in eye and vision outcomes noted in Chapter 2. Komaromy and colleagues (1996) found that African American and Hispanic primary care physicians were much more likely than primary care physicians of other ethnicities to care for African American and Hispanic patients, respectively. African American and Hispanic patients also report receiving higher quality care from African American and Hispanic physicians, respectively, than from physicians of other races (Saha et al., 1999).[10] Komaromy and colleagues (1996) found that the physician-to-population ratio was lower in areas where African Americans and Hispanics made up higher proportions of the population and that African American and Hispanic physicians were more likely than non-Hispanic white and Asian physicians to practice in these areas. Although these findings were based on primary care practice, they suggest that a lack of diversity in the ophthalmologic and optometric workforce could limit care access and quality

---

[9] Lewin Group (2014) noted, "In the 2012 National Eye Care Survey of Optometrists, responding optometrists indicated that they could provide, on average, 32 percent more visits per year than they were currently providing." Factoring in this excess capacity creates an excess in the supply of eye care for the period studied (2012 to 2025).

[10] African American patients with African American physicians were more likely to rate their physicians as excellent and to report receiving preventative care and all needed medical care. Hispanic patients with Hispanic physicians were more likely to report being satisfied with their overall health care.

among minority patients, an implication that adds emphasis to efforts to increase the diversity and cultural competency of the eye and vision care workforce.

Despite advances in the overall diversity of medical student cohorts and medical school faculties, the lack of diversity in the schools and colleges of optometry and ophthalmology remains a significant issue for the vision care workforce. The 2015 AAMC faculty roster lists 2,902 faculty members working in departments of ophthalmology. Of these, 603 (20.8 percent) are Asian, 57 (2.0 percent) are African American, and 50 (1.7 percent) are Hispanic, Latino, or of Spanish origin (AAMC, 2015b, table 16). Not surprisingly, estimates of the ethnicities of practicing ophthalmologists reflect the lack of diversity in the academic pipeline and in academia. In a 2014 AAMC report on diversity in the physician workforce, ophthalmology was among the less diverse specialties: Among ophthalmologists, African Americans, Hispanics, American Indian/Native Alaskans, and Asians, respectively made up 2.4 percent, 3.0 percent, 0.2 percent, and 14.6 percent of the workforce, compared with 4.2 percent, 4.6 percent, 0.4 percent, and 12.5 percent in the larger physician workforce (AAMC, 2015a, table 8).

The lack of diversity in schools and colleges of optometry is also a substantial problem, with only modest increases in the diversity of student enrollment during the past 5 years. Between the academic years 2009–2010 and 2014–2015, African American student enrollments increased from 2.8 percent to 3.1 percent of total enrollments, while Hispanic students increased from 4.4 percent to 5.1 percent (ASCO, 2015b). Asian enrollment also saw a modest increase, but with a considerably higher representation, going from 27.5 percent to 29.1 percent in those same 5 years (ASCO, 2015b). Female enrollment increased to 66.1 percent in 2014–2015 from 64.0 percent in 2009–2010 (ASCO, 2015b). Of the 1,569 students graduating from regular and special O.D. programs in 2014, 2.4 percent were African American, 3.4 percent were Hispanic, and 30.1 percent were Asian (ASCO, 2015b). In 2014, female graduates accounted for 64.6 percent of graduates (ASCO, 2015b). The diversity of the faculty of O.D. programs is also limited. In academic year 2014–2015, African Americans, Hispanics, and Asians accounted for, respectively, 2.8 percent, 5.2 percent, and 15.7 percent of the fulltime faculty of O.D. programs (ASCO, 2015a). The optometrist workforce mirrors student enrollment, especially for African Americans and Hispanics. Using data from the 2010–2012 American Community Survey, the National Center for Health Workforce Analysis estimated the optometrist workforce to be 2.8 percent African American, 4.9 percent Hispanic, and 13.0 percent Asian, indicating a lack of diversity (HHS, 2015). Efforts to recruit more diverse student bodies in ophthalmology and optometry schools and colleges should be emphasized as a tool to improve access for minority and underserved populations.

Community and Rural Health Services

The literature demonstrates a high prevalence of unmet vision health needs in a substantial number of communities (Chou et al., 2014; Elam and Lee, 2014; Elliott et al., 2010; MacLennan et al., 2014). Disparities in vision health between rural and urban communities have been documented and observed, with long travel distances, limited provider availability, and lower income cited as significant obstacles to the provision of appropriate health care to people living in rural settings (Richardson et al., 2013; Tsui et al., 2015). Individuals living in rural areas are significantly more likely to self-identify as having diabetic retinopathy, and they are less likely to receive an annual dilated eye examination (Hale et al., 2010). Another study found that rural primary care physicians were significantly more likely to report shortages for pediatric specialties when referring patients (Pletcher et al., 2010). Approximately 19.3 percent of the U.S. population resides in rural areas (U.S. Census Bureau, 2015). This raises questions about how to better meet the eye and vision care needs of people living in rural communities.

For many underserved and low-income communities, federally funded community and rural health centers may be the only source of eye and vision care services. Federally qualified community health centers are required by statute to provide vision screening services for pediatric patients.[11] Yet, in a survey administered by the George Washington University School of Public Health and Health Services, only 20 percent of health centers reported having an onsite optometrist or ophthalmologist who bills for comprehensive eye exams (Shin and Finnegan, 2009). Furthermore, in 2014, just 1.9 percent of health center patients used vision services from staff ophthalmologists and optometrists (HRSA, 2014). Another study found that approximately 72 percent of patients screened at a rural free community health clinic met the criteria for further ophthalmic evaluation[12] (Tsui et al., 2015). Of those who received ophthalmic referrals, approximately 89 percent of the group kept their referral appointments (Tsui et al., 2015).

The National Rural Health Association released a policy brief advocating for increased efforts to incentivize optometrists to practice in rural areas, but noted that support of funding for the NHSC (National Health Service Corps) would be necessary to place optometrists in rural and frontier areas (NRHA, 2009). Similarly, the American Public Health Association

---

[11] 42 U.S.C. § 254b(b)(1)(A)(i)(III)(ff).

[12] Criteria included: (1) two or more positive responses to a set of eight screening questions regarding past medical history; (2) less than 20/30 distance acuity despite pinhole, or less than 20/40 near acuity; (3) any distortions, blind spots, or irregularities with Amsler grid testing; (4) any abnormality of extraocular movements in the cardinal positions of gaze; and (5) any visual field defect on confrontation visual field testing.

has recommended that the U.S. Congress improve access to primary eye and vision care in medically underserved communities by "reinstating doctors of optometry in the National Health Service Corps" and by including "optometry as a named primary health care discipline in CHCs [community health centers]" (APHA, 2009).

In the absence of optometrists and ophthalmologists, primary care physicians, nurse practitioners, physician assistants, and other primary care providers can provide vision screenings at community and rural health centers. More research is needed to better understand how to use the existing infrastructure of community health organizations and established relationships with underserved and low-income communities. This research could better assess the capacity of community health centers to deliver comprehensive eye examinations, identify factors that influence whether screening programs lead to improved eye and vision health, and explore policy and funding strategies to expand the role of community health centers to improve access to eye and vision care services.

To ensure that populations, especially underserved and at-risk populations, have access to timely and high-quality eye and vision care, new strategies will be needed to expand access to eye and vision care services—beyond the offices of eye and vision care specialist. In some cases, population health efforts may have the most impact if resources are focused on geographic areas or populations that are defined in terms of eye care professional supply.

Emerging Technologies to Expand Access

With the focus on increasing value in health care, alternative technologies to expand access to providers have been explored as keys to improve access to eye and vision care. Technology options include telemedicine for the screening, evaluation, and diagnosis of eye disease and Internet technologies for patients and their families to take a greater role in the monitoring of their chronic disease conditions, thus reducing the need for more frequent follow-up visits. These technologies cannot replace key clinical services, such as in-person or comprehensive eye examinations and patient counseling, as a whole. Rather they complement existing services and can be a tool for bringing high-risk populations into the eye and vision care system.

Telemedicine

Telemedicine is "the use of medical information exchanged from one site to another via electronic communications to improve a patient's clinical health status" (ATA, 2016). Telescreening of eye disease, which is a type of telemedicine, offers a way to provide diagnostic services to populations that do not have access to adequate local eye care services. In many telescreening programs, screenings are provided in a community setting, such as a federally qualified health center, and the results are forwarded electronically to a diagnostic referral center for interpretation by an eye care provider. Patients receive a diagnosis and are referred, as necessary, for follow-up care.

Telescreening has the potential to improve population vision health and the performance of the vision care system by promoting the early detection of select eye diseases and conditions, minimizing personnel and overhead costs to the health care system, and reducing transportation and time costs to the patient (Brady et al., 2014; Li et al., 2012; Phan et al., 2014). For example, a randomized, controlled trial found that adult diabetic patients who received diabetic retinopathy telescreening in a primary care setting were significantly more likely to have a follow-up eye examination in the first 18 months of the study than patients who only received referrals for eye examinations from community eye care providers (Mansberger et al., 2013). Over 5 years of follow-up, the severity of diabetic retinopathy remained generally stable in more than 90 percent of the study's participants. In a systematic review and meta-analysis, Shi and colleagues (2015) found that the pooled sensitivity and specificity of telescreening exceeded 70 percent and 90 percent, respectively, for the detection of absence of most forms of diabetic retinopathy and macular edema.[13] A number of studies suggest that telescreening for open-angle glaucoma is effective at reducing costs, lowering barriers to access, and promoting the early detection of glaucoma among remote and medically underserved populations (Arora et al., 2014b; Thomas et al., 2014, 2015; Verma et al., 2014). A few studies have also concluded that telescreening may be used to accurately diagnose retinopathy of prematurity (Lorenz et al., 2009; Wang et al., 2015; Weaver, 2013). However, professional organizations, such as the American Academy of Ophthalmology, the American Academy of Pediatrics, and the American Association of Certified Orthoptists have stated that telemedicine-based remote digital fundus imaging cannot replace bedside binocular indirect ophthalmoscopy, despite moderate-quality evidence to support its use in

---

[13] Sensitivity for the detection of absence of diabetic retinopathy, 86 percent; mild non-proliferative diabetic retinopathy, 76 percent; moderate non-proliferative diabetic retinopathy, 72 percent; severe non-proliferative diabetic retinopathy, 53 percent; low-risk proliferative diabetic retinopathy, 84 percent; high-risk proliferative diabetic retinopathy, 81 percent; diabetic macular edema, 76 percent; and clinically significant macular edema, 75 percent. Specificity for detection of the absence of diabetic retinopathy, 95 percent, mild non-proliferative diabetic retinopathy, 89 percent; moderate non-proliferative diabetic retinopathy, 94 percent; severe non-proliferative diabetic retinopathy, 99 percent; low-risk proliferative diabetic retinopathy, 98 percent; high-risk proliferative diabetic retinopathy, 99 percent; diabetic macular edema, 95 percent; and clinically significant macular edema, 97 percent.

the identification of certain patients with clinically significant or referral-warranted retinopathy of prematurity (Fierson et al., 2015).

Telescreening programs also have the potential to reduce health care expenditures when compared to traditional eye examinations for select populations. Several studies suggest that telescreening for diabetic retinopathy can be a cost-effective means of screening some populations with diabetes. A study on diabetic patients receiving digital retinal imaging versus a standard ophthalmologic examination at a federally qualified health center found that the total per-patient costs[14] of teleretinopathy screening were $40.40, compared with $77.80 for a conventional examination. Even including the cost of a follow-up eye examination for the 12.3 percent of telescreened patients who screened positive with clinically significant disease, average per-patient costs were lower under the telescreening protocol ($49.95 versus $77.80) (Li et al., 2012). Kirkizlar and colleagues found that a telescreening program to detect diabetic retinopathy was a cost-effective (i.e., ≤$50,000/quality-adjusted life year [QALY] gained) means of screening diabetic populations that were larger than 3,500 people or whose members were younger than 80 years of age. The program was cost-saving when screened patients were younger than 50 years of age (Kirkizlar et al., 2013). In a modeling study, biennial eye exams were found to be more cost-effective than telescreening or annual eye exams at reducing visual morbidity in a hypothetical population of patients with diabetes and a low risk of progression, when it was assumed that exams could detect diabetic retinopathy, early and advanced AMD, glaucoma, and uncorrected refractive error, and that telescreening could detect diabetic retinopathy and AMD.[15] On the other hand, when the model assumed that telescreening could detect 25 percent to 75 percent of uncorrected refractive error, it was found to offer more QALYs at a lower cost than biennial exams (Rein et al., 2011). However, the high cost of imaging equipment may negatively affect return on investment, especially for short-term telescreening initiatives (Phan et al., 2014).

There are several challenges to implementing a telescreening program. First, covering equipment and facility costs, contracting with eye care

---

[14] The primary cost for digital retinal imaging per patient was the sum of costs for a medical assistant ($3.80), ophthalmologist ($15.00), capital cost of equipment and training ($17.60), equipment maintenance ($1.50), and transportation fee ($2.50). The primary direct cost for a standard examination per patient was the sum of costs for round-trip transportation ($8.70), Medicaid Physician Fee Schedule allowable for bilateral eye examination ($65.30), and medical assistant personnel ($3.80). The cost of a follow-up examination per patient was an additional $9.55 (Li et al., 2012).

[15] Low-risk individuals were defined as those who were ages 30 and older with diagnosed type 2 diabetes, had no diabetic retinopathy or only retinal microaneurysms, and visited a primary care physician in the previous 12 months.

providers, and training local caregivers to perform telescreenings all entail significant costs that some communities or clinics may have difficulty affording (Thomas et al., 2014, 2015). Second, imaging technologies may lack sufficient diagnostic sensitivity and specificity, the methods to encrypt patient data may not meet security needs or may obstruct data sharing, and training of screeners may be inadequate (Heaven et al., 1993). Furthermore, care providers must be appropriately trained and quality metrics will have to be clarified in order to create a program that provides optimal care (Li, 1999). A study that polled ophthalmologists and optometrists found that 82 percent reported that they were willing or extremely willing to participate in consultations or to interpret photographs, though the majority (71 percent) indicated they were not currently participating in any telemedicine initiatives (Woodward et al., 2015). However, 59 percent indicated that they had low confidence in making decisions for care, and 68 percent were not comfortable basing care solely on remote evaluations (Woodward et al., 2015).

The public and policy makers must be aware of the limitations of telescreenings for eye and vision health. Comprehensive eye exams, patient–provider interactions, surgical procedures, and in-patient treatments for eye disease cannot be provided through telescreening, which "does not replace optometrists or ophthalmologists, but instead complements their contribution" (Ng et al., 2009). These challenges are as relevant for public health practice as they are for clinical eye and vision care. Public health departments share similar concerns over the cost and cost-effectiveness of telescreening programs and the sensitivity and specificity of new screening technologies. Future research on telescreening will need to account for the capacity, training, and resource limitations of public health departments and other public health actors.

Other Emerging Technologies

In addition to telescreening, a number of other innovative, developing technologies may prove useful in tracking and diagnosing poor eye health or vision impairment in the future. More than two out of every three Americans owned a smartphone in 2015 (Pew Research Center, 2015). Recent studies of software and hardware designed to enable smartphones to perform some vision screening tests found that these technologies can accurately measure visual acuity and produce optic nerve images comparable in quality to those produced by desktop retinal cameras (Bastawrous et al., 2015, 2016). Similar tools currently in development may one day provide effective testing for diabetic retinopathy, macular edema, retinopathy of prematurity, and other eye diseases (Azrak et al., 2015; Ettore Giardini, 2015; Oluleye et al., 2016). Currently available applications for smartphones offer tests of visual acuity, astigmatism, and color vision, in addition to providing information on eye health and making it possible to locate nearby eye care services (Rocktime, 2016). Given the ubiquity, portability, innate connectivity, and comparatively low cost of smartphones, these innovations hold the potential to expand the availability of vision screenings and diagnostic and monitoring services in remote and medically underserved communities. Similarly, the use of specially designed video games makes it possible to quickly test threshold visual acuity in children, without the aid of medically trained examiners, and the results have been shown to concur with examinations by pediatric ophthalmologists in 87.5 percent of cases (Trivedi et al., 2010).

However, technological innovations come with their own set of challenges. Data protection is a particularly important issue. For example, researchers in the United Kingdom conducted a cross-sectional, systematic assessment of 79 mobile phone health applications certified by the National Health Service Health Apps Library. In order for an application to be featured, it must be ensured as clinically safe and compliant with the data protection principles of the United Kingdom's Data Protection Act of 1998 (Huckvale et al., 2015). The applications varied in function, scope, and breadth of information. Ninety-two percent of the applications had unencrypted data storage of some kind, with 53 percent of the applications storing unencrypted personal or sensitive information on the device (Huckvale et al., 2015). Of the sample, 89 percent of the applications transmitted the data through the Internet. Half of the applications transmitted information with strong identifiers, and of these, 66 percent of the applications sent this sensitive data without encryption (Huckvale et al., 2015).

Investing in research to speed the development of new screening tools and models of care that are Web based or carried out via smartphones have the potential to expand screening services with increasing diagnostic specificity and sensitivity at a lower cost to patients and the health care system. However, appropriate care must be taken to ensure mechanisms are in place to protect patient privacy and health information as these emerging technologies continue to evolve.

COVERAGE FOR EYE AND VISION CARE SERVICES

A lack of insurance coverage, poor access to services, and unaffordable costs are identified as major barriers to obtaining eye and vision care (CDC, 2011; Chou et al., 2014; DeVoe et al., 2007; Fudemberg et al., 2016; Levin et al., 2013; Zhang et al., 2008b). This is consistent across racial groups, with one survey reporting that approximately one-third of African Americans, Hispanics, Asians, and non-Hispanic whites having eye exams less frequently than they would like because of their insurance status (Research!America, 2014). An analysis of the 2006–2011 BRFSS data found that costs and a lack of insurance were cited by 32.3 percent of diabetic patients as the reason they did not seek an annual eye exam, with rates higher among those individuals with annual incomes less than $35,000 (Chou et al., 2014). A few studies have also described cost as a barrier to obtaining eyeglasses (Berry et al., 2012; Hodges and Berk, 1999). Data from NHANES revealed that in 2008, 16.0 percent of non-Hispanic whites, 15.3 percent of African Americans, and 26.7 percent of Hispanic adults could not afford eyeglasses when needed (Zhang et al., 2012).

A number of studies have also found that insurance coverage is an independent predictor of vision health, with a lack of insurance associated with a higher incidence of vision loss and an older mean age of diagnosis for the degenerative diseases of glaucoma and cataracts (Chan et al., 2014; Jin et al., 2013). Age-adjusted rates of service utilization are highest among those with private insurance[16] (67 percent) and lower for those with public (55 percent) or no health insurance (42 percent) (Li et al., 2013; Zhang et al., 2008b). The problems associated with the relative high cost of care, lack of insurance, and poor eye health are exacerbated by the lower income levels and education status typical for the blind and visually impaired population (Erickson et al., 2014; Kraus, 2015).

Current payment policies create access barriers for entry into and referrals within the eye and vision health system. More generally, divisions between optometry and ophthalmology or the medical establishment contributed to the development of separate insurance systems and payment policies for each profession, which continue to function largely independently. As a result, eye and vision care is bifurcated. General health insurance plans—whether public or employer-based[17]—typically offer limited or no coverage of routine and preventive eye health and vision care services and supplies (such as regular comprehensive eye examinations, eyeglasses, or contact lenses) in the absence of diagnosed risk factors for specific eye diseases or conditions, leaving beneficiaries to purchase supplemental or stand-alone vision insurance plans. In 2009, three-quarters of adults with vision insurance obtained coverage through stand-alone plans, with the rest obtaining coverage through general medical insurance (AOA, 2013). This

---

[16] Private insurance is used interchangeably in this instance alone with "employment-based" coverage to maintain consistency with the discussion from Zhang et al. (2008b). The rest of the chapter will use "employment-based" coverage to describe insurance providers from the private sector.

[17] For purposes of this report, "public insurance" is an umbrella term used to describe coverage gained as a result of eligibility for Medicare, Medicaid, or Children's Health Insurance Plan (CHIP), and may include possession of private plans as a supplement to the publicly subsidized coverage. The term "employment-based" is used to describe private insurance providers whose plans are procured through employer benefits.

practice results in additional procedural and financial burdens, especially for those populations that already experience poor health status and lower socioeconomic position—that is, for those who generally need more care but are less able to obtain it.

Overview of Costs and Coverage

In the United States, the costs of eye and vision care are typically shouldered by public programs, private insurance companies, and individuals, including patients and families. Since passage of the ACA, the size of the uninsured population in the United States has decreased and more children have access to eye and vision services, but approximately 32 million nonelderly Americans still did not have health insurance in 2014 (Kaiser Family Foundation, 2015). Those without health insurance are far less likely to have vision insurance (Zhang et al., 2008b).

A large proportion of adults in the United States do not have vision insurance that covers comprehensive eye examinations, eyeglasses, and contact lenses. The Vision Council's U.S. Optical Industry Report Card, which details the industry trends associated with vision correction usage, stated in 2015 that 76.2 percent of the adult population reported wearing some form of vision correction[18] (Vision Council, 2015, 2016). However, one 2012 survey found that 48 percent of the adults reported that they were not enrolled in any type of vision insurance plan, and another 5 percent were not sure if they were enrolled (Jobson Optical Research, 2012). This is not for lack of want: A consumer survey found that 92.9 percent of respondents identified vision coverage benefits as somewhat or very important, just slightly less than that for general medical insurance (94.5 percent) (NAVCP, 2013).

The next few sections discuss coverage of eye and vision care services through Medicare, Medicaid, and CHIP, and employer-based insurance. The purpose it to highlight inconsistencies in policies and opportunities to consider coverage decisions that can better serve a population health approach to eye and vision care, by enabling populations to access eye and vision care services that can modify or correct vision impairment, especially for underserved and low-income communities. These sections also highlight the numbers of people who would immediately be impacted by changes in payment policies governing provision of eye and vision services.

---

[18] "Vision correction" includes prescription eyeglasses, prescription sunglasses, plano sunglasses, contact lenses, and over-the-counter readers.

Medicare

In general, Medicare eligibility extends to adults over the age of 65 and to individuals with certain disabilities and diseases. In 2013, there were approximately 52.3 million Medicare part A and/or Medicare part B beneficiaries. Of these, approximately 42.5 million were eligible for Medicare on the basis of age, and 9.8 million were eligible because of disability (CMS, 2014c). Various stipulations involving Social Security benefits or disability pension eligibility qualify beneficiaries to sign up for Medicare Part A at no cost. In most cases, eligibility for social security disability benefits is a prerequisite for disability-based eligibility in Medicare.

Some Medicare beneficiaries are also dually eligible for Medicaid. The Kaiser Family Foundation estimates that approximately 9 million beneficiaries are "dual eligible," meaning they are covered by both Medicare (Parts A and B) and Medicaid or receive some assistance with Medicare cost sharing or premiums through a specific Medicare Savings Program category (CMS, 2016a; Kaiser Family Foundation, 2016a). Of these 9 million beneficiaries, an estimated 5.5 million are low-income seniors, and 3.4 million are people with disabilities under the age of 65 (Kaiser Family Foundation, 2011). All services received by dual-eligible beneficiaries are covered and paid for first by Medicare, with Medicaid seen as the "payer of last resort" (CMS, 2016a).

Overview of Medicare Coverage

Medicare benefits include four categories of medical services and supplies. These include (1) those medically necessary to treat a disease or condition in hospitals, nursing facilities, nursing homes, hospice, or through home care (Part A); (2) preventive and medically necessary inpatient and outpatient services such as clinical research, ambulance services, durable medical equipment, inpatient or outpatient hospitalization related to a condition or disease, a second opinion prior to surgery, and some prescription medications (Part B) (CMS, 2016k,m). These two parts comprise what is often referred to as traditional Medicare[19] (Kaiser Family Foundation, 2016b). Traditional Medicare benefits, or the medical services and supplies covered by Parts A and B, can alternatively be provided through a private health plan called (3) Part C or Medicare Advantage (CMS, 2016k; Kaiser Family Foundation, 2016b). Finally, (4) coverage of outpatient prescription drugs (Part D) is received through private plans that contract with Medicare, supplementing traditional Medicare (CMS, 2016d,m; Kaiser Family

---

[19] The Centers for Medicare & Medicaid Services (CMS) refers to this as "original Medicare" (CMS, 2016k).

Foundation, 2016b). Generally, Part D benefits are included in the Part C benefits package (Kaiser Family Foundation, 2016b). For those enrolled in traditional Medicare and not Part C, Medigap policies sold through private companies offer additional, supplemental coverage for copayments, coinsurance, and deductibles (CMS, 2016j).

Because Medicare Part A covers in-hospital services, medically necessary inpatient procedures to treat eye injuries, conditions, and diseases are generally covered by Medicare (CMS, 2016d,l). Federal statutes explicitly prohibit Medicare from covering expenses "for routine physical checkups, eyeglasses (other than eyewear described in section 1861(s)(8)) or eye examinations for the purpose of prescribing, fitting, or changing eyeglasses, procedures performed (during the course of any eye examination) to determine the refractive state of the eyes," along with hearing aids or examinations and immunizations, unless otherwise noted (42 U.S.C. § 1862(a)(1)(A); 42 U.S.C. § 1395y; see also CMS, 2016b). CMS has interpreted this as prohibiting coverage of any device containing a lens (including low vision optical devices, electronic magnifiers, eyeglasses, or contact lenses). Some individual preventive services are allowed by statute, including screenings associated with diabetes and personalized prevention plan services (42 U.S.C. § 1862(a)(1)(M),(K)&(L)), but there are no statutory allowances for preventive services for eye and vision health. In essence, Medicare pays only for corrective lenses implanted in the eye, with the exception of one pair of eyeglasses or one set of contact lenses following a cataract surgery that implants an intraocular lens (CMS, 2016c). Comprehensive eye exams are covered only after a specific diagnosis or identification of qualifying risk factors (CMS, 2015d). Although other congressional statutes, such as the Medicare Modernization Act (2003) and the ACA (2010), have expanded eligibility and medical services, payment for preventive or rehabilitative services specifically for eye and vision health remains limited (Blumenthal et al., 2015a,b). Table 6-1 lists examples of covered and noncovered vision services.

In 2015, there were about 17 million beneficiaries enrolled in Medicare Advantage plans (Jacobson et al., 2015). Medicare Advantage plans generally offer additional benefits, such as vision, dental, and hearing services. In the case of vision, this may include routine, yearly eye exams and eyeglasses or contact lenses every 24 months (CMS, 2015d). Alternatively, Medicare beneficiaries who enroll in supplemental Medicare insurance, may obtain additional vision benefits, though the policies vary. Medigap can cover an individual's share of the cost for Medicare-covered vision services, copayments, and deductibles. Most Medicare beneficiaries have coverage for several different vision services, but are required to pay an annual deductible, and are usually responsible for 20 percent of Medicare-approved costs for covered services (CMS, 2015d; Curtis et al., 2012). Again, these policies are only available to Medicare beneficiaries who can afford to purchase

TABLE 6-1 Examples of Covered and Noncovered Eye and Vision Items and Services Under Medicare Parts A and B

Covered Services	Noncovered Services
• Care of traumatic injury or an emergency involving the eyes • As part of cataract surgery: ○ Implantation of a conventional intraocular lens (IOL) ○ One pair of eyeglasses or contact lenses with the insertion of an IOL • Annual glaucoma screening (dilated eye examination with an intraocular pressure measurement and either a direct ophthalmoscopy examination or slit-lamp biomicroscopic examination) for these high-risk individuals: ○ Diabetes mellitus ○ Family history of glaucoma ○ African Americans ages 50 and older ○ Hispanic Americans ages 65 and older • Hydrophilic contact lenses to prevent corneal abrasions • Intraocular photography • Cataract surgery • Ocular photodynamic therapy in conjunction with verteporfin (a photosensitive drug) • Keratoplasty to treat corneal lesions • Vitrectomy incident to cataract surgery, hemorrhage, retinal detachments, proliferative retinopathy, or vitreous retraction • Purchase and routine maintenance of prosthetic eyes • Visual acuity screen as part of the "Welcome to Medicare" enrollment preventive visit	• Routine physical checkups, eyeglasses, or eye examinations to determine the refractive state of the eyes • The implantation of a presbyopia or astigmatism-correcting IOL • LASIK surgery (or any refractive keratoplasty procedures including keratomileusis, keratophakia, and radial keratotomy) to correct refractive error • Annual eye examinations to assess for diabetic retinopathy among individuals who are pre-diabetic or possess risk factors for diabetes

SOURCES: CMS, 2015a,d, 2016e–i.

supplemental insurance, which leaves many beneficiaries without coverage for basic eye and vision care or corrective lenses.

Opportunities for Action

The field of vision and eye health affords prime opportunities for value-driven initiatives that will facilitate patient-centered population health improvements in care. In particular, many opportunities exist to use payment policies as a mechanism to expand access to eye and vision care. This section explores a few of these opportunities.

Changing Medicare statute Historically, insurance coverage was designed to cover catastrophic injury and acute conditions rather than chronic conditions and prevention, which led to the exclusion of services that are essential to improving the metrics of population health. Lack of coverage contributes to out-of-pocket costs, but it also makes tracking utilization, cost by payer, and eye health outcome data difficult, not only across provider type, but also across a patient's lifespan and episodes of care. Although the costs of a comprehensive eye examination and eyeglasses to correct deficits in visual acuity may not be great in comparison to the costs of treating chronic vision impairment from conditions such as glaucoma or cataract, these expenses need to be viewed from the perspective of the patient and the potential to reduce harm to the beneficiary. This is not unique to the field, because the same divisions exist in the field of oral health.

Moreover, advances in medical treatments and technologies have greatly expanded both the cost and scope of treatment applications for lens-containing devices, and the underlying principles of insurance coverage have shifted from an indemnity system to cover large expenses to a coverage system intended to assure delivery of essential services. Because of their high cost, many Medicare beneficiaries may be unable to afford either the procedure or many types of vision assistive equipment without financial assistance in the form of insurance coverage. Under these conditions, arguments for excluding certain eye examinations related to prescription lenses, however they are defined, may no longer be valid. This is significant considering that vision impairment is highly concentrated in the Medicare population, with prevalence rates rising from 1.49 percent for 65- to 69-year-olds to 25.66 percent for individuals ages 80 and older (NEI, 2016).

CMS policies governing who is qualified to bill for specific services also restrict provision of low vision rehabilitation services. Current policy states that licensed vision rehabilitation personnel can only include ophthalmologists, optometrists, occupational/physical therapists, or social workers

(AHRQ, 2004).[20] The 2003 Medicare Prescription Drug, Improvement, and Modernization Act authorized the Medicare Low Vision Rehabilitation Demonstration Project, which was designed to "document coverage mechanisms for services provided by alternative vision rehabilitation providers," including low vision therapists, orientation and mobility specialists, and vision rehabilitation therapists (Coan, n.d.). Evaluation of the project found that the professionals were significantly underutilized, but did not make any recommendations about Medicare coverage of low vision services (Bishop et al., 2010). Some experts criticized the project design, including a lack of data necessary to identify all beneficiaries eligible for vision rehabilitation services, lack of vision rehabilitation services in some demonstration areas, and lack of "specificity, with respect to variables, data analysis, and quantitative analysis, required to pass the peer review process that is required for other federally funded research protocols" (Mogk et al., 2008). Future demonstration projects related to coverage of vision assistive equipment and to expand the definition of Medicare-approved providers working in vision rehabilitation will need to account for these issues.

Evidence-based guidelines can help inform specific payment policies related to "routine" eye examinations and corrective lenses, as well as qualified providers for rehabilitation services. As discussed in Chapter 7, professional societies for both ophthalmologists and optometrists release evidence-based guidelines as a tool to implement efficient and consistent care based on an established evidence base, though there are differences between the guidelines. Many health plans use these guidelines to make coverage decisions, which can become problematic when evidence is lacking or misinterpreted (Garber, 2001; Woolf et al., 1999). A unified set of evidence-based guidelines would be helpful to guide changes to CMS payment policies, especially those related to comprehensive eye examinations for asymptomatic patients, corrective lenses, and rehabilitation services.

"Welcome to Medicare" and the annual wellness visit Inclusion of eye and vision health as a measure of overall health is a logical fit for regular wellness examinations, preventive care, and chronic disease management already offered through the Medicare program. As defined in the Code of Federal Regulations, the initial preventive physical exam (IPPE), among other services, includes a visual acuity screen.[21] Gower and colleagues (2013) noted that broader inclusion of eye and vision care in the IPPE could lead to earlier detection of high-cost, irreversible eye diseases because

---

[20] The U.S. Code defines doctors of optometry as physicians with respect to the provision of certain items or services related to the Medicare and Medicaid programs (42 U.S.C. 1395x).

[21] Initial Preventive Physical Examination: Conditions for and Limitations on Coverage, 42 C.F.R. § 410.16 (2008).

Medicare claims show that the uptake for certain services on their own, such as glaucoma screening, is low among beneficiaries. The first visit should, in addition to the visual acuity screen, also establish a "list of risk factors and conditions for which primary, secondary or tertiary interventions are recommended or are underway for the individual, including . . . any such risk factors or conditions that have been identified through an initial preventive physical examination."[22] Under these definitions, conditions that relate to deficits in visual acuity could be included on the patient's list of risk factors and conditions.

After the first IPPE, the ACA (§ 4103) authorizes an annual wellness visit (AWV), which does not explicitly include another visual acuity test.[23] As part of the AWV, a health care provider must include a health risk assessment (HRA). The HRA allows a physician to evaluate the health status and risk of an individual through a personal prevention plan that also includes counseling, coaching, and behavior change interventions (Staley et al., 2011). Among other functions, the HRA may be used to identify chronic diseases, injury risks, modifiable risk factors, and the urgent health needs of an individual through encounters with a health care professional or community-based prevention programs (CDC, 2015b). A loss of vision is associated with negative health outcomes beyond vision impairment, including reduced quality of life, higher likelihood of falls, increased odds of nursing home placement, and unintentional mortality (Dhital et al., 2010; Klein et al., 2003; Lee et al., 2002).

Incorporating questions regarding visual function would be an appropriate short-term solution, as the questions relate to the review and potential update on functional ability and level of safety (which at a minimum includes hearing impairment, activities of daily living, falls risk, and home safety). CMS has not officially announced what the HRA must include. The sample HRA that CMS provided asks about exercise, tobacco use, alcohol use, nutrition, seat belt use, anxiety, high stress, social support, pain, depression, general support, activities of daily living, sleep, blood pressure, cholesterol, blood glucose, and height and weight (CVFP, 2016). The sample HRA does not include any questions related to the social determinants of health beyond social or emotional support, nor are there questions specific to vision, but the goals of the program parallel those goals laid out by the committee in Chapter 1 to advance a population health approach that will improve eye health in the United States (CVFP, 2016; Loeppke, 2011). The sample is not meant to be a prototype; questions included in the HRA should be prioritized, but providers should ask questions with a "capability to tailor and drill down

---

[22] Annual Wellness Visits Providing Personalized Prevention Plan Services: Conditions for and Limitations on Coverage, 42 C.F.R. § 410.15 (2011).

[23] Ibid.

with additional queries depending upon patients' responses" (Goetzel et al., 2011, p. 22). Emerging technologies have also demonstrated an initial promise for making possible rapid and portable tests for visual acuity, but these methods should be appropriately validated and tested before being widely adopted for use in the AWV (Arora et al., 2014a).

Although inclusion of vision-specific questions during the AWV would be a relatively straightforward way to incorporate eye and vision health into existing health policy without requiring statutory changes, it is limited by utilization of the benefit in general. Although the number of Medicare beneficiaries receiving an IPPE or an AWV has been increasing (CMS, 2011, 2014a, 2015b), a survey found that only 2.8 percent of eligible individuals had an IPPE and 63 percent were unaware of the benefit (Petroski and Regan, 2009). Another study found that about 96 percent of primary care physicians surveyed were aware of the AWV benefit, yet two-thirds of those physicians conducted fewer than 10 AWV visits per month (Hurley et al., 2016). Thus, the impact of the AWV on eye and vision health among Medicare beneficiaries would turn, in part, on efforts to expand utilization of the IPPE and AWV benefit.

Payment for telemedicine An Institute of Medicine (IOM) workshop on "The Role of Telehealth in an Evolving Health Care Environment" discussed the potential for telemedicine to expand access through "creating better reimbursement models" but it would be important to consider how to "remov[e] barriers for providers to take advantage of those models" (IOM, 2012, p. 38). Provider payment will be an important variable affecting the degree of accessibility to telemedicine. Literature suggests that providers may be skeptical or hesitant to adopt telemedicine technology because of a multitude of factors, one of which is difficulty procuring what providers perceive as insufficient payment for services (Brooks et al., 2013; Shimizu and Chorneau, 2009). For example, in a policy statement released by the American Academy of Pediatrics, "inadequate payment for services" is addressed as a barrier to telemedicine expansion (Burke et al., 2015).

Medicare's current payment policy has been described as "restrictive" (Horton et al., 2014, p. 196; Neufeld et al., 2015). To qualify for telemedicine payment, authorized originating sites must either fall outside a metropolitan area or be in a geographic "health professional shortage area" (HRSA, 2016). Counseling for smoking cessation and the AWV are two reimbursable telehealth services for 2016 (CMS, 2015c). In addition, Medicare Part B limits the services that can be provided, and telescreening for eye disease is not explicitly covered (CMS, 2015c). Medicare will only cover services that "mimic normal face-to-face interactions" but does not cover store-and-forward applications,[24] which are utilized in teleophthalmology and teleoptometry for retinal imaging (Horton et al., 2014; HRSA, 2016). Similar to the variations observed in scope and coverage for in-person eye and vision care services, Medicaid reimbursement is dependent on the state (CCHP, 2014). More than 40 of the individual states perform some type of reimbursement for telehealth (Quashie, 2012). California is one state that has expanded Medicaid to cover teleophthalmology for eligible beneficiaries (CDHCS, 2016).

Demonstration projects aimed at evaluating the impact of telemedicine on health care delivery, especially in the context of "high-value purchasing strategies, market power, payment reform, and benefit design," could allow for more widespread adoption across the nation, especially for ophthalmologic and optometric services (Delbanco and Tessitore, 2016). The Congressional Budget Office noted that the "results of a demonstration project conducted in the fee-for-service Medicare program could be especially valuable in light of particular challenges of controlling spending on new benefits in that program" (Housman et al., 2015). While the committee acknowledges that there are reservations regarding full substitution of telehealth services for in-person care delivery, a demonstration project to examine the cost-effectiveness and vision outcomes could serve to advise policy makers on budget considerations for the expansion of teleophthalmology and teleoptometry services for populations that may need this care the most.

At present, Medicare spending on telehealth is below projections. An analysis of Medicare spending in 2012 found that total telemedicine-related expenditures were about $5 million, or only 65.2 percent of the total budget allocated to telemedicine for that year (Neufeld and Doarn, 2015). The annual cost to each Medicare beneficiary was just $0.09, indicating that actual telemedicine expenditures have been significantly below earlier budget projections (Neufeld and Doarn, 2015). The Medicare Telehealth Parity Act of 2015[25] was introduced to the House Energy and Commerce Committee in July 2015, but was last referred to the House Subcommittee on Health with no further action. This bill, among other things, would extend qualified sites for telehealth payments to include any federally qualified health center, rural health clinic, and home telehealth sites; authorize additional telehealth providers; and develop additional payment methods. Medicare and Medicaid's payment policies have broader implications on the larger health insurance market; the responses from one 2012 survey

---

[24] "Store-and-Forward Telehealth involves the acquisition and storing of clinical information (e.g., data, image, sound, video) that is then forwarded to (or retrieved by) another site for clinical evaluation" (VA, 2015).

[25] H.R. 2948, 114th Congress (2015–2016), July 7, 2015.

of insurance providers demonstrated government rules for telemedicine payment were highly influential for determining payment policies for other insurance providers (Antoniotti et al., 2014). This compounds the need for CMS to update telemedicine payment policies to reflect the most current evidence and emerging technological capabilities.

Medicaid and the Children's Health Insurance Program

Medicaid is the largest health insurance provider in the United States, covering approximately 62 million people, or one in five Americans and one in three children (Kaiser Family Foundation, 2013). It covers low-income families, children, pregnant women, parents, seniors, people with severe disabilities, and low-income Medicare beneficiaries (Kaiser Family Foundation, 2013; Medicaid, 2016c). CHIP provides insurance coverage for children under age 19 in families with incomes too high to qualify for Medicaid (Medicaid, 2016c). CHIP operates as a distinct entity from Medicaid, an expansion of a state's Medicaid program, or as some combination of the two program types, depending on the state (Medicaid, 2016d).

In 2015, the average monthly enrollment in Medicaid among beneficiaries receiving coverage because of blindness, vision impairment, or disability was 10 million, or about 16 percent of the total Medicaid beneficiary population. By 2025, this number is projected to increase to 11 million enrollees (CBO, 2016). The unduplicated annual enrollment of blind or disabled Medicaid and CHIP beneficiaries was 10.7 million out of 72.8 million total enrollees in 2013, up from 6.5 million out of 43.3 million total enrollees in 1995 (HHS, 2013a). In 2011, individuals with vision difficulties comprised 5.8 percent of the total population of U.S. adults over age 18 who were receiving income-based government assistance through programs such as Medicaid (Boursiquot and Brault, 2013).

Overview of Medicaid and the Children's Health Insurance Program Coverage

Medicaid programs are managed individually by the states, but are jointly funded by the state and federal governments. Each state's Medicaid program must operate within federal guidelines, but the state has leeway to "determine the type, amount, duration, and scope of services within federal guidelines" (Medicaid, 2016a). As a precondition for federal funding, federal law requires state Medicaid programs to extend coverage to certain populations and allows states to individually determine whether additional populations will be covered under the program (Medicaid, 2016c). Similarly, state Medicaid programs are required to offer specific mandatory services in exchange for federal support dollars, but may expand coverage benefits to include optional services.

Mandatory vision-related services All plans that cover children and adolescents must provide basic eye care services and treatment under the early and periodic screening, diagnostic, and treatment (EPSDT) benefit (CMS, 2014b). This requirement guarantees comprehensive and preventive health care services for Medicaid-enrolled children under age 21, including the diagnosis and treatment of vision conditions or diseases as well as the provision of eyeglasses as necessary (Medicaid, 2016b). States that designate CHIP as part of the Medicaid expansion program must ensure EPSDT coverage for all CHIP beneficiaries (Medicaid, 2016a). States that operate CHIP as a separate program have the option to pick coverage options that similarly meet all federal requirements (Medicaid, 2016a). At a minimum, the vision screening component in each state must include diagnosis and treatment for vision defects. These screenings occur at "regular intervals," which may be determined by the state but should be based on current practices of pediatric care and must be reviewed by the state to ensure that the periodicity schedule reflects best practices (AAP, 2016).[26] When vision screening results require further evaluation, diagnostic services must be provided, and "necessary referrals should be made without delay and there should be follow-up to ensure the enrollee receives a complete diagnostic evaluation" (Medicaid, 2016b). Each state determines how frequently these services are provided (Medicaid, 2016b). Medically necessary services to correct problems found during vision screenings, including eyeglasses and their replacement if lost, stolen, or broken, are covered. EPSDT also includes medically necessary screenings outside of the state's screening schedule, if there is a change in the child's condition that warrants examination.

Optional vision-related services Individual states determine which optional benefits to offer under Medicaid, and those benefits may include the provision of eyeglasses and optometric, diagnostic, screening, preventive, and rehabilitative services, as well as prescription drugs, dental care, physical and occupational therapy, and podiatric services, among others (Medicaid, 2016a). As of 2012, Medicaid programs in all states and the District of

---

[26] CMS recommends Bright Futures of the American Academy of Pediatrics (AAP) as a reasonable and current periodicity schedule. Currently, AAP's vision schedule includes "risk assessments to be performed with appropriate action to follow, if positive" at regular intervals until age 3. Assessments should be performed at ages 3–6, 8, 10, 12, 15, and 18, with risk assessments at all other ages until 21 (AAP, 2016).

Columbia covered optometric services and 41 states and the District of Columbia covered the cost of eyeglasses (Kaiser Family Foundation, 2012a, 2012b). To better understand the differences in vision-related coverage under state Medicaid programs, the committee collected information from state websites and other sources to catalogue the types and scope of vision-related services offered by states for adults and for children beyond the mandatory essential health benefits (see Appendix G).[27,28]

There are wide variations among states in Medicaid coverage for vision benefits. Most states provide coverage to those over age 21 for some eye care services, including optometric examinations, eyeglasses and contact lenses, cataract surgery, and emergency medical procedures. Although many states cover periodic vision examinations for all or most adult beneficiaries (usually between every 1 and 3 years), fewer states cover eyeglasses for that same population.

Of the states that do cover eyeglasses, many cover them only for a specific population, typically post-op cataract patients, pregnant women, and long-term residents of nursing or other types of facilities. For example, Delaware, a state that has expanded Medicaid coverage, does not cover routine eye care or corrective lenses for adults, unless these supplies and services are incident to cataract surgery (DMAP, 2016; Kaiser Family Foundation, 2016c). Similarly Arkansas, a state that also has expanded coverage, limits the Medicaid benefit to "a total of twelve (12) office visits allowed per fiscal year for any combination of the following: certified nurse midwife, nurse practitioner, physician, medical services provided by a dentist, medical services furnished by an optometrist and Rural Health Clinics" (Arkansas DHS, 2012, p. 7; Kaiser Family Foundation, 2016c). Conversely, Iowa will cover routine eye examinations once every year, nonroutine eye examinations when presented with a complaint or injury, and corrective lenses (Iowa DHS, 2014). The state of Washington will cover eye examinations for asymptomatic adults every 2 years, and additionally covers vision therapy with prior authorization, including lenses,

---

[27] The committee found it difficult to locate and, sometimes, to access current information on Medicaid vision benefits, including a description of what services or benefits are covered, by whom, and how often. Some states provided a list enumerating noncovered items or services, but not all states provided such a clear-cut list. Although EPSDT services are explicitly required for state Medicaid programs, many states do not make information readily available to consumers. Similarly, some states do provide a list of covered vision benefits for adults, but the benefits listed are often vague. One state in particular listed more than 100 Current Procedural Terminology (CPT) codes as "covered services," without describing the procedure to which the codes referred (Cabinet for Health and Family Services, 2007).

[28] Individual state Medicaid offices were asked to confirm the data. States that replied are identified in the appendix.

prisms, filters, occlusion or patching, and orthoptic and pleoptic training (WSHCA, 2016).

Expanding Medicaid coverage The Omnibus Budget Reconciliation Act of 1989 expanded EPSDT benefits to encompass codified, inter-periodic screening;0 vision, dental, and hearing coverage; and all services and supplies allowable under the definition of "medical assistance,"[29] regardless of eligibility for adult coverage (Naylor, 2013; Rosenbaum and Wise, 2007). Improvements in various clinical and financial outcomes have been associated with the utilization of EPSDT benefits, including a lower rate of emergency department visits, increased care utilization in rural counties, improved navigation of the health care system, and better school readiness (Pittard et al., 2007; Schor et al., 2007; Snowden et al., 2008).

These opportunities should not be unique to children and adolescents. Individuals with an annual income of less than $20,000 are more than twice as likely as individuals with incomes above $55,000 to be visually impaired (Salman and Shirey, 2002). Compared to working-age adults without disabilities, those with vision impairment exhibit lower rates of full-time employment (26.4 percent versus 56.8 percent), lower median annual earnings ($35,300 versus $43,300), and lower median annual household income ($36,500 versus $62,000) (Erickson et al., 2014; Kraus, 2015). This restricts their opportunities for enrolling in employment-based vision plans. One study from the dental field demonstrated that Massachusetts' Medicaid expansion of dental benefits to all adults ages 19 to 64 who were below the federal poverty level increased care utilization by 11 percent; when coverage for dental services was eliminated, the state saved less than 1 percent of total MassHealth spending (Nasseh and Vujicic, 2013). State Medicaid programs do provide some coverage for adult eye and vision health services and supplies, but the scope of coverage varies considerably (see Appendix G). In addition, states face challenges balancing growing demand with decreasing budgets. However, when debating coverage determinations and qualifying individuals, states should consider the impact that improved eye and vision care services could have not only on reduced vision impairment but also on downstream health consequences (see Chapter 3).

The exclusion of stand-alone plans from the exchange As mentioned, the exclusion of vision benefits from general health insurance plans is similar to the coverage limitations for dental benefits. Although both the dental

---

[29] Defined as all items and services medically necessary to correct and ameliorate physical and mental conditions and illnesses.

and vision fields have progressed toward better coverage through Medicaid expansion and pediatric oral and vision coverage, both are similarly limited through regulatory restrictions for Medicare.[30] However, more Americans have access to some form of dental insurance coverage than have access to vision coverage, with an average of 47 percent of civilian workers reporting access to dental plans versus 26 percent for vision plans (BLS, 2015a).

As written, the ACA does not allow stand-alone vision plans to be featured on the government exchange, while dental plans are featured as either part of a bundled benefit or as a stand-alone plan (Kirkner, 2011; Tozzi, 2014). Stand-alone vision plan companies may enter the exchange only under contracts with ACA-recognized qualified health plans to provide the vision benefits in a bundled benefit package (AOA, 2014). The American Dental Association, Delta Dental Plans Association, and the National Association of Dental Plans were able to successfully advocate for the inclusion of stand-alone dental plans in the federal exchange, arguing that bundling of medical and dental benefits without stand-alone dental plans as an option would raise costs by splitting family policies to remain compliant with the ACA mandate for pediatric dental benefits (Kirkner, 2011).

Conversely, the American Academy of Ophthalmology and the American Optometric Association opposed the inclusion of stand-alone vision plans in federal exchanges (Kirkner, 2011). The organizations argued that "stand-alone vision plan companies aim to turn back the clock by continuing to segment vision from eye health, and seeking to impose misguided limits on the care that our patients—especially children—receive. Such plans are routinely mislabeled as complete or comprehensive . . . any expansion of stand-alone vision plans through health care reform would result in a continuation of non-responsive action and fractured and uncoordinated care" (AAO/AOA, 2009). The National Association of Vision Care Plans (NAVCP), which represents 17 different private plans, countered with the argument that stand-alone plans are better fit to address the barriers to eye care access and utilization (Kirkner, 2011).

A study conducted among 10 managed vision care plans submitting claims data for more than 86 million beneficiaries found individuals enrolled in stand-alone plans were twice as likely to receive an eye examination than those with bundled plans (NAVCP, 2010). The study was published by the NACVP and was not peer-reviewed. Furthermore, this association may not be causal, because intuitively beneficiaries who prioritize the purchase of a stand-alone plan would likely self-select as a group that would be more likely to use this particular benefit than beneficiaries who have access to eye care as part of a bundled plan. However, Li and colleagues (2013) found

---

[30] Limitations on Services of a Doctor of Dental Surgery or Dental Medicine, 42 C.F.R. § 410.24 (1991).

that individuals with vision insurance (as an add-on benefit) were twice as likely to have had an eye care visit in the previous year than those without, further noting that "having general health insurance was not a significant predictor of an eye care visit once vision insurance was included in the model" (p. 501).

The committee acknowledges that the provision of stand-alone vision plans on the exchange may extend access and coverage at the expense of propagating fractured and bifurcated vision and medical care; however, the better access to plans could also increase rates of care utilization and decreased financial barriers to care (see Nasseh and Vujicic, 2013; and Vujicic et al., 2014, for general examples of policies to increase coverage and utilization in oral health). However, significant consideration should be given to weighing the benefits and harms of such a decision, because further fragmenting the field in favor of suboptimal coverage lies in direct opposition to the ACA's push toward integrated and coordinated care. Opportunities to improve access through other, more preferable means should be identified.

Employment-Based Coverage

Employment-based insurance is a major source of coverage for services and supplies related to eye care for working age adults under age 65. Unfortunately, comprehensive information detailing employment-based insurance coverage for eye and vision care in the peer-reviewed literature is limited. In 2012, 17 vision insurance companies offered their products in the U.S. marketplace (AOA, 2013). Yet recent surveys suggest that about only half of American adults have some form of vision coverage through various employer-based plans (International Vision Expo East, 2015; Jobson Optical Research, 2012). Among U.S. adults ages 18 and older who had vision problems, 74.7 percent and 17.1 percent had employment-based insurance or public health insurance, respectively, whereas 8.2 percent had no general health insurance coverage (Zhang et al., 2008b). Of individuals with employment-based insurance, 58 percent also had vision insurance, compared with 44 percent of those with public insurance and 4 percent of those without health insurance (Zhang et al., 2008b).

In the United States, populations may purchase either medical or vision insurance or both to help cover expenses related to eye and vision care. A detailed breakdown of expenditures by payer can be found in Chapter 3. Employment-based vision insurance can be offered as a stand-alone insurance plan or as an add-on benefit to general health insurance plans. Most individuals, whether they have employment-based or public medical insurance, must pay additional monthly premiums for general eye examinations and corrective lenses or purchase of stand-alone vision insurance.

Yet employees may be "much more price sensitive to the out-of-pocket premium for fringe benefits other than health insurance" including vision insurance (Royalty and Hagens, 2005, p. 97). Of individuals with vision insurance in 2009, approximately 72 percent were enrolled in a stand-alone vision plan (AOA, 2013). The frequent exclusion of comprehensive vision benefits from general health insurance plans is mirrored by similar coverage limitations for dental benefits. Results from the National Compensation Survey in 2015 suggested that, if vision benefits were offered, they would be well utilized: the survey found a 79 percent take-up rate for employees offered vision care (BLS, 2015a).

Employment-based medical insurance typically covers medical payments for eye injury and various eye diseases such as cataract, glaucoma, and diabetic retinopathy as well as for related corrective lenses (Bihari, 2014; UnitedHealthcare, 2016). In some cases, elective laser surgery for vision correction may also be covered. Most employment-based medical insurance plans do not include any vision benefits related to asymptomatic eye examinations or corrective lenses absent documented risk factors for specific diseases or conditions. Similarly, health insurance exchanges established under the ACA do not cover these services for adults, although vision benefits for families and for children under age 19, as well as small group markets, are required to offer this coverage benefit. The singling out of small group markets in the ACA may reflect historical data suggesting that larger employers are more likely to provide vision insurance for their employees (Spahr, 2015).

The cost and services covered by employment-based vision insurance vary between plans. For example, the Federal Employees Dental and Vision Insurance Program (FEDVIP) offers vision insurance plans through Aetna, Blue Cross Blue Shield, UnitedHealthcare, and Vision Service Plan (VSP). The monthly rates for these plans range from $6.31 to $8.30, and copays range from $0 to $10 per eye exam. See Table 6-2 below for details. The coverage of eye exams under private vision insurance plans available to the general public is similar. For example, three private vision insurance plans offered by VSP all require beneficiaries to pay a $15 copayment for coverage of an annual comprehensive eye exam, and three plans offered by EyeMed either provide full coverage or require a $10 copay for an annual eye exam with dilation as necessary (EyeMed, 2016; VSP, 2016a,b,c). Although these rates may seem relatively low compared to medical insurance, these additional costs to people with few financial resources can serve as a barrier to critical care, especially in at-risk populations.

Employers are an important source of the provision of medical and vision insurance, though benefits vary by plan in terms of the type of coverage and the costs. A 2014 Kaiser Family Foundation survey of employers

TABLE 6-2 Costs and Coverage of Employment-Based Vision Insurance Plans

Plan Profile	Aetna Vision-Standard	FEP BlueVision-Standard	UnitedHealthcare Vision-Standard	VSP-Standard
Monthly Rates[a]				
Individual Plan	$7.11	$8.30	$6.31	$7.95
Two-Person Plan	$14.19	$16.60	$12.33	$15.88
Family Plan	$21.32	$24.87	$18.35	$23.86
Benefits	In-network/ Out-of-network	In-network only	In-network/ Out-of-network	In-network/ Out-of-network
Vision Exam	Every 12 months	Every 12 months	Every 12 months	Every 12 months
Vision Lenses Only	Every 12 months	Every 12 months	Every 12 months	Every 12 months
Frames	Every 24 months	Every 24 months	Every 12 months	Every 12 months
Copay (in-network)	$10 lenses/$0 exam, materials	0	$10 exam/$25 materials	$10 exam, $20 eyeglasses
Additional Features	Additional lens options, retinal imaging, second pair of eyeglasses, laser vision correction discount	Breakage warranty; choose eyeglasses or contact lenses; laser vision correction discount, low vision coverage	Low vision, prosthetic eye, vision therapy; choose eyeglasses or contact lenses; laser vision correction discount	Prescription eyewear, choose eyeglasses or contact lenses; laser vision correction discount

NOTES: [a] Rates are for DC area beneficiaries. Rates may vary by locality.
FEP = federal employee program; VSP = Vision Service Plan.
SOURCE: Adapted from OPM, 2016.

found that only 63 percent of large companies (defined as having 200 or more employees) and 34 percent of small companies (under 200 employees) offered stand-alone vision benefits (Claxton et al., 2014). Cost was cited as the primary reason that companies did not offer ancillary health coverage. The BLS data corroborated this trend, indicating that larger companies were more likely to offer vision benefits: Forty-two percent of companies with 500 employees or more offered vision care benefits, while only 17 percent of companies with under 49 employees offered vision benefits (BLS, 2015a).

Health savings accounts (HSAs) and flexible spending accounts (FSAs) are also offered as a benefit accompanying general medical insurance plans and are often used by consumers to cover vision and eye care expenditures (NAVCP, 2013). Consumer participation is affected by plan type, coverage, and deductibles, and available funds must be spread across competing expenses, such as prescription drugs and copayments (Konrad, 2010). Although these mechanisms are useful for increasing vision and eye care utilization, they do not substitute for general vision and eye care coverage, because FSAs and HSAs are subject to annual limits (IRS, 2016). Individuals are also responsible for most, if not all, contributions to FSA and HSAs. Given the limitation of consumers having to self-finance these accounts, these benefits may have limited value to low-income individuals (Blumberg, 2008).

The decision to subsidize medical costs and not vision costs poses an additional barrier to parity between general medical care and eye and vision care. Voluntary plans allow employers to provide ancillary benefits without significant investment, because employees pay up to the full premium at a group rate (Aetna, 2016). About 60 percent of benefit advisers identified vision insurance as a voluntary benefit plan of high interest to employers, including the federal government (Bradley, 2016). Federal enrollees are responsible for 100 percent of the premiums for the FEDVIP, in contrast to medical insurance, which was subsidized by up to 75 percent by the federal government in 2014 (Cornell, 2015). Thus, employers often subsidize care for eye diseases and conditions that affect older populations, such as glaucoma and cataract, but do not provide equal subsidies for services that are more likely to impact children and young adults, such as detection of refractive error and correction of subsequent vision impairment with eyeglasses or corrective lenses.

The committee was not able to identify robust literature documenting the potential impact of expanding employer-based medical insurance to cover comprehensive eye examinations for asymptomatic patients or corrective lenses on the cost of coverage, the number of insured people, or on access to timely and appropriate eye and vision care. The committee was not able to find any peer-reviewed literature that documents the average cost (both to the insurer and average out-of-pocket costs) for corrective lenses[31] and examinations in the private sector, although various independent sources are available that indicate variation in pricing based on a variety of factors (e.g., Aetna, 2016; Blue Cross Blue Shield, 2016; CMS, 2014b; OkCopay, 2016[32]; UnitedHealthcare, 2016; VSP, 2016d). However, basic economic theory states that reducing the cost to consumers will increase participation in insurance plans. To better understand the impacts of various coverage decisions on total health expenditure and health outcomes, especially on a national scale, it will be important for insurers and health care providers to be more transparent in the costs associated with eye and vision care. More research is needed to guide evidence-based policies

---

[31] The glossary (see Appendix C) contains the committee's definition for "corrective lenses."

[32] OkCopay provides free information on health care costs and is unaffiliated with insurance providers or health care providers. Data on eye exam cost is compiled from surveys of eye care providers performed by OkCopay, publicly available claims data, and provider websites.

that ensure higher rates of insurance coverage for comprehensive eye examinations and corrective lenses in employment-based insurance markets. This will likely include a more robust literature on the cost-effectiveness and comparative effectiveness of particular services and equipment or devices.

COST-EFFECTIVENESS RESEARCH

In *Improving the Nation's Vision Health: A Coordinated Public Health Approach*, the Centers for Disease Control and Prevention (CDC) stated that "cost-effectiveness information is . . . needed to establish that expenditures for prevention and treatment interventions are justified" (CDC, 2009, p. 24). Cost-effectiveness research has the potential to inform payment policy for eye and vision health broadly, although the existing cost-effectiveness literature related to eye and vision health tends to focus on the detection, treatment, and management of a singular eye disease or condition. For example, Brown and colleagues (2013) analyzed the cost-utility of cataract surgery and found that third-party insurer and overall societal per-QALY costs for unilateral cataract surgery were $1,636/QALY and $74,759/QALY respectively, indicating cost-effectiveness. The study also found that the 13-year return on investment for a 1-year cohort of cataract surgery patients equated to $36.4 in savings for Medicare and $48.6 billion in savings for patients (Brown et al., 2013), although aspects of the study's methodology have drawn criticism (Lee and Kymes, 2015). A modeling study of patients ages 65 and older with cataract and astigmatism found that those who received astigmatism-correcting toric intraocular lenses (IOLs), as compared to conventional IOLs with or without intraoperative refractive correction, were more likely to achieve uncorrected visual acuity of 20/25 or better (Ochoa et al., 2014). Toric IOLs were also associated with lifetime cost savings of $34 per patient and $349/QALY compared to conventional IOLs. Rein and colleagues (2009) used computer models to determine that office-based identification of glaucoma through routine eye examinations and subsequent American Academy of Ophthalmology (AAO)-recommended treatment of glaucoma is cost-effective at $28,000 to $46,000 per QALY gained compared to no treatment, depending on the assumed efficacy of treatment. The cost per QALY dropped to $11,000 to $20,000, depending on assumed efficacy of treatment, when the costs of eye examinations (which include tests and procedures unrelated to detection of glaucoma) were excluded. The probability that routine eye examination followed by recommended treatment would be cost-effective was greater than 99 percent for a willingness to pay of $14,000 per QALY (assuming high treatment efficacy and excluding examination costs) to $64,000 per QALY (assuming low treatment efficacy and including examination costs) (Rein et al., 2009).

Despite some studies finding specific instances of cost-effectiveness, overall the literature on cost-effectiveness or risk-benefit for eye and vision health remains insufficient, especially in the context of vision screenings. For instance, the U.S. Preventive Services Task Force found an inadequacy of direct evidence on the benefits and harms of glaucoma screening (Moyer, 2013; USPSTF, 2013). The Agency for Healthcare Research and Quality (AHRQ) was unable to identify studies addressing five of these six key questions when attempting to determine the predictive value and harms of glaucoma screening programs (AHRQ, 2012). Evidence on the predictive value of glaucoma screening tests was identified, but "the lack of a definitive diagnostic reference standard for glaucoma and heterogeneity in the design and conduct of the studies" prevented a coherent synthesis of the data (AHRQ, 2012, p. 15). Another systematic review found that available cost-effectiveness research was insufficient for developing glaucoma screening recommendations (Hernandez et al., 2008). Because glaucoma disproportionately impacts African Americans, the paucity of research to guide development of effective and cost-effective glaucoma screening programs may have the adverse impact of perpetuating disparities in eye and vision health. The application of some cost-effectiveness research may be further limited by a lack of generalizability to the U.S. population (Tamura et al., 2015).

Cost-effectiveness may be influenced by many factors, including the eye disease and vision impairment risk profile of the targeted population, the screening interval, the diagnostic accuracy of screening tools, the staffing models used in a screening program, the rate of follow-up after abnormal screening results, the efficacy of available clinical treatments, and numerous other factors. One review found significant variation in the cost-effectiveness of different diabetic retinopathy screening efforts, noting the influence of differences in the size and age of the screened population, whether a program employed a systematic or opportunistic model of screening, the extent of centralization of the screening processes, and the screening interval on the cost-effectiveness of the screening efforts (Jones and Edwards, 2010). Whether a particular screening is found to be cost-effective can also be influenced by whether the screening occurs alone or in combination with other treatments (e.g., Chan et al., 2015; Rein et al., 2012b). Assumptions about patients' willingness to pay also affect the range in which specific screenings are determined to be cost-effective (Rein et al., 2012a). Blumberg and colleagues (2014) found that the costs of specific types of glaucoma screening (i.e., spectral-domain optical coherence tomography), as well as its effect on visual field loss, were sensitive to assumed rates of follow-up care, suggesting that efforts to promote patient and provider adherence to follow-up and referral guidelines could improve the effectiveness and cost-effectiveness of glaucoma screening.

Cost-effectiveness may also turn on prevalence of a specific disease. For example, Burr and colleagues (2007) performed a systematic review and economic evaluation to determine the cost-effectiveness of glaucoma screening in the United Kingdom and found that the prevalence of glaucoma among adults age 40 was 0.3 percent, but would have to be approximately 3 percent to 4 percent for screening to approach cost-effectiveness. Targeted screenings of high-risk populations may be more clinically effective and cost-effective (Blumberg et al., 2014; Burr et al., 2007; Ladapo et al., 2012). Research on these and other issues is needed, but remains limited (Azuara-Blanco et al., 2016; Blumberg et al., 2014; Burr et al., 2007; Ladapo et al., 2012).

There are several government-funded initiatives to encourage cost-effectiveness research, but these are generally discrete efforts from individual agencies. For example, the CDC developed a discrete simulation model called the CDC and Research Triangle Institute (RTI) Multiple Eye Disease Simulation (CR-MEDS) to estimate the combined economic impact of major adult eye and vision disorders in the United States (CDC, 2015a). Models for diabetes, amblyopia, and comprehensive eye examinations are similarly being studied (CDC, 2015a; Hoerger et al., 2009, p. 9). Similarly, insurance providers can also participate in cost-effectiveness research, especially research that examines the impact of expanding coverage of preventive services or corrective lenses on long-term costs associated with chronic vision impairment, as part of ongoing continuous quality improvement programs (see Chapter 7). The recent passage of the Medicare Access and CHIP Reauthorization Act of 2015 (MACRA)[33] is a recent example of efforts to promote value-driven care through, for example, the creation of the quality payment program. The impact of the law cannot be assessed because its provisions are being gradually phased in through 2021, but the committee is optimistic about its potential impact for providers and patients.

Several databases exist to catalog cost-effectiveness research studies. These include the AHRQ Clinical Economics Research Database and the Cost-Effectiveness Analysis Registry (CEA Registry) (NICHSR, 2016). Two other databases have lost funding: The National Health Service (NHS) Economic Evaluation Database (EED) lost funding in early 2015, though the information can still be accessed (Cochrane Community Archive, 2015). Similarly, the Health Economic Evaluations Database ceased publication in 2014, though the articles can be accessed through the publisher (John Wiley & Sons, Inc., 2016). The databases vary in the features that they include; for example, the NHS EED includes a critical appraisal by health economists, while the others do not (NICHSR, 2016). Similarly, the CEA Registry

---

[33] P.L. 114-10, 114th Congress, April 16, 2015.

only catalogues studies that use the QALY metric (NICHSR, 2016). The AHRQ Clinical Economics Research Database is limited to publications funded by the government and only includes studies published from 1997 to 2001 (AHRQ, 2014). Unlike the Cochrane Database, the databases centered on economic evaluation do not use catalogued information to generate systematic reviews, with one exception. The CEA Registry does facilitate such studies, but they are hugely limited. For example, in 2015 only five studies were published from CEA Registry data across all subjects (CEA Registry, 2015). While these databases are critical to facilitating research and encouraging collaborative studies, they are limited in their scope by the lack of sustainable funding.

More research is needed to accurately characterize the factors affecting, and effectiveness of, different treatments and screening techniques for different eye diseases and conditions. Research should include the cost-effectiveness of vision screenings versus comprehensive eye examinations (including rates of follow-up care), the validity and reliability of the methodological techniques used to assess screening, the effectiveness and cost-effectiveness of screening models that have the capacity to detect multiple eye diseases, and what resources are necessary to facilitate access to the appropriate services. Moreover, a research program with sustainable funding sources that evaluates the cost-effectiveness of vision and eye health prevention, treatment, and management could support the development of evidence-based guidelines (see Chapter 7), value-based payment policies, and coverage determinations that better promote value-based eye and vision care.

CONCLUSION

Access to clinical services is only one determinant of eye and vision health and 1 of 10 essential public health services (see Chapter 1) that comprise an overarching population health approach to reduce the impact of vision loss and impairment in the United States. However, given the number of people at risk for and affected by uncorrectable and correctable vision impairment, especially in the context of an aging population and the long-term effects of uncorrected vision impairment in childhood, appropriate entry into the eye and vision care system becomes an elevated concern. Overarching social and political barriers, including the availablity of trained eye and vision care professionals, existing payment policies, and the availability of vision insurance, have direct implications for populations who are most in need of assistance and likely to suffer from uncorrectable or uncorrected vision impairment.

Understanding the roles of traditional eye and vision care providers can help policy makers assess the adequacy of the workforce to address growing demands and determine how best to reach underserved populations through emerging technologies, including telemedicine and telescreening, as complementary services to critical in-person examinations and treatments. It will also be important for the eye and vision field to establish clear messaging about the roles of eye and vision care professionals to communicate effectively with other health care providers and the public. Ensuring diversity within the eye and vision health workforce can help address observed inequities in vision impairment prevalence and severity among different populations. A comprehensive understanding of the distribution and needs of the workforce could help clarify the directions that policy makers should take to mitigate these disparities.

Payment policies have the ability to not only expand coverage of evidence-based services to at-risk populations, but also incorporate eye and vision health into national policy discussions about chronic conditions and how eye and vision health can help promote function and overall quality of life. Unfortunately, the bifurcation of coverage for eye and vision services between traditional health insurance and separate vision insurance exacerbates inequities in eye and vision care and reflects historical decisions and distinctions that no longer reflect available evidence and trends in payment policies for other similarly placed services. A number of currently

---

BOX 6-1
Key Research Gaps

- Determine whether or not the current workforce distribution should be maintained or expanded to meet growing need for eye care services.
- Examine disparities in access to eye and vision care for medically underserved populations and the role community health centers play in providing this care.
- Assess the current extent of vision screenings in community health centers, the factors that mediate the implementation and effectiveness of such programs, and policy and funding strategies to expand access.
- Clarify the association between diversity in the eye and vision care workforce and barriers to care for minority patients.
- Explore ways to improve upon the specificity and sensitivity of screenings (including telescreenings) and other emerging technologies especially in medically underserved areas.
- Examine the cost-effectiveness of various interventions and treatments, including teleoptometry and teleophthalmology programs and specific examinations and screenings among different populations.
- Demonstrate the effect certain payment policies on expanding access to appropriate eye and vision care and long-term outcomes, including coverage for corrective eye glasses and certain vision rehabilitation equipment.

reimbursable services could incorporate elements related to eye and vision health into existing platforms in order to improve the health and well-being of Medicare beneficiaries. There are additional opportunities to reexamine broader Medicare, Medicaid, and private coverage decisions and policies related to eye and vision care that could help reduce the impact of vision impairment (e.g., allowing Medicare to cover routine eye examinations, corrective lenses, and certain rehabilitation services, as well as expanding or reducing state variability in Medicaid benefits). These opportunities involve varying degrees of regulatory, procedural, or economic hurdles and should account for the different populations at risk for different etiologies of vision loss.

Changes in payment policies should reflect the best available evidence, including evidence-based guidelines (see Chapter 7). To better inform decision makers, additional research related to the eye and vision care workforce and payment policies is needed. Box 6-1 includes key research gaps identified in this chapter. Investment in cost-effectiveness research may help identify opportunities to reduce or shift the economic costs associated with vision impairment and strengthen clinical practice guidelines.

REFERENCES

AAMC (Association of American Medical Colleges). 2014. *2014 physician specialty data book.* Washington, DC: AAMC.

———. 2015a. *Diversity in the physician workforce: Facts & figures 2014.* Washington, DC: AAMC. http://aamcdiversityfactsandfigures.org (accessed August 15, 2016).

———. 2015b. *U.S. medical school faculty, 2015.* Washington, DC: AAMC. https://www.aamc.org/data/facultyroster/reports/453490/usmsf15.html (accessed August 15, 2016).

AAO (American Academy of Ophthalmology). 2011. Differences in education between optometrists and ophthalmologists. http://www.aao.org/about/policies/differences-education-optometrists-ophthalmologists (accessed April 7, 2016).

AAO/AOA (American Optometric Association). 2009. Letter to Senator Debbie Stabenow, October 20.

AAP (American Academy of Pediatrics). 2016. Recommendations for preventive pediatric health care. https://www.aap.org/en-us/Documents/periodicity_schedule.pdf (accessed April 7, 2016).

Aetna. 2016. Frequently asked questions. http://www.aetna.com/voluntary/faqs.html (accessed April 7, 2016).

AHRQ (Agency for Healthcare Research and Quality). 2004. *Vision rehabilitation for elderly individuals with low vision or blindness.* Rockville, MD: AHRQ.

———. 2012. *Screening for glaucoma: Comparative effectiveness.* Washington, DC: AHRQ.

———. 2014. Research Initiative in Clinical Economics. http://www.ahrq.gov/professionals/clinicians-providers/resources/rice/index.html#Projects (accessed April 7, 2016).

Antoniotti, N. M., K. P. Drude, and N. Rowe. 2014. Private payer telehealth reimbursement in the United States. *Telemedicine and e-Health* 20(6):539–543.

AOA (American Optometric Association). 2013. *An action-oriented analysis of the state of the optometric profession: 2013.* St. Louis, MO: AOA.

———. 2014. Vision plans: Myth vs. fact. http://fs.aoa.org/docs/feb-20-vision-plan-myths-and-facts.pdf (accessed May 18, 2016).

APHA (American Public Health Association). 2009. Improving access to vision care in community health centers. http://www.apha.org/policies-and-advocacy/public-health-policy-statements/policy-database/2014/07/31/08/14/improving-access-to-vision-care-in-community-health-centers (accessed April 7, 2016).

Arkansas DHS (Department of Human Services). 2012. *Arkansas Medicaid program overview.* Little Rock: Arkansas DHS.

Arora, K. S., D. S. Chang, W. Supakontanasan, M. Lakkur, and D. S. Friedman. 2014a. Assessment of a rapid method to determine approximate visual acuity in large surveys and other such settings. *American Journal of Ophthalmology* 157(6):1315–1321, e1311.

Arora, S., C. J. Rudnisky, and K. F. Damji. 2014b. Improved access and cycle time with an "in-house" patient-centered teleglaucoma program versus traditional in-person assessment. *Telemedicine and e-Health* 20(5):439–445.

ASCO (Association of Schools and Colleges of Optometry). 2009. *Annual student data report: Academic year 2008–2009.* http://www.opted.org/wp-content/uploads/2013/03/2008-2009-Student-Data-Report.pdf (accessed June 15, 2016).

———. 2015a. *Annual faculty data report: Academic year 2014–2015.* http://www.opted.org/wp-content/uploads/2015/03/2014-15-Annual-Faculty-Data-Report.pdf (accessed June 15, 2016).

———. 2015b. *Annual student data report: Academic year 2014–2015.* http://www.opted.org/wp-content/uploads/2015/03/2014-15-Annual-Faculty-Data-Report.pdf (accessed June 15, 2016).

ATA (American Telemedicine Association). 2016. What is telemedicine. http://www.americantelemed.org/about-telemedicine/what-is-telemedicine#.VwfkS_krLGg (accessed June 15, 2016).

Azrak, C., A. Palazon-Bru, M. V. Baeza-Diaz, D. M. Folgado-De la Rosa, C. Hernandez-Martinez, J. J. Martinez-Toldos, and V. F. Gil-Guillen. 2015. A predictive screening tool to detect diabetic retinopathy or macular edema in primary health care: Construction, validation and implementation on a mobile application. *PeerJ* 3:e1404.

Azuara-Blanco, A., K. Banister, C. Boachie, P. McMeekin, J. Gray, J. Burr, R. Bourne, D. Garway-Heath, M. Batterbury, R. Hernandez, G. McPherson, C. Ramsay, and J. Cook. 2016. Automated imaging technologies for the diagnosis of glaucoma: A comparative diagnostic study for the evaluation of the diagnostic accuracy, performance as triage tests and cost-effectiveness (GATE study). *Health Technology Assessment* 20(8):1–168.

Bastawrous, A., H. K. Rono, I. A. T. Livingstone, H. A. Weiss, S. Jordan, H. Kuper, and M. J. Burton. 2015. Development and validation of a smartphone-based visual acuity test (Peek Acuity) for clinical practice and community-based fieldwork. *JAMA Ophthalmology* 133(8):930–937.

Bastawrous, A., M. E. Giardini, N. M. Bolster, T. Peto, N. Shah, I. A. T. Livingstone, H. A. Weiss, S. Hu, H. Rono, H. Kuper, and M. Burton. 2016. Clinical validation of a smartphone-based adapter for optic disc imaging in Kenya. *JAMA Ophthalmology* 134(2):151–158.

Berry, J. L., L. M. Cuzzo, S. R. Bababeygy, and P. A. Quiros. 2012. Unmet need for corrective eyeglasses: Results from a Los Angeles County hospital survey. *International Ophthalmology* 32(3):245–250.

Bihari, M. 2014. Beyond medical coverage: Vision care insurance. https://www.verywell.com/vision-care-insurance-providers-and-coverage-1738489 (accessed April 29, 2016).

Bishop, C. E., W. Leutz, D. Gurewich, and M. D. Gaiser. 2010. *Evaluation of the medicare low vision rehabilitation demonstration beneficiary case study: A final report.* Waltham, MA: The Heller School for Social Policy and Management at Brandeis University.

BLS (Bureau of Labor Statistics). 2015a. Healthcare benefits: Access, participation, and take-up rates. http://www.bls.gov/ncs/ebs/benefits/2015/benefits_health.htm (accessed May 9, 2016).

———. 2015b. Optometrists. http://www.bls.gov/ooh/healthcare/optometrists.htm (accessed May 31, 2016).

Blue Cross Blue Shield. 2016. FEP BlueVision: A nationwide vision PPO plan. https://www.opm.gov/healthcare-insurance/healthcare/plan-information/plan-codes/2016/brochures/FEPBlueVi.pdf (accessed July 18, 2016).

Blumberg, D. M., R. Vaswani, E. Nong, L. Al-Aswad, and G. A. Cioffi. 2014. A comparative effectiveness analysis of visual field outcomes after projected glaucoma screening using SD-OCT in African American communities. *Investigative Ophthalmology & Visual Science* 55(6):3491–3500.

Blumberg, L. J. 2008. *Health savings accounts and high deductible health insurance plans: Implications for those with high medical costs, the low-income, and the uninsured.* Washington, DC: The Urban Institute.

Blumenthal, D., K. Davis, and S. Guterman. 2015a. Medicare at 50—Moving forward. *New England Journal of Medicine* 372(7):671–677.

———. 2015b. Medicare at 50—Origins and evolution. *New England Journal of Medicine* 372(5):479–486.

Boursiquot, B. L., and M. W. Brault. 2013. *Disability characteristics of income-based government assistance recipients in the United States: 2011.* Washington, DC: U.S. Census Bureau.

Bradley, C. 2016. Critical illness coverage a big part of voluntary benefits growth in 2016. In *The Employee Benefits Blog.* http://www.winstonbenefits.com/the-employee-benefits-blog/critical-illness-coverage-a-big-part-of-voluntary-benefits-growth-in-2016 (accessed June 15, 2016).

Brady, C. J., A. C. Villanti, O. P. Gupta, M. G. Graham, and R. C. Sergott. 2014. Teleophthalmology screening for proliferative diabetic retinopathy in urban primary care offices: An economic analysis. *Ophthalmic Surgery, Lasers, Imaging Retina* 45(6):556–561.

Brooks, E., C. Turvey, and E. F. Augusterfer. 2013. Provider barriers to telemental health: Obstacles overcome, obstacles remaining. *Telemedicine and e-Health* 19(6):433–437.

Brown, G. C., M. M. Brown, A. Menezes, B. G. Busbee, H. B. Lieske, and P. A. Lieske. 2013. Cataract surgery cost utility revisited in 2012: A new economic paradigm. *Ophthalmology* 120(12):2367–2376.

Burke, B. L., R. W. Hall, P. J. Dehnel, J. J. Alexander, D. M. Bell, M. Bunik, B. L. Burke, and J. R. Kile. 2015. Telemedicine: Pediatric applications. *Pediatrics* 136(1):e293–e308.

Burr, J. M., G. Mowatt, R. Hernandez, M. A. Siddiqui, J. Cook, T. Lourenco, C. Ramsay, L. Vale, C. Fraser, A. Azuara-Blanco, J. Deeks, J. Cairns, R. Wormald, S. McPherson, K. Rabindranath, and A. Grant. 2007. The clinical effectiveness and cost-effectiveness of screening for open angle glaucoma: A systematic review and economic evaluation. *Health Technololgy Assessment* 11(41):iii–iv, ix–x, 1–190.

Cabinet for Health and Family Services. 2007. *Kentucky Medicaid vision program manual.* Frankfort, KY: Department for Medicaid Services.

CBO (Congressional Budget Office). 2016. Detail of spending and enrollment for medicaid—CBO's March 2016 baseline. https://www.cbo.gov/sites/default/files/51301-2016-03-Medicaid.pdf (accessed March 8, 2016).

CCHP (The Center for Connected Health Policy). 2014. State telehealth policies and reimbursement schedules: A comprehensive plan of the 50 states and District of Columbia. Sacramento, CA: CCHP.

CDC (Centers for Disease Control and Prevention). 2009. *Improving the nation's vision health: A coordinated public health approach.* Atlanta, GA: CDC.

———. 2011. Reasons for not seeking eye care among adults aged ≥40 years with moderate-to-severe visual impairment—21 states, 2006–2009. *Morbidity and Mortality Weekly Report* 60(19):610–613.

———. 2015a. Economic studies. http://www.cdc.gov/visionhealth/projects/economic_studies.htm (accessed April 7, 2016).

———. 2015b. Sec. 4103: Medicare coverage of annual wellness visit providing a personalized prevention plan. http://www.cdc.gov/policy/hst/hra/4103.html (accessed April 7, 2016).

CDHCS (California Department of Health Care Services). 2016. Telehealth frequently asked questions. http://www.dhcs.ca.gov/provgovpart/Pages/TelehealthFAQ.aspx (accessed March 14, 2016).

CEA Registry (Cost-Effectiveness Analysis Registry). 2015. Publications using registry data. https://research.tufts-nemc.org/cear4/Resources/Publications.aspx (accessed April 7, 2016).

Chan, C. H., G. E. Trope, E. M. Badley, Y. M. Buys, and Y. P. Jin. 2014. The impact of lack of government-insured routine eye examinations on the incidence of self-reported glaucoma, cataracts, and vision loss. *Investigative Ophthalmology & Visual Science* 55(12):8544–8549.

Chan, C. K., R. A. Gangwani, S. M. McGhee, J. Lian, and D. S. Wong. 2015. Cost-effectiveness of screening for intermediate age-related macular degeneration during diabetic retinopathy screening. *Ophthalmology* 122(11):2278–2285.

Chou, C. F., X. Zhang, J. E. Crews, L. E. Barker, P. P. Lee, and J. B. Saaddine. 2012. Impact of geographic density of eye care professionals on eye care among adults with diabetes. *Ophthalmic Epidemiology* 19(6):340–349.

Chou, C. F., C. E. Sherrod, X. Zhang, L. E. Barker, K. M. Bullard, J. E. Crews, and J. B. Saaddine. 2014. Barriers to eye care among people aged 40 years and older with diagnosed diabetes, 2006–2010. *Diabetes Care* 37(1):180–188.

Claxton, G., M. Rae, N. Panchal, A. Damico, N. Bostick, K. Kenward, and H. Whitmore. 2014. *Employer health benefits: 2014 annual survey.* Chicago, IL: Henry J. Kaiser Family Foundation; Health Research & Educational Trust.

CMS (Centers for Medicare & Medicaid Services). 2011. Free preventive services for people in Medicare: 5.5 million Americans on Medicare have used preventive benefits. https://downloads.cms.gov/files/preventionreport.pdf (accessed June 15, 2016).

———. 2014a. Beneficiaries utilizing free preventive services by state, YTD 2013. https://downloads.cms.gov/files/Beneficiaries-Utilizing-Free-Preventive-Services-by-State-YTD2013.pdf (accessed March 9, 2016).

———. 2014b. *EPSDT—a guide for states: Coverage in the Medicaid benefit for children and adolescents.* Chicago, IL: NORC at the University of Chicago.

———. 2014c. Medicare enrollment—National trends 1966–2013. https://www.cms.gov/Research-Statistics-Data-and-Systems/Statistics-Trends-and-Reports/MedicareEnrpts/Downloads/SMI2013.pdf (accessed March 7, 2016).

———. 2015a. The ABCs of the initial preventive physical examination (IPPE). https://www.cms.gov/Outreach-and-Education/Medicare-Learning-Network-MLN/MLNProducts/Downloads/MPS_QRI_IPPE001a.pdf (accessed March 7, 2015).

———. 2015b. Beneficiaries utilizing free preventive services by state, YTD 2014. https://downloads.cms.gov/files/Beneificiaries-Utilizing-Free-Preventive-Services-by-State-YTD-2014.pdf (accessed March 9, 2016).

———. 2015c. Coverage determination process. https://www.cms.gov/Medicare/Coverage/DeterminationProcess/Downloads/8a.pdf (accessed April 7, 2016).

———. 2015d. *Medicare vision services.* Washington, DC: Medicare Learning Network.

———. 2016a. Dual eligible beneficiaries under the Medicare and Medicaid programs. https://www.cms.gov/Outreach-and-Education/Medicare-Learning-Network-MLN/MLN Products/downloads/Medicare_Beneficiaries_Dual_Eligibles_At_a_Glance.pdf (accessed May 9, 2016).

———. 2016b. Eye exams. https://www.medicare.gov/coverage/eye-exams.html (accessed March 7, 2016).

———. 2016c. Eyeglasses/contact lenses. https://www.medicare.gov/coverage/eyeglasses-contact-lenses.html (accessed March 7, 2016).

———. 2016d. Medicare advantage plans cover all Medicare services. https://www.medicare.gov/what-medicare-covers/medicare-health-plans/medicare-advantage-plans-cover-all-medicare-services.html (accessed March 6, 2016).

———. 2016e. National coverage determination (NCD) for hydrophilic contact lens for corneal bandage (80.1). https://www.cms.gov/medicare-coverage-database/details/ncd-details.aspx?NCDId=136&ver=1 (accessed October 14, 2016).

———. 2016f. National coverage determination (NCD) for intraocular photography (80.6). https://www.cms.gov/medicare-coverage-database/details/ncd-details.aspx?NCDId=56&ver=1 (accessed October 17, 2016).

———. 2016g. National coverage determination (NCD) for photodynamic therapy (OPT) (80.2). https://www.cms.gov/medicare-coverage-database/details/ncd-details.aspx?NCDId=128&ver=3 (accessed October 17, 2016).

———. 2016h. National coverage determination (NCD) for refractive keratoplasty (80.7). https://www.cms.gov/medicare-coverage-database/details/ncd-details.aspx?NCDId=72&ver=1 (accessed October 17, 2016).

———. 2016i. National coverage determination (NCD) for vitrectomy (80.11). https://www.cms.gov/medicare-coverage-database/details/ncd-details.aspx?NCDId=18&ver=2 (accessed October 17, 2016).

———. 2016j. What's Medicare supplement insurance (Medigap)? https://www.medicare.gov/supplement-other-insurance/medigap/whats-medigap.html (accessed June 21, 2016).

———. 2016k. What's Medicare? https://www.medicare.gov/sign-up-change-plans/decide-how-to-get-medicare/whats-medicare/what-is-medicare.html (accessed June 21, 2016).

———. 2016l. What Part A covers. https://www.medicare.gov/what-medicare-covers/part-a/what-part-a-covers.html (accessed March 6, 2016).

———. 2016m. What Part B covers. https://www.medicare.gov/what-medicare-covers/part-b/what-medicare-part-b-covers.html (accessed March 6, 2016).

Coan, J. n.d. Medicare low vision rehabilitation demonstration. https://www.cms.gov/Medicare/Demonstration-Projects/DemoProjectsEvalRpts/downloads/LowVisDemo_pp022206.pdf (accessed September 1, 2016).

Cochrane Community Archive. 2015. NHS economic evaluation database. http://community-archive.cochrane.org/editorial-and-publishing-policy-resource/nhs-economic-evaluation-database (accessed April 7, 2016).

Cooper, S. L. 2012. 1971–2011: Forty year history of scope expansion into medical eye care. *Optometry* 83(2):64–73.

Cornell, A. S. 2015. *Health benefits for members of Congress and designated congressional staff.* Washington, DC: Congressional Research Service.

Curtis, L. H., B. G. Hammill, L. G. Qualls, L. D. DiMartino, F. Wang, K. A. Schulman, and S. W. Cousins. 2012. Treatment patterns for neovascular age-related macular degeneration: Analysis of 284 380 Medicare beneficiaries. *American Journal of Ophthalmology* 153(6):1116–1124, e1111.

CVFP (Central Virginia Family Physicians). 2016. Health risk assessment (HRA) template for use with annual wellness visits. http://www.cvfp.net/images/PDFs/cvfp-healthrisk.pdf (accessed April 7, 2016).

Delbanco, S., and L. Tessitore. 2016. The payment reform landscape: How does telehealth fit into a high-value purchasing strategy? http://healthaffairs.org/blog/2016/02/12/the-payment-reform-landscape-how-does-telehealth-fit-into-a-high-value-purchasing-strategy-2 (accessed June 16, 2016).

DeVoe, J. E., A. Baez, H. Angier, L. Krois, C. Edlund, and P. A. Carney. 2007. Insurance + access ≠ health care: Typology of barriers to health care access for low-income families. *Annals of Family Medicine* 5(6):511–518.

Dhital, A., T. Pey, and M. R. Stanford. 2010. Visual loss and falls: A review. *Eye* 24(9):1437–1446.

DMAP (Delaware Medical Assistant Program). 2016. *General policy manual.* Dover: Delaware Health and Social Services.

Elam, A. R., and P. P. Lee. 2014. Barriers to and suggestions on improving utilization of eye care in high-risk individuals: Focus group results. *International Scholarly Research Notices* 2014:8.

Elliott, A. F., C. F. Chou, X. Zhang, J. E. Crews, J. B. Saaddine, G. L. Beckles, and M. D. Owens-Gary. 2010. Eye-care utilization among women aged ≥40 years with eye diseases—19 states, 2006–2008. *Morbidity and Mortality Weekly Report* 59(19):588–591.

Erickson, W., C. Lee, and S. von Schrader. 2014. *2013 Disability status report: United States.* Ithaca, NY: Cornell University.

Ettore Giardini, M. 2015. The portable eye examination kit: Mobile phones can screen for eye disease in low-resource settings. *IEEE Pulse* 6(6):15–17.

EyeMed. 2016. Summary of benefits. https://sasidsecure.blob.core.windows.net/pdf/171_1.pdf (accessed April 21, 2016).

Fierson, W. M., A. Capone, D. B. Granet, R. J. Blocker, G. E. Bradford, F. S. S. Lehman, S. E. Rubin, R. M. Siatkowski, and J. B. Ruben. 2015. Telemedicine for evaluation of retinopathy of prematurity. *Pediatrics* 135(1):e238–e254.

Fudemberg, S. J., D. C. Amarasekera, M. H. Silverstein, K. M. Linder, P. Heffner, L. A. Hark, and M. Waisbourd. 2016. Overcoming barriers to eye care: Patient response to a medical social worker in a glaucoma service. *Journal of Community Health* [Epub ahead of print].

Garber, A. M. 2001. Evidence-based coverage policy. *Health Affairs* 20(5):62–82.

Gibson, D. M. 2014. Eye care availability and access among individuals with diabetes, diabetic retinopathy, or age-related macular degeneration. *JAMA Ophthalmology* 132(4):471–477.

———. 2015. The geographic distribution of eye care providers in the United States: Implications for a national strategy to improve vision health. *Preventive Medicine* 73:30–36.

Goetzel, R. Z., P. Staley, L. Ogden, P. Stange, J. Fox, J. Spangler, M. Tabrizi, M. Beckowski, N. Kowlessar, R. E. Glasgow, M. V. Taylor, and C. Richards. 2011. *A framework for patient-centered health risk assessments: Providing health promotion and disease prevention services to Medicare beneficiaries.* Atlanta, GA: CDC. https://www.cdc.gov/policy/hst/hra/frameworkforhra.pdf (accessed June 15, 2016).

Gower, E. W., J. Whiteside-de Vos, S. D. Cassard, N. S. Shekhawat, and D. S. Friedman. 2013. The Medicare glaucoma screening benefit: A critical program that misses its target. *American Journal of Ophthalmology* 156(2):211–212, e212.

Hale, N. L., K. J. Bennett, and J. C. Probst. 2010. Diabetes care and outcomes: Disparities across rural America. *Journal of Community Health* 35(4):365–374.

Hall, M. A., and K. A. Schulman,. 2010. Property, privacy, and the pursuit of integrated electronic medical records. In *The fragmentation of U.S. health care: Causes and solutions*, edited by E. Elhauge. New York: Oxford University Press.

Heaven, C. J., J. Cansfield, and K. M. Shaw. 1993. The quality of photographs produced by the non-mydriatic fundus camera in a screening programme for diabetic retinopathy: A 1-year prospective study. *Eye (London)* 7(6):787–790.

Hernandez, R., K. Rabindranath, C. Fraser, L. Vale, A. A. Blanco, and J. M. Burr. 2008. Screening for open angle glaucoma: Systematic review of cost-effectiveness studies. *Journal of Glaucoma* 17(3):159–168.

HHS (U.S. Department of Health and Human Services). 2008. *The physician workforce: Projections and research into current issues affecting supply and demand.* Rockville, MD: HHS.

———. 2013a. *2013 CMS statistics.* Rockville, MD: HHS.

———. 2013b. *The U.S. health workforce chartbook: Part II: Clinicians and health administration.* Rockville, MD: HHS.

———. 2015. Sex, race, and ethnic diversity of U.S. health occupations (2010–2012). http://bhpr.hrsa.gov/healthworkforce/supplydemand/usworkforce/diversityushealth occupations.pdf (accessed June 15, 2016).

Higginbotham, E. J. 2012. The physician workforce discussion revisited: The implications for ophthalmology. *Archives of Ophthalmology* 130(5):648–649.

Higginbotham, E. J., and L. Lippa. 2010. Assessing the status of ophthalmic education 100 years after the Flexner report. *Archives of Ophthalmology* 128(12):1600–1601.

Hodges, L. E., and M. L. Berk. 1999. Unmet need for eyeglasses: Results from the 1994 Robert Wood Johnson Access to Care Survey. *Journal of the American Optometry Association* 70(4):261–265.

Hoerger, T. J., J. E. Segel, P. Zhang, and S. W. Sorensen. 2009. *Validation of the CDC-RTI diabetes cost-effectiveness model.* Research Triangle Park, NC: RTI International. http://www.rti.org/sites/default/files/resources/mr-0013-0909-hoerger.pdf (accessed June 21, 2016).

Horton, K., M.-B. Malcarney, and N. Seiler. 2014. Medicare payment rules and telemedicine. *Public Health Reports* 129(2):196–199.

Housman, L., Z. Williams, and P. Ellis. 2015. Telemedicine. https://www.cbo.gov/publication/50680 (accessed March 14, 2016).

HRSA (Health Resources and Services Administration). 2014. 2014 health center data. http://bphc.hrsa.gov/uds/datacenter.aspx (accessed April 7, 2016).

———. 2016. Medicare telehealth payment eligibilty analyzer. http://datawarehouse.hrsa.gov/tools/analyzers/geo/Telehealth.aspx (accessed March 14, 2016).

Huckvale, K., J. T. Prieto, M. Tilney, P.-J. Benghozi, and J. Car. 2015. Unaddressed privacy risks in accredited health and wellness apps: A cross-sectional systematic assessment. *BMC Medicine* 13(1):1–13.

Hurley, L. P., C. B. Bridges, R. Harpaz, M. A. Allison, O. L. ST, L. A. Crane, M. Brtnikova, S. Stokley, B. L. Beaty, A. Jimenez-Zambrano, and A. Kempe. 2016. Physician attitudes toward adult vaccines and other preventive practices, United States, 2012. *Public Health Reports* 131(2):320–330.

International Vision Expo East. 2015. MVC coverage among U.S. adults. http://www.vision expoeast.com/Press/Vision-Voice-Newsletter/MVC-Coverage-among-US-Adults (accessed April 7, 2016).

IOM (Institute of Medicine). 2012. *The role of telehealth in an evolving health care environment: Workshop summary.* Washington, DC: The National Academies Press.

Iowa DHS (Department of Human Services). 2014. *Optometrist and optician services provider manual.* Des Moines: Iowa DHS.

IRS (Internal Revenue Service). 2016. *Publication 502 (2015), medical and dental expenses.* https://www.irs.gov/publications/p502 (accessed April 7, 2016).

Jacobson, G., M. Gold, A. Damico, T. Neuman, and G. Casillas. 2015. Medicare advantage 2016 data spotlight: Overview of plan changes. http://kff.org/medicare/issue-brief/medicare-advantage-2016-data-spotlight-overview-of-plan-changes (accessed June 15, 2016).

Jin, Y.-P., Y. M. Buys, J. Xiong, and G. E. Trope. 2013. Government-insured routine eye examinations and prevalence of nonrefractive vision problems among elderly. *Canadian Journal of Ophthalmology* 48(3):167–172.

Jobson Optical Research. 2012. *2012 Consumer Perceptions of Managed Vision Care.* New York: Jobson Optical Research.

John Wiley & Sons, Inc. 2016. *HEED: Health Economic Evaluations Database.* http://onlinelibrary.wiley.com/book/10.1002/9780470510933? (accessed May 17, 2016).

Jones, S., and R. T. Edwards. 2010. Diabetic retinopathy screening: A systematic review of the economic evidence. *Diabetic Medicine* 27(3):249–256.

Kaiser Family Foundation. 2011. *Financial alignment models for dual eligibles: An update.* Menlo Park, CA: The Henry J. Kaiser Family Foundation.

———. 2012a. Medicaid benefits: Eyeglasses. http://kff.org/medicaid/state-indicator/eyeglasses (accessed March 8, 2016).

———. 2012b. Medicaid benefits: Optometrist services. http://kff.org/medicaid/state-indicator/optometrist-services (accessed March 8, 2016).

———. 2013. *Medicaid: A primer.* Menlo Park, CA: The Henry J. Kaiser Family Foundation.

———. 2015. Key facts about the uninsured population. http://kff.org/uninsured/fact-sheet/key-facts-about-the-uninsured-population (accessed March 7, 2016).

———. 2016a. Dual eligible. http://kff.org/tag/dual-eligible (accessed May 9, 2016).

———. 2016b. *An overview of Medicare.* Menlo Park, CA: Kaiser Family Foundation.

———. 2016c. Status of state action on the Medicaid expansion decision. http://kff.org/health-reform/state-indicator/state-activity-around-expanding-medicaid-under-the-affordable-care-act (accessed May 19, 2016).

Kilmer, G., L. Bynum, and A. Balamurugan. 2010. Access to and use of eye care services in rural Arkansas. *Journal of Rural Health* 26(1):30–35.

Kirkizlar, E., N. Serban, J. A. Sisson, J. L. Swann, C. S. Barnes, and M. D. Williams. 2013. Evaluation of telemedicine for screening of diabetic retinopathy in the Veterans Health Administration. *Ophthalmology* 120(12):2604–2610.

Kirkner, R. M. 2011. Vision plans hope to gain access to state insurance exchanges. http://www.managedcaremag.com/archives/2011/1/vision-plans-hope-gain-access-state-insurance-exchanges (accessed May 18, 2016).

Klein, B. E. K., S. E. Moss, R. Klein, K. E. Lee, and K. J. Cruickshanks. 2003. Associations of visual function with physical outcomes and limitations 5 years later in an older population. *Ophthalmology* 110(4):644–650.

Komaromy, M., K. Grumbach, M. Drake, K. Vranizan, N. Lurie, D. Keane, and A. B. Bindman. 1996. The role of Black and Hispanic physicians in providing health care for underserved populations. *New England Journal of Medicine* 334(20):1305–1310.

Konrad, W. 2010. Flexible spending, a little less so. *The New York Times,* April 16. http://www.nytimes.com/2010/04/17/health/17patient.html (accessed June 15, 2016).

Kraus, L. 2015. *2015 disability statistics annual report.* Durham: University of New Hampshire.

Ladapo, J. A., S. M. Kymes, J. A. Ladapo, V. C. Nwosu, and L. R. Pasquale. 2012. Projected clinical outcomes of glaucoma screening in african american individuals. *Archives of Ophthalmology* 130(3):365–372.

Lee, B. S., and S. M. Kymes. 2015. Re: Brown et al.: Cataract surgery cost utility revisited in 2012: A new economic paradigm. (Ophthalmology 2013;120:2367–2376). *Ophthalmology* 122(3):e18.

Lee, D. J., O. Gomez-Marin, B. L. Lam, and D. D. Zheng. 2002. Visual acuity impairment and mortality in us adults. *Archives of Ophthalmology* 120(11):1544–1550.

Lee, P. P., C. A. Jackson, and D. A. Relles. 1995. Estimating eye care workforce supply and requirements. *Ophthalmology* 102(12):1964–1971; discussion 1971–1972.

Lee, P. P., D. A. Relles, and C. A. Jackson. 1998. Subspecialty distributions of ophthalmologists in the workforce. *Archives of Ophthalmology* 116(7):917–920.

Lee, P. P., H. D. Hoskins Jr., and D. W. Parke III. 2007. Access to care: Eye care provider workforce considerations in 2020. *Archives of Ophthalmology* 125(3):406–410.

Levin, A. V., L. T. Pizzi, M. Snitzer, and K. M. Prioli. 2013. Barriers to follow up care in children with vision diseases: Development of a conceptual framework and parent/caregiver survey through the children's eye care adherence project. *Value in Health* 16(3):A38.

Lewin Group. 2014. *Eye care workforce study: Supply and demand projections.* Falls Church, VA: The Lewin Group.

Li, H. K. 1999. Telemedicine and ophthalmology. *Survey of Ophthalmology* 44(1): 61–72.

Li, Y., S. Xirasagar, C. Pumkam, M. Krishnaswamy, and C. L. Bennett. 2013. Vision insurance, eye care visits, and vision impairment among working-age adults in the United States. *JAMA Ophthalmology* 131(4):499–506.

Li, Z., C. Wu, J. N. Olayiwola, D. S. Hilaire, and J. J. Huang. 2012. Telemedicine-based digital retinal imaging vs standard ophthalmologic evaluation for the assessment of diabetic retinopathy. *Connecticut Medicine* 76(2):85–90.

Loeppke, R. 2011. CDC HRA briefing. http://prevent.org/data/files/hra/loeppke-cdc%20 hra%20briefing%20short%20version%202-1-11.pdf (accessed June 15, 2016).

Lorenz, B., K. Spasovska, H. Elflein, and N. Schneider. 2009. Wide-field digital imaging based telemedicine for screening for acute retinopathy of prematurity (ROP). Six-year results of a multicentre field study. *Graefe's Archives for Clinical and Experimental Ophthalmology* 247(9):1251–1262.

MacLennan, P. A., G. McGwin, K. Searcey, and C. Owsley. 2014. A survey of Alabama eye care providers in 2010–2011. *BMC Ophthalmology* 14(1):1–10.

Mansberger, S. L., K. Gleitsmann, S. Gardiner, C. Sheppler, S. Demirel, K. Wooten, and T. M. Becker. 2013. Comparing the effectiveness of telemedicine and traditional surveillance in providing diabetic retinopathy screening examinations: A randomized controlled trial. *Telemedicine and e-Health* 19(12):942–948.

Medicaid. 2016a. Benefits. https://www.medicaid.gov/medicaid-chip-program-information/ by-topics/benefits/medicaid-benefits.html (accessed October 20, 2015).

———. 2016b. Early and periodic screening, diagnostic, and treatment. https://www.medicaid. gov/medicaid-chip-program-information/by-topics/benefits/early-and-periodic-screening-diagnostic-and-treatment.html (accessed March 8, 2016).

———. 2016c. Eligibility. https://www.medicaid.gov/medicaid-chip-program-information/ by-topics/eligibility/eligibility.html (accessed October 20, 2015).

———. 2016d. Financing. https://www.medicaid.gov/chip/financing/financing.html (accessed October 20, 2015).

Mogk, L., G. R. Watson, and M. Williams. 2008. Speaker's corner: A commentary on the Medicare low vision rehabiliatation demonstration project. *Journal of Visual Impairment and Blindness* 102(2):69–75.

Moyer, V. A. 2013. Screening for glaucoma: U.S. Preventive Services Task Force recommendation statement. *Annals of Internal Medicine* 159(7):484–489.

Nasseh, K., and M. Vujicic. 2013. Health reform in Massachusetts increased adult dental care use, particularly among the poor. *Health Affairs* 32(9):1639–1645.

NAVCP (National Association of Vision Care Plans). 2010. *National Association of Vision Care Plans vision exam utilization study (Study period: 2008–2009): Executive summary.* Louisville, KY: Ingenix Consulting.

———. 2013. *Invigorating interest in the vision benefit.* Indianapolis, IN: National Association of Vision Care Plans.

Naylor, L. 2013. *Providing access to preventative health care: Child health and EPSDT.* http://patimes.org/providing-access-preventative-care-child-health-epsdt (accessed April 7, 2016).

NEI (National Eye Institute). 2016. Vision impairment tables. https://nei.nih.gov/eyedata/vision_impaired/tables (accessed May 17, 2016).

Neufeld, J. D., and C. R. Doarn. 2015. Telemedicine spending by medicare: A snapshot from 2012. *Telemedicine and e-Health* 21(8):686–693.

Ng, M., N. Nathoo, C. J. Rudnisky, and M. T. Tennant. 2009. Improving access to eye care: Teleophthalmology in Alberta, Canada. *Journal of Diabetes Science and Technology* 3(2):289–296.

NICHSR (National Information Center on Health Services Research and Health Care Technology). 2016. Module 1, part 2: Key information sources. https://www.nlm.nih.gov/nichsr/edu/healthecon/01_he_11.html (accessed April 7, 2016).

NRHA (National Rural Health Association). 2009. National Rural Health Association policy brief: Workforce series: Primary eye care—Recruitment and retention of quality health workforce in rural areas: A series of policy papers on the rural health careers pipeline. (Paper no. 8.) Alexandria, VA: NRHA.

Ochoa, F., E. Simbaqueba, M. Romero, and A. Lopez. 2014. Analysis of cost-effectiveness of use of toric intraocular lenses compared with tranditional monofocal lenses in patients with cataracts and pre-existing corenal astigmatism. *Value in Health* 17:A286.

ODPHP (Office of Disease Prevention and Health Promotion). 2016. Disparities. https://www.healthypeople.gov/2020/about/foundation-health-measures/Disparities (accessed May 31, 2016).

OkCopay. 2016. Eye exam costs in the USA. http://www.okcopay.com/map/eye-exam-cost (accessed April 21, 2016).

Oluleye, T. S., A. Rotimi-Samuel, and A. Adenekan. 2016. Mobile phones for retinopathy of prematurity screening in Lagos, Nigeria, Sub-Saharan Africa. *European Journal of Ophthalmology* 26(1):92–94.

OPM (Office of Personnel Management). 2016. Dental and vision plan search. https://www.opm.gov/healthcare-insurance/dental-vision/plan-information/compare-plans/FEDVIP Profiles.aspx?plans=VAP1SVAH1SVAJ1SVAK1S&rates=a&benefits=x&general=abcd&payperiod=a&FEDVIP (accessed March 8, 2016).

Petroski, C., and J. Regan. 2009. Use and knowledge of the new enrollee "Welcome to Medicare" physical examination benefit. *Health Care Financing Review* 30(3):71–76.

Pew Research Center. 2015. *Technology device ownership: 2015.* Washington, DC: Pew Research Center.

Phan, A.-D. T., J. J. Koczman, C.-W. Yung, A. A. Pernic, E. D. Doerr, and M. M. Kaehr. 2014. Cost analysis of teleretinal screening for diabetic retinopathy in a county hospital population. *Diabetes Care* 37(12):e252–e253.

Pittard III, W. B., J. N. Laditka, and S. B. Laditka. 2007. Early and periodic screening, diagnosis, and treatment and infant health outcomes in Medicaid-insured infants in South Carolina. *Journal of Pediatrics* 151(4):414–418.

Pletcher, B. A., M. E. Rimsza, W. L. Cull, S. A. Shipman, R. P. Shugerman, and K. G. O'Connor. 2010. Primary care pediatricians' satisfaction with subspecialty care, perceived supply, and barriers to care. *Journal of Pediatrics* 156(6):1011–1015.

Prevent Blindness. 2012. Vision problems in the U.S.: Visual impairment http://visionproblemsus.org/cgi-bin/vpus.cgi (accessed July 5, 2016).

Quashie, R. 2012. The real issue in telehealth: How can I get paid? *TechHealth Perspectives.* http://www.techhealthperspectives.com/2012/11/05/513 (accessed June 15, 2016).

Rein, D. B., J. S. Wittenborn, P. P. Lee, K. E. Wirth, S. W. Sorensen, T. J. Hoerger, and J. B. Saaddine. 2009. The cost-effectiveness of routine office-based identification and subsequent medical treatment of primary open-angle glaucoma in the United States. *Ophthalmology* 116(5):823–832.

Rein, D. B., J. S. Wittenborn, X. Zhang, B. A. Allaire, M. S. Song, R. Klein, and J. B. Saaddine. 2011. The cost-effectiveness of three screening alternatives for people with diabetes with no or early diabetic retinopathy. *Health Services Reseach* 46(5):1534–1561.

Rein, D. B., J. S. Wittenborn, X. Zhang, T. J. Hoerger, P. Zhang, B. E. Klein, K. E. Lee, R. Klein, and J. B. Saaddine. 2012a. The cost-effectiveness of Welcome to Medicare visual acuity screening and a possible alternative Welcome to Medicare eye evaluation among persons without diagnosed diabetes mellitus. *Archives of Ophthalmology* 130(5):607–614.

Rein, D. B., J. S. Wittenborn, X. Zhang, M. Song, and J. B. Saaddine. 2012b. The potential cost-effectiveness of amblyopia screening programs. *Journal of Pediatric Ophthalmology and Strabismus* 49(3):146–155; quiz 145, 156.

Research!America. 2014. *Attiudinal survey of minority populations on eye and vision health and research.* Alexandria, VA: Research!America.

Richardson, D. R., R. L. Fry, and M. Krasnow. 2013. Cost-savings analysis of telemedicine use for ophthalmic screening in a rural Appalachian health clinic. *West Virginia Medical Journal* 109(4):52–55.

Rocktime, L. 2016. Vision test. https://itunes.apple.com/us/app/vision-test/id380288414?mt=8 (accessed June 15, 2016).

Rosenbaum, S., and P. H. Wise. 2007. Crossing the Medicaid–private insurance divide: The case of EPSDT. *Health Affairs* 26(2):382–393.

Royalty, A. B., and J. Hagens. 2005. The effect of premiums on the decision to participate in health insurance and other fringe benefits offered by the employer: Evidence from a real-world experiment. *Journal of Health Economics* 24(1):95–112.

Saha, S., M. Komaromy, T. D. Koepsell, and A. B. Bindman. 1999. Patient–physician racial concordance and the perceived quality and use of health care. *Archives of Internal Medicine* 159(9):997–1004.

Salman, C., and L. Shirey. 2002. Visual impairments. https://hpi.georgetown.edu/agingsociety/pubhtml/visual/visual.html (accessed August 15, 2016).

Schor, E. L., M. Abrams, and K. Shea. 2007. Medicaid: Health promotion and disease prevention for school readiness. *Health Affairs* 26(2):420–429.

Shi, L., H. Wu, J. Dong, K. Jiang, X. Lu, and J. Shi. 2015. Telemedicine for detecting diabetic retinopathy: A systematic review and meta-analysis. *British Journal of Ophthalmology* 99(6):823–831.

Shimizu, W., and C. Chorneau. 2009. *Telehealth optimization initiative: Summary of focus group methodology and responses.* Sacramento: California Telemedicine and eHealth Center.

Shin, P., and B. Finnegan. 2009. Assessing the need for on-site eye care professionals in community health centers. Policy Brief. *George Washington University Center Health Services Research Policy,* February:1–23.

Sloan, F. A., D. S. Brown, E. S. Carlisle, G. A. Picone, and P. P. Lee. 2004. Monitoring visual status: Why patients do or do not comply with practice guidelines. *Health Services Research* 39(5):1429–1448.

Sloan, F. A., A. P. Yashkin, and Y. Chen. 2014. Gaps in receipt of regular eye exams among Medicare beneficiaries diagnosed with diabetes or chronic eye diseases. *Ophthalmology* 121(12):2452–2460.

Snowden, L. R., M. Masland, N. Wallace, K. Fawley-King, and A. E. Cuellar. 2008. Increasing California children's Medicaid-financed mental health treatment by vigorously implementing Medicaid's Early Periodic Screening, Diagnosis, and Treatment (EPSDT) program. *Medical Care* 46(6):558–564.

Soroka, M., D. M. Krumholz, M. Krasner, and J. Portello. 2000. Optimal clinical management of eye problems: The role of optometrists in managed care plans. *Optometry* 71(12):781–790.

Spahr, J. 2015. Panel 5: Perspectives on policy and system change Q&A. Paper read at Second Meeting of the Committee on Public Health Approaches to Reduce Vision Impairment and Promote Eye Health, Washington, DC.

Staley, P., P. Stange, and C. Richards. 2011. Interim guidance for health risk assessments and their modes of provision for Medicare beneficiaries. https://www.cms.gov/Medicare/Coverage/CoverageGenInfo/downloads/healthriskassessmentsCDCfinal.pdf (accessed June 15, 2016).

The State of Obesity. 2016. States with the highest type 2 diabetes rates. http://stateofobesity.org/lists/highest-rates-diabetes (accessed June 20, 2016).

Tamura, H., R. Goto, Y. Akune, Y. Hiratsuka, S. Hiragi, and M. Yamada. 2015. The clinical effectiveness and cost-effectiveness of screening for age-related macular degeneration in Japan: A Markov modeling study. *PLoS ONE* 10(7):e0133628.

Thomas, S. M., M. M. Jeyaraman, W. G. Hodge, C. Hutnik, J. Costella, and M. S. Malvankar-Mehta. 2014. The effectiveness of teleglaucoma versus in-patient examination for glaucoma screening: A systematic review and meta-analysis. *PLoS ONE* 9(12):e113779.

Thomas, S., W. Hodge, and M. Malvankar-Mehta. 2015. The cost-effectiveness analysis of teleglaucoma screening device. *PLoS ONE* 10(9):e0137913.

Tozzi, J. 2014. Obamacare mystery: Why can't you buy vision coverage? http://www.bloomberg.com/news/articles/2014-09-30/obamacare-mystery-why-cant-you-buy-vision-insurance (accessed May 18, 2016).

Trivedi, R. H., M. E. Wilson, M. M. Peterseim, K. B. Cole, and R. G. W. Teed. 2010. A pilot study evaluating the use of EyeSpy video game software to perform vision screening in school-aged children. *Journal of the American Association for Pediatric Ophthalmology and Strabismus* 14(4):311–316.

Tsui, E., A. N. Siedlecki, J. Deng, M. C. Pollard, S. Cha, S. M. Pepin, and E. M. Salcone. 2015. Implementation of a vision-screening program in rural northeastern United States. *Clinical Ophthalmology (Auckland, N.Z.)* 9:1883–1887.

UnitedHealthcare. 2016. Vision. https://www.uhc.com/employer/health-plans/ancillary-specialty-benefits/vision (accessed April 29, 2016).

U.S. Census Bureau. 2015. *2010 census urban and rural classification and urban area criteria.* https://www.census.gov/geo/reference/ua/urban-rural-2010.html (accessed May 31, 2016).

USPSTF (U.S. Preventive Services Task Force). 2013. Final recommendation statement: Glaucoma screening. http://www.uspreventiveservicestaskforce.org/Page/Document/RecommendationStatementFinal/glaucoma-screening (accessed April 25, 2016).

VA (U.S. Department of Veterans Affairs). 2015. Store-and-forward telehealth. http://www.telehealth.va.gov/sft/ (accessed June 6, 2016).

Varma, R., T. S. Vajaranant, B. Burkemper, S. Wu, M. Torres, C. Hsu, F. Choudhury, and R. McKean-Cowdin. 2016. Visual impairment and blindness in adults in the United States: Demographic and geographic variations from 2015 to 2050. *JAMA Ophthalmology.*

Verma, S., S. Arora, F. Kassam, M. C. Edwards, and K. F. Damji. 2014. Northern Alberta remote teleglaucoma program: Clinical outcomes and patient disposition. *Canadian Journal of Ophthalmology* 49(2):135–140.

Vision Council. 2015. *Vision Council: US optical industry report card december 2015.* Alexandria, VA: The Vision Council.

———. 2016. Vision Watch history and methodology. http://www.thevisioncouncil.org/members/research-history-and-methodology (accessed May 24, 2016).

VSP (Vision Service Plan). 2016a. EasyOptions plan details. https://www.vspdirect.com/plan_files/1/plan_details (accessed June 15, 2016).

———. 2016b. Enhanced plan details. https://www.vspdirect.com/plan_files/3/plan_details (accessed June 15, 2016).

———. 2016c. Standard plan details. https://www.vspdirect.com/plan_files/2/plan_details (accessed June 15, 2016).

———. 2016d. VSP vision care: A nationwide PPO vision plan. https://www.opm.gov/health care-insurance/healthcare/plan-information/plan-codes/2016/brochures/VSP.pdf (accessed July 18, 2016).

Vujicic, M., C. Yarbrough, and K. Nasseh. 2014. The effect of the Affordable Care Act's expanded coverage policy on access to dental care. *Medical Care* 52(8):715–719.

Wang, S. K., N. F. Callaway, M. B. Wallenstein, M. T. Henderson, T. Leng, and D. M. Moshfeghi. 2015. Sundrop: Six years of screening for retinopathy of prematurity with telemedicine. *Canadian Journal of Ophthalmology* 50(2):101–106.

Weaver, D. T. 2013. Telemedicine for retinopathy of prematurity. *Currents Opinions in Ophthalmology* 24(5):425–431.

Webb, J. A. 2011. Kentucky ODs win right to perform laser surgery. *Optometry Times,* April 1. http://optometrytimes.modernmedicine.com/optometrytimes/news/modern medicine/modern-medicine-now/kentucky-ods-win-right-perform-laser-surgery (accessed June 15, 2016).

Wittenborn, J., and D. Rein. 2016 (unpublished). *The potential costs and benefits of treatment for undiagnosed eye disorders.* Paper prepared for the Committee on Public Health Approaches to Reduce Vision Impairment and Promote Eye Health. http://www.nationalacademies.org/hmd/~/media/Files/Report%20Files/2016/UndiagnosedEye DisordersCommissionedPaper.pdf (accessed September 15, 2016).

Wittenborn, J. S., X. Zhang, C. W. Feagan, W. L. Crouse, S. Shrestha, A. R. Kemper, T. J. Hoerger, and J. B. Saaddine. 2013. The economic burden of vision loss and eye disorders among the United States population younger than 40 years. *Ophthalmology* 120(9):1728–1735.

Woodward, M. A., P. Ple-Plakon, T. Blachley, D. C. Musch, P. A. Newman-Casey, L. B. De Lott, and P. P. Lee. 2015. Eye care providers' attitudes towards tele-ophthalmology. *Telemedicine Journal and e-Health* 21(4):271–273.

Woolf, S. H., R. Grol, A. Hutchinson, M. Eccles, and J. Grimshaw. 1999. Potential benefits, limitations, and harms of clinical guidelines. *British Medical Journal* 318(7182):527–530.

WSHCA (Washington State Health Care Authority). 2016. *Physician-related services/Health care professional services provider guide.* Olympia: WSHCA.

Zhang, X., R. Andersen, J. B. Saaddine, G. L. Beckles, M. R. Duenas, and P. P. Lee. 2008a. Measuring access to eye care: A public health perspective. *Ophthalmic Epidemiology* 15(6):418–425.

Zhang, X., P. P. Lee, T. J. Thompson, S. Sharma, L. Barker, L. S. Geiss, G. Imperatore, E. W. Gregg, X. Zhang, and J. B. Saaddine. 2008b. Health insurance coverage and use of eye care services. *Archives of Ophthalmology* 126(8):1121–1126.

Zhang, X., M. F. Cotch, A. Ryskulova, S. A. Primo, P. Nair, C.-F. Chou, L. S. Geiss, L. Barker, A. F. Elliott, J. E. Crews, and J. B. Saaddine. 2012. Vision health disparities in the United States by race/ethnicity, education, and economic status: Findings from two nationally representative surveys. *American Journal of Ophthalmology* 154(60):S53–S62, e51.

7

Toward a High-Quality Clinical Eye and Vision Service Delivery System

Encouraging high-quality eye and vision care is one component of a comprehensive population health approach to reduce vision impairment in the United States. As defined by the Institute of Medicine (IOM), quality care must be safe, timely, effective, efficient, equitable, and patient-centered (IOM, 2001). Currently, the clinical eye and vision service delivery system faces several challenges to achieving these goals. Multiple and sometimes conflicting clinical practice guidelines create different standards from which to measure and improve quality and clear, consistent public messaging about what care is needed when. Limited integration among and between clinical and public health services, combined with insufficient cross-disciplinary training of the workforce, may negatively affect diagnosis and follow-up care. Inadequate health care services research on the vision care system further hampers the ability to improve care quality through application of continuous quality improvement programs.

This chapter focuses on improving the quality and consistency of eye and vision care in the United States. The first section discusses the importance of consistent evidence-based guidelines to inform care seeking and providing behaviors, especially in the context of vision screenings and comprehensive eye examinations. The second section examines the role of continuous quality improvement initiatives in promoting high-quality eye and vision care. The third section explores potential integrated models of care to promote detection and diagnosis of vision problems and subsequent referral to eye care providers. The state of, and need for, cross-disciplinary education of the public health, eye care, and broader clinical workforce is described in the final section, with a focus on training to promote cultural

325

competency, leadership, teamwork, and awareness of the interrelations between eye and vision health, general health, and population health.

THE NEED FOR EVIDENCE-BASED GUIDELINES: ESTABLISHING THE BASELINE

Evidence-based guidelines are an important foundational element to anchor a population health approach that advances eye and vision health. First, they provide guidance based on sound, objective evidence that a variety of care providers can use to improve the uniformity of messaging about, and the quality of, patient care. Second, they establish a baseline from which to measure improvement in care processes and patient health outcomes. Third, they promote a culture of accountability by enabling performance comparisons and encouraging the uniform adoption of best practices.

To promote clear and consistent messaging about whom needs what care and when, it is important that a single set of evidence-based guidelines be available to the public, especially in the context of vision screenings and comprehensive eye examinations. Evidence-based guidelines released by the American Academy of Ophthalmology and the American Optometric Association (AOA), which are based on a review of the literature, serve to guide the members of the respective organizations in the treatment and management of eye diseases.[1] These organizations use some of the same literature from which to develop their guidelines and, in many cases, offer consistent guidelines or recommendations. However, there are important differences, especially on topics related to the frequency of exams, specific types of treatments, and the use of screenings. These differences may be due to a confluence of factors, including guideline development processes, evidentiary standards, and professional emphasis of optometrists and ophthalmologists.

This section is intended to describe some of the current inconsistencies and challenges related to clinical practice guidelines in eye and vision health and to reiterate the standards to which clinical practice guidelines should be held. This section does not endorse any particular set of professional guidelines nor make conclusions about the quality of evidence supporting any specific guideline.

---

[1] Clinical practice guidelines developed by AAO are referred to as "Preferred Practice Pattern® guidelines," whereas clinical practice guidelines developed by AOA are referred to as "Clinical Practice Guidelines" or "Optometric Clinical Practice Guidelines." Throughout this report, AAO and AOA clinical practice guidelines will be referred to as "guidelines," or, wherever the distinction is pertinent, as "evidence-based guidelines" or "consensus-based guidelines."

Distinguishing Comprehensive Eye Examinations from Vision Screenings

A comprehensive eye examination is a dilated eye examination that may include a series of assessments and procedures to evaluate the eyes and visual system, assess eye and vision health and related systemic health conditions, characterize the impact of disease or abnormal conditions on the function and status of the visual system, and provide treatment and follow-up options (see Chapter 1). Eye examinations can detect incipient eye disease before the onset of visual symptoms. Eye examinations can also detect chronic conditions, such as diabetes and multiple sclerosis (Crews et al., 2016; Frohman et al., 2008). Schaneman and colleagues (2010) conducted a retrospective, claims-based analysis of employed adults living in the United States, and found that individuals who detected a chronic disease through an eye examination had lower first-year health plan costs and fewer missed work days and were less likely to terminate employment than individuals who did not detect chronic conditions early through eye examinations.

Eye examinations are performed by ophthalmologists and optometrists and usually include taking a patient history, assessing the patient's visual functioning (e.g., visual acuity, field of vision, eye movements), observing indicators of eye health (e.g., intraocular pressure), and examining the state of the pupil, iris, cornea, lens, optic nerve, retina, and other parts of the eye after dilation (AAO, 2012a). Eye providers may also perform the procedures listed in Box 7-1, along with cover tests, color blindness tests, depth perception tests, and other supplementary tests. Comprehensive eye examinations may last 45 to 90 minutes, and may require the use of photoropters, keratometers, tonometers, gonioscopy, diagnostic testing, and anesthetic and pupillary dilating eye drops (AAO, 2012a, 2016c; AOA, 2015d).

Vision screenings are tools that allows for the possible identification but not diagnosis of eye disease and conditions. Screenings are available for a variety of diseases and conditions, such as refractive error, eye problems in children, diabetic retinopathy, and age-related macular degeneration (AMD) (AAPOS, 2014; Garg and Davis, 2009; Jain et al., 2006). Vision screenings can be used by both optometrists and ophthalmologists, as well as by other health care professionals, as a public health tool in community settings to identify potential vision problems early and to assist in the collection of evidence-based population vision health data (AAPOS, 2014). Vision screenings are used to identify issues with visual functioning or symptoms suggestive of an eye disease or condition. Box 7-2 lists a number of examples of common vision screening tests.

There is significant debate among professional and advocacy organizations about the role of vision screenings in clinical eye and vision care. Comprehensive eye examinations and vision screenings have different

---

BOX 7-1
Common Procedures Included in Comprehensive Eye Exams

Visual acuity testing—This procedure uses an eye chart to evaluate a patient's ability to see clearly at various distances (Medline Plus, 2015e). This is the primary vision screening tool.

Ocular motility and alignment—This procedure identifies problems with eye movement and alignment. Cover tests may be used to assess eye alignment (Medline Plus, 2015a; Rupp, 2016).

Refraction—This procedure uses a phoropter (i.e., refractor) to make a final determination of refractive status, and to identify patients in need of corrective lenses (Medline Plus, 2015b; University of Michigan, 2015b). In children, refractive error may be assessed by means of cycloplegic retinoscopy (AAO, 2012b; AOA, 2002).

Examination of pupils, lids, adnexa, and anterior segment—These procedures involve observing pupil size and shape in the dark and light, using an indirect light source (Rupp, 2016). The provider will also assess the reactivity of each pupil separately and will check for an afferent pupillary defect (Rupp, 2016). The provider will use a slit lamp—a low-powered microscope combined with a high-intensity light source—to closely examine the eye for abnormalities (Medline Plus, 2015c). The slit lamp shines a high-intensity light into the eye to illuminate the eyelids, adnexa, conjunctiva, iris, lens, sclera, cornea, retina, and optic nerve (Rupp, 2016).

Visual field testing—These procedures measure the size and sensitivity of the visual field, which can be compromised in eye diseases such as glaucoma, diabetic retinopathy, and age-related macular degeneration (Cleveland Clinic, 2015; Medline Plus, 2015f). Optic nerve gliomas, stroke, multiple sclerosis, and other ocular diseases and neurological conditions can also affect the visual field.

Tonometry—This procedure provides a measure of intraocular pressure, by directing a puff of air onto the eye or by applying a pressure-sensitive tip near or against the eye after the application of fluorescein (i.e., Goldman applanation tonometry) (Medline Plus, 2015d; NEI, 2016). The latter method is considered the "gold standard" for this procedure (Rupp, 2016; Stevens et al., 2007). Anesthetic drops may be applied to the eye for these procedures (NEI, 2016).

Dilation—This procedure uses medicated drops to dilate the pupil, allowing an eye care provider to view and assess the inside of the eye with a special magnifying lens (NEI, 2016). Examined tissues include the vitreous, retina, macula, and optic nerve (AAO, 2012a; NEI, 2016).

BOX 7-2
Examples of Vision Screenings

Autorefraction—This procedure uses an autorefractor to quickly determine preliminary refractive status and to identify patients in need of corrective lenses. Research indicates that some autorefractors can accurately detect amblyopia, strabismus, significant refractive error, and reduced visual acuity in children (Schmidt et al., 2004; Ying et al., 2005, 2011).

Cover testing— In these tests, the patient focuses on an object, while the examiner covers each of the patient's eyes in turn to assess for misalignment of the eyes, which is a sign of strabismus (AAPOS, 2014; Kellogg Eye Center, 2015). This is a vision screening for pediatric patients.

Photoscreening—This rapid, automated test is used to identify eye problems in children, such as amblyogenic factors, including strabismus, media opacities, and significant refractive errors. Images of the pupillary and red reflexes are taken with a special camera and then assessed by a computer or eye care professional (AAP, 2002). Photoscreening has been found to have higher screening yield rates among 3-year-old children than screening with eye charts (Lowry et al., 2015).

Red reflex testing—This assessment uses an ophthalmoscope to observe the reflection from a light that is shone on the lining of the inside of the eye. The reflection, or "red reflex," in the two eyes should be bright and equal (AAPOS, 2014). An abnormal red reflex (e.g., asymmetries, dark spots, the presence of a white reflex, a diminished red reflex) can be caused by cataracts, unequal or high refractive error, strabismus, iris or retinal abnormalities, and corneal, aqueous, or vitreous opacities (AAP, 2008d). This is a vision screening for pediatric patients.

Visual acuity testing—This procedure uses an eye chart (i.e., Snellen chart, LEA symbols test, or other letter or symbol chart) to evaluate a patient's ability to see clearly at various distances (Medline Plus, 2015e). This is the primary vision screening test.

---

strengths and weaknesses, and each serves a different role in the promotion of eye and vision health. In general, the findings of eye examinations are more complete, accurate, precise, and broader in scope than the results of vision screening. A comprehensive eye exam is more sensitive and specific and can precisely measure the extent—and identify the cause—of decreased visual acuity and the presence of eye disease and disorders and conditions of the eye and visual system, in addition to providing other assessments of eye health and functioning. The costs of comprehensive eye examinations are briefly mentioned in Chapter 6.

On the other hand, vision screenings have the potential to improve eye and vision health through potentially less expensive and resource-intensive means of identifying specific vision problems, especially in children. For example, visual acuity tests using a letter or symbol chart, autorefractor, or photoscreener can be performed in a few minutes by a school nurse at no cost to the patient, or by primary care providers as part of a comprehensive physical examination. However, the effectiveness of vision screening as a diagnostic tool varies among patient populations, and depends on the screening tools used and the diseases or conditions targeted by screening (Chou et al., 2016a,b; USPSTF, 2011). Furthermore, studies have reported low or inconsistent rates of referral and follow-up care for individuals with abnormal screening results (Hartmann et al., 2006; Hered and Wood, 2013; Kemper et al., 2011).

The cost-effectiveness of screening can be sensitive to the eye disease or conditions and vision impairment risk profile of the targeted population, the screening interval, the diagnostic accuracy of screening tools, the staffing models used in a screening program, the rate of follow-up after abnormal screening results, the efficacy of available clinical treatments, and numerous other factors. Research on these and other issues is needed, but remains limited (Azuara-Blanco et al., 2016; Blumberg et al., 2014; Burr et al., 2007; Ladapo et al., 2012). The cost-effectiveness of vision screenings and comprehensive eye examinations is considered further in Chapter 6.

Conflicting study results and relatively limited research on the cost-effectiveness of vision screenings for specific eye diseases and conditions and comprehensive eye examinations for asymptomatic patients can also impede efforts to align existing guidelines (see, e.g., AHRQ, 2012; Burr et al., 2007; Gangwani et al., 2014; Jones and Edwards, 2010; Karnon et al., 2008; Rein et al., 2012a,b).

Advancing Evidence-Based Guidelines

Guidelines for Comprehensive Eye Examinations

Although comprehensive eye examinations are generally accepted as the gold standard in clinical vision care to most accurately identify and diagnose eye and vision problems, different professional groups often disagree on the age and frequency at which different patient groups should specific services. Both the American Academy of Ophthalmology and AOA recommend that at-risk populations receive more frequent eye exams. For example, the American Academy of Ophthalmology and AOA guidelines and/or policy statements both indicate that the frequency of age-related eye examinations should increase with advancing age, but AOA supports shorter intervals for testing at each age (AAO, 2015a; AOA, 2015d). In addition, AOA recommends that persons ages 18 to 39 without symptoms or risk factors be seen at least every 2 years, whereas the American

Academy of Ophthalmology states that "a routine comprehensive annual adult eye examination in individuals under age 40 unnecessarily escalates the cost of eye care" and is not indicated without specific risk factors or symptoms (AAO, 2015a; AOA, 2015d). Table 7-1 compares AAO and AOA guidelines on the frequency of comprehensive eye examinations for patients by age group with and without risk factors or symptoms.

TABLE 7-1 Comparison of AAO and AOA Guidelines for Frequency of Comprehensive Eye Examinations for Adults

AAO			AOA		
Ages	Without Risk Factors or Symptoms[a]	Higher Risk Groups[b]	Ages	Without Risk Factors or Symptoms[c]	At-Risk Groups[d]
Adults under age 40	5–10 years[e]	Every 1–2 years	18–39	At least every 2 years[f]	At least annually or as recommended
40–54	Every 2–4 years[g]	Every 1–3 years	40–64	At least every 2 years[h]	At least annually or as recommended
55–64	Every 1–3 years	Every 1–2 years			
65 and older	Every 1–2 years	Every 1–2 years	65 and older	Annually[h]	At least annually or as recommended

[a] Intervals in this column apply to individuals who lack "symptoms or other indications following the initial comprehensive medical eye evaluation." These intervals account for "the relationship between increasing age and the risk of asymptomatic or undiagnosed disease" (AAO, 2016c).

[b] Intervals in this column apply to individuals with glaucoma risk factors. The recommended frequency of eye exams varies among eye disease risk factors (AAO, 2016c).

[c] Intervals in this column apply to "asymptomatic, low risk" individuals (AOA, 2015d).

[d] Intervals in this column apply to "[p]ersons who notice vision changes, those at higher risk for the development of eye and vision problems, and individuals with a family history of eye disease." AOA states that "adult patients should be advised by their doctor to seek eye care more frequently than the recommended re-examination interval if new ocular, visual, or systemic health problems develop" (AOA, 2015d).

[e] AAO states that "routine comprehensive annual adult eye examination in individuals under the age of 40 unnecessarily escalates the cost of eye care" and is not indicated without specific risk factors or symptoms (AAO, 2015a).

[f] AOA Consensus-Based Action Statement (AOA, 2015d).

[g] AAO states that "[a]dults with no signs or risk factors for eye disease should receive a comprehensive medical eye evaluation at age 40 if they have not previously received one" (AAO, 2016c).

[h] AOA Evidence-Based Action Statement (AOA, 2015d).

SOURCES: AAO, 2015a, 2016c; AOA, 2015d.

Guidelines for pediatric populations may also differ. For example, AOA guidelines on pediatric eye and vision examinations recommend comprehensive eye examinations for both asymptomatic/risk-free and at-risk pediatric patients. Table 7-2 details AOA recommendations on the frequency of pediatric eye examinations. By comparison, the American Academy of Ophthalmology states that "[c]omprehensive eye examinations are not necessary (but can be performed) for healthy asymptomatic children who have passed an acceptable vision screening test, have no subjective visual symptoms, and have no personal or familial risk factors for eye disease" (AAO, 2012b). It further recommends eye examinations for children who "fail a vision screening, are untestable, have a vision complaint or an observed abnormal visual behavior, or are at risk for the development of eye problems" and, where appropriate, for children with learning disabilities to rule out the presence of eye and vision problems, and for children with intellectual disabilities, neuropsychological conditions, or behavioral issues that cause them to be otherwise untestable (AAO, 2012b).

The American Academy of Ophthalmology and AOA guidelines for the evaluation and treatment of specific eye diseases may also vary in terms of the recommended frequency of eye care. For example, the American Academy of Ophthalmology guidelines on primary open-angle glaucoma

TABLE 7-2 AOA Recommended Frequency of Comprehensive Eye Examinations for Pediatric Patients

Age	Asymptomatic/Risk-Free	At-Risk
Birth to 24 months	At 6 months of age	At 6 months of age or as recommended
2–5 years	At 3 years of age	At 3 years of age or as recommended
6–18 years	Before first grade and every 2 years thereafter	Annually or as recommended

NOTES: AOA states that "[t]he extent to which a child is at risk for the development of eye and vision problems determines the appropriate re-evaluation schedule. Individuals with ocular signs and symptoms require prompt examination. Furthermore, the presence of certain risk factors may necessitate more frequent examinations, based on professional judgement" (AOA, 2002). According to AOA, the factors placing an infant, toddler, or child at significant risk for visual impairment include "prematurity, low birth weight, prolonged supplemental oxygen, or grade III or IV intraventricular hemorrhage; a family history of retinoblastoma, congenital cataracts, or metabolic or genetic disease; infection of mother during pregnancy (e.g., rubella, toxoplasmosis, venereal disease, herpes, cytomegalovirus, or human immunodeficiency virus); difficult or assisted labor, which may be associated with fetal distress or low Apgar scores; high refractive error; strabismus; anisometropia; known or suspected central nervous system dysfunction evidenced by developmental delay, cerebral palsy, dysmorphic features, seizures, or hydrocephalus" (AOA, 2002).
SOURCE: AOA, 2002.

recommend follow-up evaluations for glaucoma patients from every 1 to 2 months to at least once every 12 months, depending on the duration of control of intraocular pressure (IOP), the extent of progression of glaucomatous damage, and whether the patient's target IOP is reached (AAO, 2015b). By comparison, the frequency of follow-up glaucoma evaluations recommended by AOA varies by patient status and the stability and severity of disease, ranging from weekly or biweekly evaluations for new glaucoma patients or patients with unstable IOP, progressing optic nerve damage, or visual field loss, to once every 6 to 12 months for suspected cases of glaucoma, depending on a particular patient's risk (AOA, 2011).[2]

Vision Screening Guidelines

Guidelines specific to vision screenings may also differ and, in some instances, even contradict one another. In a joint policy statement on pediatric vision screenings in community, school, and primary care settings, the American Academy of Ophthalmology and the American Association for Pediatric Ophthalmology and Strabismus (AAPOS) stated that "routine comprehensive professional eye examinations performed on normal asymptomatic children have no proven medical benefit" (AAO, 2013, p. 3). Instead, the American Academy of Pediatrics (AAP), the American Association of Certified Orthoptists (AACO), AAPOS, and the American Academy of Ophthalmology jointly recommended that pediatricians assess the visual system beginning in infancy and continuing at regular intervals throughout childhood and adolescence. They also suggested that serial visual system screenings in the medical home, using validated techniques, could provide an effective mechanism for the detection and subsequent referral of potentially treatable visual system disorders (AAP et al., 2016). Table 7-3 details the joint pediatric vision screening recommendations.

Conversely, AOA does not generally recommend vision screenings (AOA, 2015d, 2016c). AOA argues that screening is not effective in detecting eye and vision health problems (AOA, 2016c). Moreover, AOA argues

---

[2] According to the American Academy of Ophthalmology and AOA guidelines on primary open-angle glaucoma, care of patients with glaucoma includes initial and follow-up glaucoma evaluations (AAO, 2015b; AOA, 2011). Initial glaucoma evaluations include many of components of a comprehensive eye examination in addition to procedures or tests specific to diagnosis of glaucoma. For follow-up glaucoma evaluations, the American Academy of Ophthalmology guidelines state that evaluation involves "clinical examination of the patient, including optic nerve head assessment (with periodic color stereophotography or computerized imaging of the optic nerve and retinal nerve fiber layer structure) and visual field assessment" (AAO, 2015b, p. 76). AOA guidelines state that follow-up evaluations are similar to the initial evaluation and may include patient history, visual acuity, blood pressure and pulse, biomicroscopy, tonometry, gonioscopy, optic nerve assessment, nerve fiber layer assessment, fundus photography, and automated perimetry, among other procedures (AOA, 2011).

TABLE 7-3 AAP, AAO, AAPOS, and AACO Joint Recommendations on Frequency of Visual System Assessment in Asymptomatic Infants, Children, and Young Adults by Pediatricians

Assessment	Newborn to 6 Months	6–12 Months	1–3 Years	4–5 Years	6 Years and Older
Ocular history	X	X	X	X	X
External inspection of lids and eyes	X	X	X	X	X
Red reflex testing	X	X	X	X	X
Pupil examination	X	X	X	X	X
Ocular motility assessment		X	X	X	X
Instrument-based screening when available		X[a]	X	X	X[b]
Visual acuity fixate and follow response	X[c]	X	X		
Visual acuity age-appropriate optotype assessment			X[d]	X	X

[a] AAO recommends instrument-based screening at age 6 months. However, the rate of false-positive results is high for this age group, and the likelihood of ophthalmic intervention is low. A future AAO policy statement will likely reconcile what appears to be a discrepancy.
[b] Instrument-based screening at any age is suggested if the care provider is unable to test visual acuity monocularly with age-appropriate optotypes.
[c] The development of fixating on and following a target should occur by 6 months of age; children who do not meet this milestone should be referred.
[d] Visual acuity screening may be attempted in cooperative 3-year-old children.
SOURCE: AAP et al., 2016.

that vision screening promotes a "false sense of security" and delays treatment for individuals with eye diseases or conditions (AOA, 2016c). Draft guidelines on pediatric eye and vision examination currently available on AOA's website for comment state that "age-appropriate examination strategies should be used" for infants and toddlers, whereas preschool-age and school-age children are more cooperative with traditional eye and vision tests, although some modifications may still be necessary (AOA, 2016, p. 13). AOA guidelines on the care of patients with amblyopia state that "screening for causes of form deprivation amblyopia should be conducted by the infant's primary care physician within the first 4 to 6 weeks after birth, and children at risk should be monitored yearly throughout the sensitive developmental period (birth to 6 to 8 years of age)" (AOA, 2004, p. 12). AOA is currently updating its clinical practice guidelines, many of which are almost 15 years old, to better reflect recent research.[3] Again, the import of these examples is not to endorse or criticize a particular set of

---

[3] Personal communication, R. Peele, American Optometric Association, September 6, 2016.

guidelines, but rather to highlight conflicting information available to the public and health care providers.

Lack of guideline consistency is exacerbated by separate guidelines for primary care providers and related evidentiary standards. The U.S. Preventive Services Task Force (USPSTF) issues evidence-based recommendations that assess the balance of benefits and harms of preventative services provided to asymptomatic patients in a primary care setting or by a primary care clinician (USPSTF, 2016a).[4] In 2013, the USPSTF concluded that current evidence "was insufficient to assess the balance of benefits and harms of screening for primary open-angle glaucoma (POAG) in adults," citing the inadequacy of available evidence (USPSTF, 2013).[5] USPSTF found no studies that directly evaluated the impact of glaucoma screening on the prevention of visual field loss, vision impairment, or worsened quality of life, nor any direct evidence demonstrating screening-related harm. Evidence on the accuracy of glaucoma screening was inadequate, and the risks of inaccurate diagnosis associated with glaucoma screening were recognized (Moyer, 2013; USPSTF, 2013). Similar conclusions were reached regarding visual acuity screening of asymptomatic adults ages 65 and older (USPSTF, 2016a). The USPSTF concluded that "evidence [was] insufficient to assess the balance of benefits and harms of screening for impaired visual acuity in older adults" (USPSTF, 2016c, p. 908). In particular, although evidence supporting the benefits of early treatment of refractive error, cataracts, and AMD was deemed adequate, three randomized controlled trials (RCTs) found no association between visual acuity screening of adults ages 65 and older and improved clinical outcomes (Chou et al., 2016b; USPSTF, 2016c).

In contrast, visual acuity screening by a primary care provider of all children ages 3 to 5 years to detect amblyopia or amblyopia risk factors received a B grade recommendation (USPSTF, 2011). The USPSTF found adequate evidence that the early treatment of amblyopia is associated with improved vision outcomes and that vision screening tools are reasonably

---

[4] USPSTF recommendations are graded according to the strength of evidence identified by literature review. Grade A recommendations are used when "[t]here is high certainty that the net benefit is substantial." Grade B recommendations are used when "[t]here is high certainty that the net benefit is moderate or there is moderate certainty that the net benefit is moderate to substantial." Grade C and D recommendations are used when there is moderate certainty that the net benefit is small or there is evidence of harm or lack of benefit (USPSTF, 2016b). The Patient Protection and Affordable Care Act of 2010 permits the secretary of the U.S. Department of Health and Human Services to authorize Medicare coverage of preventative services that receive an A or B grade from the USPSTF. Therefore, although the USPSTF does not account for the cost of a service when assessing its benefits and harms, its recommendations nevertheless have consequences for Medicare payment policy and care access (Lesser et al., 2011).

[5] USPSTF I statements are used when "[e]vidence is lacking, of poor quality, or conflicting, and the balance of benefits and harms cannot be determined" (USPSTF, 2016b).

accurate at detecting refractive error, strabismus, and amblyopia. There was limited evidence on the harms of screening. Although a literature review found limited direct evidence supporting the comparative benefit of screening over not screening in pediatric populations, USPSTF noted that good evidence supporting the accuracy of screening methods and the effectiveness of treatments suggests that screening is more likely to lead to improved eye health than no screening (Chou et al., 2011; USPSTF, 2011). USPSTF I statements include information on clinical considerations (e.g., potential preventable burden, potential harm of the intervention, costs, and current practice) in an effort to provide guidance to primary care providers in the absence of a recommendation (Petitti et al., 2009).

Some experts have criticized the USPSTF methodology, especially when rigorous evidentiary standards contribute to the proliferation of I statements that provide limited clinical guidance. For example, Lee (2016) noted that the methodological and financial challenges of conducting an RCT on the impact of visual acuity screening among asymptomatic older adults poses a barrier to the production of evidence that could lead to a conclusive recommendation. Parke and colleagues (2016), commenting on the same recommendation, noted that the review discounted strong evidence on the negative health consequences of vision impairment. Others have noted that the high standards for evidence quality and the narrow focus of questions informing USPSTF literature reviews limit the scope of recommendations and their value as tools to guide clinical decisions (Donahue and Ruben, 2011; Sommer, 2016).

Developing a unified set of evidence-based clinical and rehabilitation guidelines could serve to guide payment policies and address inconsistencies, coverage gaps, and duplicative or wasteful spending. Recent initial attempts by the American Academy of Ophthalmology, the American Society of Cataract and Refractive Surgery, and the American Academy of Optometry to foster such unification through joint educational initiatives or integrated care delivery have highlighted the opportunity for providers to engage one another and promote quality, efficient care (AAO/AAO, 2013; Bailey, 2013).

Assessing the Quality of Guidelines for Eye and Vision Care

In its 2011 report *Clinical Practice Guidelines We Can Trust*, the IOM highlighted the need for a set of standards that clinical guidelines must meet in order to be trustworthy and serve as a framework for provider decision making (IOM, 2011b). This will require systematic reviews of the evidence, including research question identification, adherence to evidentiary standards, and a compilation of all findings that meets the standard (IOM, 2011a,b). According to the IOM, the evidence should be used to

---

BOX 7-3
The Standards for Development of Trustworthy
Clinical Practice Guidelines

- Establishing transparency
- Management of conflict of interest
- Guideline development group composition
- Clinical practice guideline–systematic review intersection
- Establishing evidence foundations for and rating strength of recommendations
- Articulation of recommendations
- External review
- Updating

SOURCE: IOM, 2011a.

---

establish guidelines, which are reviewed and updated every 3 to 5 years (IOM, 2011a). This will require an ongoing commitment to a rigorous evidence-based guideline development process and greater collaboration among professional groups. Box 7-3 includes a list of specific standards from which to assess guideline quality.

Unfortunately, limited research suggests that many existing guidelines, in general, do not meet these standards. For example, a 2012 review of 114 guidelines found that only 49.1 percent met more than half of 18 selected IOM standards (Kung et al., 2012). Other assessment tools, such as the Appraisal of Guidelines for Research and Evaluation II instrument, can be used to assess the quality of guidelines in terms of their scope and purpose, stakeholder involvement, rigor of development, clarity of presentation, applicability, and editorial independence.[6] Several peer-reviewed evaluations of the quality of AAO guidelines are available (Wu et al., 2015a,b,c,d; Young et al., 2015). The committee did not find any similar assessments of AOA guidelines in the published literature. Although the committee was not constituted to evaluate or identify the most effective tools for evaluating guidelines for eye and vision health, it is important that the development of evidence-based guidelines adhere to particular standards, to the extent possible, to ensure robust and comprehensive support for recommended actions.

---

[6] The Appraisal of Guidelines for Research and Evaluation (AGREE) and AGREE II instruments are frequently used in clinical practice guideline (CPG) evaluations. All CPG evaluations referred to in this report use AGREE or AGREE II. See Brouwers et al. (2010) for a description and comparison of the tools.

The committee acknowledges efforts within the eye and vision field to improve professional guidelines. The American Academy of Ophthalmology and AOA have made efforts to improve and ensure the quality of their respective guidelines. According to Lum and colleagues (2016), the American Academy of Ophthalmology guidelines are "based on the best available scientific data as interpreted by panels of knowledgeable physicians and methodologists"—in cases where data are not persuasive, guideline development groups must "rely on both their collective experience and the evaluation of current evidence" (p. 928). The American Academy of Ophthalmology guideline development process includes the identification, limitation, and management of conflicts of interest through an adherence to codes set by the Council of Medical Specialty Societies, and review by several medical societies and relevant patient organizations. The American Academy of Ophthalmology guidelines use standardized methods to grade the quality of individual studies, the quality of the body of evidence supporting recommendations, and the strength of recommendations.[7] Barring revisions, the American Academy of Ophthalmology guidelines are valid for 5 years after their release date (AAO, 2016e). As of May 2016, 22 AAO Preferred Practice Pattern® guidelines were listed on the AAO website (AAO, 2016a).

AOA has developed 18 consensus-based guidelines and two evidence-based guidelines, Eye Care of the Patient with Diabetes Mellitus, and the Comprehensive Adult Eye and Vision Examination (AOA, 2014, 2015d).[8] AOA has created a 14-step process for developing evidence-based guidelines and states that its Evidence-Based Optometry Committee is revising optometric guidelines in response to the IOM standards for trustworthy guidelines (AOA, 2015c, 2016a). AOA evidence-based guidelines use scales to grade the strength of evidence and recommendations and offer a guideline development process that includes steps to manage conflicts of interest and allow for peer and public review (AOA, 2014, 2015d).[9] AOA evidence-based guidelines state that the guidelines should be revised every 2 to 5 years (AOA, 2014, 2015d). Unfortunately, statements in AOA consensus-

---

[7] AAO uses the Scottish Intercollegiate Guideline Network and the Grading of Recommendations Assessment, Development and Evaluation methods for grading evidence quality and recommendation strength. For details, see the Methods and Key to Ratings section of an AAO Preferred Practice Pattern guideline.

[8] At the time of writing, a third clinical practice guideline (Comprehensive Pediatric Eye and Vision Examination) was under revision, and a draft version of the document was available for peer and public review.

[9] The evidence and recommendation grading tools as described in the AOA evidence-based guidelines on Eye Care of the Patient with Diabetes Mellitus and on Comprehensive Adult Eye and Vision Examination are not identical. For details, see the How to Use This Guideline sections of these guidelines.

based guidelines, such as the guidelines on Pediatric Eye and Vision Examination, do not always provide information on the graded strength of this evidence or of the statements it supports (AOA, 2002). Similarly, the AOA consensus guidelines on Pediatric Eye and Vision Examination do not include information on the guideline development process, including methods of literature review, management of conflicts of interest, or external review (AOA, 2002). AOA consensus-based guidelines, such as the guidelines on Pediatric Eye and Vision Examination, state that the guidelines will be reviewed periodically and revised as needed (AOA, 2002).[10]

Improving the Consistency of Eye and Vision Care Guidelines

Coming to consensus on recommended care is critical to create clear messaging that targets both patients and non–eye care providers about the need for regular eye care services. From a population health perspective, prioritizations for guideline development should be influenced by the number of people affected, the severity and reversibility of vision loss that can occur, the diversity with which the condition is currently managed, the number of health care professionals who typically engage with patients about a specific disease or condition, and the breadth of the literature currently available. This might be of most relevance for guidance on the frequency of eye examinations and may be supported by federal guidance on what factors (e.g., frequency, severity, preventability, treatability, difference between current and optimal practice) should be used in consensus-based and evidence-based recommendations.

A collaborative and inclusive working group would be useful to establish a single set of guidelines that are coherent, comprehensive, and clear about what services are required at what intervals, and how best to connect patients to necessary follow-up care. The process for conducting a systematic review of existing evidence and distilling guidelines from that evidence is a lengthy process, and collaboration throughout the eye and vision care field (including federal and state governmental entities that focus on eye and vision health) will be paramount. This collaborative process can also help identify research gaps to promote a shared research agenda.

---

[10] The AOA consensus-based guideline on Care of the Patient with Learning Related Vision Problems states that the guideline "will be reviewed periodically" (AOA, 2008, p. ii). All other consensus-based guidelines state that the guideline will be "will be reviewed periodically and revised as needed."

ASSESSING QUALITY AND IMPROVEMENT INITIATIVES

Focusing on quality improvement as an overarching goal can help standardize and promote high-quality care; in turn, high-quality care can address factors that contribute to poor and inequitable eye and vision health care. Continuous quality improvement (CQI) is a "process-based, data-driven approach to improving the quality of a product or service through iterative cycles of action and evaluation" (RWJF, 2012, p. 1). Rather than a short-term, single-issue quality improvement and assurance initiative, CQI focuses on correcting the root causes of systemic issues through an iterative quality improvement process. This process complements the public health wheel (see Chapter 1), which depicts population health as an iterative process of assessment, policy development, and assurance.

Figure 7-1 presents a common CQI framework adapted for eye and vision care. In this figure, the CQI process is a five-step process: guideline development, practice change, performance monitoring, surveillance and data analysis, and identification of opportunities for improvement. An adherence to established guidelines provides the baseline from which to

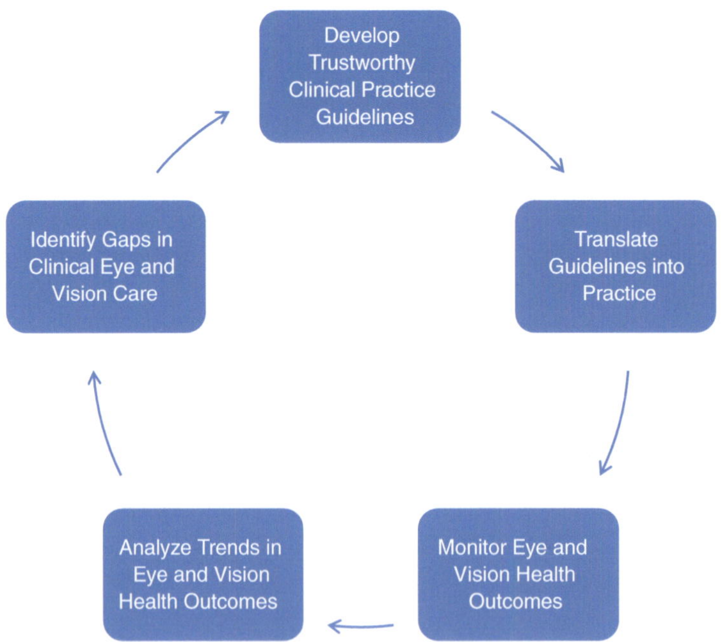

FIGURE 7-1 Continuous quality improvement framework.
SOURCE: Adapted from Kneib, 2009.

measure impact on health outcomes and improvement over time. Development of evidence-based guidelines requires sufficient research and data. The rapid and accurate translation of guidelines into daily practice may require the development and provision of educational materials and training programs informed by translational and implementation science. Tracking patient outcomes and process and performance measures of the health care system requires a broad set of surveillance and monitoring tools, including electronic health records (EHRs). Data analysis may require the expertise of statisticians, epidemiologists, health informaticians, and other public health and quality improvement specialists. Identifying opportunities for improved patient outcomes and health care system performance can then inform revisions of evidence-based guidelines, which can help accelerate policy changes that better support eye and vision health.

An effective CQI process requires organizational champions and committed leadership. A number of government agencies, educational organizations, and professional groups are involved in CQI activities or efforts that could facilitate a CQI process, to improve the quality of eye and vision care. The Health Resources and Services Administration (HRSA) is one of a number of agencies and organizations that provide guidance and tools to help stakeholders design, implement, sustain, and spread quality improvement within a health care system (HRSA, 2011). Toolkits have been developed to promote CQI in eye and vision health (Brien Holden Vision Institute, 2016). AOA and the American Academy of Ophthalmology have launched patient registries as part of larger quality improvement efforts (AAO, 2016b; AOA, 2015b).[11] Patient registries can promote improvements in care quality by enabling providers to assess the effectiveness of treatment, analyze their performance for improvement opportunities, and monitor patient outcomes. Data from patient registries may also be used to inform policy, monitor the effectiveness of treatments across populations, and identify public health issues (Kent, 2015). The U.S. Department of Veterans Affairs (VA) has employed its Quality Enhancement Research Initiative to identify opportunities for improving eye care and preventing vision loss among veterans with diabetes (Krein et al., 2008). The Diabetes Recognition Program of the National Committee for Quality Assurance (NCQA) recognizes physicians for complying with diabetes care quality measures, which include the appropriate referral of diabetic patients for eye examination (NCQA, 2016b). In January 2016, HRSA announced a funding opportunity for rural providers to participate in a Small Health Care Provider Quality Improvement Program, and it listed eye exams for diabetic patients as an optional quality measure (HRSA, 2016b). Although evidence

---

[11] See Chapter 4 for further detail on the AOA and American Academy of Ophthalmology registries.

on the impact of these efforts and programs on eye care quality and patient outcomes is limited, their existence points to an increased emphasis on CQI in eye and vision care. These efforts can be used as a foundation from which to implement subsequent CQI initiatives.

Quality improvement is also being explicitly built into grants that support eye and vision health in communities. For example, the National Institute for Children's Health Quality has partnered with the National Center for Children's Vision & Eye Health at Prevent Blindness on a 3-year, HRSA-funded project to support the development of comprehensive and coordinated approaches to children's vision and eye health in five states (NICHQ, 2015). The project will employ quality improvement (QI) principles and practices to strengthen statewide partnerships and stakeholder coordination, increase accessibility of eye care in remote communities, increase early detection and treatment of eye diseases, establish state-level surveillance, and implement accountability measures (NICHQ, 2015). As more eye and vision professionals participate in accountable care organizations or other pay-for-performance initiatives in the value-driven health care landscape, CQI will play an increasingly important role in clinical eye and vision care.

A number of organizations, including the National Quality Forum (NQF), Physician Consortium for Performance Improvement, NCQA, and Agency for Healthcare Research and Quality, have identified and developed, or evaluated and endorsed, quality improvement measures and metrics that can be used for CQI activities (AHRQ, 2016a; AMA, 2016; NCQA, 2016a; NQF, 2016c). The NQF has endorsed several quality measures related to counseling and eye examinations for patients with AMD, eye examination and follow-up care for patients with diabetic retinopathy, examination of the optic nerve head and treatment outcomes for patients with glaucoma, and complications and outcomes after cataract surgery.[12] Unfortunately, NQF has not endorsed—and the National Quality Measures Clearinghouse does not list—other measures related to eye and vision care, including those pertaining to vision screening and the subsequent referral and follow-up of adult patients, referral to vision rehabilitation and support services for patients with irreversible vision impairment, correction of identified

---

[12] NQF-endorsed, eye care–related quality measures include Primary Open-Angle Glaucoma: Optic Nerve Evaluation (NQF-0086); Age-Related Macular Degeneration: Dilated Macular Examination (NQF-0087); Diabetic Retinopathy: Documentation of Presence or Absence of Macular Edema and Level of Severity of Retinopathy (NQF-0088); Diabetic Retinopathy: Communication with the Physician Managing Ongoing Diabetes Care (NQF-0089); Primary Open-Angle Glaucoma: Reduction of Intraocular Pressure by 15% or Documentation of a Plan of Care (NQF-0563); Cataracts: Complications Within 30 Days Following Cataract Surgery Requiring Additional Surgical Procedures (NQF-0564); Cataracts: 20/40 or Better Visual Acuity Within 90 Days Following Cataract Surgery (NQF-0565); and Age-Related Macular Degeneration: Counseling on Antioxidant Supplement (NQF-0566).

refractive error, or patient counseling on modifiable risk factors for eye disease. To support the CQI process, research to build the evidence base informing these and other quality these measures will need to be pursued.

Pursuing a CQI research agenda will require collaboration among investigators working in multiple areas, as well as the dedication of funding, tools, and facilities. It will also require a population health surveillance system capable of collecting data on myriad facets of the vision care system and the populations and communities it serves (see Chapter 4). These surveillance data are necessary for the implementation of a successful CQI program to improve the performance of the vision care system.

PROMOTING DIAGNOSIS AND FOLLOW-UP CARE TRANSITIONS THROUGH INTEGRATION

Identifying who needs what care at what time is only part of the equation to promoting appropriate eye care. In many cases, especially in the context of vision screening, additional follow-up care will be necessary to provide prescription lenses or other types of clinical treatments or monitoring. Despite advances in the clinical treatments for major eye diseases that have dramatically improved population eye and vision health, many barriers to care delivery remain. Structural separations between optometry, ophthalmology, and primary care may contribute to inconsistent referral practices, poor communication, inappropriate or delayed referrals, and interruptions in care continuity, as reported in studies assessing the state of primary care–specialty referrals (Mehrotra et al., 2011; Wiggins et al., 2013). The integration of primary care and eye and vision care, as modeled in the patient-centered medical home and accountable care organizations, holds potential as a strategy for improving coordination and communication between providers in primary care and those in eye and vision care. EHRs and other health informatics tools can contribute to integration by enabling secure data sharing among providers.

Referrals Within and Across Professional Lines

According to the World Health Organization (WHO), collaborative practice occurs when "multiple health workers from different professional backgrounds provide comprehensive services by working with patients, their families, caregivers, and communities to deliver the highest quality of care across settings" (WHO, 2010, p. 13). Beyond simply raising public awareness about the roles, competencies, and services of eye and vision care professionals and ensuring an adequate workforce to meet patient needs (see Chapter 6), it is important to recognize that eye and vision health is the domain of all types of health care providers. For example, eye and vision care providers can help identify risk factors as well as detect and help manage many chronic diseases. For example, comprehensive dilated eye exams can detect retinal vascular changes that may suggest hypertension or diabetes, reveal cholesterol plaques within retinal arteries that indicate risk of stroke, and detect tumors, among other things (Chous and Knabel, 2014). Similarly, by providing vision screenings and referring patients as appropriate to eye and vision care providers, primary care providers can help identify potentially vision-threatening problems and refer patients to an ophthalmologist or optometrist for a comprehensive eye examination to make a definitive diagnosis, establishing productive and ongoing professional relationships. An investigation of the referral patterns of 136 family physicians found that referrals to ophthalmologists were more likely than referrals to other medical specialties to result in long-term (as compared to short-term) referrals or consultations and in the transfer of patient management (Starfield et al., 2002). However, the study also found that family physicians referred patients with diabetes to ophthalmologists in only 27 of 56 cases, with remaining referrals directed primarily to endocrinologists and nutritionists.

Eye and vision health is also relevant to health care providers beyond primary care physicians. Often, vision impairment is a manifestation or consequence of a disease that requires the expertise of other health care specialists involved in the coordination of care. For example, visual impairment is a key symptom of multiple sclerosis (Balcer et al., 2015). The American Academy of Neurology's current practice parameter on the diagnostic assessment of children with cerebral palsy notes that vision impairment and disorders of ocular motility occur in 28 percent of children with cerebral palsy and recommends that this patient population receive vision screenings (Ashwal et al., 2004). Endocrinology is another specialty that frequently intersects with vision care, particularly in diabetes management.

Physician assistants and nurse practitioners provide at least 11 percent of all outpatient medical services in the United States, and are more likely to practice in rural areas than primary care physicians (16 percent versus 11 percent) (AHRQ, 2014a; Hooker and Everett, 2012). The inclusion of nurse practitioners and physician assistants in patient care is associated with decreased health care costs, higher-quality care, and improved patient outcomes (Hooker and Everett, 2012; Reuben et al., 2013; Roblin et al., 2004). However, research indicates that nurse practitioners or physician assistants seldom practice in ophthalmology. The 2013 Annual Survey Report of the American Academy of Physician Assistants found that only 10 out of 15,798 responding physician assistants worked in ophthalmology as a primary specialty (AAPA, 2014). A report by the American Association of Nurse Practitioners (AANP) on nurse practitioner practice environments did not include ophthalmology as a subspecialty in which nurse practitioners actively practiced (AANP, 2015). In addition, specialty certification and postgraduate training focused on ophthalmology is not available for nurse practitioners or physician assistants. The AANP Certification Program does not offer certification in ophthalmic care (AANPCP, 2016). The National Commission on Certification of Physician Assistants offers specialty certifications, but not in ophthalmology (NCCPA, 2016). The Association of Postgraduate Physician Assistant Programs compiles a list of current postgraduate programs; although none of these programs focuses specifically on ophthalmology, several programs include clinical or surgical rotations in ophthalmology (APPAP, 2016).[13] For registered nurses specializing in ophthalmic care, certification through the National Certifying Board for Ophthalmic Registered Nurses is available but not required (ASORN, 2016).

Unfortunately, referrals to ophthalmologists and optometrists from other health care professionals remain suboptimal, for various reasons. Holley and Lee (2010) interviewed focus groups of nurse practitioners, physician assistants, and rural and academic primary care physicians in order to identify barriers to referring patients to eye care. The three most commonly cited barriers were "no/little feedback from eye care providers" (27.5 percent of comments), followed by "patient's lack of finances/insurance coverage" (25.5 percent), and "difficulty in scheduling ophthalmology appointments" (15.7 percent) (p. 1867).[14] The most common suggestions for improving referral to eye care involved implementing shared electronic medical records (26.5 percent of comments), improving eye care provider communication and feedback (22.4 percent), and having ophthalmologists in primary care clinics on an intermittent basis (18.4 percent) (Holley and Lee, 2010).[15] Thus, there is an opportunity for both eye care professionals and the medical establishment to capitalize on shared interests and concern for patients. By considering referrals to be part of whole patient care, health care providers contribute to practices that may lead to improvements across multiple measures of health.

---

[13] The Emergency Medicine physician assistant (PA) residency at Johns Hopkins University, the PA Postgraduate Fellowship in Emergency Medicine at Albany Medical Center, the Emergency Medicine PA Residency at the University of California, San Francisco (UCSF) Fresno, the Surgery Physician Assistant Fellowship at the Texas Children's Hospital, and the Emergency Medicine PA/Nurse Practitioner (NP) Residency Program at Yale New Haven Hospital all include clinical or surgical rotations in ophthalmology (APPAP, 2016).

[14] Percentages are calculated. Out of 51 total comments, 14 were categorized as "No/little feedback from eye care providers" [(14/51) × 100 = 27.5 percent], 13 were categorized as "Patient's lack of finances/insurance coverage" [(13/51) × 100 = 25.5 percent], and 8 were categorized as "Difficulty in scheduling ophthalmology appointment" [(8/51) × 100 = 15.7 percent].

[15] Percentages are calculated. Out of 49 total comments, 13 were categorized as "Implement electronic medical records" [(13/49) × 100 = 26.5 percent], 11 were categorized as "Better communication/feedback from ECPs" [(11/49) × 100 = 22.4 percent], and 9 were categorized as "Have ophthalmologists in primary care clinic on certain days" [(9/49) × 100 = 18.4 percent].

Models of Integrated Eye and Vision Care in the United States

Integrated models of care improve efficiencies within the medical establishment to facilitate coordinated, patient-centered care across multiple providers in a time when the increasing prevalence of chronic conditions, such as chronic vision impairment, and age-related diseases require more value-conscious health care systems. For purposes of this report, the term "integrated care" refers to any model of care designed to promote collaborative practice for the purposes of improving eye and vision care access and quality.

Unfortunately, the research on the distribution, frequency, cost, effectiveness, and cost-effectiveness of models of integrated vision care in the United States is limited. A number of studies have documented international efforts to improve referral patterns between general practitioners, ophthalmologists, and optometrists and to implement referral-only diagnostic services for patients with common eye diseases in order to improve the referral process and reduce costs and patient load on secondary and tertiary services. These efforts have met with some success (Bourne et al., 2010; Jamous et al., 2015; Mandalos et al., 2012; Voyatzis et al., 2014). Several of these studies have highlighted the need for new or additional training to effectively implement referral centers. Although these studies can be instructional in identifying factors to consider when designing interventions within the United States, they have limited applicability in the United States because of the differences in how health care systems are structured.

Several recent international investigations have highlighted the success of integrated care models at decreasing the costs of health care, increasing the efficiency of health systems, and improving patient outcomes. For example, an RTC conducted in the Netherlands compared different methods of monitoring glaucoma patients and found that eye care provided to stable glaucoma patients and patients at risk of glaucoma by ophthalmic technicians and optometrists working in hospital-based glaucoma follow-up units was equal in quality and lower in cost than care provided by hospital-based residents and ophthalmologists specializing in glaucoma care (Holtzer-Goor et al., 2010).[16] Compared to monitoring of stable glaucoma patients and patients at-risk of glaucoma by glaucoma specialists (i.e., ophthalmologists specializing in glaucoma) and residents, monitoring of these patients by a

---

[16] Care quality was measured in terms of provider compliance to a predetermined care protocol; multiple indicators of patient satisfaction; the stability of the patient according to practitioner, as measured by changes in the duration of intervals between patient visits; difference between IOP at baseline and at study conclusion; examination results; and the number of treatment changes. There were no statistically significant differences between the care provided by glaucoma specialists or residents and the care provided by optometrists and ophthalmic technicians for any of the care quality measures. Patients randomized to receive care from the glaucoma follow-up unit were seen by an ophthalmologist every third visit, or sooner if necessary.

glaucoma follow-up unit staffed by optometrists and ophthalmic technicians was associated with a high probability of reduced costs of care to the patient (78 percent probability of reduced costs of care), to the hospital (98 percent probability of reduced costs of care), to the health care system (87 percent probability of reduced costs of care), and to society as a whole (84 percent to 89 percent probability of reduced costs of care) (Holtzer-Goor et al., 2010). A subsequent study of the same integrated care model found that care provided in the glaucoma follow-up unit adhered closely to treatment protocols and was preferred by patients (Holtzer-Goor et al., 2016).

A study performed in Belgium compared the efficiency and efficacy of "lean" care pathways for cataract surgery and perioperative care, where the management of uncomplicated cases was shared by ophthalmologists, optometrists, and nurses, to the efficiency and efficacy of traditional pathways, where ophthalmologists managed nearly all elements of care (van Vliet et al., 2010). In the traditional care pathway, the eye examination and pre-assessment (e.g., health check, patient-reported medical history) were performed during separate patient visits to the hospital, and the formulation of the surgical care plan and the next-day post-surgery review required visits by all patients. In the "lean" care pathway, the eye examination and pre-assessment were performed in a single patient visit to the hospital, and the formulation of the surgical plan and next-day post-surgery review did not require patient visits in cases where ocular comorbidities and perioperative complications were not present. The minimum number of patient visits to the hospital decreased from five in the traditional care pathway to three in the lean care pathway. Compared to patients in the traditional pathway, those in the "lean" care pathway required on average significantly fewer hospital visits. Compared to the traditional care pathway, the "lean" care pathway also allowed ophthalmologists to treat significantly more patients in the same amount of time, and the authors suggest that further gains in efficiency might be achieved through greater adherence to the design of the "lean" care pathway (van Vliet et al., 2010).

In the United Kingdom, the National Health Service's Chronic Eye Care Services Programme supported eight pilot projects that sought to improve care pathways for the treatment of glaucoma, AMD, and vision impairment through better integration of the eye care workforce (McLeod et al., 2006). Together, these findings suggest that the integration of clinical eye and vision care services holds promise for lowering costs, improving patient satisfaction, promoting adherence to guidelines, and ensuring efficient and effective care. It is important to note that while these studies can serve as examples, they may have limited applicability to the U.S. system because of differences in the health care systems, in the scopes of practices of eye care providers, and in the patient populations in these countries compared to those in the United States. The committee was unable to identify peer-reviewed studies that described how U.S.-based integrated optometrist-ophthalmologist models are organized or operated, their associated costs and cost-effectiveness, or their impact on eye and vision health care and patient outcomes. Existing articles in trade publications only acknowledge that these models exist and are viable from a business perspective, although evidence supporting these claims may be insufficient. This is a much needed area of research. One potential strategy for developing an evidence base would be to conduct demonstration projects testing different models of eye and vision care organization, operation, and payment.

Incorporating Vision and Eye Health into Emerging Medical Models of Care

According to the American College of Physicians, the patient-centered medical home (PCMH) is a "care delivery model whereby patient treatment is coordinated through their primary care physician to ensure they receive the necessary care when and where they need it, in a manner they can understand" (ACP, 2016). The model emphasizes services that are comprehensive, patient-centered, coordinated, accessible, safe, and of high quality (AHRQ, 2016b). A review of peer-reviewed studies, government reports, industry studies, and independent federal program evaluations found that PCMH programs have been associated with reductions in cost and in the unnecessary use of health care services, and may also lead to improvements in patient satisfaction, quality-of-care metrics, and access to primary care services (Nielsen et al., 2016). Examples of PCMH programs that have resulted in improved patient health and care quality, reduced readmissions rates, reduced care costs, and/or short-term return on investments include the New York-Presbyterian Regional Health Collaborative, the Pennsylvania Chronic Care Initiative, and Illinois Medicaid's Illinois Health Connect and Your Healthcare Plus program (Carrillo et al., 2014; Friedberg et al., 2014; Phillips et al., 2014).

The Veterans Health Administration (VHA) has developed a unique PCMH model called the Patient Aligned Care Team (PACT). The provider team includes a primary care provider, a nurse care manager, a clinical associate, and an administrative clerk. Specialty care, including vision care, is provided through referral (VA, 2016). Studies of the PACT program suggest that PACT implementation is associated with significant improvements in the proportion of acute care patients contacted within 2 days of hospital discharge (Werner et al., 2014). PACT implementation has also been associated with a significant increase in the overall rate of telephone-based encounters between providers and patients, in the proportion of patients seen within 7 days of desired appointment date, and in the proportion of same day appointment requests accommodated (Rosland et al.,

2013). Among 913 VHA primary care clinics, greater progress in the PACT implementation process was associated with higher patient satisfaction, lower staff burnout rates, lower hospital admission rates for some ambulatory conditions, lower emergency department usage rates, and improved performance on 41 of 48 clinical quality measures (Nelson et al., 2014).

Despite the success of PACT and other PCMH models at reducing health care costs and improving some measures of care quality and access, it is not clear what impact these models have had on eye health, as research on the impact of the PCMH model on eye care is limited. However, studies on the impact of the PCMH model on comprehensive diabetes care—a component of which is annual dilated eye exams—can provide clues to the quality of eye care received within a PCMH. Kern and colleagues (2014) compared quality of patient care provided by physicians practicing in PCMHs established over the course of a 3-year study to that provided by physicians not practicing in a PCMH and who used either paper-based patient health records or an EHR. Quality of care was assessed using 10 quality measures, including provision of dilated eye examinations for patients with diabetes. At baseline, no significant differences in the percentage of patients with diabetes who were receiving dilated eye examinations existed between groups. By the end of the study, the proportion of patients with diabetes receiving dilated eye examinations was significantly higher among those receiving care from physicians practicing in a PCMH compared to those receiving care from physicians not practicing in a PCMH. Over the course of the study, performance on the dilated eye examination quality measure was 3–4 percent higher for physicians practicing in PCMHs than for physicians not practicing in PCMHs (Kern et al., 2014). A follow-up study found that although the overall care quality was similar between physician groups, patients with diabetes who were receiving care from physicians in PCMHs were still more likely to have eye exams than patients with diabetes who were receiving care from other physicians (Kern et al., 2016). Another study found that diabetic patients of primary care physicians who did not formally practice within a PCMH but who adhered closely to key features of the PCMH model were more likely to have received an eye exam in the previous year than diabetic patients of primary care physicians who adhered less closely to the PCMH model (Stevens et al., 2014).[17] These studies demonstrate the positive impact of the PMCH model of care on the provision of diabetic eye exams, and suggest the possibility that the PCMH model's emphasis on coordinated, team-based care

---

[17] Physician adherence to features of PCMH was based on patient responses to the Primary Care Assessment Tools (PCAT) Adult Expanded. A one-point increase in a physician's overall PCAT score was associated with 1.88 higher odds of his or her patients having received an eye exam in the previous year (Stevens et al., 2014).

that is comprehensive, patient-centered, and high-quality could also benefit other aspects of eye care.

The PCMH model may not always promote the quality of eye and vision care. Among a core set of clinical quality measures recommended by the Patient-Centered Medical Home Evaluators' Collaborative for evaluating and comparing the effectiveness of PCMH programs, the sole vision-related measure was the percentage of patients ages 18 to 75 with type 1 or 2 diabetes who received a retinal eye exam as a component of comprehensive diabetes care (Rosenthal et al., 2012).[18] The 2014 Standards and Guidelines for NCQA's Patient-Centered Medical Home, which provide guidance for assessing the quality of care offered by practices using the PCMH model, do not explicitly require the collection of vision-related clinical data, the inclusion of vision-specific components within the patient health assessment, or the use of vision screenings except where recommended by major public health agencies or organizations (NCQA, 2014b). Thus, while the PCMH model of care represents an opportunity for improved integration of eye and primary care, the inclusion of more eye care services and additional eye care professionals on the team should be studied to determine how it would affect the quality of eye and vision care in PCMH programs.

Providing high-quality, accessible, and patient-centered care requires coordination between primary care providers practicing in the PCMH and clinical and nonclinical providers and services operating outside the medical home.[19] The concept of the "medical neighborhood" was developed to account for the role that this broader set of services plays in achieving the goals of the PMCH, and the NCQA Patient-Centered Specialty Practice (PCSP) Recognition Program was developed to recognize and support specialty practices that seek to improve the quality of specialty care through coordination with primary care, performance measurement, and

---

[18] In addition to the core set of clinical quality measures, the collaborative also recommended that PCMH program evaluators select a group of clinical quality measures from a list that included measures related to adolescent well-child visits, well-child visits in the first 15 months of life, and well-child visits in the third, fourth, fifth, and sixth years of life. American Academy of Pediatrics guidelines require eye care to be included as part of the physical exam component of these visits (AAP, 2008a,b,c).

[19] AHRQ has conceived the medical neighborhood as a "PCMH and the constellation of other clinicians providing health care services to patients within it, along with community and social service organizations and State and local public health agencies" (AHRQ, 2011, p. 5). NCQA has identified specialty practices, accountable care organizations, behavioral health, public health, work site and retail clinics, and pharmacies as members of the medical neighborhood (NCQA, 2014a).

other means (Fisher, 2008; Huang and Rosenthal, 2014; NCQA, 2016d).[20] Ophthalmologists, but not optometrists, are eligible to participate in the PCSP Recognition Program (NCQA, 2016c).[21] Excluding optometrists from participating in the PCSP program may eliminate the contribution of a critical cohort of eye care providers and may limit the degree to which eye and vision care can be easily incorporated into specific PCMH models and medical neighborhoods.

Accountable care organizations (ACOs) offer another path to integration of primary care and specialty medical services. The Centers for Medicare & Medicaid Services (CMS) describes ACOs as "groups of doctors, hospitals, and other health care providers, who come together voluntarily to give coordinated high quality care" (CMS, 2015b). Initiatives such as the Medicare Shared Savings Program and the Pioneer and Next Generation ACO Models seek to improve the quality of patient care while lowering health care costs (CMS, 2015c,d, 2016b). Achieving these twin goals may require extensive data sharing, transitioning to value-based payment policies, using quality measures to monitor provider performance and patient outcomes, and the coordination of providers and services, among other strategies.

The fact that there is a limited amount of research on the impacts of ACOs on eye and vision health may in part be the consequence of limitations in the reporting requirements for ACOs. ACOs participating in the Medicare Shared Savings Program are required to report quality data, and they must meet established quality performance standards set by CMS in order to be eligible to receive shared savings (CMS, 2016a). Since performance year 2012, quality measures related to diabetes care have been included among the quality performance measures CMS requires ACOs to report; however, a measure related to the provision of diabetic eye exams was not included among these until performance year 2015 (CMS, 2011, 2012, 2014, 2015a, 2016a). For performance years 2015 and 2016, ACO performance on the provision of diabetic eye exams will be reported as a composite measure with ACO performance on control of hemoglobin A1c

---

[20] The objectives of the PCSP Recognition Program are to enhance coordination between primary care and specialty care, strengthen relationships between primary care clinicians and clinicians outside the primary care specialties, improve the experience of patients accessing specialty care, align requirements with processes demonstrated to improve quality and eliminate waste, encourage practices to use performance measurement and results to drive improvement; and identify requirements appropriate for various specialty practices seeking recognition for excellent care integration within the medical home (NCQA, 2016e).

[21] Other clinicians who are eligible to participate in the PCSP Recognition Program include nurse practitioners, physician assistants, and certified nurse midwives, as well as doctoral or master's-level psychologists, social workers, and marriage and family counselors who are state licensed or certified (NCQA, 2016c).

levels among diabetic patients.[22] Data for ACO performance on this composite measure were not available at the time of writing. The addition of eye care–related quality measures to the set of measures that CMS requires ACOs to report could provide useful data on how ACOs affect eye care quality and access.

As the population ages, and chronic eye disease and other vision problems become increasingly prevalent, demand for models of care capable of meeting national eye and vision health needs will continue to grow. More research is needed to understand how the medical field can work as a cohesive and coordinated unit, achieving better value and health outcomes. For example, it is important to determine how PCMHs, ACOs, and other integrated models of care that promote collaborative practice—as well as the policies that inform their organization, adoption, and performance monitoring and quality improvement activities—can be adapted to best meet current and future eye and vision health needs. Strategies and actions to better support integration of clinical eye and vision services with vision rehabilitation, social services, public health departments, and other stakeholders are also needed. More health services research and evaluation of existing programs will be essential to guide these efforts.

Role of Health Informatics

Advances in health information technology, particularly the implementation of EHRs, have the potential to optimize care delivery, enhance quality and safety in a number of ways, and ultimately improve patient outcomes (Blumenthal and Tavenner, 2010). Implementing EHR systems can ensure that providers have access to up-to-date, relevant clinical patient information at the point of care (Chiang et al., 2011). It can also facilitate information exchange across care settings, thereby improving communication and coordination between primary care providers and eye care providers (e.g., optometrists, ophthalmologists) or other specialists treating comorbidities. This would theoretically reduce the duplication of various laboratory tests or imaging and lessen the risk of treatment errors. The data in EHRs can also be used to prioritize, justify, and analyze public health activities by identifying and tracking eye disease and vision impairment—and interventions to prevent and reduce the same—at the population level.

---

[22] CMS-required quality performance measures on diabetic eye exams and control of hemoglobin A1c levels are based on NQF-endorsed quality measures. NQF-0055: "The percentage of members 18 to 75 years of age with diabetes (type 1 and type 2) who had an eye exam (retinal) performed" (NQF, 2016a). NQF-0059: "The percentage of patients 18–75 years of age with diabetes (type 1 and type 2) whose most recent HbA1c level during the measurement year was greater than 9.0% (poor control) or was missing a result, or if an HbA1c test was not done during the measurement year" (NQF, 2016b).

For this reason, EHRs can be powerful tools for informing public health practice and improving public health.

EHR use has grown considerably in recent years. From 2001 to 2014 the proportion of office-based physicians who used any type of EHR system increased from 18.0 percent to 82.8 percent, and the proportion of office-based physicians who reported having an EHR system that met the criteria for a basic EHR system increased significantly from 11.0 percent in 2006 to 50.5 percent in 2014 (CDC, 2015; Hsiao, 2014).[23] However, EHR use among ophthalmologists is low compared with most other medical specialties, with only 15.0 percent and 34.7 percent of ophthalmologists reporting EHR use in 2003 and 2010, respectively, compared with 13.7 percent and 64.2 percent in 2003 and 2010 for general or family medicine. In multivariate analysis, ophthalmologists had lower odds of using EHRs than any other of 13 specialties except psychiatry and dermatology (Kokkonen et al., 2013). A 2012 survey of 492 ophthalmologists found that 32 percent of ophthalmology practices in the United States had adopted EHR systems, and another 31 percent planned to do so within 2 years (Boland et al., 2013). A 2015 survey by AOA found that 17 percent and 49 percent of responding optometrists planned to achieve criteria for, respectively, stage 1 and stage 2 meaningful use in 2015. The survey also found that 66 percent of responding optometrists used complete EHRs, as defined by the AOA (AOA, 2015a).[24] Adoption among both groups is increasing: EHR adoption among surveyed ophthalmologists doubled from 2007 to 2011 and increased by 3 percent from 2014 to 2015 among surveyed optometrists (AOA, 2015a; Boland et al., 2013).

The adoption of EHRs by eye care specialists may be impeded by concerns about its effects on the quality of clinical documentation. Sanders and colleagues (2013) compared the effects of a paper-based health record system to those of an EHR system on the clinical documentation habits of ophthalmologists assessing patients with AMD, glaucoma, and pigmented choroidal lesions. For all three diseases, the paper-based system was associated with significantly fewer complete examination findings and critical

---

[23] According to Hsiao (2014), a basic EHR system is one that has each of the following features: "patient history and demographics, patient problem lists, physician clinical notes, [a] comprehensive list of patients' medications and allergies, computerized orders for prescriptions, and [the] ability to view laboratory and imaging results electronically."

[24] Complete EHRs were defined as those that included both practice management and patient health information systems. Practice management systems were defined as "electronic software packages that track and maintain information such as: patient demographics, scheduling, billing, insurance, and recall." Patient health information systems were defined as "electronic software packages that maintain health information such as: exam data, testing, images and prescriptions" (AOA, 2015a, p. 1).

clinical findings (Sanders et al., 2013).[25] Sanders and colleagues (2014) found that EHR implementation in an ophthalmic surgical practice was associated with significant short-term increases in the portion of total procedure time spent on the documentation of cataract, vitreoretinal, and extraocular procedures and with significant increases in the number of circulating operating room nurses present for cataract and vitreoretinal procedures. These values returned to baseline after 3 months for most, but not all, procedures (Sanders et al., 2014).[26] Chan and colleagues (2013) investigated the impact of three different methods (i.e., keyboard-based, mouse-based, and paper-based documentation) of recording patient data on the accuracy and speed of clinical documentation of ophthalmology residents and fellows and found that sensitivity was highest for the keyboard-based method, while paper-based documentation performed better than the other methods in terms of positive ratio and documentation speed.[27] Other studies have found associations between EHR implementation in some eye care practices and significantly longer nonclinical documentation times, as well as increases in the amount of time that eye care providers spend on clinical examinations (Chiang et al., 2013; Pandit and Boland, 2013). Finally, transitioning to an EHR system can have negative impacts on the ability of eye care providers to include drawings in patient records. The rate of drawing in EHRs is low, and EHR adoption can dramatically decrease the proportion of clinical records that include drawings (Lim et al., 2015; Sanders et al., 2013). Ophthalmologists have reported difficulties in using existing EHR drawing programs and have identified the inability to include drawings in patient records as a moderate to significant barrier to EHR adoption (Boland et al., 2013; Chiang et al., 2008, 2011).

Research also suggests that EHR adoption among eye care practices is associated with measurable, but rarely significant, economic impacts. A large multispecialty ophthalmic practice saw only nonsignificant changes in mean net monthly revenue and mean patient visits per month after

---

[25] Complete examination includes general examination, slit-lamp examination, and fundus examination. Critical clinical findings were defined as the subset of ophthalmic examination elements believed to be required documentation for clinical evaluation of that disease.

[26] Circulating operating room nurses and documentation time as a percentage of total procedure time remained elevated for cataract procedures, and the total documentation time remained significantly higher for all but the cornea- and glaucoma-related procedures.

[27] Sensitivity was calculated by dividing the number of findings identified by subject that were truly present in the actual case by the total number of actual findings in the case. Positive ratio was calculated by dividing the number of findings identified by subject that were truly present in the actual case by the number of positive findings reported by subject. Documentation speed was calculated by dividing the documentation time of the entire case by the number of examination findings identified by subject (Chan et al., 2013).

transitioning to EHRs (Singh et al., 2015).[28] EHR implementation in an academic medical center resulted in nonsignificant changes in the average number of ophthalmic surgical procedures per month and in operating room turnover time (Read-Brown et al., 2013).[29] Other studies confirm the absence of statistically significant changes in clinical volume associated with EHR implementation in ophthalmology practices (Chiang et al., 2013; Redd et al., 2014). Lim and colleagues (2015) reported that EHR implementation in an academic ophthalmology practice resulted in a significant decrease in annual transcription costs and related cost-savings but that changes to annual clinical revenue per provider and to the number of patients per provider per year were nonsignificant, leading the authors to conclude that the study had not demonstrated a clear financial gain associated with EHR implementation.[30]

According to a national survey, a majority of physicians consider the large initial costs and uncertain return on investment (ROI) to be barriers to EHR adoption (DesRoches et al., 2008). These concerns are not unfounded. For example, the costs associated with implementation of a customized EHR system at the Cole Eye Institute included $1,571,864 in capital costs as well as $1,160,694 in personnel and ongoing costs and $1,514,334 in operating costs in 2011 (Chiang et al., 2013). Adler-Milstein and colleagues (2013) found that just 27 to 33 percent of specialty practices participating in the Massachusetts eHealth Collaborative projected a positive 5-year ROI; on average, the participating specialty practices expected to lose $50,722 per physician over 5 years. However, ROI varied considerably with practice size and type, with primary care practices showing smaller losses, practices with six or more physicians showing positive ROI, and ROI improving for all practices over longer periods. Other studies have found that EHR implementation in general and also the particular functions of an EHR system (e.g., computerized provider order entry), are associated with long-term cost-savings, improvements in medication safety, reductions in medical error, and benefits to society (Charles et al., 2014; Forrester et al., 2014; Grieger et al., 2007; Kaushal et al., 2006; Nuckols et al., 2014; Patil et al., 2008).

Increasingly, EHR systems designed for general use by health care institutions are becoming able to support the unique requirements of vision care, which previously hindered widespread implementation (Chiang et al.,

---

[28] Total net fiscal revenue declined by $44,372 per month (median value) over the 24-month study period. Total patient volume increased by 217 visits per month (mean value).

[29] Ophthalmic surgical procedures per month decreased after EHR implementation (14.9 to 14.2 among 25 stable providers), while operating room turnover time decreased (17.3 minutes to 15.6 minutes for the 4- to 12-month period after implementation).

[30] Reduced transcription costs resulted in cost-savings of $188,951 over a 4-year post-EHR implementation period.

2011). For example, some current EHR systems can incorporate images or add sketches of the eye, which many ophthalmologists and optometrists rely on in assessing patient records. Health information technology can also simplify care delivery and patient adherence to treatment protocols. For example, one study found that embedding a referrals tool into EHR systems can improve the quality and frequency of referral-related communications between primary care providers and specialists (Gandhi et al., 2008). It can potentially encourage at-risk patients to seek preventive eye care and adhere to recommended guidelines for receiving comprehensive eye examinations. There are also other strategies for improving patient care; for example, electronic dosing aids with audiovisual reminders, provided as part of a multifaceted intervention, can increase patient adherence to glaucoma medication regimens, and telephone and text message reminders can improve adherence to follow-up care (Lin and Wu, 2014; Okeke et al., 2009).

Although health informatics has the potential to improve the delivery of eye care and thus improve patient outcomes, a number of challenges have limited the adoption of these tools, especially in solo practices. Key among these is the limited interoperability among EHRs and other sources of patient data.[31] The Office of the National Coordinator for Health Information Technology (ONC) has reported that claimed barriers to interoperability include the "use of different technical standards, lack of business incentives that can lead vendors and providers to block the transmission of health information to other vendors and providers, deficits in trust, and differences in state laws and regulations that make it difficult to share health information across state lines" (ONC, 2015). Other barriers to interoperability can include negative impacts of EHR use on provider workflow, and challenges in maintaining the security of patient information (HITPC, 2015). The potential of interoperable EHRs to enhance care coordination and collaboration may hold special value for eye and vision care, where several providers—including ophthalmologists and optometrists, primary care providers, multidisciplinary vision rehabilitation teams, and public health workers—can contribute to a single patient treatment plan. Research is needed to identify strategies to promoting interoperability of EHR systems and other sources of patient data used by providers involved in eye and vision care.

---

[31] Interoperability is "the ability of two or more systems to exchange information and the ability of those systems to use the information that has been exchanged without special effort" (HITPC, 2015, p. 4).

WORKFORCE TRAINING AND EDUCATION TO PROMOTE EYE AND VISION HEALTH

Improving access to high-quality care requires well-educated workforces across a variety of fields that are familiar with each other's expertise and capabilities. Eye care providers must be able to communicate with, educate, counsel, and treat a racially, ethnically, and culturally diverse patient population whose members speak multiple languages, occupy various socioeconomic positions, have different professional and educational backgrounds, possess diverse beliefs about health and health care, and suffer from eye diseases and comorbid conditions of varying complexity and severity. Unfortunately, a lack of trust, communication, and coordination among different primary medical personnel and ophthalmologists and optometrists may lead to miscommunication, poor health care decisions, medical errors, the unnecessary duplication of services, lost continuity, excess costs, low-quality (e.g., inappropriate and untimely) care, and suboptimal outcomes in health care (Elhauge, 2010; Enthoven, 2009; IOM, 2001).

In order to cultivate the practices and knowledge needed to meet the multidisciplinary needs of eye care patients and address fragmentation of the vision care system, eye care providers, medical professionals working in primary care and medical specialties, allied health professionals, social workers, and members of the public health workforce must all be aware of the services offered by other health care and public health disciplines and must engage cooperatively with professionals in those disciplines on the development and implementation of treatment plans. Achieving high levels of health care system performance and improved patient outcomes through changes to the culture, practices, and processes of the vision care system and workforce will also require exceptional leadership, ongoing and effective teamwork, and commitment to the principles and purpose of quality improvement. Thus, positive change demands a workforce that is culturally competent and diverse, trained in cross-disciplinary and integrative approaches to care, predisposed to both teamwork and leadership, and inclined to lead quality improvement efforts.

Interprofessional Education

Optometrists, ophthalmologists, and primary care clinicians who can collaborate with one another and with other professionals in allied health, public health, social services, and other relevant fields, are essential to integrated models of eye and vision care. Interprofessional education (IPE) is one strategy for developing a workforce with the competencies necessary to meet the demands of integrated care. According to WHO, "[i]nterprofessional education occurs when students from two or more professions learn about, from and with each other to enable effective collaboration and improve health outcomes" (WHO, 2010, p. 10). This training is a "key step in moving health systems from fragmentation to a position of strength" (WHO, 2010, p. 10). IPE can take place during formal professional training, as part of continuing education or professional development or quality programs.

A review of studies comparing IPE modules in health professional education programs found a wide range of instructional models, objectives, and reported outcomes (Abu-Rish et al., 2012). Reeves and colleagues (2010) performed a synthesis of systematic reviews and found that, despite heterogeneity among interventions, IPE was frequently well received by students and had a positive impact on care quality patient outcomes. A systematic review found limited evidence that IPE improves patient outcomes, provider adherence to clinical guidelines, patient satisfaction, or clinical processes. However, the differences among interventions and a limited number of high-quality studies made it impossible to make broader conclusions about the value of IPE (Reeves et al., 2013). Studies on the impacts of IPE on students or practitioners of optometry or ophthalmology are very limited, but they indicate that IPE can have positive impacts on attitudes toward collaborative practice (Sheppard et al., 2015).

Despite uncertainty regarding their optimal design and implementation, IPE programs are broadly supported by numerous stakeholders in health care. The IOM report *Health Professions Education: A Bridge to Quality* asserts that interdisciplinary education is a key to fostering interdisciplinary practice (IOM, 2003a).[32] WHO and the American Public Health Association (APHA) have identified interprofessional education as essential to promoting collaborative practice (APHA, 2008; WHO, 2010). IPE programs have been implemented by HRSA, the VA, and several medical centers (Bridges et al., 2011; Remington et al., 2006). The Liaison Committee on Medical Education (LCME) requires the curricula of M.D. programs to include training in "interprofessional collaborative skills" (LCME, 2015, p. 11).[33] The Council on Education for Public Health requires public health

---

[32] Working in interdisciplinary teams was described as involving cooperation, collaboration, and integration of care. Interdisciplinary education was defined as "a group of students from the health-related occupations with different educational backgrounds learn[ing] and interact[ing] together during certain periods of their education in order to collaborate in providing health-related services" (IOM, 2003a, p. 79).

[33] LCME Standard 7.9: "The faculty of a medical school ensure that the core curriculum of the medical education program prepares medical students to function collaboratively on health care teams that include health professionals from other disciplines as they provide coordinated services to patients. These curricular experiences include practitioners and/or students from the other health professions" (LCME, 2015, p. 11).

schools to "function as a collaboration of disciplines" and to "provide a special learning environment that supports interdisciplinary communication" (CEPH, 2011, p. 2). The Accreditation Council on Optometric Education (ACOE) does not explicitly require O.D. programs to include training in interprofessional education or other competencies to support collaborative practice (ACOE, 2014). Inclusion of training in interprofessional education in ACOE accreditation standards for O.D. programs could potentially foster collaboration in the eye care workforce.

Eye and Vision Health in Medical and Population Health Education

All physicians are generally trained in the fundamentals of ophthalmic diseases and examination. A recent survey by Shah and colleagues reported that 95 percent, or 104 of the 109 osteopathic and allopathic schools of medicine who responded to the survey, conduct preclinical didactics within the first 2 years and 84 percent, or 92 schools, provide specific training related to the ophthalmic examination (Shah et al., 2014). However, additional training beyond this initial exposure varies with only 18 percent of schools requiring a clinical rotation in ophthalmology (Shah et al., 2014).

There is documented erosion in ophthalmic training in general medical education (Quillen et al., 2005; Shah et al., 2014). The accrediting body for schools of medicine, the Liaison Committee on Medical Education, does not specify ophthalmic training in its guidelines, making it difficult for ophthalmologists to increase their presence in the curriculum. The Centers for Disease Control and Prevention (CDC) notes a need to emphasize ophthalmic education in the medical curriculum (CDC, 2009). A survey conducted by residency program directors in primary care fields found that 64 percent of directors in family practice, 87.5 percent in internal medicine, and 86.3 percent in pediatrics believed that additional training in ophthalmology should be incorporated into their residency programs (Stern, 1995). Additionally, 90 percent of directors believed that less than 50 percent of entering residents met the minimum standard on medical student education set by the Association of University Professors of Ophthalmology (AUPO) (Stern, 1995). See Box 7-4 for AUPO policy on medical student education. Requiring a rotation in ophthalmology during medical school training could be proposed as a solution.

Some medical and dental schools are incorporating coursework with a focus on interprofessional competencies into their curriculums. For example, dental students at Harvard University participate in a primary care medical rotation, dental and medical students at the University of Michigan can elect to take interprofessional education courses, and dental and medical students at the University of Connecticut and Harvard Medical School follow identical curriculums during their first 2 years of study (HSDM,

---

BOX 7-4
Association of University Professors of Ophthalmology (AUPO) Policy Statement on Medical Student Education

The AUPO Policy Statement on Medical Student Education states that all physicians should be able to:

1. Measure and record a visual acuity
2. Evaluate a red eye
3. Evaluate a traumatized eye
4. Detect strabismus and abnormal eye movements
5. Detect abnormal pupillary responses
6. Perform direct ophthalmoscopy to detect abnormalities of the optic nerve and fundus
7. Initiate management and/or referral for detected or suspected abnormalities of the eye and visual system

SOURCE: Stern, 1995.

2016; Kirk, 2011; University of Michigan, 2015a). To support integration efforts, many schools have also developed programs on interprofessional collaboration and education (e.g., University of Michigan, 2015a).

Because the public health workforce is responsible for a range of activities to support eye and vision health (see Chapter 5), public health professionals need to be knowledgeable about eye and vision health. To support efforts to improve eye and vision health, public health professionals need to be able to ascertain and communicate information about community health to providers, understand the roles that different eye care specialists and other health care providers play in advancing vision and eye health, and have a reasonable appreciation for the types of effective treatments or interventions that are available.

Population Health Training in Clinical Medicine

Over the past decade, the general landscape affecting health within communities has changed dramatically, emphasizing the health of individuals *and* populations. In 2008, Berwick and colleagues at the Institute for Healthcare Improvement (IHI) introduced the "Triple Aim," which altered thinking about how to improve the U.S. health care system by suggesting three interdependent goals: improving the experience of care, improving the health of populations, and reducing per-capita costs of health care (Berwick et al., 2008). To achieve the "Triple Aim," health care professionals will need to understand the types of patient experiences and data that are relevant to population health activities and population health practitioners will need to understand the demands placed on health care providers and what they need in order to provide high-quality care. In terms of eye health, this means that health care providers need to understand what types of eye diseases and conditions pose the greatest risk of vision impairment within their communities, how to eliminate the most significant risk factors and foster the most significant protective factors (including health literacy and social determinants of health), and how this shapes patient interactions.

Some medical schools and other health professional curricula and practicums already expose students to population health theory and practices. For example, seven schools in 2003 received grants to become regional medicine-public health education centers and are expected to partner with local or state public health departments to improve population health and public health practice for current medical students (Maeshiro, 2008). The program has since expanded with a second cohort of medical schools in 2006 and then into other graduate medical education programs in 2008 (AAMC, 2015). Numerous medical schools offer dual degree programs in medicine and public health; a program in public health ophthalmology at Johns Hopkins University seeks to enable eye care professionals to apply public health concepts to blindness prevention (Johns Hopkins Medicine, 2016).

HRSA supports interprofessional education through grants to consortiums or partnerships identified in the Public Health Service Act (HRSA, 2016a). Grant-winning programs are supported by the Coordinating Center for Interprofessional Education and Practice, which serves as a focal point for efforts to increase collaborative, team-based care through program coordination, research, and data collection (HRSA, 2016a). Funded by the HRSA grant program, the National Center for Interprofessional Practice and Education (National Center) collects and offers educational resources on interprofessional education; manages a network of researchers, educators, and practitioners engaged in interprofessional education; and partners with researchers across the country to develop and evaluate interprofessional education programs (NCIPE, 2016a). Currently, only a few of the research efforts and educational materials available through the National Center concern the interprofessional education of eye care providers (NCIPE, 2016b,c). An increased emphasis by the National Center or other HRSA grant awardees on the education of the vision care workforce could provide valuable support for actions to improve the quality of eye care through workforce integration.

There are also growing links among educational institutions in public health, optometry, and ophthalmology. The schools and colleges of optometry include various aspects of public health (e.g., epidemiology, biostatistics, health policy, ethics) in their curricula, and public health content is included on Part II of the National Board of Examiners in Optometry exam. In addition, education on public health is included in the curricula of medical schools and ophthalmology residencies. The American Board of Ophthalmology includes content about public health on the written and oral examinations of ophthalmologists for board certification. APHA's Vision Care Section, whose members include optometrists, ophthalmologists, and other public health practitioners, was established to promote health and well-being with an emphasis on vision and eye health through interdisciplinary partnerships (APHA, 2016).

The American Optometric Student Association has partnered with Salus University to offer a scholarship to optometry students seeking to earn a master's degree in public health at Salus University, and the Massachusetts College of Pharmacy and Health Sciences offers a dual degree program in optometry and public health (AOSA, 2016; MCPHS, 2016). The University of California, Los Angeles (UCLA), provides the opportunity for ophthalmology residents to obtain a doctorate in the UCLA Fielding School of Public Health during residency, and Johns Hopkins University offers a program in public health ophthalmology. Additionally, the emergence of initiatives in support of IPE signal new opportunities for enhancing interprofessional collaboration and improving population health.

Cultivating Leadership and Teamwork

Beyond knowledge of clinical and population health management, health care personnel and public health practitioners will need leadership abilities that allow them to cultivate trust between different groups and sectors and the capacity to form and articulate a shared vision to unite different stakeholders. Leadership programs exist for public health workers, optometrists, and ophthalmologists. For example, the Center for Health Leadership and Practice promotes leadership within the public health workforce through its National Leadership Academy programs (CHLP, 2016). AOA and the American Academy of Ophthalmology both offer professional leadership programs or training (AAO, 2016d; AOA, 2016b). The Robert Wood Johnson Foundation's Interdisciplinary Research Leaders program provides interdisciplinary research teams with the leadership and technical skills necessary to pursue research to improve community health and promote health equity (RWJF, 2016). The successful cultivation of leadership and teamwork skills can positively impact patient and population health outcomes, by developing a workforce with the competencies necessary to pursue the difficult work of change and improvement at the level of health care systems.

Promoting Cultural Competency

Cultural competency helps build concordance between patients and health care providers by challenging providers to think outside of their strict biomedical constructs and respond to the cultural barriers that are inherent in their patients' diverse belief systems and views about health, health care, and health care providers. For example, religious and spiritual beliefs, culturally traditional healing rituals, denial, and conflicting perspectives about the etiology of disease and the efficacy of long-term therapies can create roadblocks to the biomedical management of clinical conditions. The use of community health centers has been linked to improved health outcomes, through addressing health needs with culturally and linguistically appropriate services (Torres et al., 2014).[34]

The Association of American Medical Colleges, the Association of Schools and Colleges of Optometry, and the Association of Schools of Public Health have made efforts to incorporate cultural competency components into the curricula of member institutions. The Liaison Committee on Medical Education has required the faculty and students of medical schools to "demonstrate an understanding of the manner in which people of diverse cultures and belief systems perceive health and illness and respond to various symptoms, diseases, and treatments," and it requires medical students to "recognize and appropriately address gender and cultural biases in health care delivery, while considering first the health of the patient" (AAMC, 2005, p. 1). Similarly, the Association of Schools and Colleges of Optometry have developed guidelines for culturally competent eye and vision care (ASCO, 2008); the Interprofessional Education Collaborative Expert Panel identified "embrac[ing] the cultural diversity and individual differences that characterize patients, populations, and the health care team" as a specific competency in health professional education (Interprofessional Education Collaborative Expert Panel, 2011, p. 19); and the Expert Panel on Cultural Competence Education for Students in Medicine and Public Health developed a set of common cultural competencies that medical and public health schools can use to "standardize curricula, benchmark student performance, and better prepare graduates for culturally competent practice" (Expert Panel on Cultural Competence Education for Students in Medicine and Public Health, 2012, p. 1).

Despite these broader gains, many gaps in the cultural competency of eye care remain. For example, only limited attempts have been made

---

[34] Torres et al. (2014) describe community health workers (CHWs) as front-line health workers who are members of the communities and provide community outreach programs or practices. The authors state that "CHWs are considered to have a deep understanding of the issues faced by these communities in accessing health and social services, and are able to offer linguistically and culturally appropriate assistance" (Torres et al., 2014, p. 75).

to tailor vision interventions to the unique cultural characteristics of the patient. Typically, these efforts in the past have been integrated into other programs. For example, a study utilizing the Spoken Knowledge in Low Literacy in Diabetes survey measured baseline knowledge of low-literate Hispanic-speaking individuals with diabetes. Diabetes baseline knowledge was weak in understanding the relationship to eye health, with only 31.5 percent of the study cohort correctly identifying the importance of seeing an eye doctor (Pena-Purcell and Boggess, 2014). The use of a 5-week diabetes education series conducted with pictorial materials and spoken Spanish significantly improved awareness, with 74.6 percent of participants identifying the importance of seeing an eye doctor post-intervention (Pena-Purcell and Boggess, 2014).

The continuing development, implementation, and evaluation of cultural competence programs, training modules, and educational tools designed to improve the affective dimensions of communication and clinical behavior along with increasing the diversity in the health care workforce can help increase patient–provider concordance, reduce implicit bias, and not only address the public health challenge of eliminating ethnic and cultural disparities, but also address contributors to the health outcomes, affecting the health of vulnerable populations (Elam and Lee, 2013; IOM, 2003b; Sabin and Greenwald, 2012). Including training in cultural competency in all medical, optometric, allied health, and public health educational programs could be an effective strategy for improving health system quality across all specialties and professions. Finally, while this discussion has focused on the development and training of the clinical eye and vision care workforce, similar interventions may be necessary to develop a patient-centered and culturally proficient public health workforce.

CONCLUSION

A comprehensive population health approach to reducing vision impairment and promoting eye and vision health requires, among other important components, the ability to deliver and measure high-quality care. Establishing clear messaging about who should receive what care and when is essential to educating not only the public, but also health care and population health fields. A single set of evidence-based guidelines, especially in the context of vision screenings and comprehensive eye examinations, that adhere to specific development standards can improve the uniformity and quality of patient care, establish a consistent baseline from which to measure improvement, and promote accountability for eye and vision health outcomes and care processes.

Quality improvement initiatives are important to help standardize care and address factors that contribute to unnecessary vision impairment and inequitable health outcomes. Numerous governmental and health care entities are engaged in various CQI activities, but the evidence generated thus far has only led to a handful of nationally endorsed quality measures for specific diseases and conditions. Other measures related to vision screenings, general eye examinations, and vision rehabilitation are still lacking. Addressing the key research gaps and opportunities (see Box 7-5) could lead to additional improvements in the quality of eye and vision care. However, this research will require a broad set of surveillance and monitoring tools, which are currently limited (see Chapter 4).

Integrated models of care have the potential to improve detection and diagnosis of vision problems and subsequent referral to eye care providers. Patient-centered medical homes, ACOs, and other integrated care models provide lessons in collaboration and coordination that can inform efforts to integrate vision care, medicine, and public health. Investment in emerging technologies may also increase the accessibility of vision care for underserved populations. There is a need for cross-disciplinary education and training in the public health, eye and vision care, and broader clinical workforces, emphasizing cultural competency, leadership, teamwork, and awareness of the interrelations between eye and vision health, general health, and population health. The alignment of professional guidelines for eye and vision care, investment in CQI activities, and the integrated delivery of eye and vision care with the general field of medicine will require collaboration and commitment from a wide range of complementary, yet sometimes competing, stakeholders. Although this will be challenging, it

---

BOX 7-5
Key Research Gaps and Opportunities

- Identify and characterize current models of integrated eye and vision care to assess the potential of ACOs and PCMHs to improve eye and vision health and to promote the development of cost-effective integrated models for eye and vision care.
- Assess the benefits and harms of existing vision screening programs, improve the sensitivity and specificity of current and emerging vision screening tools, and develop methods of vision screening that are cost-effective.
- Identify, assess, and improve training programs to promote collaborative practices and shared knowledge of eye and vision health among health care providers and public health professionals.
- Develop health information technologies that meet the needs of clinical eye and vision care providers, and identify and address barriers to adoption of these technologies among stakeholders in eye and vision care.

can be done and is necessary to improve the quality of eye and vision care and to promote the overall health of populations in the United States.

REFERENCES

AAMC (Association of American Medical Colleges). 2005. *Cultural competence education.* Washington, DC: AAMC. https://www.aamc.org/download/54338/data/culturalcomped. pdf (accessed June 21, 2016).

———. 2015. Regional medicine-public health education centers. https://www.aamc.org/initiatives/diversity/portfolios/cdc/aamcbased/rmphec (accessed April 7, 2016).

AANP (American Association of Nurse Practitioners). 2015. 2013–14 national nurse practitioner practice site census. https://www.aanp.org/press-room/press-releases/166-press-room/2015-press-releases/1694-2013-14-national-nurse-practitioner-practice-site-census (accessed June 21, 2016).

AANPCP (AANP Certification Program). 2016. AANP certification program: Program description. http://www.aanpcert.org/ptistore/control/certs/program (accessed April 27, 2016).

AAO (American Academy of Ophthalmology). 2012a. Eye exams 101. http://www.aao.org/eye-health/tips-prevention/eye-exams-101 (accessed March 29, 2016).

———. 2012b. Pediatric eye evaluations Preferred Practice Pattern® guidelines. http://www.aao.org/Assets/7364f939-97b3-4c2e-948f-e6c3d78cb45d/636009832100970000/pediatric-eye-evaluations-ppp-pdf (accessed July 18, 2016).

———. 2013. Vision screening for infants and children. http://www.aao.org/clinical-statement/vision-screening-infants-children--2013 (accessed April 7, 2016).

———. 2015a. Policy statement: Frequency of ocular examinations. http://www.aao.org/clinical-statement/frequency-of-ocular-examinations--november-2009 (accessed June 21, 2016)

———. 2015b. Primary open-angle glaucoma Preferred Practice Pattern® guidelines. http://www.aaojournal.org/article/S0161-6420(15)01276-2/pdf (accessed July 18, 2016).

———. 2016a. AAO guidelines. http://www.aao.org/guidelines-browse?filter=preferredpractice patternsguideline (accessed April 7, 2016).

———. 2016b. About the IRIS® registry. http://www.aao.org/iris-registry/about (accessed April 7, 2016).

———. 2016c. Comprehensive adult medical eye evaluation Preferred Practice Pattern® guidelines. http://www.aaojournal.org/article/S0161-6420(15)01269-5/pdf (accessed July 18, 2016).

———. 2016d. Leadership development program. http://www.aao.org/about/leadership-development/overview (accessed April 7, 2016).

———. 2016e. Preferred Practice Pattern® guidelines. http://www.aao.org/about-preferred-practice-patterns (accessed May 16, 2016).

AAO/AAO (American Academy of Ophthalmology/American Academy of Optometry). 2013. American Academy of Ophthalmology and American Academy of Optometry to explore educational opportunities to advance quality eye care. December 4. http://www.aao.org/newsroom/news-releases/detail/american-academy-of-ophthalmology-optometry-to-exp (accessed June 15, 2016).

AAP (American Academy of Pediatrics). 2002. Use of photoscreening for children's vision screening. *Pediatrics* 109(3):524–525.

———. 2008a. Bright futures guidelines: Adolescence 11 to 21 years. https://brightfutures. aap.org/Bright%20Futures%20Documents/18-Adolescence.pdf (accessed July 18, 2016).

———. 2008b. Bright futures guidelines: Early childhood 1 to 4 years. https://brightfutures. aap.org/Bright%20Futures%20Documents/16-Early_Childhood.pdf (accessed July 18, 2016).

———. 2008c. Bright futures guidelines: Middle childhood 5 to 10 years. https://brightfutures. aap.org/Bright%20Futures%20Documents/17-Middle_Childhood.pdf (accessed July 18, 2016).

———. 2008d. Red reflex examination in neonates, infants, and children. *Pediatrics* 122(6): 1401–1404.

AAP, Committee on Practice and Ambulatory Medicine, Section on Ophthalmology, American Association of Certified Orthoptists, American Association for Pediatric Ophthalmology and Strabismus, and American Academy of Opthalmology. 2016. Visual system assessment in infants, children, and young adults by pediatricians. *Pediatrics* 137(1):1–3. http://pediatrics.aappublications.org/content/pediatrics/early/2015/12/07/peds. 2015-3596.full.pdf (accessed June 20, 2016).

AAPA (American Academy of Physician Assistants). 2014. 2013 AAPA annual survey report. https://www.aapa.org/WorkArea/DownloadAsset.aspx?id=2902 (accessed June 21, 2016).

AAPOS (American Association for Pediatric Ophthalmology and Strabismus). 2014. Vision screening. http://www.aapos.org/terms/conditions/107 (accessed March 29, 2016).

Abu-Rish, E., S. Kim, L. Choe, L. Varpio, E. Malik, A. A. White, K. Craddick, K. Blondon, L. Robins, P. Nagasawa, A. Thigpen, L. L. Chen, J. Rich, and B. Zierler. 2012. Current trends in interprofessional education of health sciences students: A literature review. *Journal of Interprofessional Care* 26(6):444–451.

ACOE (Accreditation Council on Optometric Education). 2014. *Accreditation manual: Professional optometric degree programs*. St. Louis, MO: ACOE. http://www.aoa.org/ Documents/students/od_manual_08_2014.pdf (accessed July 19, 2016).

ACP (American College of Physicians). 2016. What is the patient-centered medical home? https://www.acponline.org/practice-resources/business/payment/models/pcmh/ understanding/what-pcmh (accessed June 21, 2016).

Adler-Milstein, J., C. E. Green, and D. W. Bates. 2013. A survey analysis suggests that electronic health records will yield revenue gains for some practices and losses for many. *Health Affairs* 32(3):562–570.

AHRQ (Agency for Healthcare Research and Quality). 2011. *Coordinating care in the medical neighborhood: Critical components and available mechanisms*. Washington, DC: AHRQ.

———. 2012. *Screening for glaucoma: Comparative effectiveness*. Washington, DC: AHRQ.

———. 2014a. Primary care workforce facts and stats no. 3. http://www.ahrq.gov/research/ findings/factsheets/primary/pcwork3/index.html (accessed January 8, 2016).

———. 2014b. Research Initiative in Clinical Economics. http://www.ahrq.gov/professionals/ clinicians-providers/resources/rice/index.html#Projects (accessed April 7, 2016).

———. 2016a. AHRQuality indicators—Introduction. http://www.qualityindicators.ahrq.gov (accessed May 5, 2016).

———. 2016b. Defining the PCMH. https://pcmh.ahrq.gov/page/defining-pcmh (accessed June 21, 2016).

AMA (American Medical Association). 2016. About the PCPI. https://www.ama-assn.org/ama/ pub/physician-resources/physician-consortium-performance-improvement/about-pcpi. page? (accessed May 5, 2016).

AOA (American Optometric Association). 2002. Pediatric eye and vision examination. https:// www.aoa.org/documents/CPG-2.pdf (accessed June 21,2016).

———. 2004. Care of the patient with amblyopia. http://www.aoa.org/documents/CPG-4.pdf (accessed July 18, 2016).

————. 2008. Care of the patient with learning related vision problems. http://www.aoa.org/documents/optometrists/CPG-20.pdf (accessed July 18, 2016).

————. 2011. Care of the patient with open angle glaucoma. http://www.aoa.org/documents/optometrists/CPG-9.pdf (accessed July 18, 2016).

————. 2014. Eye care of the patient with diabetes mellitus. http://www.aoa.org/Documents/EBO/EyeCareOfThePatientWithDiabetesMellitus%20CPG3.pdf (accessed July 18, 2016).

————. 2015a. 2015 AOA new technology & EHR survey. https://www.aoa.org/Documents/ric/2015%20EHR%20Executive%20Summary_FINAL.pdf (accessed July 18, 2016).

————. 2015b. AOA MORE. http://www.aoa.org/more?sso=y (accessed April 7, 2016).

————. 2015c. AOA optometric clinical practice guidelines. http://www.aoa.org/patients-and-public/caring-for-your-vision/clinical-practice-guidelines?sso=y (accessed May 18, 2016).

————. 2015d. Comprehensive adult eye and vision examination. https://www.aoa.org/documents/CPG-1.pdf (accessed June 21, 2016).

————. 2016a. AOA's 14 steps to evidence-based clinical practice guideline development. http://www.aoa.org/Documents/EBO/APPENDIX%20A-1%20AOA%2014%20Steps%20form.pdf (accessed June 1, 2016).

————. 2016b. Education & training. http://www.aoa.org/optometrists/education-and-training?sso=y (accessed April 7, 2016).

————. 2016c. Limitations of Vision Screening Programs. http://www.aoa.org/patients-and-public/caring-for-your-vision/comprehensive-eye-and-vision-examination/limitations-of-vision-screening-programs?sso=y (accessed July 18, 2016).

AOSA (American Optometric Student Association). 2016. Optometry education and public health. http://theaosa.org/about/optometry-education-and-public-health (accessed April 7, 2016).

APHA (American Public Health Association). 2008. Promoting interprofessional education. http://www.apha.org/policies-and-advocacy/public-health-policy-statements/policy-database/2014/07/23/09/20/promoting-interprofessional-education (accessed June 21, 2016).

————. 2016. Vision care. https://www.apha.org/apha-communities/member-sections/vision-care (accessed June 21, 2016).

APPAP (Association of Postgraduate Physician Assistant Programs). 2016. Post graduate PA programs listings. http://appap.org/post-graduate-pa-programs/programs (accessed April 27, 2016).

ASCO (Association of Schools and Colleges of Optometry). 2008. Guidelines for culturally competent eye and vision care. Diversity Task Force, Association of Schools and Colleges of Optometry. http://opted.org/files/Guidelines_CulturallyCompetentEyeAndVisionCare.pdf (accessed June 21, 2016).

Ashwal, S., B. S. Russman, P. A. Blasco, G. Miller, A. Sandler, M. Shevell, and R. Stevenson. 2004. Practice parameter: Diagnostic assessment of the child with cerebral palsy: Report of the Quality Standards Subcommittee of the American Academy of Neurology and the Practice Committee of the Child Neurology Society. *Neurology* 62(6):851–863.

ASORN (American Society of Ophthalmic Registered Nurses). 2016. Why Certification for Registered Nurse in Ophthalmology (CRNO)? http://www.asorn.org/certification (accessed April 27, 2016).

Azuara-Blanco, A., K. Banister, C. Boachie, P. McMeekin, J. Gray, J. Burr, R. Bourne, D. Garway-Heath, M. Batterbury, R. Hernandez, G. McPherson, C. Ramsay, and J. Cook. 2016. Automated imaging technologies for the diagnosis of glaucoma: A comparative diagnostic study for the evaluation of the diagnostic accuracy, performance as triage tests and cost-effectiveness (GATE study). *Health Technology Assessment* 20(8):1–168.

Bailey, G. M. 2013. Certain ODs welcome to participate in new ASCRS integrated program. http://ophthalmologytimes.modernmedicine.com/ophthalmologytimes/news/user-defined-tags/ophthalmology/certain-ods-welcome-participate-new-ascrs-in (accessed May 17, 2016).

Balcer, L. J., D. H. Miller, S. C. Reingold, and J. A. Cohen. 2015. Vision and vision-related outcome measures in multiple sclerosis. *Brain* 138(1):11–27.

Berwick, D. M., T. W. Nolan, and J. Whittington. 2008. The triple aim: Care, health, and cost. *Health Affairs* 27(3):759–769.

Blumberg, D. M., R. Vaswani, E. Nong, L. Al-Aswad, and G. A. Cioffi. 2014. A comparative effectiveness analysis of visual field outcomes after projected glaucoma screening using SD-OCT in African American communities. *Investigative Ophthalmology & Visual Science* 55(6):3491–3500.

Blumenthal, D., and M. Tavenner. 2010. The "meaningful use" regulation for electronic health records. *New England Journal of Medicine* 363(6):501–504.

Boland, M. V., M. F. Chiang, M. C. Lim, L. Wedemeyer, K. D. Epley, C. A. McCannel, D. E. Silverstone, and F. Lum. 2013. Adoption of electronic health records and preparations for demonstrating meaningful use: An American Academy of Ophthalmology survey. *Ophthalmology* 120(8):1702–1710.

Bourne, R. R., K. A. French, L. Chang, A. D. Borman, M. Hingorani, and W. D. Newsom. 2010. Can a community optometrist-based referral refinement scheme reduce false-positive glaucoma hospital referrals without compromising quality of care? The Community and Hospital Allied Network Glaucoma Evaluation Scheme (CHANGES). *Eye (London)* 24(5):881–887.

Bridges, D. R., R. A. Davidson, P. S. Odegard, I. V. Maki, and J. Tomkowiak. 2011. Interprofessional collaboration: Three best practice models of interprofessional education. *Medical Education Online* 16:6035. doi: 10.3402/meo.v16i0.6035.

Brien Holden Vision Institute. 2016. Eye & vision care toolkit. https://academy.brienholdenvision.org/browse/resources/courses/eye-toolkit (accessed June 21, 2016).

Brouwers, M. C., M. E. Kho, G. P. Browman, J. S. Burgers, F. Cluzeau, G. Feder, B. Fervers, I. D. Graham, J. Grimshaw, S. E. Hanna, P. Littlejohns, J. Makarski, and L. Zitzelsberger. 2010. GREE II: Advancing guideline development, reporting and evaluation in health care. *Canadian Medical Association Journal* 182(18):E839–E842.

Burr, J. M., G. Mowatt, R. Hernandez, M. A. Siddiqui, J. Cook, T. Lourenco, C. Ramsay, L. Vale, C. Fraser, A. Azuara-Blanco, J. Deeks, J. Cairns, R. Wormald, S. McPherson, K. Rabindranath, and A. Grant. 2007. The clinical effectiveness and cost-effectiveness of screening for open angle glaucoma: A systematic review and economic evaluation. *Health Technololgy Assessment* 11(41):iii–iv, ix–x, 1–190.

Carrillo, J. E., V. A. Carrillo, R. Guimento, J. Mucaria, and J. Leiman. 2014. The New York-Presbyterian Regional Health Collaborative: A three-year progress report. *Health Affairs* 33(11):1985–1992.

CDC (Centers for Disease Control and Prevention). 2009. A public health approach to vision loss. http://www.cdc.gov/visionhealth/about/approach.htm (accessed October 7, 2015).

———. 2015. 2014 NEHRS data on electronic health record adoption and use among office-based physicians in the U.S., by state. http://www.cdc.gov/nchs/data/ahcd/nehrs/2015_web_tables.pdf (accessed July 18, 2016).

CEPH (Council on Education for Public Health). 2011. *Accreditation criteria: Schools of public health.* Silver Spring, MD: CEPH. http://ceph.org/assets/SPH-Criteria-2011.pdf (accessed June 21, 2016).

Chan, P., P. J. Thyparampil, and M. F. Chiang. 2013. Accuracy and speed of electronic health record versus paper-based ophthalmic documentation strategies. *American Journal of Ophthalmology* 156(1):165–172, e162.

Charles, K., M. Cannon, R. Hall, and A. Coustasse. 2014. Can utilizing a computerized provider order entry (CPOE) system prevent hospital medical errors and adverse drug events? *Perspectives in Health Information Management* 11:1b.

Chiang, M. F., M. V. Boland, J. W. Margolis, F. Lum, M. D. Abramoff, and P. L. Hildebrand. 2008. Adoption and perceptions of electronic health record systems by ophthalmologists: An American Academy of Ophthalmology survey. *Ophthalmology* 115(9):1591–1597; quiz 1597, e1591–e1595.

Chiang, M. F., M. V. Boland, A. Brewer, K. D. Epley, M. B. Horton, M. C. Lim, C. A. McCannel, S. J. Patel, D. E. Silverstone, L. Wedemeyer, and F. Lum. 2011. Special requirements for electronic health record systems in ophthalmology. *Ophthalmology* 118(8):1681–1687.

Chiang, M. F., S. Read-Brown, D. C. Tu, D. Choi, D. S. Sanders, T. S. Hwang, S. Bailey, D. J. Karr, E. Cottle, J. C. Morrison, D. J. Wilson, and T. R. Yackel. 2013. Evaluation of electronic health record implementation in ophthalmology at an academic medical center. *Transactions of the American Ophthalmological Society* 111:70–92.

CHLP (Center for Health Leadership & Practice). 2016. Home page: Center for Health Leadership & Practice. http://healthleadership.org (accessed August 15, 2016).

Chou, R., T. Dana, and C. Bougatsos. 2011. Screening for visual impairment in children ages 1–5 years: Update for the USPSTF. *Pediatrics* 127(2):e442–e479.

Chou, R., T. Dana, C. Bougatsos, S. Grusing, and I. Blazina. 2016a. *Screening for impaired visual acuity in older adults: A systematic review to update the 2009 U.S. Preventive Services Task Force recommendation.* Rockville, MD: AHRQ.

———. 2016b. Screening for impaired visual acuity in older adults: Updated evidence report and systematic review for the U.S. Preventive Services Task Force. *JAMA* 315(9):915–933.

Chous, L. M., and T. L. Knabel. 2014. Impact of eye exams in identifying chronic conditions. https://www.uhc.com/content/dam/uhcdotcom/en/Employers/PDF/EyeExamsChronic Conditions.pdf (accessed July 18, 2016).

Cleveland Clinic. 2015. Diseases and conditions. https://my.clevelandclinic.org/health/diseases_ conditions/hic_ocular_health/hic_visual_field_testing (accessed March 31, 2016).

CMS (Centers for Medicare & Medicaid Services). 2011. Accountable care organization 2012 program analysis: Quality performance standards narrative measure specification: Final report. https://www.cms.gov/medicare/medicare-fee-for-service-payment/shared savingsprogram/downloads/aco_qualitymeasures.pdf (accessed June 21, 2016).

———. 2012. Accountable care organization 2013 program analysis quality performance standards narrative measure specifications. https://www.cms.gov/medicare/medicare-fee-for-service-payment/sharedsavingsprogram/downloads/aco_qualitymeasures.pdf (accessed June 21, 2016).

———. 2014. Accountable care organization 2014 program analysis quality performance standards narrative measure specifications. http://www.healthreform.ct.gov/ohri/lib/ohri/ work_groups/quality/2014-09-03/aco_narrative_measures_specs_1.pdf (accessed June 21, 2016).

———. 2015a. Accountable care organization 2015 program analysis quality performance standards narrative measure specifications. https://www.cms.gov/medicare/medicare-fee-for-service-payment/sharedsavingsprogram/downloads/ry2015-narrative-specifications. pdf (accessed June 21, 2106).

———. 2015b. Accountable care organizations (ACO). https://www.cms.gov/Medicare/ Medicare-Fee-for-Service-Payment/ACO/index.html?redirect=/Aco (accessed March 29, 2016).

———. 2015c. Next generation ACO model. https://innovation.cms.gov/initiatives/Next-Generation-ACO-Model (accessed April 7, 2016).

———. 2015d. Shared Savings Program. https://www.cms.gov/Medicare/Medicare-Fee-for-Service-Payment/sharedsavingsprogram/index.html (accessed March 29, 2016).

———. 2016a. Accountable care organization 2016 program quality measure narrative specifications. https://www.cms.gov/Medicare/Medicare-Fee-for-Service-Payment/sharedsavings program/Downloads/2016-ACO-NarrativeMeasures-Specs.pdf (accessed June 21, 2016).

———. 2016b. Pioneer ACO models. https://innovation.cms.gov/initiatives/Pioneer-ACO-Model/index.html (accessed April 29, 2016).

Crews, J. E., C. F. Chou, M. M. Zack, X. Zhang, K. M. Bullard, A. R. Morse, and J. B. Saaddine. 2016. The association of health-related quality of life with severity of visual impairment among people aged 40–64 years: Findings from the 2006-2010 Behavioral Risk Factor Surveillance System. *Ophthalmic Epidemiology* 23(3):145–153.

DesRoches, C. M., E. G. Campbell, S. R. Rao, K. Donelan, T. G. Ferris, A. Jha, R. Kaushal, D. E. Levy, S. Rosenbaum, A. E. Shields, and D. Blumenthal. 2008. Electronic health records in ambulatory care—A national survey of physicians. *New England Journal of Medicine* 359(1):50–60.

Donahue, S. P., and J. B. Ruben. 2011. U.S. Preventive Services Task Force vision screening recommendations. *Pediatrics* 127(3):569–570.

Elam, A. R., and P. P. Lee. 2013. High-risk populations for vision loss and eye care underutilization: A review of the literature and ideas on moving forward. *Survey of Ophthalmology* 58(4):348–358.

Elhauge, E. 2010. Why we should care about health care fragmentation and how to fix it. In *The fragmentation of U.S. health care: Causes and solutions*, edited by E. Elhauge. New York: Oxford University Press.

Enthoven, A. C. 2009. Integrated delivery systems: The cure for fragmentation. *American Journal of Managed Care* 15(10 Suppl):S284–S290.

Expert Panel on Cultural Competence Education for Students in Medicine and Public Health. 2012. *Cultural competence education for students in medicine and public health: Report of an expert panel*. Washington, DC: Association of American Medical Colleges and Association of Schools of Public Health.

Fisher, E. S. 2008. Building a medical neighborhood for the medical home. *New England Journal of Medicine* 359(12):1202–1205.

Forrester, S. H., Z. Hepp, J. A. Roth, H. S. Wirtz, and E. B. Devine. 2014. Cost-effectiveness of a computerized provider order entry system in improving medication safety ambulatory care. *Value Health* 17(4):340–349.

Friedberg, M. W., E. C. Schneider, M. B. Rosenthal, K. G. Volpp, and R. M. Werner. 2014. Association between participation in a multipayer medical home intervention and changes in quality, utilization, and costs of care. *JAMA* 311(8):815–825.

Frohman, E. M., J. G. Fujimoto, T. C. Frohman, P. A. Calabresi, G. Cutter, and L. J. Balcer. 2008. Optical coherence tomography: A window into the mechanisms of multiple sclerosis. *Nature Clinical Practice Neurology* 4(12):664–675.

Gandhi, T. K., N. L. Keating, M. Ditmore, D. Kiernan, R. Johnson, E. Burdick, and C. Hamann. 2008. Improving referral communication using a referral tool within an electronic medical record. In *Advances in patient safety: New directions and alternative approaches*, edited by K. Henriksen, J. B. Battles, M. A. Keyes, and M. L. Grady. Rockville, MD: Agency for Healthcare Research and Quality.

Gangwani, R., W. W. Lai, R. Sum, S. M. McGhee, C. W. Chan, A. J. Hedley, and D. Wong. 2014. The incidental findings of age-related macular degeneration during diabetic retinopathy screening. *Graefe's Archive for Clinical and Experimental Ophthalmology* 252(5):723–729.

Garg, S., and R. M. Davis. 2009. Diabetic retinopathy screening update. *Clinical Diabetes* 27(4):140–145.

Grieger, D. L., S. H. Cohen, and D. A. Krusch. 2007. A pilot study to document the return on investment for implementing an ambulatory electronic health record at an academic medical center. *Journal of the American College of Surgeons* 205(1):89–96.

Hartmann, E. E., G. E. Bradford, P. K. Chaplin, T. Johnson, A. R. Kemper, S. Kim, and W. Marsh-Tootle. 2006. Project Universal Preschool Vision Screening: A demonstration project. *Pediatrics* 117(2):e226–e237.

Hered, R. W., and D. L. Wood. 2013. Preschool vision screening in primary care pediatric practice. *Public Health Reports* 128(3):189–197.

HITPC (Health IT Policy Committee). 2015. Report to congress: Challenges and barriers to interoperability. https://www.healthit.gov/facas/sites/faca/files/HITPC_Final_ITF_Report_2015-12-16%20v3.pdf (accessed July 19, 2016).

Holley, C. D., and P. P. Lee. 2010. Primary care provider views of the current referral-to-eye-care process: Focus group results. *Investigative Ophthalmology & Visual Science* 51(4):1866–1872.

Holtzer-Goor, K. M., E. van Sprundel, H. G. Lemij, T. Plochg, N. S. Klazinga, and M. A. Koopmanschap. 2010. Cost-effectiveness of monitoring glaucoma patients in shared care: An economic evaluation alongside a randomized controlled trial. *BMC Health Services Research* 10(1):1–11.

Holtzer-Goor, K. M., E. J. van Vliet, E. van Sprundel, T. Plochg, M. A. Koopmanschap, N. S. Klazinga, and H. G. Lemij. 2016. Shared care in monitoring stable glaucoma patients: A randomized controlled trial. *Journal of Glaucoma* 25(4):e392–e400.

Hooker, R. S., and C. M. Everett. 2012. The contributions of physician assistants in primary care systems. *Health & Social Care in the Community* 20(1):20–31.

HRSA (Health Resources and Services Administration). 2011. Redesigning a system of care to promote QI. http://www.hrsa.gov/quality/toolbox/methodology/redesigningasystemof care (accessed June 21, 2016).

———. 2016a. Interprofessional Education Coordinating Center for Interprofessional Education and Collaborative Practice. http://bhpr.hrsa.gov/grants/interprofessional/index.html (accessed April 7, 2016).

———. 2016b. Small Health Care Provider Quality Improvement Program. Funding opportunity number: HRSA-16-019. http://www.hrsa.gov/ruralhealth/programopportunities/fundingopportunities/?id=b5c3a786-4ffc-4e0a-bb2e-e7e3cc6b29a6 (accessed June 21, 2016).

HSDM (Harvard School of Dental Medicine). 2016. Case for action. http://oralhealth.hsdm.harvard.edu/home (accessed July 18, 2016).

Hsiao, C-J., E. Hing. 2014. Use and characteristics of electronic health record systems among office-based physician practices: United States, 2001–2013. NCHS Data Brief No. 143, January. http://www.cdc.gov/nchs/products/databriefs/db143.htm (accessed June 21, 2016).

Huang, X., and M. B. Rosenthal. 2014. Transforming specialty practice—The patient-centered medical neighborhood. *New England Journal of Medicine* 370(15):1376–1379.

Interprofessional Education Collaborative Expert Panel. 2011. *Core competencies for interprofessional collaborative practice: Report of an expert panel.* Washington, DC: Interprofessional Education Collaborative. https://www.aamc.org/download/186750/data/core_competencies.pdf (accessed July 18, 2016).

IOM (Institute of Medicine). 2001. *Crossing the quality chasm: A new health system for the 21st century.* Washington, DC: National Academy Press.

———. 2003a. *Health professions education: A bridge to quality.* Washington, DC: The National Academies Press.

———. 2003b. *Unequal treatment: Confronting racial and ethnic disparities in health care.* Washington, DC: The National Academies Press.

————. 2011a. *Clinical practice guidelines we can trust.* Washington, DC: The National Academies Press.

————. 2011b. Report brief: Clinical practice guidelines we can trust. http://www.national academies.org/hmd/~/media/Files/Report%20Files/2011/Clinical-Practice-Guidelines-We-Can-Trust/Clinical%20Practice%20Guidelines%202011%20Report%20Brief.pdf (accessed April 7, 2016).

Jain, S., S. Harnada, W. L. Membrey, and V. Chong. 2006. Screening for age-related macular degeneration using nonstereo digital fundus photographs. *Eye* 20(4):471–475.

Jamous, K. F., M. Kalloniatis, M. P. Hennessy, A. Agar, A. Hayen, and B. Zangerl. 2015. Clinical model assisting with the collaborative care of glaucoma patients and suspects. *Clinical & Experimental Ophthalmology* 43(4):308–319.

Johns Hopkins Medicine. 2016. Public Health Ophthalmology (PHO) program. http://www.hopkinsmedicine.org/wilmer/education/dana.html (accessed April 7, 2016).

Jones, S., and R. T. Edwards. 2010. Diabetic retinopathy screening: A systematic review of the economic evidence. *Diabetic Medicine* 27(3):249–256.

Karnon, J., C. Czoski-Murray, K. Smith, C. Brand, U. Chakravarthy, S. Davis, N. Bansback, C. Beverley, A. Bird, S. Harding, I. Chisholm, and Y. C. Yang. 2008. A preliminary model-based assessment of the cost-utility of a screening programme for early age-related macular degeneration. *Health Technology Assessment* 12(27):iii–iv, ix–124.

Kaushal, R., A. K. Jha, C. Franz, J. Glaser, K. D. Shetty, T. Jaggi, B. Middleton, G. J. Kuperman, R. Khorasani, M. Tanasijevic, and D. W. Bates. 2006. Return on investment for a computerized physician order entry system. *Journal of the American Medical Informatics Association* 13(3):261–266.

Kellogg Eye Center. 2015. Strabismus (misaligned eyes, crossed eyes, or wall eyes). http://www.kellogg.umich.edu/patientcare/conditions/strabismus.html (accessed March 29, 2016).

Kemper, A. R., A. Helfrich, J. Talbot, N. Patel, and J. E. Crews. 2011. Improving the rate of preschool vision screening: An interrupted time-series analysis. *Pediatrics* 128(5):e1279–e1284.

Kent, C. 2015. The IRIS registry: The first 18 months. *The Review of Ophthalmology.* November 5. http://www.reviewofophthalmology.com/content/c/58132 (accessed June 21, 2016).

Kern, L. M., A. Edwards, and R. Kaushal. 2014. The patient-centered medical home, electronic health records, and quality of care. *Annals of Internal Medicine* 160(11):741–749.

————. 2016. The patient-centered medical home and associations with health care quality and utilization: A 5-year cohort study. *Annals of Internal Medicine* 164(6):395–405.

Kirk, N. 2011. The curriculum: "A model for other schools to follow." *UConn Today,* April 25. http://today.uconn.edu/2011/04/the-curriculum-a-model-for-other-schools-to-follow (accessed July 18, 2016).

Kneib, B. A. 2009. AOA Continuous Quality Improvement Process.

Kokkonen, E. W. J., S. A. Davis, H.-C. Lin, T. S. Dabade, S. R. Feldman, and A. B. Fleischer. 2013. Use of electronic medical records differs by specialty and office settings. *Journal of the American Medical Informatics Association* 20(e1):e33–e38.

Krein, S. L., S. J. Bernstein, C. E. Fletcher, F. Makki, C. L. Goldzweig, B. Watts, S. Vijan, and R. A. Hayward. 2008. Improving eye care for veterans with diabetes: An example of using the QUERI steps to move from evidence to implementation: QUERI series. *Implementation Science* 3:18.

Kung, J., R. R. Miller, and P. A. Mackowiak. 2012. Failure of clinical practice guidelines to meet Institute of Medicine standards: Two more decades of little, if any, progress. *Archives of Internal Medicine* 172(21):1628–1633.

Ladapo, J. A., S. M. Kymes, J. A. Ladapo, V. C. Nwosu, and L. R. Pasquale. 2012. Projected clinical outcomes of glaucoma screening in African American individuals. *Archives of Ophthalmology* 130(3):365–372.

LCME (Liaison Committee on Medical Education). 2015. Functions and structure of a medical school: Standards for accreditation of medical education programs leading to the M.D. degree. http://umsc.org.uic.edu/documents/LCME_standards.pdf (accessed June 21, 2016).

Lee, P. 2016. Visual acuity screening among asymptomatic older adults. *JAMA* 315(9):875–876.

Lesser, L. I., A. H. Krist, D. B. Kamerow, and A. W. Bazemore. 2011. Comparison between U.S. Preventive Services Task Force recommendations and Medicare coverage. *Annals of Family Medicine* 9(1):44–49.

Lim, M. C., R. P. Patel, V. S. Lee, P. D. Weeks, M. K. Barber, and M. R. Watnik. 2015. The long-term financial and clinical impact of an electronic health record on an academic ophthalmology practice. *Journal of Ophthalmology* 2015:329819.

Lin, H., and X. Wu. 2014. Intervention strategies for improving patient adherence to follow-up in the era of mobile information technology: A systematic review and meta-analysis. *PLoS ONE* 9(8):e104266.

Lowry, E. A., W. Wang, and O. Nyong'o. 2015. Objective vision screening in 3-year-old children at a multispecialty practice. *Journal of the American Association for Pediatric Ophthalmology and Strabismus* 19(1):16–20.

Lum, F., R. S. Feder, S. D. McLeod, and D. W. Parke, II. 2016. The preferred practice pattern guidelines in ophthalmology. *Ophthalmology* 123(5):928–929.

Maeshiro, R. 2008. Responding to the challenge: Population health education for physicians. *Academic Medicine* 83(4):319–320.

Mandalos, A., R. Bourne, K. French, W. Newsom, and L. Chang. 2012. Shared care of patients with ocular hypertension in the Community and Hospital Allied Network Glaucoma Evaluation Scheme (CHANGES). *Eye* 26(4):564–567.

McLeod, H., H. Dickinson, I. Williams, S. Robinson, and J. Coast. 2006. *Evaluation of the chronic eye care services programme: Final report.* Birmingham, UK: Health Services Management Centre, University of Birmingham. www.eyecare.nhs.uk/uploads/Chronic EyecareServicesProgramme.doc (accessed June 21, 2016).

MCPHS (Massachusetts College of Pharmacy and Health Sciences). 2016. Optometry/public health (O.D./M.P.H.). http://www.mcphs.edu/Academics/Programs/Optometry%20 OD%20MPH (accessed April 7, 2016).

Medline Plus. 2015a. Extraocular muscle function testing. https://www.nlm.nih.gov/med lineplus/ency/article/003397.htm (accessed April 20, 2016).

———. 2015b. Refraction test. https://www.nlm.nih.gov/medlineplus/ency/article/003844.htm (accessed April 20, 2016).

———. 2015c. Slit-lamp exam. https://www.nlm.nih.gov/medlineplus/ency/article/003880.htm (accessed April 20, 2016).

———. 2015d. Tonometry. https://www.nlm.nih.gov/medlineplus/ency/article/003447.htm (accessed April 20, 2016).

———. 2015e. Visual acuity test. https://www.nlm.nih.gov/medlineplus/ency/article/003396. htm (accessed April 20, 2016).

———. 2015f. Visual field. https://www.nlm.nih.gov/medlineplus/ency/article/003879.htm (accessed April 20, 2016).

Mehrotra, A., C. B. Forrest, and C. Y. Lin. 2011. Dropping the baton: Specialty referrals in the United States. *The Milbank Quarterly* 89(1):39–68.

Moyer, V. A. 2013. Screening for glaucoma: U.S. Preventive Services Task Force recommendation statement. *Annals of Internal Medicine* 159(7):484–489.

NCCPA (National Commission on Certification of Physician Assistants). 2016. Specialty Certificates of Added Qualification (CAQs). http://www.nccpa.net/Specialty-CAQs (accessed April 27, 2016).

NCIPE (National Center for Interprofessional Practice and Education). 2016a. Home page: National Center for Interprofessional Practice and Education. https://nexusipe.org (accessed June 21, 2016).

———. 2016b. Interprofessional professionalism collaborative. https://nexusipe.org/informing/resource-center/interprofessional-professionalism-collaborative (accessed June 21, 2016).

———. 2016c. University of Alabama at Birmingham: The role of interprofessional faculty development in improving collaborative practice behavior competencies. https://nexusipe.org/advancing/nexus-innovations-network/university-alabama-birmingham-role-interprofessional-faculty (accessed June 21, 2016).

NCQA (National Committee for Quality Assurance). 2014a. The future of patient-centered medical homes. Foundation for a Better Health Care System. https://www.ncqa.org/Portals/0/Public%20Policy/2014%20Comment%20Letters/The_Future_of_PCMH.pdf (accessed June 21, 2016).

———. 2014b. Standards and guidelines for NCQA's patient-centered medical home (PCMH) 2014. http://www.acofp.org/acofpimis/Acofporg/Apps/2014_PCMH_Finals/Tools/1_PCMH_Recognition_2014_Front_Matter.pdf (accessed June 21, 2016).

———. 2016a. About NCQA. http://www.ncqa.org/about-ncqa (accessed May 5, 2016).

———. 2016b. Diabetes Recognition Program (DRP). http://www.ncqa.org/tabid/139/Default.aspx (accessed April 7, 2016).

———. 2016c. Patient-centered specialty practice (PCSP) clinician eligibility. http://www.ncqa.org/programs/recognition/practices/patient-centered-medical-home-pcmh/during-earn-it-pcmh/other-pcmh-resources/pcsp-clinician-eligibility (accessed March 29, 2016).

———. 2016d. Patient-centered specialty practice recognition. http://www.ncqa.org/programs/recognition/practices/patient-centered-specialty-practice-pcsp (accessed April 29, 2016).

———. 2016e. *Standards and guidelines for PCSP 2016 recognition.* Washington, DC: NCQA.

NEI (National Eye Institute). 2016. What is a comprehensive dilated eye exam? https://nei.nih.gov/healthyeyes/eyeexam (accessed March 29, 2016).

Nelson, K. M., C. Helfrich, H. Sun, P. L. Hebert, C. F. Liu, E. Dolan, L. Taylor, E. Wong, C. Maynard, S. E. Hernandez, W. Sanders, I. Randall, I. Curtis, G. Schectman, R. Stark, and S. D. Fihn. 2014. Implementation of the patient-centered medical home in the Veterans Health Administration: Associations with patient satisfaction, quality of care, staff burnout, and hospital and emergency department use. *JAMA Internal Medicine* 174(8):1350–1358.

NICHQ (National Institute for Children's Health Quality). 2015. Reducing vision impairment in young children is focus of new initiative. http://www.nichq.org/news%20and%20events/news/vision_impairment_project (accessed April 7, 2016).

Nielsen, M., L. Buelt, K. Patel, and L. M. Nichols. 2016. *The patient-centered medical home's impact on cost and quality: Annual review of evidence 2014-2015.* Washington, DC: Patient-Centered Primary Care Collaborative.

NQF (National Quality Forum). 2016a. Comprehensive diabetes care: Eye exam (retinal) performed. http://www.qualityforum.org/QPS/0055 (accessed April 29, 2016).

———. 2016b. Comprehensive diabetes care: Hemoglobin a1c (hba1c) poor control (>9.0%). http://www.qualityforum.org/QPS/0059 (accessed April 29, 2016).

———. 2016c. Improving healthcare quality. http://www.qualityforum.org/Setting_Priorities/Improving_Healthcare_Quality.aspx (accessed May 5, 2016).

Nuckols, T. K., C. Smith-Spangler, S. C. Morton, S. M. Asch, V. M. Patel, L. J. Anderson, E. L. Deichsel, and P. G. Shekelle. 2014. The effectiveness of computerized order entry at reducing preventable adverse drug events and medication errors in hospital settings: A systematic review and meta-analysis. *Systematic Reviews* 3:56.

Okeke, C. O., H. A. Quigley, H. D. Jampel, G. S. Ying, R. J. Plyler, Y. Jiang, and D. S. Friedman. 2009. Interventions improve poor adherence with once daily glaucoma medications in electronically monitored patients. *Ophthalmology* 116(12):2286–2293.

ONC (Office of the National Coordinator for Health Information Technology). 2015. Federal health IT strategic plan 2015–2020. https://www.healthit.gov/sites/default/files/9-5-federal healthitstratplanfinal_0.pdf (accessed July 18, 2016).

Pandit, R. R., and M. V. Boland. 2013. The impact of an electronic health record transition on a glaucoma subspecialty practice. *Ophthalmology* 120(4):753–760.

Parke, D. W., Ii, M. X. Repka, and F. Lum. 2016. The US Preventive Services Task Force recommendation on vision screening in older adults: A narrow view. *JAMA Ophthalmology* 134(5):485–486.

Patil, M., L. Puri, and C. M. Gonzalez. 2008. Productivity and cost implications of implementing electronic medical records into an ambulatory surgical subspecialty clinic. *Urology* 71(2):173–177.

Pena-Purcell, N. C., and M. M. Boggess. 2014. An application of a diabetes knowledge scale for low-literate Hispanic/Latinos. *Health Promotion Practice* 15(2):252–262.

Petitti, D. B., S. M. Teutsch, M. B. Barton, G. F. Sawaya, J. K. Ockene, and T. DeWitt. 2009. Update on the methods of the U.S. Preventive Services Task Force: Insufficient evidence. *Annals of Internal Medicine* 150(3):199–205.

Phillips, R. L., M. Han, S. M. Petterson, L. A. Makaroff, and W. R. Liaw. 2014. Cost, utilization, and quality of care: An evaluation of Illinois' Medicaid primary care case management program. *Annals of Family Medicine* 12(5):408–417.

Quillen, D. A., R. A. Harper, and B. G. Haik. 2005. Medical student education in ophthalmology: Crisis and opportunity. *Ophthalmology* 112(11):1867–1868.

Read-Brown, S., D. S. Sanders, A. S. Brown, T. R. Yackel, D. Choi, D. C. Tu, and M. F. Chiang. 2013. Time-motion analysis of clinical nursing documentation during implementation of an electronic operating room management system for ophthalmic surgery. *AMIA Annual Symposium Proceedings* 2013:1195–1204.

Redd, T. K., S. Read-Brown, D. Choi, T. R. Yackel, D. C. Tu, and M. F. Chiang. 2014. Electronic health record impact on pediatric ophthalmologists' productivity and efficiency at an academic center. *Journal of the American Association for Pediatric Ophthalmology and Strabismus* 18(6):584–589.

Reeves, S., J. Goldman, A. Burton, and B. Sawatzky-Girling. 2010. Synthesis of systematic review evidence of interprofessional education. *Journal of Allied Health* 39(Suppl 1):198–203.

Reeves, S., L. Perrier, J. Goldman, D. Freeth, and M. Zwarenstein. 2013. Interprofessional education: Effects on professional practice and healthcare outcomes (update). *Cochrane Database of Systematic Reviews* 3:Cd002213.

Rein, D. B., J. S. Wittenborn, X. Zhang, T. J. Hoerger, P. Zhang, B. E. Klein, K. E. Lee, R. Klein, and J. B. Saaddine. 2012a. The cost-effectiveness of Welcome to Medicare visual acuity screening and a possible alternative Welcome to Medicare eye evaluation among persons without diagnosed diabetes mellitus. *Archives of Ophthalmology* 130(5):607–614.

Rein, D. B., J. S. Wittenborn, X. Zhang, M. Song, and J. B. Saaddine. 2012b. The potential cost-effectiveness of amblyopia screening programs. *Journal of Pediatric Ophthalmology and Strabismus* 49(3):146–155; quiz 145, 156.

Remington, T. L., M. A. Foulk, and B. C. Williams. 2006. Evaluation of evidence for interprofessional education. *American Journal of Pharmaceutical Education* 70(3):66.

Reuben, D. B., D. A. Ganz, C. P. Roth, H. E. McCreath, K. D. Ramirez, and N. S. Wenger. 2013. The effect of nurse practitioner co-management on the care of geriatric conditions. *Journal of the American Geriatrics Society* 61(6):857–867.

Roblin, D. W., D. H. Howard, E. R. Becker, E. Kathleen Adams, and M. H. Roberts. 2004. Use of midlevel practitioners to achieve labor cost savings in the primary care practice of an MCO. *Health Services Research* 39(3):607–626.

Rosenthal, M. B., M. K. Abrams, A. Bitton, and The Patient Centered Medical Home Evaluators' Collaborative. 2012. Recommended core measures for evaluating the patient-centered medical home: Cost, utilization, and clinical quality. http://www.commonwealthfund.org/~/media/Files/Publications/Data%20Brief/2012/1601_Rosenthal_recommended_core_measures_PCMH_v2.pdf (accessed June 20, 2016).

Rosland, A. M., K. Nelson, H. Sun, E. D. Dolan, C. Maynard, C. Bryson, R. Stark, J. M. Shear, E. Kerr, S. D. Fihn, and G. Schectman. 2013. The patient-centered medical home in the Veterans Health Administration. *American Journal of Managed Care* 19(7): e263–e272.

Rupp, J. D. 2016. The 8 point eye exam. American Academy of Ophthamology, May 24. http://www.aao.org/young-ophthalmologists/yo-info/article/how-to-conduct-eight-point-ophthalmology-exam (accessed April 20, 2016).

RWJF (Robert Wood Johnson Foundation). 2012. Improving the science of continuous quality improvement program and evaluation: An RWJF national program. http://www.rwjf.org/content/dam/farm/reports/program_results_reports/2012/rwjf73230 (accessed July 18, 2016).

———. 2016. Interdisciplinary research leaders. http://www.rwjf.org/en/library/funding-opportunities/2016/interdisciplinary-research-leaders.html (accessed April 7, 2016).

Sabin, J. A., and A. G. Greenwald. 2012. The influence of implicit bias on treatment recommendations for 4 common pediatric conditions: Pain, urinary tract infection, attention deficit hyperactivity disorder, and asthma. *American Journal of Public Health* 102(5):988–995.

Sanders, D. S., D. J. Lattin, S. Read-Brown, D. C. Tu, D. J. Wilson, T. S. Hwang, J. C. Morrison, T. R. Yackel, and M. F. Chiang. 2013. Electronic health record systems in ophthalmology: Impact on clinical documentation. *Ophthalmology* 120(9):1745–1755.

Sanders, D. S., S. Read-Brown, D. C. Tu, W. E. Lambert, D. Choi, B. M. Almario, T. R. Yackel, A. S. Brown, and M. F. Chiang. 2014. Impact of an electronic health record operating room management system in ophthalmology on documentation time, surgical volume, and staffing. *JAMA Ophthalmology* 132(5):586–592.

Schaneman, J., A. Kagey, S. Soltesz, and J. Stone. 2010. The role of comprehensive eye exams in the early detection of diabetes and other chronic diseases in an employed population. *Population Health Management* 13(4):195–199.

Schmidt, P., M. Maguire, V. Dobson, G. Quinn, E. Ciner, L. Cyert, M. T. Kulp, B. Moore, D. Orel-Bixler, M. Redford, and G. S. Ying. 2004. Comparison of preschool vision screening tests as administered by licensed eye care professionals in the Vision in Preschoolers Study. *Ophthalmology* 111(4):637–650.

Shah, M., D. Knoch, and E. Waxman. 2014. The state of ophthalmology medical student education in the United States and Canada, 2012 through 2013. *Ophthalmology* 121(6):1160–1163.

Sheppard, K. D., C. R. Ford, P. Sawyer, K. T. Foley, C. N. Harada, C. J. Brown, and C. S. Ritchie. 2015. The interprofessional clinical experience: Interprofessional education in the nursing home. *Journal of Interprofessional Care* 29(2):170–172.

Singh, R. P., R. Bedi, A. Li, et al. 2015. The practice impact of electronic health record system implementation within a large multispecialty ophthalmic practice. *JAMA Ophthalmology* 133(6):668–674.

Sommer, A. 2016. The USPSTF position on vision screening of adults—Seeing is believing? *JAMA Internal Medicine* 176(4):438–439.

Starfield, B., C. B. Forrest, P. A. Nutting, and S. von Schrader. 2002. Variability in physician referral decisions. *Journal of the American Board of Family Practice* 15(6):473–480.

Stern, G. A. 1995. Teaching ophthalmology to primary care physicians. The Association of University Professors of Ophthalmology Education Committee. *Archives of Ophthalmology* 113(6):722–724.

Stevens, G. D., L. Shi, C. Vane, and A. L. Peters. 2014. Do experiences consistent with a medical-home model improve diabetes care measures reported by adult Medicaid patients? *Diabetes Care* 37(9):2565–2571.

Stevens, S., C. Gilbert, and N. Astbury. 2007. How to measure intraocular pressure: Applanation tonometry. *Community Eye Health* 20(64):74–75.

Torres, S., R. Labonté, D. L. Spitzer, C. Andrew, and C. Amaratunga. 2014. Improving health equity: The promising role of community health workers in Canada. *Healthcare Policy* 10(1):73–85.

UnitedHealthcare. 2016. UnitedHealthcare vision plan. https://www.opm.gov/healthcare-insurance/healthcare/plan-information/plan-codes/2016/brochures/UnitedHealth.pdf (accessed April 21, 2016).

University of Michigan. 2015a. Interprofessional education. https://interprofessional.umich.edu/about/courses/ (accessed April 7, 2016).

———. 2015b. Vision tests. http://www.uofmhealth.org/health-library/hw235693#aa24248 (accessed March 31, 2016).

USPSTF (U.S. Preventive Services Task Force). 2011. Visual impairment in children ages 1-5: Screening. http://www.uspreventiveservicestaskforce.org/Page/Document/UpdateSummaryFinal/visual-impairment-in-children-ages-1-5-screening (accessed April 7, 2016).

———. 2013. Final recommendation statement: Glaucoma screening. http://www.uspreventiveservicestaskforce.org/Page/Document/RecommendationStatementFinal/glaucoma-screening (accessed April 25, 2016).

———. 2016a. About the USPSTF. http://www.uspreventiveservicestaskforce.org/Page/Name/about-the-uspstf (accessed September 1, 2016).

———. 2016b. Grade definitions: Grade definitions after July 2012. http://www.uspreventiveservicestaskforce.org/Page/Name/grade-definitions (accessed July 19, 2016).

———. 2016c. Screening for impaired visual acuity in older adults: U.S. Preventive Services Task Force recommendation statement. *JAMA* 315(9):908–914.

VA (U.S. Department of Veterans Affairs). 2016. Team-based care: PACT. http://www.va.gov/HEALTH/services/primarycare/pact/team.asp (accessed June 30, 2016).

van Vliet, E. J., W. Sermeus, C. M. van Gaalen, J. C. Sol, and J. M. Vissers. 2010. Efficacy and efficiency of a lean cataract pathway: A comparative study. *Quality & Safety in Health Care* 19(6):e13.

Voyatzis, G., H. W. Roberts, J. Keenan, and M. S. Rajan. 2014. Cambridgeshire cataract shared care model: Community optometrist-delivered postoperative discharge scheme. *British Journal of Ophthalmology* 98(6):760–764.

Werner, R. M., A. Canamucio, J. A. Shea, and G. True. 2014. The medical home transformation in the Veterans Health Administration: An evaluation of early changes in primary care delivery. *Health Services Research* 49(4):1329–1347.

WHO (World Health Organization). 2010. *Framework for action on interprofessional education & collaborative practice*. Geneva: WHO. Available at http://apps.who.int/iris/bitstream/10665/70185/1/WHO_HRH_HPN_10.3_eng.pdf?ua=1 (accessed June 21, 2016).

Wiggins, M. N., R. D. Landes, S. D. Bhaleeya, and S. H. Uwaydat. 2013. Primary care physician's knowledge of the ophthalmic effects of diabetes. *Canadian Journal of Ophthalmology* 48(4):10.1016/j.jcjo.2013.1003.1011.

Wu, A. M., C. M. Wu, B. K. Young, D. J. Wu, A. Chen, C. E. Margo, and P. B. Greenberg. 2015a. Evaluation of primary open-angle glaucoma clinical practice guidelines. *Canadian Journal of Ophthalmology* 50(3):192–196.

Wu, A. M., C. M. Wu, B. K. Young, D. J. Wu, C. E. Margo, and P. B. Greenberg. 2015b. Critical appraisal of clinical practice guidelines for age-related macular degeneration. *Journal of Ophthalmology* 2015:1–5.

Wu, C. M., A. M. Wu, B. K. Young, D. Wu, A. Chen, C. E. Margo, and P. B. Greenberg. 2015c. An evaluation of cataract surgery clinical practice guidelines. *British Journal of Ophthalmology* 99(3):401–404.

Wu, C. M., A. M. Wu, B. K. Young, D. J. Wu, C. E. Margo, and P. B. Greenberg. 2015d. An appraisal of clinical practice guidelines for diabetic retinopathy. *American Journal of Medical Quality* 31(4):370–375.

Ying, G. S., M. T. Kulp, M. Maguire, E. Ciner, L. Cyert, and P. Schmidt. 2005. Sensitivity of screening tests for detecting vision in preschoolers-targeted vision disorders when specificity is 94%. *Optometry & Vision Science* 82(5):432–438.

Ying, G. S., M. Maguire, G. Quinn, M. T. Kulp, and L. Cyert. 2011. ROC analysis of the accuracy of noncycloplegic retinoscopy, retinomax autorefractor, and suresight vision screener for preschool vision screening. *Investigative Ophthalmology & Visual Science* 52(13):9658–9664.

Young, B. K., C. M. Wu, A. M. Wu, C. E. Margo, and P. B. Greenberg. 2015. Are clinical practice guidelines for cataract and glaucoma trustworthy? *American Journal of Medical Quality* 30(2):188–190.

Meeting the Challenge of Vision Loss in the United States: Improving Diagnosis, Rehabilitation, and Accessibility

Vision impairment can adversely affect an individual's health, functioning, and quality of life (QOL) in numerous ways. "Low vision adversely affects many daily activities, such as writing a check, telling time, looking for daily items, using a phone, managing medications, and preparing a meal" (Liu et al., 2013, p. 280). Vision impairment may comprise a patient's mobility, as well as his or her ability to read and drive (Brown et al., 2014; Owsley and McGwin, 2010; Swenor et al., 2015). Vision impairment in children and young adults affects development and academic performance, with a long-term, detrimental impact on QOL (Davidson and Quinn, 2011). Vision impairment is also associated with reduced mental and physical health (Crews et al., 2006, 2016b; Zhang et al., 2013a) and with increased risk of falls, injury, and mortality (Christ et al., 2014; Crews et al., 2016a; Patino et al., 2010). Vision impairment is associated with less education, lower income, and lower employment rates (Erickson, 2016). Chapter 3 discusses in further detail the adverse effects of vision impairment on QOL, independence, mobility, falls and injuries, mental health, cognition, and mortality.

A considerable portion of vision impairment can be prevented, mitigated, or reversed through public health intervention and clinical treatment. For example, estimates of uncorrected refractive error range from 8.2 million to 15.9 million (Varma et al., 2016; Wittenborn and Rein, 2016). However, even if all preventable cases of vision impairment were eliminated, millions of Americans would still live with vision impairment because of limits in the ability to prevent and manage eye disease. In 2015, 4.24 million U.S. adults ages 40 and older were affected by uncorrectable vision impairment, including blindness; this number is projected to rise to almost 8.96 million by 2050 (Varma et al., 2016).[1] Given the magnitude of this burden, meeting the health care needs of visually impaired populations is a challenge—a challenge that will only grow over time. Yet, with appropriate access to high-quality care and interventions that effectively manage vision loss, individuals with chronic vision impairment can gain significant advantages in facing this major health obstacle. Lacking these services and interventions, however, the consequences of vision impairment on one's life can be substantial and broad ranging.

Congenital, genetic, and acquired eye diseases and conditions, such as untreated amblyopia, retinitis pigmentosa, and Stargardt's disease can lead to chronic vision impairment in children and young adults (Bradfield, 2013; NEI, 2014, 2015). Chronic vision impairment in these populations can impose a considerable public health burden by adversely affecting health and socioeconomic outcomes across the lifespan. The greatest burden of eye disease, however, falls on older populations, who are at increased risk for age-related eye disease (CDC, 2009; Gilbert and Foster, 2001). In their advanced forms, age-related eye diseases such as glaucoma and diabetic retinopathy can result in irreversible vision loss, and the aging of the U.S. population means the prevalence of these diseases and the vision impairment they can entail is projected to increase in the coming decades (NEI, 2010).

For individuals with vision impairment that cannot be corrected by available refractive, medical, or surgical treatments, vision rehabilitation has the potential to prevent depression and emotional distress and to improve or maintain QOL, the ability to perform daily activities, and overall visual ability (Brody et al., 2005; Goldstein et al., 2015; Lamoureux et al., 2007; Walter et al., 2007).[2] According to an Agency for Healthcare Research and Quality (AHRQ) report, the aim of vision rehabilitation is "to maximize the use of any residual vision that an individual might have and provide practical adaptations that reduce the disabilities associated with low vision or blindness" (AHRQ, 2004, p. 36). Desired outcomes of vision

---

[1] In 2015, 3.22 million adults ages 40 and older had vision impairment (visual acuity worse than 20/40, but better than 20/200), and 1.02 million were blind (visual acuity of 20/200 or worse, based on visual acuity in the best-corrected, better-seeing eye). In 2050, 6.95 million adults ages 40 and older are projected to have vision impairment and 2.01 million are projected to be blind (Varma et al., 2016).

[2] Vision rehabilitation and low vision rehabilitation refer to the same care processes and models. As noted in Chapter 1, this report will use the term vision impairment, rather than low vision, to describe patients with functional limitations of the eye(s) or visual system that result from vision loss. In keeping with this decision, vision rehabilitation—rather than low vision rehabilitation—will be used throughout the report. See Chapter 1 for further information on terminology.

rehabilitation include increased functional ability, independence, and QOL (AHRQ, 2004). However, achieving these outcomes is made challenging by the existence of several impediments to the provision of accessible and high-quality vision rehabilitation services.

Awareness of the benefits of vision rehabilitation may be limited among providers and patients, which creates missed opportunities for improving health outcomes (Casten et al., 2005; Lam and Leat, 2013; O'Connor et al., 2008). Limitations in the eye and vision care workforce and in the availability of some vision rehabilitation services may prevent patients from accessing needed care (Goldstein et al., 2012; Owsley et al., 2009). Minority race and ethnicity and lower socioeconomic position pose barriers to accessing primary eye and vision care and could potentially compromise access to vision rehabilitation services as well (Zhang et al., 2012, 2013b). Inadequate research on the cost, effectiveness, and cost-effectiveness of vision rehabilitation services constrains treatment options that providers may consider or confidently recommend.

This chapter explores the role of vision rehabilitation in promoting the health, functioning, and QOL of people in the United States living with chronic vision impairment. The vision rehabilitation process as well as key interventions and unique care models will be discussed. Major barriers to vision rehabilitation quality and access will be explored, as well as strategies to overcome them. The chapter will also highlight opportunities and innovative directions related to models of care that hold great promise for lessening the impacts and consequences of chronic vision impairment.

VISION REHABILITATION INTERVENTIONS AND MODELS

Overview of the Vision Rehabilitation Process

Vision rehabilitation services comprise a wide array of models of care and interventions and services provided by numerous professionals working in varied clinical settings to accomplish a diverse range of goals. According to the National Eye Health Education Program of the National Eye Institute (NEI):

> Vision rehabilitation helps people adapt to vision loss and maintain their current lifestyle. A vision rehabilitation program offers a wide range of services, including training in the use of magnifiers and other adaptive devices, ways to complete daily living skills safely and independently, guidance on modifying residences, and information on where to locate resources and support. These programs typically include a team of professionals consisting of a primary eye care professional and an optometrist or ophthalmologist specializing in low vision. Occupational therapists,

orientation and mobility specialists, certified low vision therapists, counselors, and social workers may also be a part of this team. (NEHEP, n.d.)

Binns et al. (2012) states that "vision rehabilitation services conform
to a variety of different models" that vary in the number and type of
services they emphasize and offer (p. 36). Vision rehabilitation models of
care include hospital-based vision rehabilitation services, multidisciplinary
outpatient and community-based services, and self-management education
programs (Ryan, 2014). Other current and proposed models offer a range
of tiered, increasingly comprehensive services designed to meet the needs
of patients with different needs and degrees of vision impairment (Leat,
2016; VA, 2015). In addition to optometrists and ophthalmologists, vision
rehabilitation can involve opticians, occupational therapists, physical therapists, vision rehabilitation therapists, vision rehabilitation teachers, social
workers, orientation and mobility specialists, psychologists, and counselors,
among others (Binns et al., 2012; Markowitz, 2006b). Vision rehabilitation services can be provided in specialized vision centers, general or rehabilitation hospitals, outpatient clinics, extended care facilities, private and
university-based optometry and ophthalmology practices, private homes,
community-based health centers, and facilities operated by government
agencies, nonprofit organizations, or community groups (Deremeik et al.,
2007; Owsley et al., 2009; Ryan, 2014).

Despite this heterogeneity in the provision, organization, setting, and
scope of care, vision rehabilitation services share a common, overarching
model of care. This overarching model describes vision rehabilitation as a
process of care that begins with examination and diagnosis, followed by
development of a treatment plan, and then proceeds to management of
vision impairment (Markowitz, 2006b). Reevaluation of the patient leads
to adjustments as necessary to the treatment plan until the patient's needs
have been addressed or treatment options have been exhausted. Below,
Figure 8-1 depicts the vision rehabilitation process in the context of the
larger continuum of eye and vision care.

Clinical practice guidelines (guidelines) developed by the American Academy of Ophthalmology and American Optometric Association
(AOA) recommend comprehensive eye exams as the initial step in the
vision rehabilitation process (AAO, 2013; AOA, 2007). Initial care of
the vision rehabilitation patient may include an initial assessment to
determine the patient's medical history, a brief examination to confirm the
medical history, determination of cognitive function, and identification of
priority tasks for rehabilitation, followed by comprehensive assessment
of residual visual function and residual functional vision (Markowitz,
2006b). Assessment of residual visual function can include assessment of
refractive error, visual acuity, visual fields, oculomotor functions, cortical

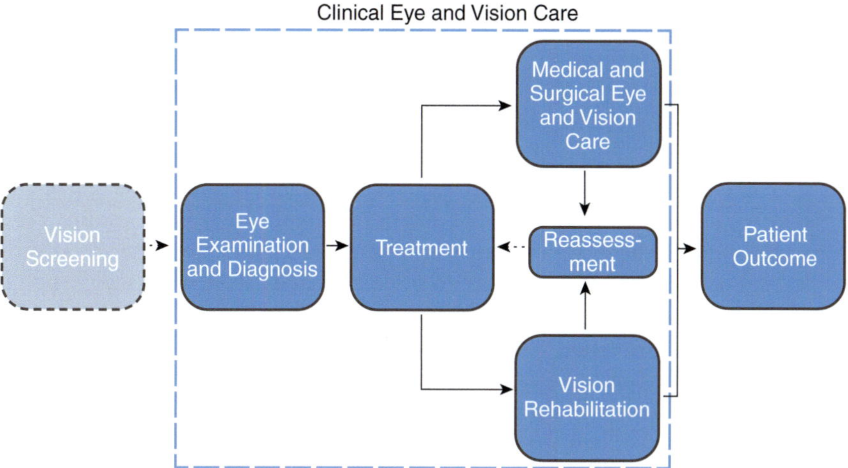

FIGURE 8-1 Conceptual framework of vision rehabilitation.

visual integration, and light characteristics affecting visual (Markowitz, 2006b). The assessment of residual functional vision is used to determine "how well a patient uses residual visual function to perform routine tasks in different places, using different items, and throughout the day," and its results inform the development of the treatment plan (Markowitz, 2006b, p. 299).

Vision rehabilitation treatment plans are guided by the concept of patient-centered care, and therefore account for the unique preferences, goals, priorities, and relevant contextual factors (e.g., health status, social and educational supports, presence of stakeholder networks) of the individual patient when addressing the consequences of vision loss (IOM, 2001). Among U.S. adults referred to vision rehabilitation services, such consequences often include difficulty reading, driving, using assistive devices, performing daily activities inside and outside the home, walking, watching television, and performing work- and school-related activities (Brown et al., 2014).

To address these problems, vision rehabilitation treatment plans may include prescription of, and training in the use, of low vision aids and devices, orientation and mobility training, modification of home and work environments to promote functioning and safety, training in adaptive strategies and skills, and counseling, among other interventions and services (Binns et al., 2012; Markowitz, 2006b; Mogk and Goodrich, 2004; Ryan, 2014). The effectiveness and scope of vision rehabilitation models of care and services and interventions are explored below.

The Effectiveness of Vision Rehabilitation

Although evidence for the effectiveness of vision rehabilitation is still emerging, some available research does indicate that vision rehabilitation helps improve health and visual functioning for patients in numerous age groups and with different degrees and causes of vision impairment. One prospective, observational study measured the effects of vision rehabilitation on overall visual ability and on performance in four domains: reading, mobility, visual motor function, and visual information processing (Goldstein et al., 2015). Among 468 adult patients seeking vision rehabilitation services, 47 percent achieved a minimum clinically important difference in overall visual ability between baseline and reevaluation at 6 to 9 months. Over the same 6- to 9-month period, 27 percent to 44 percent of participants experienced minimum clinically important differences in their performance in a functional domain (Goldstein et al., 2015). A randomized controlled trial (RCT) compared the effects of vision rehabilitation to no treatment on reading ability, mobility, visual information processing, and visual motor skills among 126 adults with vision impairment (Stelmack et al., 2008).[3] Over 4 months, participants receiving vision rehabilitation achieved significant improvements in all functional domains, while those receiving no treatment experienced declines in all functional domains. A survey of 105 patients who reported receipt of vision rehabilitation found that these services were associated with significant improvements in the ability to perform near-vision activities (e.g., reading ordinary and small print, performing near-vision work, self-grooming, ambulating down stairs during full- and low-light conditions) and distance-vision activities (e.g., reading street signs, recognizing people, watching television). Patients also reported nonsignificant improvements in perceived ability to perform vision-related social activities (Walter et al., 2007).[4] Specific vision rehabilitation programs and interventions have been associated with increased social participation and overall QOL, as well as decreased emotional distress and increased vision-related functioning, especially among patients with visual impairments who were depressed prior to receiving vision rehabilitation (Berger et al., 2013; Brody et al., 2002, 2005; Lamoureux et al., 2007).

---

[3] Vision impairment was defined as visual acuity of worse than 20/100 and better than 20/500 in the better-seeing eye. Participants had diagnosis in the better-seeing eye of macular degeneration, macular dystrophy, macular hole, or inflammation of the macula. Vision rehabilitation included examination, education on the eye disease diagnosis and prognosis, prescription of low vision devices, five weekly sessions of low vision therapy, and one home visit.

[4] Vision rehabilitation included comprehensive low vision examinations and functional vision assessments, assessments of daily activities, referrals to community services, orientation and mobility evaluations, counseling, and device funding.

Although most patients in vision rehabilitation are adults, these services also appear to confer gains in visual functioning on children and adolescents. An observational study on the effects of vision rehabilitation among 183 children ages 8 to 16 with vision impairment who were living in India found that visual disability was significantly decreased 3 to 4 months after baseline for participants with mild, moderate, and severe vision impairment (Gothwal et al., 2015). Among children ages 6 to 16 with vision impairment, prescription of, and training on, low vision aids significantly improved near and distance visual acuity and self-reported ability to perform activities such as reading textbooks and copying from a blackboard (Ganesh et al., 2013).[5] However, a systematic review found that vision rehabilitation in children is severely understudied, most investigations are descriptive case series with small sample sizes, and these limitations permit few conclusions to be drawn from the available literature (Chavda et al., 2014).

Research suggests that patients with vision impairment consequent to eye diseases, including age-related macular degeneration (AMD), glaucoma, diabetic retinopathy, and amblyopia can all benefit from rehabilitation (Demers-Turco, 1999; Ganesh et al., 2013; Hooper et al., 2008; Luo et al., 2011; Nilsson, 1986). However, the extent of the benefits of vision rehabilitation may vary among patient groups, measures of visual functioning, and rehabilitation interventions and models. Wang et al. (2012) found that multidisciplinary vision rehabilitation led to significantly greater improvements in overall visual ability among visually impaired patients than in legally blind patients at 30 days and 3 months follow-up (p. 1403). Patients ages 85 and older saw significantly greater improvements in overall visual ability than patients ages 84 and younger, as did patients without glaucoma versus those with the disease (Wang et al., 2012).[6] Another study found that the impact of vision rehabilitation on visual ability varies among functional domains. Specifically, a greater proportion of patients receiving vision rehabilitation achieved minimum clinically important differences in reading ability (44 percent), than in vision motor function (38 percent), vision information processing (33 percent), or mobility (27 percent) (Goldstein et al., 2015). A study comparing two methods of training adult patients

---

[5] Vision rehabilitation included examination, educational guidance and counseling, training in use of assistive software, and prescription of, and training in, low vision aids.

[6] Vision impairment replaces the term "low vision," defined as a visual acuity of <20/60, but ≥20/200. Legally blind was defined as best-corrected visual acuity of <20/200 or constriction of visual field to within 10 degrees of fixation, irrespective of visual acuity. Intergroup differences in the impact of vision rehabilitation are based on the U.S. Department of Veterans Affairs Low-Vision Visual Functioning Questionnaire (VA LV VFQ-48) scores. Scores from the Impact of Vision Impairment Questionnaire showed no significant intergroup differences in the impact of vision rehabilitation.

with vision impairment in the use of low vision aids for reading found that extended training (i.e., five weekly 1-hour sessions) as compared to standard training (i.e., one weekly 1-hour session) was associated with significantly greater improvements in reading speed and accuracy at 5 and 12 weeks from baseline. At 12 weeks from baseline, compared to participants who received standard training, those who received extended training reported less difficulty performing common vision-related tasks and rated their eyesight higher (Scanlan and Cuddeford, 2004). As discussed below, clinical outcomes achieved by different models of care in vision rehabilitation also vary, though differences in study methodologies and patient populations make it difficult to compare the clinical effectiveness of these models.

These and other research findings suggest that generalizations about the effectiveness of vision rehabilitation services may not be applicable to a particular intervention, model of care, or treatment plan in vision rehabilitation. Similarly, the diversity in the limitations, needs, and priorities of vision rehabilitation patients mean that those interventions and models of care found to be effective for one patient or patient group may be of limited therapeutic value to another. A systematic review concluded that while research suggests that vision rehabilitation can benefit patients with vision impairment, the available evidence is insufficient to make more specific claims about the characteristics of an effective rehabilitation program, the patient populations most likely to benefit from rehabilitation, the value of rehabilitation for children, or the cost-effectiveness of vision rehabilitation (Binns et al., 2012). Future research on vision rehabilitation will need to employ a standardized methodology and prioritize investigations that identify the effectiveness of specific interventions and care models in achieving the unique treatment goals of a given population.

Vision Rehabilitation Services and Interventions

As described above, accomplishing the many individualized goals of vision rehabilitation will require an array of interventions and many providers. Optometrists and ophthalmologists may prescribe low vision optical systems that improve functionality in activities ranging from reading and writing to driving and social events (AAO, 2013; AOA, 2007). Orientation and mobility specialists can provide training in the use of white mobility canes, guide dogs, and other techniques that help preserve mobility in the home and community (ACVREP, 2014a). To improve productivity and functioning in the workplace and beyond, occupational therapists teach patients with vision impairment adaptive strategies, including the use of sensory techniques that rely on touch and hearing to perform tasks (Markowitz, 2006a). Low vision therapists and vision rehabilitation therapists may assist patients with vision impairment in adapting their work and home environments to promote functioning and safety, or train patients in the use of low vision aids and devices, as well as techniques to maximize remaining visual function (ACVREP, 2014b). It is important to note that the individuals involved in the care of patients with vision impairment may also be informal caregivers who are not trained in vision rehabilitation. Furthermore, several types of providers, including low vision therapists and orientation and mobility specialists, are not recognized as providers by Medicare and, as a result, cannot be compensated by Medicare for the care of beneficiaries with vision impairment. The following section describes in greater detail the interventions that clinicians, therapists, and specialists provide in the course of treatment.

Optical Low Vision Aids

An impaired ability to read is a common complaint among patients seeking vision rehabilitation. Among 819 new patients at 28 vision rehabilitation centers in the United States, 66.4 percent reported difficulty reading (Brown et al., 2014). In another study, 69 of 87 participants identified improved reading ability as a goal of vision rehabilitation. Moreover, 89.9 percent of those who identified improved reading ability as a goal ranked this goal as very important (Renieri et al., 2013). Prescription and training in the use of optical low vision aids is one strategy for improving reading ability and other measures of visual functioning. Non-electronic optical low vision aids include spectacle-mounted and hand-held microscopes and telescopes for near and distance magnification, prisms for field enhancement, and selective absorption filters and occlusion for contrast and glare control (AOA, 2007; Minto and Butt, 2004). Electronic optical low vision aids include electronic video magnification (e.g., hand-held "camera," closed circuit television [CCTV]) and computer-based magnification (AOA, 2007; Minto and Butt, 2007). A systematic review to assess the effectiveness of occupational therapy interventions for improving reading ability in older adults with vision impairment found moderately strong evidence to support the use of electronic magnifiers, while the evidence supporting the use of optical magnifiers was limited. One study reported that vision rehabilitation including training in the use of magnifying devices and vision aids resulted in significant improvements in self-estimated reading ability (Renieri et al., 2013). Another study investigated the effect of low vision aids on the reading ability of 530 adults ages 52 to 98 and diagnosed with AMD (Nguyen et al., 2009). Without low vision aids, reading speed was less than 30 words per minute (wpm) for almost all participants. After training in the use of electronic and non-electronic low vision aids, reading speed increased significantly from 20 ± 30 wpm to 72 ± 35 wpm. Improvements in reading speed were significantly greater for individuals with best-corrected distance visual acuity of ≥20/200 or better in the better-seeing eye compared to those with best-corrected distance visual acuity of <20/200 in the better-seeing eye (Nguyen et al., 2009).

By comparison with these promising findings, several systematic reviews have found the evidence supporting the use of low vision aids to be insufficient or of low quality. For example, a systematic review examining the evidence for the impact of conventional hand-held magnification, optical telescopes, and stand-mounted or hand-held electronic magnification on reading ability in people with vision impairment, concluded that there was insufficient evidence due to the small size and moderate to low quality of available studies, and the outdated research on electronic magnification in particular (Virgili et al., 2013). Two other systematic reviews found no RCTs or quasi-RCTs comparing optical low vision aids to standard refractive correction or exploring the use of assistive technologies (e.g., CCTV, electronic vision enhancement systems, tablet computers, screen readers, screen magnifiers, optical character recognition programs) among children ages 5 to 16 with vision impairment (Barker et al., 2015; Thomas et al., 2015). The discrepancies observed among studies regarding the effect of optical low vision aids on reading ability and other measures of visual functioning may be the result of several differences in the characteristics of study cohorts, the types of optical low vision aids provided, and the duration and quality of training in the use of these aids. For example, studies suggest that difficulty using visual assistive equipment is a common concern among patients in rehabilitation programs, and that extended training in low vision aids is correlated with an improved reading ability and increased QOL (Brown et al., 2014; Scanlan and Cuddeford, 2004). As indicated by the findings of systematic reviews, more research is needed to determine how training, patient characteristics, and other factors mediate the impact of low vision aids on visual functioning.

Orientation and Mobility Training

Performance in mobility-related activities is a common concern among patients seeking vision rehabilitation services. In the Low Vision Rehabilitation Outcomes Study, 16.3 percent of participants reported difficulty with walking or with daily activities outside the home (Brown et al., 2014). A survey of older adults seeking vision rehabilitation in the United States found that 52 percent of 564 responding participants reported a fall in the previous 2 years, and that 23 percent and 16 percent of 699 responding participants reported using a straight cane or a walker/rollator, respectively (Goldstein et al., 2012). Defined as "a sequential process in which visually impaired individuals are taught to utilize their remaining senses to determine their position within their environment and to negotiate safe movement from one place to another," orientation and mobility is a strategy for improving the functional status of individuals with vision impairments (ACVREP, 2015, p. 5).

Techniques to improve mobility include the use of white mobility canes, guide dogs, human guides, and mental mapping. Research to assess the effectiveness of these techniques is limited. For example, a recent systematic review discovered very few studies or other documents on the development, content, feasibility, or effectiveness of white cane training programs (Ballemans et al., 2011). More generally, a 2010 systematic review was unable to reach any conclusions regarding the effectiveness of mobility and orientation training in general, and it recommended carrying out RCTs to compare the effectiveness of different training methods (Virgili, 2010). Another systematic review found insufficient evidence to support multidisciplinary vision rehabilitation, driving simulator training, or driver education programs as effective interventions for improving or maintaining community mobility (Justiss, 2013).

Zijlstra et al. (2013) report on the development of a structured and theory-based approach to white cane training that includes two in-person meetings and one telephone conference that emphasize problem-solving and addressing psychosocial issues related to the use of the cane, in addition to practical training (pp. 7, 17). An initial study comparing the effectiveness of this novel training program approach with regular training programs among 68 older adults with vision impairment found no significant differences (89 percent versus 84 percent) in the proportion of participants reporting that training was beneficial, although participant ratings of overall training, trainer performance, and participant engagement were higher for the standardized programs than for the regular program (Ballemans et al., 2012).

Environmental Modifications

Among the 819 patients recruited for the Low Vision Rehabilitation Outcomes Study, 11.7 percent reported problems with glare and lighting, 15.1 percent reported problems with performing in-home activities, and 10.3 percent reported vision-related difficulties in recognizing faces and interacting in social situations (Brown et al., 2014). Modifications to the home and work environment can help address these issues. Interventions include marking the edges of stairs with brightly colored tape, using large print reading materials, placing raised or fluorescent markings on the dials and buttons of appliances, and placing drapes and lamps to decrease glare and increase luminescence (AHRQ, 2002). Research into the impact of these interventions is limited: a recent systematic review of environmental interventions for individuals with vision impairment found no RCTs or quasi-RCTs that compared the effect of environmental and/or behavioral interventions to other environmental and/or behavioral interventions or controls on adults ages 60 and older with vision impairment (Skelton et al., 2013). An AHRQ report observes that the paucity of controlled trials may be due to the individualized nature of these interventions, and the fact that third-party payors have not pursued or called for research to support these interventions because they "have not typically been subject to reimbursement" (AHRQ, 2002).

Nonetheless, some evidence exists to support specific modifications. For example, one study found that reading performance among study participants with vision impairment consequent to AMD was significantly improved under optimal lighting levels as compared to the lighting level found inside most homes and other buildings (Bowers et al., 2001). Lighting improvements have also been shown to improve QOL and also the performance of some activities of daily living (ADLs) among individuals with vision impairment (Brunnström et al., 2004). An RCT assessed the impact of a home safety assessment and modifications to improve safety in the home environment on falls and fall-related injuries in adults ages 75 and older with vision impairment and found that among participants who received the home safety assessment as compared to those who did not receive the assessment, the incidence rate ratio of falls and injurious falls was 0.59 and 0.81, respectively (Campbell et al., 2005). Another RCT assessed the impact of an intervention to remove home hazards on falls in older adults with and without vision impairments (Day et al., 2002). In combination with an intervention to improve vision and/or an intervention to improve strength and balance through an exercise program, reduction of home hazards significantly reduced the rate ratio of falls in comparison to participants who received no interventions (Day et al., 2002). Further research is needed on the effectiveness and cost-effectiveness of single- and multi-component environmental modifications in home, work, and academic environments for promoting safety and functioning in individuals with vision impairment.

Adaptive Strategies: Knowledge, Skills, and Tools

In the context of vision rehabilitation, adaptive strategies may include learned behaviors and skills that allow individuals with vision impairment to independently, effectively, and safely perform daily activities as well as the broader range of activities required to fully participate in social, political, economic, educational, and recreational activities. At their most basic, these strategies help individuals with vision impairment bathe, dress, and eat without assistance. For example, patients may be advised to place a finger just inside the lip of a cup while pouring liquid into it in order to avoid spills (VisionAware, 2016b). Patients with difficulty distinguishing colors may be taught to label their clothing (e.g., "navy" or "black") to help identify items that match (VisionAware, 2016a). More complex or particular strategies aid individuals with vision impairment in their ability to shop for food, cook meals, clean their homes, manage finances, communicate with friends and family, and move freely in the community.

Some adaptive strategies involve maximizing remaining visual function. For example, eccentric viewing is a technique in which patients learn to use portions of the retina that have not been damaged by disease. Training in eccentric viewing is included as a strategy for managing central visual field defects in the AOA guidelines for vision rehabilitation and is listed as an occupational therapy and reading rehabilitation intervention in the American Academy of Ophthalmology guidelines for vision rehabilitation (AAO, 2013; AOA, 2007). A systematic review of the effectiveness of eccentric viewing training for improving performance of daily visual activities in individuals with vision impairment consequent to AMD included five studies that had reported statistically significant improvements in reading speed, maximal reading speed, duration of reading, reading comprehension, and performance in daily activities (Hong et al., 2014). The review authors concluded that eccentric viewing training has a moderate-sized effect on the ability of the studied populations to perform daily visual activities (Hong et al., 2014). Another systematic review found that moderate quality evidence supported eccentric viewing training incorporating or in conjunction with steady eye training as a method to improve near visual acuity, reading speed, and the ability to perform ADLs in patients with central vision loss (Gaffney et al., 2014). Further research is needed to ascertain the effect of eccentric viewing training on distance visual acuity and QOL, and the comparative effectiveness and cost-effectiveness of different training programs.

Other adaptive strategies use hearing and touch to promote functioning. For example, a growing body of research has documented the ability of blind individuals to use echolocation for navigation, with studies demonstrating the ability of echolocation experts to assess with considerable accuracy the position, size, distance, and shape of objects in space, as well as the distance and location of sounds (Kolarik et al., 2014; Kondo et al., 2012; Milne et al., 2014; Schenkman and Nilsson, 2010; Schornich et al., 2012, 2013; Teng et al., 2012; Vercillo et al., 2015; Wallmeier and Wiegrebe, 2014a,b). Teng and Whitney (2011) demonstrated that, even without feedback or formal training, some normally sighted individuals can rapidly learn to determine the size and position of objects in space by means of echolocation, suggesting that echolocation training could be pursued as a strategy to promote mobility in individuals with vision impairment.

The use of low vision aids and devices, Braille typewriters and dynamic readers, white mobility canes, and environmental modifications are also examples of adaptive strategies even though these strategies use tools in addition to learned behaviors and skills to enhance functioning. Emerging technologies, such as self-driving cars, text-to-speech and speech-to-text software, electronic personal navigation systems, and a broad range of smartphone applications offering services for individuals with vision impairment hold potential for expanding opportunities for increased independence, functioning, and participation among populations with vision impairment.

Models of Vision Rehabilitation

Although the majority of existing vision rehabilitation programs share an overarching care process (i.e., examination, diagnosis and development of treatment plan, vision rehabilitation services and interventions), broad variation exists in the organization and delivery of vision rehabilitation services. For example, highly integrated vision rehabilitation programs, such the U.S. Department of Veterans Affairs' (VA's) Vision Impairment Services in Outpatient Rehabilitation (VISOR) Program, provide individualized care in a residential setting staffed by multidisciplinary teams that offer a range of services (VA, 2016). Other programs offer self-management education in short, weekly classes provided in a community setting.

These models of care differ in the setting, cost, duration, scope, emphasis, and organization of the services they provide. These differences can affect program effectiveness in unpredictable ways. For example, one study comparing conventional vision rehabilitation services (i.e., examination and provision of low vision aids and support services by a multidisciplinary team) to enhanced services (usual care plus an 8-week self-management program to develop problem-solving and coping skills) found no significant differences between the programs in terms of impacts on the vision-specific QOL, emotional well-being, adaption to vision loss, or self-efficacy of patients (Rees et al., 2015). Other studies confirm that more comprehensive care does not necessarily lead to better outcomes. Several systematic reviews have identified evidence indicating that multidisciplinary or multicomponent interventions are effective at promoting independent functioning in the home and community, and for maintaining or enhancing social participation (Justiss, 2013; Liu et al., 2013; Smallfield et al., 2013). Individual and group-based problem-solving—in which participants identify problems, establish goals, develop and implement solutions, and assess outcomes—was strongly supported by the evidence as an effective method for improving social participation among older adults with vision impairment (Berger et al., 2013). The following section will describe both common and unique models of vision rehabilitation, and explore how variation in the scope, organization, and delivery of services relates to patient health outcomes.

VA Blind Rehabilitation Services

The VA Blind Rehabilitation Services provide a continuum of vision rehabilitation services to improve the functional status and QOL of veterans with any degree of vision impairment (VA, 2015). Intermediate vision impairment clinics "focus on effective use of remaining vision through the development and use of visual motor and visual perceptual skills" and include training in the use of low vision aids (VA, 2015). Advanced vision impairment clinics offer orientation and mobility training, including instruction on the use of white mobility canes, sensory training, and mental mapping. The VISOR Program provides short-term training to improve communication skills, access to technology, and the ability to perform daily activities. Inpatient Blind Rehabilitation Centers (BRCs) provide "comprehensive adjustment to blindness training," including individual counseling and group therapy to support emotional and behavioral health. Complementing BRCs are Vision Impairment Centers to Optimize Remaining Sight (VICTORS) programs that offer interdisciplinary rehabilitation services for veterans with severe vision impairment. Together, these programs offer a range of increasingly comprehensive vision rehabilitation services (VA, 2015).

Available research suggests that several of these programs can improve the functional status and QOL of patients with vision impairment. The VA Low Vision Intervention Trial (LOVIT) assessed the effect of a 2-month vision rehabilitation program that included an initial examination, five weekly sessions to teach adaptive strategies and provide training in the use of low vision aids, as well as a home visit to assess the home environment (Stelmack et al., 2007b, 2008). Among older adults with moderate to severe vision impairment consequent to macular disease, compared to those who did not receive vision rehabilitation, those who did experienced significant improvements in mobility, reading ability, visual motor skill, visual information processing, and overall visual ability at 4 months post-baseline (Stelmack et al., 2008).[7] In a follow-up study, standard low vision therapy (i.e., examination, education on eye disease, training in

---

[7] Moderate to severe vision impairment was defined as visual acuity worse than 20/100 and better than 20/500 in the better-seeing eye.

eccentric viewing and the use of low vision aids, psychological counseling, and social work services) was offered to the original control group, and the original experimental group received no additional care (Stelmack et al., 2012a). Twelve months after baseline, the original treatment group experienced significant losses in mean scores for reading ability and visual information processing compared to performance on these outcome measures at 4 months, while the original control group experienced significant improvements in mean scores for all outcome measures compared to performance at 4 months. For both the control and treatment groups, mean scores for overall visual ability improved significantly after 12 months compared to performance at baseline, although the improvement was significantly greater for the treatment group than for the control group (Stelmack et al., 2012a).

An economic evaluation found that the average cost per patient was significantly lower for the LOVIT program ($404.70) than for comparable care in a BRC ($43,681.70). However, mobility, visual motor skills, and overall visual ability—but not reading ability or visual information processing—improved more in the BRC than in the LOVIT program (Stroupe et al., 2008). A second LOVIT trial to compare the effectiveness and cost-effectiveness of basic care (i.e., examination, provision of low vision aids) and vision rehabilitation (i.e., examination, provision of low vision aids, two to three low vision therapy sessions) is planned (Stelmack et al., 2012b). Another study investigated the effect of a BRC inpatient blind rehabilitation program on vision-specific QOL among 206 legally blind veterans (Kuyk et al., 2008). Program interventions included examination, assessment of psychological and social needs, training in the use of low vision aids, and instruction in mobility, performance of ADLs, communication, and adaptive strategies. Compared to performance at baseline, mean composite score on the National Eye Institute Visual Function Questionnaire (NEI VFQ) was significantly higher at 2 and 6 months post-rehabilitation, although the 6-month post-rehabilitation composite score was significantly lower than the 2-month post-rehabilitation composite score. Rehabilitation also significantly improved performance on measures of social function, mental health, and vision function (Kuyk et al., 2008). A prospective observational study of patients who participated in a BRC inpatient rehabilitation program found that visual ability decreased between 3 and 12 months post-rehabilitation, but remained significantly improved over performance at baseline (Stelmack et al., 2007a). Further research is needed to assess the effectiveness and cost-effectiveness of other components of the VA blind rehabilitation services, including intermediate and advanced vision impairment clinics.

Self-Management Education Programs

Self-management education programs help patients manage chronic conditions, such as uncorrectable or irreversible vision impairment. Compared to traditional patient education programs that place the health care provider in the role of educator and focus on dissemination of disease-specific technical skills and information in order to promote patient compliance with a treatment plan, self-management education programs emphasize self-efficacy by placing the patient in charge of identifying issues related to their chronic condition and teaching problem-solving skills to address those problems (Bodenheimer et al., 2002). Available evidence suggests that self-management education programs can improve functioning and emotional distress among individuals with vision impairment.

A systematic review found that self-management education programs can "improve emotional distress, functional ability[,] and self-efficacy in elderly people with AMD," but stated that additional studies with robust methodologies were required to substantiate these findings (Lee et al., 2008, p. 174). An RCT assessed the effects of a self-management education program on 231 adults ages 60 and older with vision impairment consequent to AMD. The program involved six weekly 2-hour sessions of didactic presentations and group problem-solving, and cognitive and behavioral skills training presented to groups of 8 to 10 patients. Patients in the self-management education program experienced significant improvements in emotional distress and functioning; by comparison, changes in emotional distress and functioning were not significant for patients in the control group receiving no care (Brody et al., 2002). At 6-month follow-up, patients in the self-management education program reported significantly less emotional distress, significantly better functioning, and significantly increased self-efficacy as compared to patients in the control groups receiving either no care or 12 hours of recorded health lectures (Brody et al., 2005). In addition, among patients with depression, those randomized to the self-management education group experienced significantly greater reductions in depressive symptoms than did patients randomized to either of the control groups (Brody et al., 2006).

Studies on populations outside the United States suggest that self-management education programs can improve perceived security in the performance of several daily activities among patients with vision impairment consequent to AMD, and can increase awareness of low vision aids and practical strategies to optimize use of remaining vision among caregivers of patients with vision impairment (Dahlin Ivanoff et al., 2002; Larizza et al., 2011). Less promisingly, an RCT examining the impact of a self-management education program in addition to usual vision rehabilitation services on vision-specific QOL, emotional well-being, self-efficacy, and adaptation to vision loss among Australian adults ages 55 and older with vision impairment found no significant difference between the outcomes of patients in the usual care group and those in the usual care plus self-management education group (Rees et al., 2015). The authors called for further research to identify the patients most likely to benefit from self-management education programs and from specific components of such programs, in order to better target these interventions.

Models of Vision Rehabilitation in Australia and the United Kingdom

Lamoureux et al. (2007) investigated the effect of a multidisciplinary vision rehabilitation service on Australian adults ages 18 and older with visual acuity <6/12 or >6/12 with restricted visual fields (p. 1477).[8] Rehabilitation included an assessment by a member of a multidisciplinary team to determine the patient's needs and goals. Subsequently, an optometrist performed an examination and offered low vision aids or rehabilitation services (e.g., occupational therapy, orientation and mobility, peer support, community services) as appropriate. A care plan, including referral pathways, is developed and considered complete when the patient "feels satisfied that the desired outcomes have been met and cannot identify any further service needs" (Lamoureux et al., 2007, p. 1477). Compared to participant scores at baseline, emotional well-being and the ability to read and access information were significantly improved 3 to 6 months after rehabilitation. Nonsignificant improvements in orientation and mobility were also observed (Lamoureux et al., 2007). Another study investigated an Australian multidisciplinary vision rehabilitation service involving an initial assessment to determine patient needs, develop a unique treatment plan, and prescribe low vision aid, followed by a review appointment within 30 days to assess the need for interventions related to orientation and mobility, independent living, recreation, adaptive technologies and devices, and counseling, among others (Wang et al., 2012). The reported effectiveness of these services depended on the assessment tool used. According to the VA Low-Vision Visual Functioning Questionnaire (VA LV VFQ-48), mean scores on measures of reading ability, visual information, visual motor, and overall visual ability had improved significantly at 30 days—but not at 3 months—compared to performance at baseline. By comparison, according to the Impact of Vision Impairment questionnaire, mean scores on measures of mobility and independence at 30 days and 3 months were significantly improved over performance at baseline, and overall mean score was significantly improved at 3 months—but not at 30 days—compared to performance at baseline. In addition, mean scores

---

[8] A visual acuity of 6/12 (meters) converts to a visual acuity of 20/40 (feet).

on the VA LV VFQ-48 indicate that the benefits of vision rehabilitation were more pronounced for patients with best-corrected visual acuity of <20/60 and ≥20/200 compared to patients who were legally blind (i.e., best-corrected visual acuity <20/200 or constriction of visual field to within 10 degrees of fixation) for all mean scores, for patients ages 86 and older compared to those ages 85 and younger, and for patients without glaucoma compared to those with glaucoma (Wang et al., 2012). Further research is needed to determine how to adapt vision rehabilitation services to better meet the needs of all patient populations, and to develop standardized methods for assessing outcomes from vision rehabilitation.

In the United Kingdom, interdisciplinary low vision service (ILVS) programs staffed by multidisciplinary teams working out of general hospital clinics provide examination, diagnosis, and low vision aid provision and training. Home visits can involve training in mobility, independent living skills, and education on available social services. Six months after the initiation of vision rehabilitation, Hinds et al. (2003) found a significant decrease in patient anxiety regarding safety at home, coping ability, and further vision loss (p. 1393). Among 71 study participants ages 34 and older with vision impairment, 53 (75 percent) claimed to use the aid to read books, newspapers, or magazines, and 36 (51 percent) stated that they use the aids several times per day (Hinds et al., 2003).

The Welsh Low Vision Service expanded access to vision rehabilitation services in Wales by training community-based optometrists, ophthalmic medical practitioners, and dispensing opticians to provide vision rehabilitation services in a primary care setting. Based on the National Health Service Hospital Eye Service model, the Welsh Low Vision Service includes assessment of patient needs and goals, provision of low vision aids, patient education on vision rehabilitation services and interventions, referral to other services, and follow-up care (Ryan et al., 2010). Comparing access-related parameters 1 year before and 1 year after implementation of the Welsh Low Vision Service, the number of appointments for vision rehabilitation services increased by 51.7 percent, the proportion of patients waiting less than 2 months for an initial vision rehabilitation assessment increased from 11 percent to 60 percent, and 81 percent of patients traveled a shorter distance to reach their service provider than they would have if the Welsh Low Vision Service had not been implemented. Visual disability scores 3 months after rehabilitation were significantly improved over scores before rehabilitation, and nearly all patients (97.4 percent) reported that the service was useful (Ryan et al., 2010). A follow-up study found that visual disability scores 18 months after rehabilitation remained significantly higher than at baseline, and that 79 percent of study participants continued to use low vision aids (Ryan et al., 2013).

It is important to note that health care systems in Australia, the United Kingdom, and elsewhere serve different populations and are organized and funded differently than in the United States. As a result, vision rehabilitation models employed in these countries may perform differently if implemented in the United States. While these models can provide important lessons for U.S. policy makers and health care organizations, their direct applicability to vision rehabilitation services in the United States may be limited.

BARRIERS AND OPPORTUNITIES IN VISION REHABILITATION

There are several potential barriers to developing a universally high-quality and accessible vision rehabilitation system. A lack of awareness of the purpose and effectiveness of vision rehabilitation among medical providers, public health workers, and patients may unnecessarily limit the utilization of vision rehabilitation services by patients with vision impairment. Issues related to workforce education and capacity may pose barriers to accessing vision rehabilitation services. Racial, ethnic, and socioeconomic disparities in clinical eye and vision care exist and may negatively affect access and utilization of vision rehabilitation services. This section will briefly discuss barriers to achieving high-quality and accessible vision rehabilitation services in the United States and will identify strategies for eliminating these barriers.

Lack of Awareness and Knowledge of Vision Rehabilitation Services

Patients, medical providers, and public health actors often lack an awareness of the goals, content, effectiveness, and availability of vision rehabilitation. Patients may simply be unaware of vision rehabilitation services, or they may misunderstand their purpose. The stigma surrounding blindness or individuals' failure to acknowledge deficits in visual functioning may also contribute to less-than-optimal use of vision rehabilitation by populations with vision impairment. A lack of knowledge and inadequate communication between clinical care providers and public health officials prevents the larger population health workforce from addressing the issue of limited patient awareness. This section will discuss the gaps in knowledge of vision rehabilitation among patients and providers, and will suggest corrective strategies.

Knowledge Gaps Among Patients

The limited available evidence suggests that the knowledge and awareness of vision rehabilitation among the U.S. population is poor. The 2005 Survey of Public Knowledge, Attitudes, and Practices Related to Eye Health and Disease found that among 3,180 U.S. adults ages 18 and older, 16 percent reported having heard the term "low vision" (NEI/LCIF, 2008, p. v).[9] Of the 2 percent of surveyed adults who reported that an eye care provider had diagnosed them with vision impairment, only 31 percent had been recommended to a low vision specialist (NEI/LCIF, 2008).[10] One study assessed the knowledge of, experience with, and interest in vision rehabilitation services and devices among U.S. adults ages 65 and older who were diagnosed with AMD (Casten et al., 2005). More participants were interested in, than were aware of, vision rehabilitation (83 percent versus 24 percent), and for the majority of vision rehabilitation services or devices, the proportion of participants who were aware of a particular service or device was lower than the proportion of participants who were interested in that service or device. For example, participants were more likely to be interested in than aware of support groups (50 percent versus 31 percent), home modifications (54 percent versus 15 percent), and mobility training (49 percent versus 11 percent) (Casten et al., 2005).

Studies on the awareness of vision rehabilitation among populations in Canada and Australia suggest that the lack of awareness can vary among groups and that numerous gaps in patient knowledge may exist. Two studies of adult Canadians with vision impairment found that individuals of African descent were significantly less likely to be aware of vision rehabilitation services than individuals of other surveyed ancestries (Mwilambwe et al., 2009; Overbury and Wittich, 2011).[11] Another study reported that among 749 Canadian adults with vision impairment, 32.3 percent lacked information about vision rehabilitation services (Fraser et al., 2015). Compared to study participants who attended vision rehabilitation services, or who did not attend but were aware of such services, a greater proportion of those who lacked information about vision rehabilitation services reported great difficulty or inability to read traffic, street, or store signs, as well as being unable to perform fine handiwork (e.g., sewing, knitting). Males were also less likely than females to be aware of vision rehabilitation services (Fraser et al., 2015). Other studies have shown that patients with vision impairment may not attend vision rehabilitation services because they may not believe that vision rehabilitation will be helpful or may not identify themselves as having an impairment, or may believe that vision rehabilitation is only for

---

[9] The survey defined low vision as a visual impairment that is not corrected by standard eyeglasses, contact lenses, medication, or surgery and that interferes with the ability to perform everyday activities.

[10] "Vision impairment" replaces the term "low vision" used in the survey.

[11] Overbury and Wittich (2011) define vision impairment as a best-corrected visual acuity in the better-seeing eye of <20/60 [6/18] or a visual field of <60 degrees in either the horizontal or vertical meridian. Mwilambwe et al. (2009) define vision impairment as best-corrected visual acuity worse than 20/70 in the better-seeing eye.

blind patients (Matti et al., 2011; Pollard et al., 2003). Although these findings do not necessarily apply to populations in the United States, the implications they have for developing targeted health education activities strongly suggest the need for similar research in the United States.

Improving public awareness of vision rehabilitation begins with ensuring that health care providers are knowledgeable about vision rehabilitation and that they consistently share this knowledge with visually impaired patients. Health education campaigns implemented by stakeholders within vision rehabilitation and the clinical vision care system represent another strategy for promoting knowledge of vision rehabilitation among patients. To the extent that vision rehabilitation can mitigate the high societal and health care costs associated with vision impairment and blindness, all groups that directly or indirectly bear these costs (e.g., governments, nonprofit organizations, insurance providers, and health care organizations) also have a stake in promoting awareness of vision rehabilitation.

Knowledge Gaps Among Health Care Providers

Providers must be aware of vision rehabilitation services in order to refer patients to, and educate them about, these services. Studies from Australia and Canada support the claim that patient counseling on vision rehabilitation is essential for promoting patient awareness of these services and that failure to provide such counseling is a prominent barrier to access and utilization of vision rehabilitation services. For example, one study found that among Australian patients with vision impairment who followed up on a referral to vision rehabilitation services, 85.4 percent cited receiving a referral to and/or information about vision rehabilitation services as a facilitating factor in the decision to attend vision rehabilitation (O'Connor et al., 2008). In another study, peer workers and patients at vision rehabilitation centers in Australia reported that patients arriving at vision rehabilitation centers may have no understanding of why they are there or the nature of the service, that referral for vision rehabilitation often came late in the care process, and that patients with limited vision impairments are sometimes less likely than patients with total blindness to receive information on vision rehabilitation services (Pollard et al., 2003). In Australia, health professionals working in eye and vision care have identified a lack of knowledge of vision rehabilitation services among health professionals and poor communication between patients and providers as barriers to use of vision rehabilitation services (O'Connor et al., 2008). In the United States, patients with vision impairment have identified the quality of communication between patients and providers as the most important factor affecting the quality of care and have reported difficulties accessing health-related information (O'Day et al., 2004). As mentioned above, caution must be exercised when assessing studies performed in Canada and Australia, because these findings may not necessarily apply to populations in the United States.

Potential strategies exist for promoting the consistency and quality of patient–provider communications concerning vision rehabilitation, as well as to ensure that all health care professionals are knowledgeable about these services. For example, modules on vision rehabilitation services could be incorporated into the formal education and post-professional training of optometrists, ophthalmologists, primary care physicians, and other health care professionals who interact with visually impaired patient populations. In one study, an online continuing education program significantly improved knowledge of assessment and the treatment of vision impairment among generalist occupational therapists. After completing the program, an increased number of occupational therapists reported that they frequently screened for vision impairment, frequently provided environmental modifications to enhance visual functioning, and felt comfortable providing interventions for patients with vision impairment (Nipp et al., 2014). The need for these kinds of professional training programs has been demonstrated. For example, in a survey of 100 occupational therapists that did not specialize in vision rehabilitation, researchers found that only 52 percent believed that they had received adequate training in occupational therapy school to address the unique rehabilitation needs of patients with vision impairment (Winner et al., 2014).

Medical professional groups could also collaboratively pursue the development of guidelines describing best practices for interprofessional referral to assist care providers in the identification and appropriate referral of patients with vision impairment. Finally, health care organizations, professional groups, policy makers, and other stakeholders could promote the integration of vision rehabilitation service providers into clinical settings to better develop interprofessional trust and lines of communication and to encourage the sharing of knowledge and best practices.

These actions could be pursued as part of a larger effort to promote collaborative care and the adoption of integrated models of care in which medical, surgical, and rehabilitation interventions and services together improve the quality and accessibility of eye and vision care. Figure 8-2 depicts how the relationship between vision rehabilitation services and the surgical and medical services described in Chapter 7 could evolve toward an integrated model in which vision rehabilitation gradually assumes priority over medical and surgical care as functional limitations associated with chronic vision impairment increase.

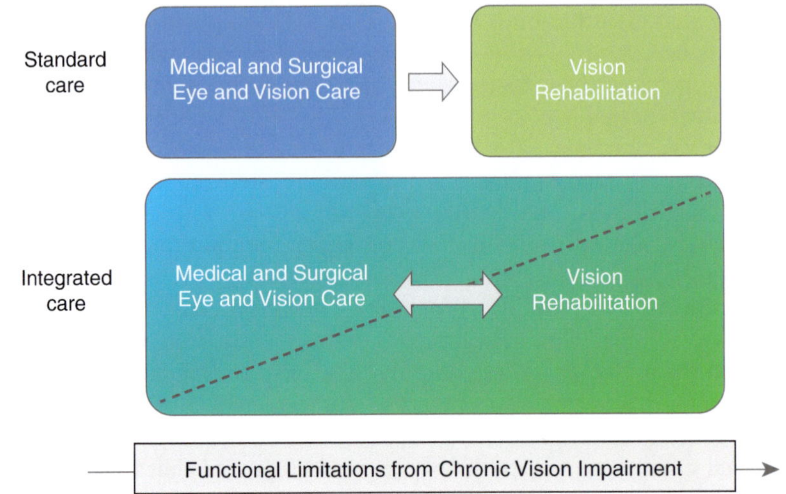

FIGURE 8-2 Evolution of the dynamic between clinical and rehabilitative care.

Knowledge Gaps Among Population Health Actors

In addition to patients and providers, members of the population health workforce also need to be knowledgeable about vision rehabilitation services. This workforce includes public health officials; epidemiologists; health policy analysts; nonprofit groups working in health care, vision care, or patient advocacy; insurance providers; administrators of health care organizations; research organizations; and health economists. The potential benefit derived from imparting knowledge about vision rehabilitation to the population health workforce is that members of each class of actor could use this information in accordance with their own interests, competencies, and professional obligations. Insurance providers could provide coverage for vision rehabilitation care and treatment under major medical insurance plans; epidemiologists could assess the impact of discrete components of vision rehabilitation on patient health outcomes; nonprofit organizations could improve care access and continuity by strengthening relationships between providers of vision rehabilitation and other community health services; health economists could assess a range of rehabilitation models to determine which provide the most cost-effective care; and health policy analysts could investigate which social policies support vision rehabilitation.

If the value of educating the population health workforce about vision rehabilitation is clear, the most appropriate means of doing so is not. Developing and running individual health education campaigns targeted to each of these groups would incur considerable costs. On the other hand, general awareness campaigns would likely have diminished penetration in at least some target groups. One strategy would be to focus health education efforts on public health departments and to rely on their unique role as conveners and coordinators to ensure that, through their dissemination activities, the population health workforce as a whole is made aware of the effectiveness of vision rehabilitation and its role in the clinical vision services system.

Workforce Education and Capacity

In considering ways to improve the value and increase the uptake of vision rehabilitation services for an increasing number of Americans with chronic vision impairment, the potential barriers related to the development of a competent multidisciplinary workforce should be addressed. The relatively limited number of optometric or ophthalmic residency or fellowship programs focused on vision rehabilitation may be one such barrier. As of academic year 2014–2015, there were no ophthalmology subspecialty residency programs in vision rehabilitation accredited by the Accreditation Council for Graduate Medical Education (ACGME), and the American Board of Ophthalmology does not currently offer specialty or subspecialty certification in vision rehabilitation (ABMS, 2016; ACGME, 2015). However, ACGME does require that physician faculty members of ophthalmology residency programs have expertise in a broad range of ophthalmic disciplines, including vision rehabilitation, and that residents must demonstrate competence in their knowledge of vision rehabilitation (ACGME, 2012). According to the American Council on Optometric Education, there were 34 accredited optometric residency programs with a focus or partial focus on vision rehabilitation in 2016 (ACOE, 2016), and the Association of Schools and Colleges of Optometry lists 20 residency programs affiliated with 12 colleges of optometry that offered focused training in vision rehabilitation in academic year 2015–2016 (ASCO, 2016).[12]

Occupational therapists have a number of opportunities for developing knowledge of or competency in vision rehabilitation. Doctoral programs are available in occupational therapy with specialty tracks or areas of concentration in vision rehabilitation and a graduate certificate in vision rehabilitation

---

[12] The 14 programs included those with a focus on low vision/ocular disease, primary care and vision rehabilitation, ocular disease and low vision rehabilitation, geriatrics and low vision, low vision rehabilitation, vision therapy and rehabilitation, vision therapy/low vision rehabilitation, low vision/primary care, vision therapy/low vision rehabilitation, geriatric and low vision rehabilitative optometry, ocular disease/low vision rehabilitation, and primary care/ low vision rehabilitation. Three additional programs offer training in vision rehabilitation (neuro-optometric rehabilitation), brain injury vision rehabilitation, and brain injury vision rehabilitation and ocular disease. An additional program in primary care optometry included training in low vision (ASCO, 2016).

(AOTA, 2016c,d). American Occupational Therapy Association (AOTA) offers a specialty certification in low vision, as well as a continuing education course on vision rehabilitation, and several AOTA-approved continuing education providers offer courses in vision rehabilitation (AOTA, 2015, 2016b). There are currently no AOTA-approved occupational therapy residency programs focused on vision rehabilitation (AOTA, 2016a). Research is needed to determine whether expanding the vision rehabilitation workforce through the development of additional training and education opportunities for optometrists, ophthalmologists, and occupational therapists can improve access to vision rehabilitation services.

Another potential barrier to access may be the distribution of the burden of care across providers and the limited availability of specific rehabilitative services. A census to determine the characteristics of vision rehabilitation patients, providers, and services in the United States found that although government agencies and independent services for visually impaired persons accounted for just 7.5 percent and 11.2 percent of all service entities, respectively, they were responsible for the provision of 28.4 percent and 22.7 percent of all vision rehabilitation services (Owsley et al., 2009). By comparison, private optometry and ophthalmology practices together comprised 60.1 percent of service entities, but provided only 22.6 percent of vision rehabilitation services. General hospitals, rehabilitation hospitals, and outpatient rehabilitation centers were more likely than private optometry and ophthalmology practices to offer several types of vision rehabilitation services (e.g., psychological services, support groups, social work services, driving rehabilitation, home visits, orientation and mobility training, eccentric viewing training, advanced/intensive training in device use), but they comprised only 2.6 percent, 1.5 percent, and 2.6 percent of service entities, respectively (Owsley et al., 2009). Research is needed to determine how the scope of practice of service entities and the distribution of the burden of care across service entities affect the quality of and access to care.

A study to assess the baseline traits of 764 patients seeking vision rehabilitation at 28 outpatient clinical centers found that 42 percent, 23 percent, and 22 percent of patients described their current emotional state as "frustrated," "anxious," and "depressed," respectively, while 85 percent reported that they limited their driving in some way (Goldstein et al., 2012, p. 1031). Another study found that 44.9 percent of vision rehabilitation patients had problems with emotional or psychological adjustments related to vision impairment and that 67.7 percent had problems or difficulties with driving (Owsley et al., 2009). Yet only a minority of service entities had a psychologist on staff (4.9 percent) or offered psychological services (21.1 percent), and only 11.4 percent offered driving rehabilitation (Owsley et al., 2009). Research is needed to ascertain whether this apparent misalignment between the needs of patients seeking vision rehabilitation and the types of interventions offered by vision rehabilitation service entities affects patient outcomes.

Finally, Medicare policies that do not recognize some members of the vision rehabilitation team, such as orientation and mobility specialists and low vision therapists, may create a barrier to care access, by failing to incentivize the growth of these professional groups or their involvement in vision rehabilitation. To address these barriers to access, policy makers could support intelligently designed vision rehabilitation demonstration projects that evaluate the efficacy and cost-effectiveness of models of care and payment and that promote and appropriately incentivize team-based vision rehabilitation services. Professional education programs could be expanded to include metrics that ensure an adequate, well-trained workforce and that address misperceptions related to vision rehabilitation. Policy makers could consider loan forgiveness and other incentives for those interested in pursuing careers in vision rehabilitation.

Racial, Ethnic, Socioeconomic, and Geographic Barriers to Accessing Vision Rehabilitation

Members of minority groups and populations living in lower socioeconomic groups access and utilize clinical eye and vision care less frequently than whites and populations in higher socioeconomic groups. Studies have found an association between lower income or less education and reduced rates of clinical eye and vision care (Zhang et al., 2012, 2013b). Other studies and reviews have reported disparities among racial and ethnic groups in access to and utilization of clinical eye and vision care (Chou et al., 2012, 2014; Elam and Lee, 2013). Because eye exams are the entry point into the vision rehabilitation process of care, it is reasonable to infer that groups that are less likely to use those services are also less likely to use vision rehabilitation services. However, there is limited direct evidence to support this inference.

There are few peer-reviewed studies on racial, ethnic, or socioeconomic barriers to vision rehabilitation access and utilization in the United States. However, studies on vision rehabilitation in Canada and Australia show that these barriers do exist in these other countries' health care systems. Among 702 Canadian adults ages 26 to 100 with vision impairment, those individuals with more education were more likely to be aware of and use vision rehabilitation services (Overbury and Wittich, 2011).[13] Lack of awareness of vision rehabilitation—which can pose a barrier to utilization— varies among racial and socioeconomic groups in Canada and is discussed above (Mwilambwe et al., 2009; Overbury and Wittich, 2011). Lack of

---

[13] Vision impairment was defined as best-corrected visual acuity in the better-seeing eye of <20/60 [6/18], or a visual field of <60 degrees in either the horizontal or vertical meridian.

transportation, which is often associated with lower socioeconomic status, is also cited as a barrier to accessing vision rehabilitation. For example, one study found that among 98 Australian patients with vision impairment who were referred to vision rehabilitation services, only 49 percent attended the service. Of those who declined or did not comply with the referral, respectively 33.3 percent and 50.0 percent cited transportation difficulties or the lack of an accompanying person as a reason for non-attendance (O'Connor et al., 2008).[14] It is important to note that differences among health care systems and patient populations mean that access barriers to vision rehabilitation in Australia and Canada may differ from those in the United States. However, the evidence of the existence of racial, ethnic, and socioeconomic barriers to accessing vision rehabilitation in other countries can be used to spur and guide efforts to determine whether such barriers also exist in the United States, and to eliminate them if they do.

In the United States, geographic variation in vision rehabilitation entities may affect the accessibility of vision rehabilitation services. One study found that the density of vision rehabilitation service entities varied among states, with higher density in some Northeastern states, and in Montana, Nebraska, North Dakota, South Dakota, and Wyoming, while many states across the southern part of the country (e.g., Alabama, Arizona, California, Georgia, Mississippi, Oklahoma, Texas) had lower densities of service entities (Owsley et al., 2009). Another study found that Alabama, Florida, Mississippi, and other states in the Southeast were among the states with the highest per capita prevalence of blindness in 2015, while several states in the Southeast, Midwest, and Northeast are among the states projected to have the highest per capita prevalence of blindness in 2050 (Varma et al., 2016). Research is needed to determine whether and how regional variations in the prevalence of vision impairment and blindness, and in the per capita density of vision rehabilitation service entities, affect, or are projected to affect, access to vision rehabilitation and demands on services.

NOVEL TECHNOLOGIES, NEW THERAPIES, AND PROMISING RESEARCH

Between technological advances that increase the effectiveness of low vision aids, an urgent push to integrate counseling and other QOL interventions into models of vision rehabilitation, and research efforts to improve the quality of care, vision rehabilitation is undergoing dramatic and beneficial changes. This section will explore how technological advance, innovative clinical care and care models, and promising research are currently

---

[14] All patients with worse than 6/12 visual acuity, or who reported functional or emotional difficulties because of their vision, were eligible to attend vision rehabilitation services.

improving health outcomes among people with vision impairment. Challenges to optimizing the impact of these powerful new tools, methods, and scientific findings will be discussed, as will strategies for overcoming those challenges.

Novel Technologies and Advances

Products and technologies that enhance the functioning and mobility of populations with vision impairment are a key component of effective vision rehabilitation services. These include products that are designed to meet the specific needs of individuals with vision impairment (e.g., dynamic Braille readers, large-print books), as well as products for use by the general public (e.g., smartphones, text-to-speech software) that also meet—or can be adapted to meet—a need common to individuals with vision impairment. This section explores the current and emerging technologies that promote QOL among populations with vision impairment and discusses the role of intentional design in supporting the development of such technologies.

Current and Emerging Technologies

As discussed above, compromised reading ability is a common complaint of patients referred to vision rehabilitation services (Brown et al., 2014; Renieri et al., 2013). Technologies to improve reading ability or otherwise provide access to written materials are numerous. Refreshable Braille displays can convert text on a digital display into Braille, though currently the available models can be prohibitively expensive (Russomanno et al., 2015). Electronic book readers with refreshable Braille displays and other devices with dynamic tactile displays are under development (Moore, 2015; Motto Ros et al., 2014). Smartphones and tablet computers have enhanced the convenience and accessibility of audiobooks, can magnify text and other images, and are increasingly equipped with speech-activated functions and text-to-speech software. A survey of 132 individuals with vision impairment found that among the 81 percent of respondents that used smartphones, 34 percent used the device to listen to audiobooks, 51 percent used the integrated camera to see an image more clearly, and 59 percent found the speech functions useful (Crossland et al., 2014). Other products and tools are designed to aid individuals with vision impairment in the performance of common activities such as cooking, exercising, and cleaning (AFB, 2014; NFB, 2016). There is a need for sustained research to continue the development of products and technologies that are accessible and that expand options for social participation, employment, and education among populations with vision impairment.

Several emerging technologies hold promise for enhancing the mobility of populations with vision impairment. For example, technology companies and car manufacturers are developing and testing self-driving cars that may create new transportation options for individuals who are otherwise unable to drive due to vision impairment (Stenquist, 2014). Difficulty with driving is a common complaint of individuals referred for vision rehabilitation (Brown et al., 2014), and individuals with some types of vision impairment (e.g., reduced contrast sensitivity) may restrict their driving habits (Fraser et al., 2013; Sandlin et al., 2014). Moreover, Owsley and McGwin (2010) note that available evidence points to an association between impaired driving performance and reduced visual acuity, visual field, or contrast sensitivity (Owsley and McGwin, 2010). These findings suggest that self-driving cars could address a documented need. Navigation systems that use smartphones and other mobile devices to provide users with real-time information about their surroundings hold potential for improving the safety and mobility of individuals with vision impairment and are being developed for use in public transportation systems, indoor settings, and other areas (Basulto, 2015; Legge et al., 2013; Pym, 2015). Mobility devices that use lasers, infrared sensors, and/or echolocation to convey information about the environment to the user via vibrational and auditory cues have also been developed and have outperformed white mobility canes in tests of hazard avoidance (Bhatlawande et al., 2014; Maidenbaum et al., 2014). Ongoing research is needed to support the development of new products and technologies that safely and effectively enhance the functioning and mobility of populations with vision impairment.

Intentional Technological Advancement and Research Needs and Opportunities

It is important to note that both existing and emerging technologies are in themselves value neutral regarding the well-being of people with vision loss. Technology can be a tool to promote or a barrier to prevent health and independent functioning. Once a luxury item, now a necessary tool, the endless adaptability of smartphones allows developers to constantly expand their uses and capabilities, and their ubiquity encourages employers, social groups, and merchants to assume every employee, acquaintance, and consumer has access to one. If accessibility remains a concern for developers of smartphones and their applications, individuals with vision impairment will have a highly portable tool with flexibility to support independence. However, if developers do not ensure their products are accessible to populations with vision impairment, these groups will have limited ability to utilize an increasingly large and crucial set of services and opportunities.

It is therefore of signal importance that entrepreneurs, developers, and innovators develop their products with the vision impairment population in mind. Moreover, the embrace of accessibility as a design principle should not be construed as a regulation that threatens business prospects and hampers creative impulse, but as an opportunity to offer goods and services to a broader set of consumers and as an engineering problem that encourages the development of technological solutions valuable in their own right.

Ensuring the universal accessibility of current and emerging technologies is one method of leveraging technological advance for the benefit of those with vision impairment. A more direct method is to invest in research and technologies that cater exclusively to this population. As part of its ongoing strategic planning activities, the NEI has previously identified the need to "[d]evelop assistive devices, environmental modifications, and rehabilitation strategies to minimize the impact of visual impairment in everyday life and reduce disability and societal limitations in visually impaired persons" (NEI, 2004, p. 28). More recently and specifically, the NEI identified the need for research to inform development of visual prostheses; tools that improve access to the internet, print materials, and navigation aids; and technologies that effectively translate key aspects of visual information into tactile and auditory information. The NEI also noted that developers of assistive technologies need to account for the unique needs and limitations of visually impaired populations that are also "elderly, cognitively impaired, or technologically naive" (NEI, 2012, p. 59). Addressing these research gaps and opportunities could accelerate development of new assistive technologies that improve independence, functioning, and QOL among individuals with vision impairment.

New Therapies and Models of Care

New Therapies for Comorbid Depression

As discussed above and in Chapter 3, several studies have found an association between vision impairment and depression (Evans et al., 2007; Horowitz et al., 2005b; Kempen et al., 2012; Nollett et al., 2016). Vision rehabilitation has been shown to be effective at mitigating depression in populations with vision impairment. An RCT compared the effects of vision rehabilitation combined with either behavior activation or supportive therapy on the prevention of depressive symptoms among patients older than 65 with bilateral AMD, functional deficits consequent to visual acuity of <20/70 in the better-seeing eye, and subthreshold depression or depressed mood.[15] After 4 months, 12.6 percent and 23.4 percent of patients in the behavioral activation and supportive therapy groups, respectively, had developed a depressive disorder. Patients in the supportive therapy group were significantly more likely to have developed a depressive disorder (Rovner et al., 2014). Another study evaluated the effects of vision rehabilitation interventions on patients ages 65 and older with vision impairment. Two years into the study, the prevalence of significant depressive symptoms had declined from 33.7 percent to 25.3 percent, and the receipt of vision rehabilitation services and skills training was associated with significantly fewer depressive symptoms. In total, vision rehabilitation interventions accounted for 10 percent of the variance in the prevalence of depression after controlling for baseline depression and other variables (Horowitz et al., 2005a).

These findings support the American Academy of Ophthalmology and AOA guidelines on vision rehabilitation, which recommend assessing the cognitive/psychological status of patients with vision impairment (AAO, 2013; AOA, 2007). The U.S. Preventive Services Task Force (USPSTF) has recommended that primary care providers screen adult patients ages 18 and older—including older adults and pregnant and postpartum women—for depression, and states that primary care providers should consider patient "risk factors, comorbid conditions, and life events to determine if additional screening of high-risk patients is warranted" (USPSTF, 2016).

Provider adherence to these guidelines and recommendations may promote early identification, and subsequent diagnosis and treatment, of depression in populations with vision impairment. Research findings suggest that novel vision rehabilitation treatment plans and training programs for providers working in vision rehabilitation may also improve clinical outcomes and care quality for patients with vision impairment and comorbid depression (Rees et al., 2012; van der Aa et al., 2015). Further research is needed to develop interventions that improve the mental health of populations with vision impairment.

New Therapies for Comorbid Cognitive Impairment

Compared to younger adults with vision impairment, cognitive impairment is more prevalent and progresses more rapidly in older adults with vision impairment (Lin et al., 2004; Reyes-Ortiz et al., 2005; Rogers and

---

[15] Behavioral activation "emphasized the link between action, mood, and mastery, and promoted self-efficacy and social connection as ways to improve mood and function and counter self-defeating behaviors" (Rovner et al., 2014, p. 3). Supportive therapy "facilitated personal expression about vision loss and disability and, in this trial, controlled for the nonspecific effects of attention" (Rovner et al., 2014, p. 4).

Langa, 2010; Tay et al., 2006; Whitson et al., 2007). Both cognitive impairment and vision impairment are disabling in their own right, but their co-occurrence has been associated with staggeringly high rates of disability and low self-rated health (Whitson et al., 2007, 2012a). Cognitive deficits were detected in about 40 percent of older adults with macular disease who were referred to an outpatient vision rehabilitation clinic (Whitson et al., 2010). Considering that rehabilitation typically entails education and training on new techniques and devices, it is easy to imagine that deficits in short-term memory, language processing, or executive function could limit a patient's progress in the program. Indeed, among patients receiving customary vision rehabilitation services, the patient and caregiver experience as well as functional outcomes were all found to be negatively affected by comorbid cognitive impairment (Lawrence et al., 2009; Whitson et al., 2012b). However, efforts are under way to evaluate and implement programs specifically designed to detect and accommodate comorbid cognitive deficits. In a pilot study of one such program, Memory or Reasoning Enhanced Low Vision Rehabilitation, participants experienced subjective and objective improvements in several measures of visual function after participation in the 6-week program (Whitson et al., 2013). Additional work is needed to evaluate the sustainability of these effects and determine whether the new models are superior to "usual care" services for individuals with co-existing vision and cognitive impairment.

New Therapies for General Medical Comorbidity

Because most of the diseases that cause chronic vision impairment are age-related, many individuals who need vision rehabilitation have a host of other medical problems. An analysis of participants in the Medicare Expenditure Panel Survey found that "eye disorders" rarely occurred in isolation: more than 80 percent of beneficiaries with eye disorders also had at least one of the four other chronic conditions assessed (heart disease, diabetes, arthritis, or hypertension) (Anderson and Horvath, 2004). Vision rehabilitation services can be highly beneficial for individuals with comorbid medical conditions, by enabling them to overcome vision-related barriers to chronic disease management. Many important activities related to self-care for medical disease (e.g., medication administration, foot checks for diabetics, blood pressure monitoring, daily weight checks for heart failure) rely on vision. However, medical comorbidities (aside from depression and cognitive deficits) can interfere with vision rehabilitation. One study analyzed more than 600 interviews with patients and their companions and identified five broad themes related to how the patients' experience in vision rehabilitation was affected by comorbid conditions (Whitson et al., 2011). For example, patients with multiple chronic conditions frequently experienced "good days and bad days," with fluctuations in symptoms such as pain or shortness of breath. When the appointments fell on "bad days," these medically complex patients were less able to focus and subsequently perceived less benefit. While the study identified many such challenges related to comorbidity, it also identified potential solutions for each challenge. For example, the issue of "good days, bad days" might be addressed through flexible scheduling options that allow patients to stack appointments on "good days" or through Web-based or take-home materials that can supplement learning that may have suffered on a "bad day."

CONCLUSION

Vision rehabilitation is essential to maximizing the independence, functioning, participation, safety, and overall QOL of people with chronic vision impairment. Yet there are numerous barriers to high-quality and universally accessible vision rehabilitation services. A lack of awareness among patients and providers of the purpose, methods, and effectiveness of vision rehabilitation; the lack of interprofessional guidelines on the clinical findings that should trigger referral of patients to vision rehabilitation; limited research, and limited resources for research, on the cost, effectiveness, and cost-effectiveness of interventions and models of care in vision rehabilitation; and barriers to access based on socioeconomic position and race all detrimentally impact care quality, access, and health outcomes. Improving the state of vision rehabilitation services and population vision health will require correcting each of these issues through a collaborative development of interprofessional guidelines, review and revision of the Centers for Medicare & Medicaid Services policy regarding coverage of vision services, design and funding of a health care services research agenda, and implementation of other strategies discussed above. In addition, stakeholders should continue to support and foster successes in vision rehabilitation related to emerging technologies and advancing medical knowledge and treatments.

This chapter identifies numerous information gaps. Box 8-1 lists these research gaps. Although this list is not comprehensive, it represents a starting point for developing a concrete set of prioritized research goals that may be fruitfully and collaboratively pursued by academic researchers, government centers, nonprofit research groups, and other stakeholders in eye and vision health.

Too often, the need for high-quality, equitable, and accessible vision rehabilitation services is lost in the focus on early detection and curative treatment of eye disease through surveillance and clinical care. Rather than treating vision rehabilitation as a last resort to be pursued only when "nothing else can be done," optometrists and ophthalmologists should integrate

---

BOX 8-1
Key Research Gaps and Opportunities

- Research is needed to determine and compare the cost, effectiveness, and cost-effectiveness of different vision rehabilitation models of care, and to ascertain the effect of greater integration of vision rehabilitation services on patient outcomes and care access and quality.
- Research is needed to determine and compare the cost, effectiveness, and cost-effectiveness of vision rehabilitation services and interventions including optical and non-optical low vision aids, mobility aids, environmental modifications, and adaptive strategies, and to develop effective, evidence-based training programs on the use of these and other interventions and services.
- Research is needed to identify the vision rehabilitation needs of children, minority groups, developmentally disabled populations, individuals with common comorbidities of vision impairment, and populations living in medically underserved areas, and to develop vision rehabilitation services and interventions that address these needs.
- Research in needed to determine the extent of awareness of vision rehabilitation among patients, providers, and the public health workforce in the United States, and to develop effective health education campaigns and other programs to eliminate lack of awareness of vision rehabilitation.
- Research is needed to assess how the organization, distribution, and scope of vision rehabilitation services affects care access and quality, and to determine how vision rehabilitation services at the national, state, and local levels could be designed to best meet patient needs.

---

discussions of vision rehabilitation services into the earliest stages of clinical care, where they can improve QOL and visual functioning throughout the care process. This shift will require both the concrete measures described above and the conceptual and cultural work of rethinking the purposes and priorities of eye and vision care.

REFERENCES

AAO (American Academy of Optometry). 2013. Vision rehabilitation—Preferred Practice Pattern® guideline. http://www.aao.org/preferred-practice-pattern/vision-rehabilitation-ppp--2013 (accessed April 5, 2016).

ABMS (American Board of Medical Specialties). 2016. Specialty and subspecialty certificates. http://www.abms.org/member-boards/specialty-subspecialty-certificates (accessed May 27, 2016).

ACGME (Accreditation Council for Graduate Medical Education). 2012. ACGME program requirements for graduate medical education in ophthalmology. http://www.acgme.org/portals/0/pfassets/programrequirements/240_ophthalmology_2016.pdf (accessed June 6, 2016).

———. 2015. ACGME data resource book academic year 2014–2015. http://www.acgme.org/Portals/0/PFAssets/PublicationsBooks/2014-2015_ACGME_DATABOOK_DOCUMENT.pdf (accessed June 6, 2016).

ACOE (American Council on Optometric Education). 2016. Accredited optometric residency programs. http://www.aoa.org/Documents/students/residency_Directory_3_18_2016.pdf (accessed June 6, 2016).

ACVREP (Academy for Certification of Vision Rehabilitation and Education Professionals). 2014a. Orientation and mobility specialist certification handbook. https://www.acvrep.org/certifications/coms (accessed June 6, 2016).

———. 2014b. Vision rehabilitation therapist certification handbook. https://www.acvrep.org/certifications/cvrt (accessed June 6, 2016).

———. 2015. Certified orientation and mobility specialist. https://www.acvrep.org/ascerteon/control/certifications/coms (accessed March 31, 2016).

AFB (American Foundation for the Blind). 2014. Products for people who are blind or visually impaired. http://www.afb.org/prodmain.asp (accessed April 2, 2016).

AHRQ (Agency for Healthcare Research and Quality). 2002. Vision rehabilitation: Care and benefit plan models: Literature review. Applying the framework to vision rehabilitation. http://www.ahrq.gov/professionals/clinicians-providers/resources/vision/vision2.html (accessed June 6, 2016).

———. 2004. Vision rehabilitation for elderly individuals with low vision or blindness. https://www.cms.gov/Medicare/Coverage/InfoExchange/downloads/rtcvisionrehab.pdf (accessed June 6, 2016).

Anderson, G., and J. Horvath. 2004. The growing burden of chronic disease in America. *Public Health Reports* 119(3):263–270.

AOA (American Optometric Association). 2007. Care of the patient with visual impairment (low vision rehabilitation). http://www.aoa.org/documents/optometrists/CPG-14.pdf (accessed June 6, 2016).

AOTA (American Occupational Therapy Association). 2015. AOTA specialty certification in low vision occupational therapist candidate application. https://www.aota.org//media/Corporate/Files/EducationCareers/BSC/initial/SCLV-A-OTA-APPLICATION.pdf (accessed June 6, 2016).

———. 2016a. Approved & candidate residency sites. http://www.aota.org/Education-Careers/Advance-Career/Residency/ResidencySites.aspx (accessed May 27, 2016).

———. 2016b. Online course: Low vision in older adults: Foundations for rehabilitation, 2nd edition. https://myaota.aota.org/shop_aota/prodview.aspx?TYPE=D&PID=165106646&SKU=OL37?sc_camp=6970EB610A00413DAD32FA9102E6A366 (accessed May 27, 2016).

———. 2016c. Postprofessional programs in OT—Doctoral level programs. http://www.aota.org/Education-Careers/Find-School/Postprofessional/PostprofessionalOT-D.aspx (accessed May 27, 2016).

———. 2016d. Postprofessional programs in OT—Masters degree programs. http://www.aota.org/Education-Careers/Find-School/Postprofessional/PostprofessionalOTM.aspx (accessed May 27, 2016).

ASCO (Association of Schools and Colleges of Optometry). 2016. Optometry residency programs in AY 2015-2016. http://www.opted.org/wp-content/uploads/2016/05/Optometry-Residency-Programs-2015-16-updated-5-23.pdf (accessed May 27, 2016).

Ballemans, J., G. I. J. M. Kempen, and G. A. R. Zijlstra. 2011. Orientation and mobility training for partially-sighted older adults using an identification cane: A systematic review. *Clinical Rehabilitation* 25(10):880–891.

Ballemans, J., G. R. Zijlstra, G. H. van Rens, J. S. Schouten, and G. I. Kempen. 2012. Usefulness and acceptability of a standardised orientation and mobility training for partially-sighted older adults using an identification cane. *BMC Health Services Research* 12(1):1–14.

Barker, L., R. Thomas, G. Rubin, and A. Dahlmann-Noor. 2015. Optical reading aids for children and young people with low vision. *Cochrane Database of Systematic Reviews* 3:CD010987.

Basulto, D. 2015. The new app that serves as eyes for the blind. *Washington Post*. October 22. https://www.washingtonpost.com/news/innovations/wp/2015/10/22/the-new-app-that-serves-as-eyes-for-the-blind (accessed September 1, 2016).

Berger, S., J. McAteer, K. Schreier, and J. Kaldenberg. 2013. Occupational therapy interventions to improve leisure and social participation for older adults with low vision: A systematic review. *American Journal of Occupational Therapy* 67(3):303–311.

Bhatlawande, S., M. Mahadevappa, J. Mukherjee, M. Biswas, D. Das, and S. Gupta. 2014. Design, development, and clinical evaluation of the electronic mobility cane for vision rehabilitation. *IEEE Transactions on Neural Systems and Rehabilitation Engineering* 22(6):1148–1159.

Binns, A. M., C. Bunce, C. Dickinson, R. Harper, R. Tudor-Edwards, M. Woodhouse, P. Linck, A. Suttie, J. Jackson, J. Lindsay, J. Wolffsohn, L. Hughes, and T. H. Margrain. 2012. How effective is low vision service provision? A systematic review. *Survey of Ophthalmology* 57(1):34–65.

Bodenheimer, T., K. Lorig, H. Holman, and K. Grumbach. 2002. Patient self-management of chronic disease in primary care. *JAMA* 288(19):2469–2475.

Bowers, A. R., C. Meek, and N. Stewart. 2001. Illumination and reading performance in age-related macular degeneration. *Clinical and Experimental Optometry* 84(3):139–147.

Bradfield, Y. S. 2013. Identification and treatment of amblyopia. *American Family Physician* 87(5):348–352.

Brody, B. L., A. C. Roch-Levecq, A. C. Gamst, K. Maclean, R. M. Kaplan, and S. I. Brown. 2002. Self-management of age-related macular degeneration and quality of life: A randomized controlled trial. *Archives of Ophthalmology* 120(11):1477–1483.

Brody, B. L., A. C. Roch-Levecq, R. G. Thomas, R. M. Kaplan, and S. I. Brown. 2005. Self-management of age-related macular degeneration at the 6-month follow-up: A randomized controlled trial. *Archives of Ophthalmology* 123(1):46–53.

Brody, B. L., A. C. Roch-Levecq, R. M. Kaplan, C. Y. Moutier, and S. I. Brown. 2006. Age-related macular degeneration: Self-management and reduction of depressive symptoms in a randomized, controlled study. *Journal of the American Geriatrics Society* 54(10):1557–1562.

Brown, J. C., J. E. Goldstein, T. L. Chan, R. Massof, and P. Ramulu. 2014. Characterizing functional complaints in patients seeking outpatient low-vision services in the United States. *Ophthalmology* 121(8):1655–1662, c1651.

Brunnström, G., S. Sörensen, K. Alsterstad, and J. Sjöstrand. 2004. Quality of light and quality of life—The effect of lighting adaptation among people with low vision. *Ophthalmic and Physiological Optics* 24(4):274–280.

Campbell, A. J., M. C. Robertson, S. J. La Grow, N. M. Kerse, G. F. Sanderson, R. J. Jacobs, D. M. Sharp, and L. A. Hale. 2005. Randomised controlled trial of prevention of falls in people aged ≥75 with severe visual impairment: The VIP trial. *British Medical Journal* 331(7520):817.

Casten, R. J., E. K. Maloney, and B. W. Rovner. 2005. Knowledge and use of low vision services among persons with age-related macular degeneration. *Journal of Visual Impairment & Blindness* 99(11):720–724.

CDC (Centers for Disease Control and Prevention). 2009. The burden of vision loss. http://www.cdc.gov/visionhealth/basic_information/vision_loss_burden.htm (accessed March 24, 2016).

Chavda, S., W. Hodge, F. Si, and K. Diab. 2014. Low-vision rehabilitation methods in children: A systematic review. *Canadian Journal of Ophthalmology* 49(3):e71–e73.

Chou, C. F., L. E. Barker, J. E. Crews, S. A. Primo, X. Zhang, A. F. Elliott, K. McKeever Bullard, L. S. Geiss, and J. B. Saaddine. 2012. Disparities in eye care utilization among the United States adults with visual impairment: Findings from the Behavioral Risk Factor Surveillance System 2006–2009. *American Journal of Ophthalmology* 154(6 Suppl):S45–S52, e41.

Chou, C. F., C. E. Sherrod, X. Zhang, L. E. Barker, K. M. Bullard, J. E. Crews, and J. B. Saaddine. 2014. Barriers to eye care among people aged 40 years and older with diagnosed diabetes, 2006–2010. *Diabetes Care* 37(1):180–188.

Christ, S. L., D. D. Zheng, B. K. Swenor, B. L. Lam, S. K. West, S. L. Tannenbaum, B. E. Muñoz, and D. J. Lee. 2014. Longitudinal relationships among visual acuity, daily functional status, and mortality: The Salisbury Eye Evaluation Study. *JAMA Ophthalmology* 132(12):1400–1406.

Crews, J. E., G. C. Jones, and J. H. Kim. 2006. Double jeopardy: The effects of comorbid conditions among older people with vision loss. *Journal of Visual Impairment & Blindness* 100:824.

Crews, J. E., C. F. Chou, J. A. Stevens, and J. B. Saaddine. 2016a. Falls among persons aged ≥65 years with and without severe vision impairment—United States, 2014. *Morbidity and Mortality Weekly Report* 65(17):433–437.

Crews, J. E., C. F. Chou, M. M. Zack, X. Zhang, K. M. Bullard, A. R. Morse, and J. B. Saaddine. 2016b. The association of health-related quality of life with severity of visual impairment among people aged 40-64 years: Findings from the 2006–2010 Behavioral Risk Factor Surveillance System. *Ophthalmic Epidemiology* 23(3):145–153.

Crossland, M. D., R. S. Silva, and A. F. Macedo. 2014. Smartphone, tablet computer and e-reader use by people with vision impairment. *Ophthalmic and Physiological Optics* 34(5):552–557.

Dahlin Ivanoff, S., U. Sonn, and E. Svensson. 2002. A health education program for elderly persons with visual impairments and perceived security in the performance of daily occupations: A randomized study. *American Journal of Occupational Therapy* 56(3):322–330.

Davidson, S., and G. E. Quinn. 2011. The impact of pediatric vision disorders in adulthood. *Pediatrics* 127(2):334–339.

Day, L., B. Fildes, I. Gordon, M. Fitzharris, H. Flamer, and S. Lord. 2002. Randomised factorial trial of falls prevention among older people living in their own homes. *British Medical Journal* 325(7356):128.

Demers-Turco, P. 1999. Providing timely and ongoing vision rehabilitation services for the diabetic patient with irreversible vision loss from diabetic retinopathy. *Journal of the American Optometric Association* 70(1):49 62.

Deremeik, J., A. T. Broman, D. Friedman, S. K. West, R. Massof, W. Park, K. Bandeen-Roche, K. Frick, and B. Muñoz. 2007. Low vision rehabilitation in a nursing home population: The seeing study. *Journal of Visual Impairment & Blindness* 101(11):701–714.

Elam, A. R., and P. P. Lee. 2013. High-risk populations for vision loss and eye care underutilization: A review of the literature and ideas on moving forward. *Survey of Ophthalmology* 58(4):348–358.

Erickson, W., C. Lee, S. von Schrader. 2016. *Disability statistics from the 2014 American Community Survey (ACS)*. Ithaca, NY: Cornell University Yang Tan Institute (YTI).

Evans, J. R., A. E. Fletcher, and R. P. Wormald. 2007. Depression and anxiety in visually impaired older people. *Ophthalmology* 114(2):283–288.

Fraser, M. L., L. B. Meuleners, A. H. Lee, J. Q. Ng, and N. Morlet. 2013. Which visual measures affect change in driving difficulty after first eye cataract surgery? *Accident Analysis and Prevention* 58:10–14.

Fraser, S. A., A. P. Johnson, W. Wittich, and O. Overbury. 2015. Critical success factors in awareness of and choice towards low vision rehabilitation. *Ophthalmic Physiological Optics* 35(1):81–89.

Gaffney, A. J., T. H. Margrain, C. V. Bunce, and A. M. Binns. 2014. How effective is eccentric viewing training? A systematic literature review. *Ophthalmic Physiological Optics* 34(4):427–437.

Ganesh, S., S. Sethi, S. Srivastav, A. Chaudhary, and P. Arora. 2013. Impact of low vision rehabilitation on functional vision performance of children with visual impairment. *Oman Journal of Ophthalmology* 6(3):170–174.

Gilbert, C., and A. Foster. 2001. Childhood blindness in the context of vision 2020: The right to sight. *Bulletin of the World Health Organization* 79(3):227–232.

Goldstein, J. E., R. W. Massof, J. T. Deremeik, S. Braudway, M. L. Jackson, K. B. Kehler, S. A. Primo, J. S. Sunness, and the Low Vision Research Network Study Group. 2012. Baseline traits of low vision patients served by private outpatient clinical centers in the United States. *Archives of Ophthalmology* 130(8):1028–1037.

Goldstein, J. E., M. Jackson, S. M. Fox, J. T. Deremeik, and R. W. Massof, for the Low Vision Research Network Study Group. 2015. Clinically meaningful rehabilitation outcomes of low vision patients served by outpatient clinical centers. *JAMA Ophthalmology* 133(7):762–769.

Gothwal, V. K., R. Sumalini, and S. Bharani. 2015. Assessing the effectiveness of low vision rehabilitation in children: An observational study. *Investigative Ophthalmology & Visual Science* 56(5):3355–3360.

Hinds, A., A. Sinclair, J. Park, A. Suttie, H. Paterson, and M. Macdonald. 2003. Impact of an interdisciplinary low vision service on the quality of life of low vision patients. *British Journal of Ophthalmology* 87(11):1391–1396.

Hong, S. P., H. Park, J. S. Kwon, and E. Yoo. 2014. Effectiveness of eccentric viewing training for daily visual activities for individuals with age-related macular degeneration: A systematic review and meta-analysis. *NeuroRehabilitation* 34(3):587–595.

Hooper, P., J. W. Jutai, G. Strong, and E. Russell-Minda. 2008. Age-related macular degeneration and low-vision rehabilitation: A systematic review. *Canadian Journal of Ophthalmology* 43(2):180–187.

Horowitz, A., J. P. Reinhardt, and K. Boerner. 2005a. The effect of rehabilitation on depression among visually disabled older adults. *Aging and Mental Health* 9(6):563–570.

Horowitz, A., J. P. Reinhardt, and G. J. Kennedy. 2005b. Major and subthreshold depression among older adults seeking vision rehabilitation services. *American Journal of Geriatric Psychiatry* 13(3):180–187.

IOM (Institute of Medicine). 2001. *Crossing the quality chasm: A new health system for the 21st century*. Washington, DC: National Academy Press.

Justiss, M. D. 2013. Occupational therapy interventions to promote driving and community mobility for older adults with low vision: A systematic review. *American Journal of Occupational Therapy* 67(3):296–302.

Kempen, G. I., J. Ballemans, A. V. Ranchor, G. H. van Rens, and G. A. Zijlstra. 2012. The impact of low vision on activities of daily living, symptoms of depression, feelings of anxiety and social support in community-living older adults seeking vision rehabilitation services. *Quality of Life Research* 21(8):1405–1411.

Kolarik, A. J., S. Cirstea, S. Pardhan, and B. C. Moore. 2014. A summary of research investigating echolocation abilities of blind and sighted humans. *Hearing Research* 310:60–68.

Kondo, H. M., D. Pressnitzer, I. Toshima, and M. Kashino. 2012. Effects of self-motion on auditory scene analysis. *Proceedings of the National Academy of Sciences of the United States of America* 109(17):6775–6780.

Kuyk, T., L. Liu, J. L. Elliott, H. E. Grubbs, C. Owsley, G. McGwin, R. L. Griffin, and P. S. Fuhr. 2008. Health-related quality of life following blind rehabilitation. *Quality of Life Research* 17(4):497–507.

Lam, N., and S. J. Leat. 2013. Barriers to accessing low-vision care: The patient's perspective. *Canadian Journal of Ophthalmology* 48(6):458–462.

Lamoureux, E. L., J. F. Pallant, K. Pesudovs, G. Rees, J. B. Hassell, and J. E. Keeffe. 2007. The effectiveness of low-vision rehabilitation on participation in daily living and quality of life. *Investigative Ophthalmology & Visual Science* 48(4):1476–1482.

Larizza, M. F., J. Xie, E. Fenwick, E. L. Lamoureux, J. E. Keeffe, and G. Rees. 2011. Impact of a low-vision self-management program on informal caregivers. *Optometry & Visual Science* 88(12):1486–1495.

Lawrence, V., J. Murray, D. Ffytche, and S. Banerjee. 2009. "Out of sight, out of mind": A qualitative study of visual impairment and dementia from three perspectives. *International Psychogeriatrics* 21(3):511–518.

Leat, S. J. 2016. A proposed model for integrated low-vision rehabilitation services in Canada. *Optometry & Visual Science* 93(1):77–84.

Lee, L., T. L. Packer, S. H. Tang, and S. Girdler. 2008. Self-management education programs for age-related macular degeneration: A systematic review. *Australasian Journal on Ageing* 27(4):170–176.

Legge, G. E., P. J. Beckmann, B. S. Tjan, G. Havey, K. Kramer, D. Rolkosky, R. Gage, M. Chen, S. Puchakayala, and A. Rangarajan. 2013. Indoor navigation by people with visual impairment using a digital sign system. *PLoS ONE* 8(10):e76783.

Lin, M. Y., P. R. Gutierrez, K. L. Stone, K. Yaffe, K. E. Ensrud, H. A. Fink, C. A. Sarkisian, A. L. Coleman, and C. M. Mangione. 2004. Vision impairment and combined vision and hearing impairment predict cognitive and functional decline in older women. *Journal of the American Geriatrics Society* 52(12):1996–2002.

Liu, C.-J., M. A. Brost, V. E. Horton, S. B. Kenyon, and K. E. Mears. 2013. Occupational therapy interventions to improve performance of daily activities at home for older adults with low vision: A systematic review. *American Journal of Occupational Therapy* 67(3):279–287.

Luo, R.-J., S.-R. Liu, Z. Tian, W.-H. Zhu, Y.-H. Zhuo, and R.-D. Liao. 2011. Rehabilitation of vision disorder and improved quality of life in patients with primary open angle glaucoma. *Chinese Medical Journal* 124(17):2687–2691.

Maidenbaum, S., S. Hanassy, S. Abboud, G. Buchs, D. R. Chebat, S. Levy-Tzedek, and A. Amedi. 2014. The "eyecane," a new electronic travel aid for the blind: Technology, behavior & swift learning. *Restorative Neurology and Neuroscience* 32(6):813–824.

Markowitz, M. 2006a. Occupational therapy interventions in low vision rehabilitation. *Canadian Journal of Ophthalmology* 41(3):340–347.

Markowitz, S. N. 2006b. Principles of modern low vision rehabilitation. *Canadian Journal of Ophthalmology* 41(3):289–312.

Matti, A. I., K. Pesudovs, A. Daly, M. Brown, and C. S. Chen. 2011. Access to low-vision rehabilitation services: Barriers and enablers. *Clinical and Experimental Optometry* 94(2):181–186.

Milne, J. L., M. A. Goodale, and L. Thaler. 2014. The role of head movements in the discrimination of 2-D shape by blind echolocation experts. *Attention, Perception & Psychophysics* 76(6):1828–1837.

Minto, H., and Butt, I. A. 2004. Low vision devices and training. *Community Eye Health* 17(49):67.

Mogk, L., and G. Goodrich. 2004. The history and future of low vision services in the United States. *Journal of Visual Impairment & Blindness* 98(10):585–600.

Moore, N. C. 2015. Bringing Braille back with better display technology. http://www.engin.umich.edu/college/about/news/stories/2015/december/bringing-braille-back-with-a-better-display-technology (accessed June 30, 2016).

Motto Ros, P., V. Dante, L. Mesin, E. Petetti, P. Del Giudice, and E. Pasero. 2014. A new dynamic tactile display for reconfigurable Braille: Implementation and tests. *Frontiers in Neuroengineering* 7:6.

Mwilambwe, A., W. Wittich, and E. E. Freeman. 2009. Disparities in awareness and use of low-vision rehabilitation. *Canadian Journal of Ophthalmology* 44(6):686–691.

NEHEP (National Eye Health Education Program). n.d. Vision rehabilitation: Helping people with low vision. https://nei.nih.gov/sites/default/files/nehep-pdfs/Low_Vision_Fact_Sheet_v3.pdf (accessed June 5, 2016).

NEI (National Eye Institute). 2004. National plan for eye and vision research. https://nei.nih.gov/sites/default/files/nei-pdfs/nationalplan1.pdf (accessed June 30, 2016).

———. 2010. Vision impairment tables. https://nei.nih.gov/eyedata/vision_impaired/tables (accessed March 25, 2016).

———. 2012. Vision research needs, gaps, and opportunities. https://nei.nih.gov/sites/default/files/nei-pdfs/VisionResearch2012.pdf (accessed February 22, 2016).

———. 2014. Facts about retinitis pigmentosa. https://nei.nih.gov/health/pigmentosa/pigmentosa_facts (accessed June 15, 2016).

———. 2015. Facts about Stargardt disease. https://nei.nih.gov/health/stargardt/star_facts (accessed June 15, 2016).

NEI/LCIF (National Eye Institute/Lions Club International Foundation). 2008. 2005 survey of public knowledge, attitudes, and practices related to eye health and disease. https://nei.nih.gov/kap (accessed June 6, 2016).

NFB (National Federation of the Blind). 2016. Technology resource list. https://nfb.org/technology-resource-list (accessed April 2, 2016).

Nguyen, N. X., M. Weismann, and S. Trauzettel-Klosinski. 2009. Improvement of reading speed after providing of low vision aids in patients with age-related macular degeneration. *Acta Ophthalmologica* 87(8):849–853.

Nilsson, U. L. 1986. Visual rehabilitation of patients with advanced diabetic retinopathy. A follow-up study at the low vision clinic, Department of Ophthalmology, University of Linkoping. *Documenta Ophthalmologica* 62(4):369–382.

Nipp, C. M., L. K. Vogtle, and M. Warren. 2014. Clinical application of low vision rehabilitation strategies after completion of a computer-based training module. *Occupational Therapy in Health Care* 28(3):296–305.

Nollett, C. L., N. Bray, C. Bunce, R. J. Casten, R. T. Edwards, M. T. Hegel, S. Janikoun, S. E. Jumbe, B. Ryan, J. Shearn, D. J. Smith, M. Stanford, W. Xing, and T. H. Margrain. 2016. High prevalence of untreated depression in patients accessing low-vision services. *Ophthalmology* 123(2):440-441.

O'Connor, P. M., L. C. Mu, and J. E. Keeffe. 2008. Access and utilization of a new low-vision rehabilitation service. *Clinical and Experimental Ophthalmology* 36(6):547–552.

O'Day, B. L., M. Killeen, and L. I. Iezzoni. 2004. Improving health care experiences of persons who are blind or have low vision: Suggestions from focus groups. *American Journal of Medical Quality* 19(5):193–200.

Overbury, O., and W. Wittich. 2011. Barriers to low vision rehabilitation: The Montreal Barriers Study. *Investigative Ophthalmology & Visual Science* 52(12):8933–8938.

Owsley, C., and G. McGwin. 2010. Vision and driving. *Vision Research* 50(23):2348–2361.

Owsley, C., G. McGwin, Jr., P. P. Lee, N. Wasserman, and K. Searcey. 2009. Characteristics of low-vision rehabilitation services in the United States. *Archives of Ophthalmology* 127(5):681–689.

Patino, C. M., R. McKean-Cowdin, S. P. Azen, J. C. Allison, F. Choudhury, and R. Varma. 2010. Central and peripheral visual impairment and the risk of falls and falls with injury. *Ophthalmology* 117(2):199–206, e191.

Pollard, T. L., J. A. Simpson, E. L. Lamoureux, and J. E. Keeffe. 2003. Barriers to accessing low vision services. *Ophthalmic Physiological Optics* 23(4):321–327.

Pym, H. 2015. Technology helps visually impaired navigate the tube. *BBC*. March 5. http://www.bbc.com/news/health-31754365 (accessed June 30, 2016).

Rees, G., E. E. Holloway, G. Craig, N. Hepi, S. Coad, J. E. Keeffe, and E. L. Lamoureux. 2012. Screening for depression: Integrating training into the professional development programme for low vision rehabilitation staff. *Clinical and Experimental Ophthalmology* 40(9):840–848.

Rees, G., J. Xie, P. P. Chiang, M. F. Larizza, M. Marella, J. B. Hassell, J. E. Keeffe, and E. L. Lamoureux. 2015. A randomised controlled trial of a self-management programme for low vision implemented in low vision rehabilitation services. *Patient Education and Counseling* 98(2):174–181.

Renieri, G., S. Pitz, N. Pfeiffer, M. E. Beutel, and R. Zwerenz. 2013. Changes in quality of life in visually impaired patients after low-vision rehabilitation. *International Journal of Rehabilitation Research* 36(1):48–55.

Reyes-Ortiz, C. A., Y. F. Kuo, A. R. DiNuzzo, L. A. Ray, M. A. Raji, and K. S. Markides. 2005. Near vision impairment predicts cognitive decline: Data from the Hispanic Established Populations for Epidemiologic Studies of the Elderly. *Journal of the American Geriatrics Society* 53(4):681–686.

Rogers, M. A. M., and K. M. Langa. 2010. Untreated poor vision: A contributing factor to late-life dementia. *American Journal of Epidemiology* 171(6):728–735.

Rovner, B. W., R. J. Casten, M. T. Hegel, R. W. Massof, B. E. Leiby, A. C. Ho, and W. S. Tasman. 2014. Low Vision Depression Prevention Trial in Age-Related Macular Degeneration: A randomized clinical trial. *Ophthalmology* 121(11):2204–2211.

Russomanno, A., S. O'Modhrain, R. B. Gillespie, and M. W. Rodger. 2015. Refreshing refreshable Braille displays. *IEEE Transactions on Haptics* 8(3):287–297.

Ryan, B. 2014. Models of low vision care: Past, present and future. *Clinical and Experimental Optometry* 97(3):209–213.

Ryan, B., S. White, J. Wild, H. Court, and T. H. Margrain. 2010. The newly established primary care based Welsh Low Vision Service is effective and has improved access to low vision services in Wales. *Ophthalmic Physiological Optics* 30(4):358–364.

Ryan, B., J. Khadka, C. Bunce, and H. Court. 2013. Effectiveness of the community-based low vision service Wales: A long-term outcome study. *British Journal of Ophthalmology* 97(4):487–491.

Sandlin, D., G. McGwin, Jr., and C. Owsley. 2014. Association between vision impairment and driving exposure in older adults aged 70 years and over: A population-based examination. *Acta Ophthalmologica* 92(3):e207–e212.

Scanlan, J., and J. E. Cuddeford. 2004. Low vision rehabilitation: A comparison of traditional and extended teaching programs. *Journal of Visual Impairment & Blindness* 98(10):601–610.

Schenkman, B. N., and M. E. Nilsson. 2010. Human echolocation: Blind and sighted persons' ability to detect sounds recorded in the presence of a reflecting object. *Perception* 39(4):483–501.

Schornich, S., A. Nagy, and L. Wiegrebe. 2012. Discovering your inner bat: Echo-acoustic target ranging in humans. *Journal of the Association for Research in Otolaryngology* 13(5):673–682.

Schornich, S., L. Wallmeier, N. Gessele, A. Nagy, M. Schranner, D. Kish, and L. Wiegrebe. 2013. Psychophysics of human echolocation. *Advances in Experimental Medicine and Biology* 787:311–319.

Skelton, D. A., T. E. Howe, C. Ballinger, F. Neil, S. Palmer, and L. Gray. 2013. Environmental and behavioural interventions for reducing physical activity limitation in community-dwelling visually impaired older people. *Cochrane Database of Systematic Reviews* 6:CD009233.

Smallfield, S., K. Clem, and A. Myers. 2013. Occupational therapy interventions to improve the reading ability of older adults with low vision: A systematic review. *American Journal of Occupational Therapy* 67(3):288–295.

Stelmack, J. A., D. Moran, D. Dean, and R. W. Massof. 2007a. Short- and long-term effects of an intensive inpatient vision rehabilitation program. *Archives of Physical Medicine and Rehabilitation* 88(6):691–695.

Stelmack, J. A., X. C. Tang, D. J. Reda, D. Moran, S. Rinne, R. M. Mancil, R. Cummings, G. Mancil, K. Stroupe, N. Ellis, and R. W. Massof. 2007b. The Veterans Affairs Low Vision Intervention Trial (LOVIT): Design and methodology. *Clinical Trials* 4(6):650–660.

Stelmack, J. A., X. C. Tang, D. J. Reda, S. Rinee, R. M. Mancil, R. W. Massof, for the LOVIT Study Group. 2008. Outcomes of the Veterans Affairs Low Vision Intervention Trial (LOVIT). *Archives of Ophthalmology* 126(5):608–617.

Stelmack, J. A., X. C. Tang, Y. Wei, and R. W. Massof, for the Low-Vision Intervention Trial Study Group. 2012a. The effectiveness of low-vision rehabilitation in 2 cohorts derived from the Veterans Affairs Low Vision Intervention Trial. *Archives of Ophthalmology* 130(9):1162–1168.

Stelmack, J. A., X. C. Tang, D. J. Reda, K. T. Stroupe, S. Rinne, and R. W. Massof. 2012b. VA LOVIT II: A protocol to compare low vision rehabilitation and basic low vision. *Ophthalmic Physiological Optics* 32(6):461–471.

Stenquist, P. 2014. In self-driving cars, a potential lifeline for the disabled. *New York Times*. November 7. http://www.nytimes.com/2014/11/09/automobiles/in-self-driving-cars-a-potential-lifeline-for-the-disabled.html?_r=0 (accessed June 30, 2016).

Stroupe, K. T., J. A. Stelmack, X. C. Tang, D. J. Reda, D. Moran, S. Rinne, R. Mancil, Y. Wei, R. Cummings, G. Mancil, N. Ellis, and R. W. Massof. 2008. Economic evaluation of blind rehabilitation for veterans with macular diseases in the Department of Veterans Affairs. *Ophthalmic Epidemiology* 15(2):84–91.

Swenor, B. K., E. M. Simonsick, L. Ferrucci, A. B. Newman, S. Rubin, and V. Wilson, for the the Health, Aging, and Body Composition Study. 2015. Visual impairment and incident mobility limitations: The Health ABC Study. *Journal of the American Geriatrics Society* 63(1):46–54.

Tay, T., J. J. Wang, A. Kifley, R. Lindley, P. Newall, and P. Mitchell. 2006. Sensory and cognitive association in older persons: Findings from an older Australian population. *Gerontology* 52(6):386–394.

Teng, S., and D. Whitney. 2011. The acuity of echolocation: Spatial resolution in the sighted compared to expert performance. *Journal of Visual Impairment & Blindness* 105(1):20–32.

Teng, S., A. Puri, and D. Whitney. 2012. Ultrafine spatial acuity of blind expert human echo-locators. *Experimental Brain Research* 216(4):483–488.

Thomas, R., L. Barker, G. Rubin, and A. Dahlmann-Noor. 2015. Assistive technology for children and young people with low vision. *Cochrane Database of Systematic Reviews* 6:CD011350.

USPSTF (U.S. Preventive Services Task Force). 2016. Screening for depression in adults: U.S. Preventive Services Task Force recommendation statement. *JAMA* 315(4): 380–387.

VA (U.S. Department of Veterans Affairs). 2015. Rehabilitation and prosthetic services: About blind rehabilitation services. http://www.prosthetics.va.gov/blindrehab/BRS_Coordinated_Care.asp (accessed March 31, 2016).

———. 2016. Kansas City VA Medical Center. http://www.kansascity.va.gov/services/Vision_Impairment_Rehabilitation.asp (accessed May 27, 2016).

van der Aa, H. P. A., G. H. van Rens, H. C. Comijs, T. H. Margrain, F. Gallindo-Garre, J. W. Twisk, and R. M. van Nispen. 2015. Stepped care for depression and anxiety in visually impaired older adults: Multicentre randomised controlled trial. *British Medical Journal* 351:h6127.

Varma, R., T. S. Vajaranant, B. Burkemper, S. Wu, M. Torres, C. Hsu, F. Choudhury, and R. McKean-Cowdin. 2016. Visual impairment and blindness in adults in the United States: Demographic and geographic variations from 2015 to 2050. *JAMA Ophthalmology* 134(7):802–809.

Vercillo, T., J. L. Milne, M. Gori, and M. A. Goodale. 2015. Enhanced auditory spatial localization in blind echolocators. *Neuropsychologia* 67:35–40.

Virgili, G., and G. Rubin, 2010. Orientation and mobility training for people with low vision. *Cochrane Database of Systematic Reviews* 5:CD003925.

Virgili, G., R. Acosta, L. L. Grover, S. A. Bentley, and G. Giacomelli. 2013. Reading aids for adults with low vision. *Cochrane Database of Systematic Reviews* 10:CD003303.

VisionAware. 2016a. Organizing and labeling clothing when you are blind or have low vision. http://www.visionaware.org/section.aspx?FolderID=8&SectionID=115&TopicID=485&DocumentID=5814&rewrite=0 (accessed June 17, 2016).

———. 2016b. Safe cooking techniques for cooks who are blind or have low vision. http://www.visionaware.org/info/everyday-living/cooking/safe-cooking-techniques/135 (accessed June 17, 2016).

Wallmeier, L., and L. Wiegrebe. 2014a. Ranging in human sonar: Effects of additional early reflections and exploratory head movements. *PLoS ONE* 9(12):e115363.

———. 2014b. Self-motion facilitates echo-acoustic orientation in humans. *Royal Society Open Science* 1(3):140185.

Walter, C., R. Althouse, H. Humble, W. Smith, and J. V. Odom. 2007. Vision rehabilitation: Recipients' perceived efficacy of rehabilitation. *Ophthalmic Epidemiology* 14(3):103–111.

Wang, B. Z., K. Pesudovs, M. C. Keane, A. Daly, and C. S. Chen. 2012. Evaluating the effectiveness of multidisciplinary low-vision rehabilitation. *Optometry and Visual Science* 89(9):1399–1408.

Whitson, H. E., S. W. Cousins, B. M. Burchett, C. F. Hybels, C. F. Pieper, and H. J. Cohen. 2007. The combined effect of visual impairment and cognitive impairment on disability in older people. *Journal of the American Geriatrics Society* 55(6):885–891.

Whitson, H. E., D. Ansah, D. Whitaker, G. Potter, S. W. Cousins, H. MacDonald, C. F. Pieper, L. Landerman, D. C. Steffens, and H. J. Cohen. 2010. Prevalence and patterns of comorbid cognitive impairment in low vision rehabilitation for macular disease. *Archives of Gerontolology and Geriatrics* 50(2):209–212.

Whitson, H. E., K. Steinhauser, N. Ammarell, D. Whitaker, S. W. Cousins, D. Ansah, L. L. Sanders, and H. J. Cohen. 2011. Categorizing the effect of comorbidity: A qualitative study of individuals' experiences in a low-vision rehabilitation program. *Journal of the American Geriatric Society* 59(10):1802–1809.

Whitson, H. E., R. Malhotra, A. Chan, D. B. Matchar, and T. Ostbye. 2012a. Comorbid visual and cognitive impairment: Relationship with disability status and self-rated health among older Singaporeans. *Asia Pacific Journal of Public Health* 26(3):310–319.

Whitson, H. E., D. Whitaker, L. L. Sanders, G. G. Potter, S. W. Cousins, D. Ansah, E. McConnell, C. F. Pieper, L. Landerman, D. C. Steffens, and H. J. Cohen. 2012b. Memory deficit associated with worse functional trajectories in older adults in low-vision rehabilitation for macular disease. *Journal of the American Geriatric Society* 60(11):2087–2092.

Whitson, H. E., D. Whitaker, G. Potter, E. McConnell, F. Tripp, L. L. Sanders, K. W. Muir, H. J. Cohen, and S. W. Cousins. 2013. A low-vision rehabilitation program for patients with mild cognitive deficits. *JAMA Ophthalmology* 131(7):912–919.

Winner, S., H. K. Yuen, L. K. Vogtle, and M. Warren. 2014. Factors associated with comfort level of occupational therapy practitioners in providing low vision services. *American Journal of Occupational Therapy* 68(1):96–101.

Wittenborn, J., and D. Rein. 2016 (unpublished). *The potential costs and benefits of treatment for undiagnosed eye disorders.* Paper prepared for the Committee on Public Health Approaches to Reduce Vision Impairment and Promote Eye Health. http://www.national academies.org/hmd/~/media/Files/Report%20Files/2016/UndiagnosedEyeDisorders CommissionedPaper.pdf (accessed September 15, 2016).

Zhang, X., M. F. Cotch, A. Ryskulova, S. A. Primo, P. Nair, C.-F. Chou, L. S. Geiss, L. Barker, A. F. Elliott, J. E. Crews, and J. B. Saaddine. 2012. Vision health disparities in the United States by race/ethnicity, education, and economic status: Findings from two nationally representative surveys. *American Journal of Ophthalmology* 154(6 Suppl):S53–S62, e51.

Zhang, X., K. M. Bullard, M. F. Cotch, M. R. Wilson, B. W. Rovner, G. McGwin, C. Owsley, L. Barker, J. E. Crews, and J. B. Saaddine. 2013a. Association between depression and functional vision loss in persons 20 years of age or older in the United States, NHANES 2005–2008. *JAMA Ophthalmology* 131(5):573–581.

Zhang, X., G. L. Beckles, C. F. Chou, J. B. Saaddine, M. R. Wilson, P. P. Lee, N. Parvathy, A. Ryskulova, and L. S. Geiss. 2013b. Socioeconomic disparity in use of eye care services among U.S. adults with age-related eye diseases: National Health Interview Survey, 2002 and 2008. *JAMA Ophthalmology* 131(9):1198–1206.

Zijlstra, G. A. R., J. Ballemans, and G. I. J. M. Kempen. 2013. Orientation and mobility training for adults with low vision: A new standardized approach. *Clinical Rehabilitation* 27(1):3–18.

9

Eye and Vision Health:
Recommendations and a Path to Action

The long-term goal of a population health approach for eye and vision health would be to transform vision impairment from an exceedingly common to a rare condition, at the same time reducing the associated health inequities. A population health approach comprises multiple actors who work separately and cooperatively to influence multiple determinants of health. These collaborations also allow governmental public health entities to fulfill their core functions: assessment (i.e., monitoring communities to identify and characterize public health needs and priorities); policy development (i.e., the use of scientific evidence to guide decisions about, and the design and implementation of, actions and policies that address population health issues); and assurance (i.e., ensuring that stakeholders have the resources necessary to achieve established process and outcome goals) (IOM, 1988). However, as discussed in Chapter 5, implementing population-level improvements is the responsibility of the entire population health system, including all the healthy system's stakeholders. Figure 5-1 in particular highlighted the relevant partners that are critical to the effort of advancing population health objectives, including the community, other government agencies, the education sector, nonprofit organizations, the media, employers and businesses, and the clinical care system.

There are steps that can be taken right now to significantly reduce the burden of vision impairment within the next few years, based on current knowledge and available treatments. To ensure that populations, especially underserved and at-risk populations, know to seek and have access to timely and high-quality eye and vision care, coordinated efforts are needed to expand the footprint of eye care and vision services beyond the offices

427

of eye and vision care providers. There are also actions that individuals and communities can take to create social and built environments that actively and passively promote healthy eye behaviors.

But current knowledge is not enough to produce optimal eye and vision health. At present, there is no long-term investment in surveillance and research to identify the most at-risk populations, associated risk and protective factors, cost-effective treatments, and efficient health care and public health system models to expand access to care. Moreover, the emphasis in eye and vision care research has shifted away from more population-based studies that focus on the translation of clinical research into effective practice and the evaluation of specific interventions and programs to promote population health to research that focuses on the pathophysiology of disease and new treatments. While this is an important aspect of biomedical research, it must be balanced against the need for interventions that have a larger population health impact.

Achieving the twin goals of improving eye and vision health and increasing health equity will require progress along multiple fronts and, in particular, national and state efforts to ensure that resources and knowledge are available and communicated to help implement actions within communities. A population health strategy to promote eye and vision health will have many layered components that influence behaviors across the human lifespan and policies and environments across an array of topics and settings. Some components will target changes that require minimal investment, such as wearing sunglasses or protective eyewear in hazardous work environments or certain recreational activities. Other changes will require sustained support from extensive partnerships that capitalize on the different strengths of the public and private sectors. Developing support for the policies, programs, and resources to generate these changes at the federal, state, and local levels will necessitate a different mindset about the role of eye and vision health promotion in daily activities and formal prioritization in national, state, and local population health strategic goals and programs.

This chapter presents a roadmap to advancing eye health. In particular, it proposes recommendations that represent key steps along the path to optimal eye and vision health of populations and to the long-term functionality of those with vision impairment. This chapter concludes by providing examples of the types of activities that different stakeholders can pursue. The examples flow from the committee's recommendations to advance sustained progress toward a culture of eye and vision health.

TRANSLATING A CONCEPTUAL FRAMEWORK
INTO ACTION: RECOMMENDATIONS

In its statement of task, the committee was asked to "examine the core principles and public health strategies to reduce visual impairment and promote eye health in the United States," including short- and long-term strategies to prioritize eye and vision health through collaborative actions across a variety of topics, settings, and different sectors of communities and levels of government (see Box 1-1, Chapter 1). At its heart, the committee's statement of task assumes that there is an unmet need that exists for individuals, families, and communities to improve eye and vision health across the lifespan of individuals. By default, the task also assumes a need to establish the conditions that will allow community participants and leaders to evaluate and weigh vision impairment in their communities against other health priorities and also consider how programs that focus on vision impairment could enhance programs aimed at other health issues.

To guide its deliberations, the committee developed a conceptual framework for action to achieve the ultimate outcome—improved population eye and vision health and health equity (see Figure 9-1). The committee's recommendations are organized by the five core action areas: (1) facilitating public awareness through timely access to accurate and locally relevant information; (2) generating evidence to guide policy decisions and evidence-based actions; (3) expanding access to clinical care; (4) enhancing public health capacities to support vision-related activities; and (5) promoting community actions that encourage eye and vision healthy environments. These action areas, which are described below, provide the framework by which the committee introduces its recommendations. The eight guiding principles defined in Chapter 1 should guide all actions within the framework for action—that is, they should be population-centered, collaborative, culturally competent, community-tailored, evidence-based, integrated, standardized, and adequately resourced.

Many of the following nine recommendations are broadly framed but are critical to establishing conditions that will support a sustainable population health initiative that achieves a long-term reduction in vision impairment and its consequences. These recommendations provide the foundational support for other, more specific actions by stakeholder groups, as described in the concluding section of this chapter and throughout this report. The result could establish new policies and practices that will have an impact on other dimensions of health and quality of life (QOL) in the United States.

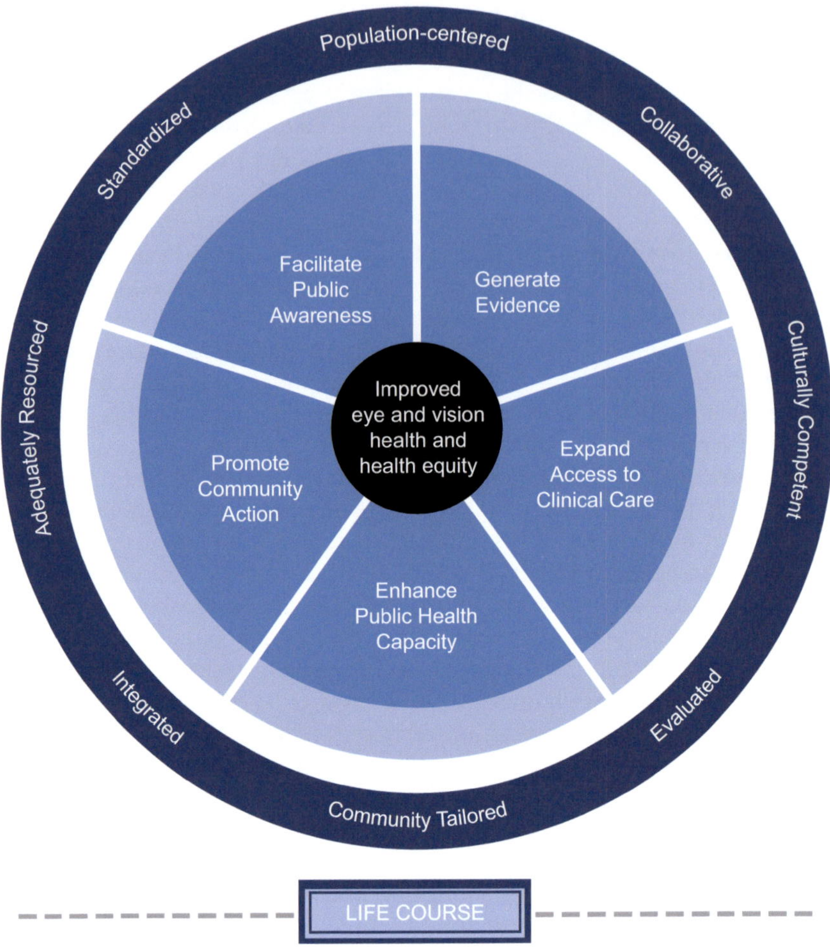

FIGURE 9-1 Components of a population health model for action to improve eye and vision health across the lifespan.

FACILITATE PUBLIC AWARENESS THROUGH TIMELY ACCESS TO ACCURATE AND LOCALLY RELEVANT INFORMATION

The public should have accessible, transparent, and easily understood information about eye and vision health prevalence, incidence, and impact (on both an individual and community level) and also information about the stakeholders that influence eye and vision health locally and nationally.

Establish Eye and Vision Health as a National Priority

The process of vision loss can affect anyone at any time and may occur suddenly and completely—for example, from injury—or may progress over time, with permanent structural damage leading to progressive changes in eye function until more pronounced deficits become noticeable. The resulting vision impairment—the functional limitation of the eye or visual system that results from vision loss—remains an unmet and urgent public health threat in the United States (HHS, 2015; NEI/NIH, 2004; USPSTF, 2009). In the United States, more than 4.24 million adults ages 40 and older suffer from uncorrectable vision impairment and blindness (Varma et al., 2016), and more than 2.155 million children and young adults have uncorrectable vision impairment (Wittenborn et al., 2013). Millions more experience vision impairment from uncorrected refractive error and cataracts (CDC, 2015c; Varma et al., 2016; Wittenborn and Rein, 2016). In 2011, the total estimated direct and indirect costs of vision impairment and eye disease were $138 billion (Wittenborn and Rein, 2013). These costs will only increase as the United States' population ages, and these costs are projected to consume an ever greater proportion of the gross domestic product (Varma et al., 2016).

According to a recent online poll, 88 percent of the 2,044 respondents surveyed identified good vision as vital to maintaining overall health, and 47 percent rated losing their vision compared to loss of limb, memory, hearing, or speech as "potentially having the greatest effect on their day-to-day life" (Scott et al., 2016, p. E3). Despite the public's perception of the importance of good vision, millions of people continue to grapple with undiagnosed or untreated vision impairment (CDC, 2015d; Varma et al., 2016; Wittenborn and Rein, 2016). The U.S. Department of Health and Human Services (HHS) supports a number of federal programs and institutes, such as the Centers for Disease Control and Prevention's (CDC's) Vision Health Initiative (VHI) and the National Eye Institute's (NEI's) National Eye Health and Education Program (NEHEP), that focus on vision loss and fund various activities to combat the effects of poor eye and vision health on at-risk populations (CDC, 2015a). Yet, eye and vision health remain relatively absent from national health priority lists, including efforts to stem the impact of chronic diseases.

A number of factors contribute to the absence of focused and sustained programmatic investment that translates into widespread action. Historically, eye care was considered separate from the more general field of medicine, and various tensions between different eye care professionals continue to contribute to the fragmentation of eye care, which excludes eye health from conversations about broader strategies to improve and measure the overall health of populations. The lack of coordination within or across federal agencies further dissipates the presence of eye and vision health as a public health issue on the national stage. Greater national and directed attention is needed to raise awareness among public health practitioners, health professionals, policy makers, and the public about the importance of eye and vision health as an indicator of health equity and overall health and as a key factor affecting QOL.

A Call to Action "is a science-based document to stimulate action nationwide to solve a major public health problem" (U.S. Surgeon General, n.d.). HHS, most often through the Office of the Surgeon General, uses calls to action to draw attention to important public health issues, including promotion of walking and walkable communities, the prevention of skin cancer and suicide, improving the health and wellness of persons with disabilities, promoting oral health, and the reduction of underage drinking (U.S. Surgeon General, n.d.). These documents, along with other reports, are often used to establish a baseline from which to measure improvement in particular areas (e.g., Anstev et al., 2011; Mertz and Mouradian, 2009; U.S. Surgeon General, 2014).

Vision loss and impairment qualify as a public health problem, based on the CDC's definition, in that they: (1) affect a large number of people; (2) impose large morbidity, QOL, and cost burdens; (3) the severity of the problem is increasing and is predicted to continue increasing; (4) the public perceives the problem to be a threat; and (5) community or public health-level interventions are feasible (CDC, 2009). Similarly, the NEI, the U.S. Preventive Services Task Force (USPSTF), and the World Health Organization have identified vision impairment in various populations as national or global public health problems (HHS, 2015; NEI/NIH, 2004; WHO, 2015). Moreover, most causes of vision impairment are chronic, continuously present, and require ongoing management over the lifespan of an individual to maintain the activities of daily living. A greater federal presence, is needed to elevate eye and vision health as a population health focus among the general public and different sectors of society.

Recommendation 1

The Secretary of the U.S. Department of Health and Human Services should issue a Call to Action to motivate nationwide action toward achieving a reduction in the burden of vision impairment across the lifespan of people in the United States. Specifically, this Call to Action should establish goals to:

- **Eliminate correctable and avoidable vision impairment by 2030,**
- **Delay the onset and progression of unavoidable chronic eye diseases and conditions,**
- **Minimize the impact of chronic vision impairment, and**

- **Achieve eye and vision health equity by improving care in underserved populations.**

A Call to Action is needed to harness the collective voice of the nation's population health system (including the governmental public health systems, clinical care systems, employers and businesses, media, nonprofit organizations, education sectors, other government agencies, and communities) to initiate nationwide actions that emphasize eye and vision health promotion. In pursing the Call to Action, the Secretary should leverage the expertise of the Surgeon General of the United States. These Calls to Action usually include a description of the public health problem, a vision statement, general goals, and key actions to support these goals. They also usually summarize the scientific evidence currently available to support behavior change, and they may include additional resources, such as checklists and guides for different stakeholders (U.S. Surgeon General, n.d.). At a minimum, the highlighted actions in a Call to Action should reflect the goals articulated by the committee and should focus on changing perceptions; overcoming barriers; building a science base around primordial, primary, secondary, and tertiary prevention; increasing clinical and public health diversity, capacity, and flexibility; and increasing collaboration.

The specificity provided in the committee's recommendation is meant to fuel conversations about what should be technically possible and what is feasible at what stage. For example, by definition, correctable and avoidable vision impairment should be something that can be eliminated. There are, of course, limitations in resources that may affect the ability to reach this goal. Similar considerations exist for slowing the progression of vision loss or improving the function of people with vision impairment through access to high-quality treatments or services. However, in setting this high bar against which to measure success, the committee hopes to stimulate innovative thinking about how to use the available resources more wisely and to encourage debate about the role that eye and vision health should play in broader initiatives to support healthy environments and reduce health inequities in the United States. This Call to Action sets the stage for the remaining recommendations.

Promoting Greater Public Awareness

Enhancing public knowledge about a health threat is a fundamental first step in informing discussions that promote behavior change across multiple determinants of health and aligning health policies with general public health interests. Unfortunately, lack of awareness of vision and eye health issues remains "a major public health concern," especially in the context of linking patients into care and attempting to make population-level changes in behavior and health practice (Bailey et al., 2006; Zhang et al., 2012). Individuals are often unaware of what the most common threats to vision are, how the physiological progression of many eye diseases occurs, early signs of vision loss, and what steps can be taken to reduce the risk of vision-threatening eye disease, conditions, and events and the impact of subsequent vision loss (Alexander et al., 2008; Chou et al., 2014; Lam and Leat, 2015; NEI/LCIF, 2008; Varano et al., 2015). Combined with the asymptomatic nature of many eye diseases and conditions, this lack of awareness can have significant ramifications on overall health.

Although rarely adequate by themselves, public awareness campaigns can be an effective tool for improving knowledge about key messages related to health within populations (Bray et al., 2015; Oto et al., 2011) and are one essential part of an effective population health strategy. Zambelli-Weiner and colleagues (2012) state that public health strategies, which include efforts "to enhance awareness, to promote education, and to increase access to successful prevention, treatment, and rehabilitation services among populations at risk for poor vision outcomes can improve vision health in the United States and globally" (pp. S23–S24). Many current education initiatives and programs focus on particular etiologies of vision impairment among the most at-risk populations. For example, the NEHEP includes vision education programs focusing on people living in Hispanic/Latino communities; people at risk for glaucoma, diabetic eye disease, and age-related conditions; and people living with low vision (NEI/NIH, 2015). Although these topics and populations are important, elevating the status of eye and vision health at a national level will require much broader messaging that emphasizes eye and vision health across the lifespan.

Achieving the goals outlined in Recommendation 1 will require having reliable, consistent, evidence-based information that is available and accessible by a variety of stakeholders to increase overall knowledge and to support policies, practices, and behaviors that promote good eye and vision health, encourage appropriate care to correct or slow progression of a vision-threatening disease or condition, or improve function when vision impairment is uncorrectable. This approach must target various audiences and consider a wide range of factors affecting eye and vision health in communities, including individual-directed strategies, mass media campaigns, and environmental and policy changes across multiple settings within defined geographic areas (e.g., city, state, province, or country).

<u>Recommendation 2</u>
The Secretary of the U.S. Department of Health and Human Services, in collaboration with other federal agencies and departments, nonprofit and for-profit organizations, professional organizations, employers, state and

local public health agencies, and the media, should launch a coordinated public awareness campaign to promote policies and practices that encourage eye and vision health across the lifespan, reduce vision impairment, and promote health equity. This campaign should target various stakeholders including the general population, care providers and caretakers, public health practitioners, policy makers, employers, and community and patient liaisons and representatives.

A coordinated public awareness campaign should focus on topics such as the various risk and protective factors across the lifespan for the major causes of vision loss, the link between eye and vision health and other measures of health (such as chronic conditions, subsequent injury, and psychological issues), vision loss as a chronic condition, when and how to access eye care and rehabilitative and support services (see Recommendation 5), and the impact of the social and built environments on one's ability to maintain optimal health and visual function following significant vision loss. For example, messages could target private businesses to convince them to cultivate healthy workplace design and practices that take into account screen time, lighting conditions, or other interventions and accommodations that can improve or preserve eye health and visual functioning. Moreover, the public awareness campaign should also target eye care professionals and public health practitioners, emphasizing the connection between eye and vision health and public health practice and how to translate clinical language into evidence-based policies, including those that eliminate the artificial divide that exists between eye and vision health and general medical care. These messages could be combined with similar messages about other sensory health issues, such as hearing loss.

To meet the goals outlined in recommendation 1, a successful public awareness campaign must emphasize a variety of activities, coordinated and supported by various groups, to enhance public awareness around specific needs for knowledge about eye and vision health across the lifespan. For example:

- The CDC and the NEI, in consultation with professional organizations, state and local public health departments, and patient advocacy groups, should enhance the development and impact of vision health education materials that appear in multiple formats and are tailored to diverse audiences.
- National and state departments of labor, national and local labor unions, and nonprofit organizations working in the sphere of labor and worker rights should incorporate educational programs on eye safety and vision-related employee rights into larger advocacy and worker education agendas.

- Governmental public health departments and population health research centers, in collaboration with the American Public Health Association and the Association of Schools and Programs of Public Health, should jointly fund and develop post-professional training on eye and vision health for public health practitioners and researchers involved in public health surveillance activities; such training is needed to augment the capacity of public health actors and surveillance systems to address eye and vision health issues.
- HHS and the Equal Employment Opportunity Commission, in collaboration with experts in the field of vision rehabilitation, should develop educational materials and provide technical assistance for private and public employers to prioritize the vision health of employees, support work practices and environments that are conducive to preservation of visual functioning, and ensure that workplace accommodations for visually impaired employees meet Americans with Disabilities Act standards.
- Nonprofit organizations dedicated to eye health and disease should partner with HHS and other agencies to support a public awareness campaign and use the campaign to springboard additional efforts in at-risk and disease-specific communities.
- Nonprofit organizations providing resources for at-risk individuals (who are at risk due to socioeconomic reasons, cognitive, physical or mental health issues, or geographic reasons) should participate in the dissemination of material about the importance of eye and vision health from the public awareness campaign in an effort to target populations that are often not reached by the efforts of most campaigns.

GENERATE EVIDENCE TO GUIDE POLICY DECISIONS AND EVIDENCE-BASED ACTIONS

Evidence-based decision making should guide population health actions. Without data, population health tools cannot characterize affected populations, identify risk and protective factors (including health care access), establish evidence-based guidelines, or quantify the effectiveness of health care systems and community-based interventions. True accountability requires good data, but less than perfect data should not be an excuse for inaction.

Enhancing Vision Surveillance

Surveillance is "the ongoing systematic collection, analysis and interpretation of health-related data essential to the planning, implementation, and evaluation of public health practice, closely integrated with the timely dissemination of these data to those who need to know" (Thacker and Berkelman, 1988, p. 164). By this definition, no system for the surveillance of eye disease or vision impairment and blindness exists.

Vision impairment and blindness are appropriate targets for surveillance because they adversely affect a large portion of the population, affect populations unequally, can be improved by treatment and preventive efforts, and will become an increasing burden as the population ages (NEI/NIH, 2004; Saaddine et al., 2003). A comprehensive, nationally representative surveillance system for eye and vision health is needed to make it possible to better understand the epidemiological patterns, risk factors, comorbidities, and costs associated with vision loss. Such data will allow health care professionals and public health decision makers to better characterize the nature and extent of the public health burden; risk factors and at-risk populations; disparities in access, care, and outcomes; and successful interventions (West and Lee, 2012).

The absence of a comprehensive, sustainably implemented and funded surveillance system with validated measures, verifiable data, and interoperable databases creates challenges for population vision health. Key among these is the inability to determine the prevalence and costs of eye disease and vision impairment; to identify at-risk groups, barriers to care access, and health disparities; and to assess the effectiveness of treatments and therapies and the availability and adequacy of vision care system resources at the national, state, and local levels.

<u>Recommendation 3</u>
The Centers for Disease Control and Prevention (CDC) should develop a coordinated surveillance system for eye and vision health in the United States. To advise and assist with the design of the system, the CDC should convene a task force comprising government, nonprofit and for-profit organizations, professional organizations, academic researchers, and the health care and public health sectors. The design of this system should include, but not be limited to:

- Developing and standardizing definitions for population-based studies, particularly definitions of clinical vision loss and functional vision impairment;

- Identifying and validating surveillance and quality-of-care measures to characterize vision-related outcomes, resources, and capacities within different communities and populations;
- Integrating eye-health outcomes, objective clinical measures, and risk/protective factors into existing clinical-health and population-health data collection forms and systems (e.g., chronic disease questionnaires, community health assessments, electronic health records, national and state health surveys, Medicare's health risk assessment, and databases); and
- Analyzing, interpreting, and disseminating information to the public in a timely and transparent manner.

Implementing a coherent surveillance system of eye and vision health will require a long-term commitment from the CDC and its partners. Most existing national vision surveillance activities consist of modules that supplement pre-existing surveys. These surveys are not ideal (e.g., they are reliant on self-report items rather than objective clinical data, and they fail to capture key populations of interest), but they are a good place from which to begin enhanced surveillance efforts. Currently, material specific to eye and vision health is under consideration for inclusion in the National Health and Nutrition Examination Survey and the Behavioral Risk Factor Surveillance System. The committee encourages inclusion of an eye-specific component within the next versions of these surveys.

In the long term, a more comprehensive approach to eye and vision health surveillance is needed to allow for a better and more accurate characterization of the population burden of eye disease and conditions and resulting vision impairment in the United States, with special emphasis on the need to identify the most at-risk and burdened populations. Surveillance efforts should be real-time and include a focus on at-risk communities and populations and should identify the root causes of disparities in vision health and care and the trends in vision health and care over time. Using a "big data" approach, the CDC should also gather eye and vision data in the various disease-specific registries managed by nonprofits, clinicians, companies, and government entities.

The CDC has already taken steps toward this goal by funding a grant that will "develop, test, and implement a vision and eye health surveillance system, using existing surveys, as well as administrative and electronic data sources" (CDC, 2015b). The grant was awarded in summer 2015, and the research it is funding is currently in the planning stages. The committee applauds these efforts and urges government contractors to inform the deliberations and consider the conclusions of the recommended task force. The task force should focus on the development of standardized definitions for all relevant terms used in surveillance, including "vision impairment," "visual functioning," and "vision-related quality of life," among others. Information technology should also focus on the development of standardized, validated, and verifiable measures; a strategy for transitioning from subjective and self-reported measures to objective measures; and the identification of existing data collection efforts, such as the community health risk assessments developed by nonprofit and public hospitals and health risk assessments performed by providers, that could incorporate standardized eye health metrics into existing forms and databases. The use of standardized vision health modules as supplements to existing surveys and surveillance efforts should also be promoted. Opportunities to develop and implement an eye disease registry capitalizing on the growing power and availability of electronic health records should be explored along with the specification of metrics for quality of care improvement.

Expanding Knowledge Related to Eye and Vision Health

Understanding the factors that affect the risk of vision impairment for different populations, the barriers to accessing care, interventions to prevent visual impairment and maintain eye function, and ways to improve the quality of care is fundamental to designing and identifying opportunities that minimize vision loss now and that will result in new knowledge and strategies to further reduce the long-term impact of vision impairment. HHS supports a number of federal programs and institutes that focus on vision loss and fund various activities to combat the effects of poor eye and vision health on at-risk populations (CDC, 2015a). The CDC and the NEI, as well as many other federal agencies, departments, and institutes have supported programs and initiatives to improve eye and vision health in different capacities and populations (ACL, n.d.; CDC, 2009; CMS, 2015; DoD, 2016; DOL, n.d.; ED, n.d.; HHS, 2015; HUD, 2016; Indian Health Service, 2008; NEI/NIH, 2015; Office of Head Start, 2015; USDA, 2015; VA, n.d.). Nonprofit organizations, professional groups, and private entities have bolstered these efforts through their own research and activities, including important and considerable collaborations with federal and state governments.

Despite these activities, eye and vision health are insufficiently represented as a programmatic focus in federal government programs overall, and existing research programs lack coordination within and across federal agencies and institutes. Moreover, significant research and knowledge gaps persist concerning eye and vision health, as documented throughout this report. This is particularly true about nonclinical research areas, i.e., more traditional public health focused research on primordial and primary prevention. Establishing a unified research agenda with larger financial and programmatic support to develop and advance knowledge about eye and vision health can maximize efficiencies and build on the strengths of established programs across a broad portfolio of topics and programs, which must include more than basic and clinical research.

The fundamental need to understand how upstream determinants of health affect the development of vision loss and impairment and how best to diagnose and treat eye diseases and conditions within different populations requires a more comprehensive approach to eye and vision health research, which in turn should strengthen both the public health and clinical response to vision loss in the long term. Moreover, knowledge about the prevalence of, incidence of, causes of, and risk and protective factors for vision impairment is severely lacking, as is an understanding of the impact of specific interventions to improve outcomes from vision impairment. Many entities have made notable efforts to enhance research to inform eye and vision health practice and outcomes, including the CDC's VHI, the NEI, Research to Prevent Blindness, Prevent Blindness, and many other national and state-level programs (see Chapter 3). However, these efforts lack coordination and a single research agenda that explains how these efforts as a whole can be used to enhance understanding and inform decisions related to eye and vision health at the federal, state, and local levels (CDC, 2009; NEI/NIH, 2015; Prevent Blindness, 2016; Research to Prevent Blindness, 2016).

<u>Recommendation 4</u>
The U.S. Department of Health and Human Services should create an inter-agency workgroup, including a wide range of public, private, and community stakeholders, to develop a common research agenda and coordinated eye and vision health research and demonstration grant programs that target the leading causes, consequences, and unmet needs of vision impairment. This research agenda should include, but not be limited to:

- **Population-based epidemiologic and clinical research on the major causes and risks and protective factors for vision impairment, with a special emphasis on longitudinal studies of the major causes of vision impairment;**
- **Health services research, focused on patient-centered care processes, comparative-effectiveness and economic evaluation of clinical interventions, and innovative models of care delivery to improve access to appropriate diagnostics, follow-up treatment, and rehabilitation services, particularly among high-risk populations;**
- **Population health services research to reduce eye and vision health disparities, focusing on effective interventions that promote eye healthy environments and conditions, especially for underserved populations; and**

- **Research and development on emerging preventive, diagnostic, therapeutic, and treatment strategies and technologies, including efforts to improve the design and sensitivity of different screening protocols.**

A research agenda that supports population health efforts to promote eye and vision health necessarily will include a broad portfolio of topics and programs, which must include more than basic and clinical research. An understanding of (1) the factors that affect the risk of vision impairment for different populations, (2) the barriers to accessing care, (3) effective interventions to prevent visual impairment and maintain eye function, and (4) ways to improve the quality of care is fundamental to designing and identifying opportunities that will minimize vision loss now and produce new knowledge and strategies to further reduce the long-term impact of vision impairment.

A common research agenda would allow for maximum efficiencies and reduce duplicative efforts and investments in research across diverse disciplines and focus areas. This will be essential at the beginning of a national effort to reprioritize eye and vision health because sustained and larger financial and programmatic support for such research is more likely to occur in the long term with better evidence. Although the committee believes that both sufficient evidence, as documented throughout this report, and also common sense support the conclusion that eye and vision health is an essential underpinning of the overall health of communities, more robust and recent research can help clarify the most important risk and protective factors associated with specific eye diseases, conditions, and injuries in order to guide decision making and programmatic emphasis at various levels and in different settings to enhance the value of future investments in eye and vision health. Demonstration projects are needed to test the most cost-effective ways to meet the eye care needs of underserved areas (e.g., testing incentives for provider practice, specialized training for providers already in the area, and the use of novel screening technologies). Vision rehabilitation is another area where significant evidence gaps were identified (see Chapter 8); filling in these gaps is a high priority in order to guide policies and community efforts intended to reduce the societal cost of chronic vision impairment.

Population health services research should focus on barriers to performance on the part of local and state health departments and should explore methods used in jurisdictions where public health agency efforts have been successful (and have failed) in advancing eye and vision health. Health services research should include programs and support to promote the interpretation and dissemination of research findings to various audiences. This could include tests of models of dissemination of information and best practices, including administrative best practices and funding procedures, to determine which are the speediest at improving the adoption of new methods, processes, and outcomes. To this end, the interagency workforce should include expertise on translational research and implementation science in order to improve the vision care system's response to the findings of new health services and public health services and epidemiological research and to speed the adoption of novel treatments, therapies, and technologies and models of care and reimbursement.

The committee suggests that research on examination and screening should prioritize the development of evidence to support guideline formation (see Recommendation 5) for high-risk groups, including children in age groups with a high prevalence of risk factors for amblyopia and strabismus and individuals diagnosed with diabetes. Similarly, research on best-practice guidelines should prioritize referral patterns of primary care and primary eye care provider groups, because these groups see the greatest number of patients and represent the first step in the continuum of care.

The committee acknowledges that the research agenda as outlined is very broad and that priorities under each bullet should be set based on available resources and greatest need in terms of research gaps. However, it is important that each bullet be addressed as part of a comprehensive approach to eye and vision health. Consideration should be given to innovative research methodologies and strategies to improve efficiency.

EXPAND ACCESS TO APPROPRIATE CLINICAL CARE

> Timely, appropriate, and equitable access to and the delivery of effective care in all settings is an important component of a population health approach to improve eye and vision health. Inequitable barriers to effective treatments and therapies should be eliminated. Heightened attention is needed to reduce vision loss and cement its importance in relation to other chronic conditions and overall health.

Establishing Unified, Evidence-Based Clinical Guidelines

Professional guidelines are an important tool to advance policies and practices that promote high-quality care for everyone. As discussed in Chapter 7, guidelines are often used to educate the public as well as public health and health care professionals about the foundational elements of value-driven payment policies, and they are used as baselines from which to measure quality improvement and enhanced accountability for care processes and patient health outcomes. Unfortunately, no single set of clinical practice guidelines or measures in eye and vision care exists, and there are marked discrepancies in the current screening and eye examination guidelines for asymptomatic people. This often reflects the absence of robust research and political tensions within the field of eye and vision health. Available guidelines provide inconsistent recommendations concerning essential measures. For example, the American Academy of Ophthalmology and the American Optometric Association disagree on the appropriate frequency of eye examinations, with the former recommending less frequent eye examinations (e.g., AAO, 2015; AOA, 2015). In the case of vision screening, evidence-based recommendations from USPSTF, which focuses on primary care practice, calls for vision screening of children ages 3 to 5 only (USPSTF, 2009), whereas consensus-based recommendations from the American Academy of Ophthalmology, the American Association for Pediatric Ophthalmology and Strabismus (AAPOS), and the National Expert Panel recommend screening for additional age groups (AAO, 2014; AAPOS, 2014; Cotter et al., 2015; Hartmann et al., 2015). The American Academy of Ophthalmology and AAPOS, but not USPSTF, recommend specific screening tests (AAO, 2012; AAPOS, 2014). Uncertainty as to the appropriate frequencies of testing may lead to either unnecessary or inadequate care, while discrepancies and contradictions among recommendations contribute to patient and provider confusion concerning the standards of care.

<u>Recommendation 5</u>

The U.S. Department of Health and Human Services should convene one or more panels—comprising members of professional organizations, researchers, public health practitioners, patients, and other stakeholders—to develop a single set of evidence-based clinical and rehabilitation practice guidelines and measures that can be used by eye care professionals, other care providers, and public health professionals to prevent, screen for, detect, monitor, diagnose, and treat eye and vision problems. These guidelines and supporting evidence should be used to drive payment policies, including coverage determinations for corrective lenses and visual assistive devices following a diagnosed medical condition (e.g., refractive error).

Evidence-based guidelines provide guidance based on objective evidence for a variety of care providers to improve the uniformity and quality of the care they deliver to patients. For example, the recommended guidelines should be used to guide decisions related to payment policies, and health insurance coverage determinations for comprehensive eye examinations,[1] preventive services and treatments (including corrective

---

[1] The committee defines a comprehensive eye examination as a dilated eye examination that may include a range of other tests, in addition to the dilation of the pupil to see the retinal structures (or back of the eye).

lenses), and rehabilitation (including assistive devices). Particular attention needs to be paid to assuring that essential services and treatments are affordable, particularly for the most vulnerable populations. Recommended guidelines would also establish a uniform baseline from which to measure improvement in care processes and patient health outcomes. This should include an evaluation of health care provider adherence to guidelines. Finally, the guidelines promote accountability by a multitude of factors by enabling performance comparisons and the appropriate use of evidence-based technology by including health care system, provider, geographic area, and population characteristics.

Guidelines should include, but not be limited to (1) the schedule and components of comprehensive eye examinations; (2) the appropriateness of particular diagnostic, treatment, and management strategies for specific eye diseases and conditions; and (3) criteria to facilitate appropriate follow-up care, both within and external to eye and vision care, and to ensure a continuum of health care that is focused on the specific eye health needs and the overall health of populations. These guidelines should apply to both the general practice of medicine and to eye care specifically, with an emphasis on steps to increase the integration of services to promote both eye and vision health and overall health. Updates to the guidelines should occur periodically, and the process should include a mechanism by which critical data findings can be incorporated into or recognized in addendums to guidelines prior to the formal guideline updates.

It is important that the development of evidence-based guidelines adhere to particular standards, to the extent possible, so as to ensure robust and comprehensive support for recommended actions. These standards can include the Institute of Medicine standards for trustworthy guidelines (IOM, 2011a) or other assessment tools (see Brouwers et al., 2010, for a description and comparison of some available tools). Assessment can include stakeholder involvement (including patient representatives), rigor of development, clarity of presentation, applicability, editorial independence, disclosed external review methods, economic considerations, the roles of the guideline development group members, disclosed search terms and inclusion/exclusion criteria for the evidence review, or the outcomes of public input.

There will be challenges in implementing this recommendation. Part of the problem in advancing eye health, as pointed out in report text, is that the professional groups involved in eye and vision care have differences in guidelines. This recommendation represents a necessary and essential first step to align the interests of the eye and vision field through an exercise that will not only improve clarity for the public, but also provide an evidence-based platform from which to advocate for necessary and overdue payment policies and research that can reduce disparities in eye and vision health for the most vulnerable members of society.

Enhancing Eye and Vision Health in Professional Training and Education

Historical divisions within the vision care system, combined with the specialization of eye care to the extent that it essentially operates as a "siloed" service rather than an incorporated component of primary health care, has led to a lack of vision health–related content in traditional health care professional training, public health education, and quality monitoring. Similarly, cross-disciplinary training in public health is generally under-represented in formal education and certification programs for providers working in optometry, ophthalmology, and vision rehabilitation. Limited knowledge of the roles and competencies of other vision health professions and tensions surrounding the scope of practice undermine efforts to integrate vision care with other health care services, diminish the timeliness and quality of care by hindering appropriate referral practices, and generally inhibit an interprofessional culture of collaboration and coordination among ophthalmologists, optometrists, primary care physicians, and providers working in vision rehabilitation. Thus, fragmentation is both a cause and consequence of the lapses in the health care and public health education system.

To cultivate professional relationships and collaboration that will advance eye and vision health across medicine and beyond clinical care, it will be important to establish common expertise that can align overarching objectives and action among health professionals. The CDC has noted the need to elevate ophthalmic education in medical curriculums (CDC, 2009; Shah et al., 2014). With a greater focus on population health in clinical care (Berwick et al., 2008), new skills will be needed to ensure that health care professionals understand the types of patient experiences and data that are relevant to population health activities, including the moral imperative to reduce inequities in both health and health care. Moreover, population health practitioners should be familiar with eye and vision health, its risk factors, and the relationship between vision loss and other chronic health conditions. Translating this knowledge into meaningful patient interactions will require cultivating trust among different patient populations, providers, and public health practitioners.

Cultural competency helps build concordance between patients and health care providers by challenging providers to think outside of their strict biomedical constructs and respond to the cultural barriers that inevitably arise because of patients' diverse belief systems and views about health, health care, and health care providers. The continuing development, implementation, and evaluation of cultural competence programs, training modules, and educational tools designed to improve the affective dimensions of communication and clinical behavior, combined with an increasing diversity in the health care workforce, can help increase patient–provider concordance and reduce implicit bias, which will not only help with the public health challenge of eliminating ethnic and cultural disparities but also address various contributors to health outcomes that affect the health of vulnerable populations (Elam and Lee, 2013; IOM, 2003b; Sabin and Greenwald, 2012).

Recommendation 6

To enable the health care and public health workforce to meet the eye care needs of a changing population and to coordinate responses to vision-related health threats, professional education programs should proactively recruit and educate a diverse workforce and incorporate prevention and detection of visual impairments, population health, and team care coordination as part of core competencies in applicable medical and professional education and training curricula. Individual curricula should emphasize proficiency in culturally competent care for all populations.

In essence, this recommendation is about creating a common language that can help advance communication and strategic planning among groups that have not traditionally worked together in the same capacity as with other public health priority areas. There are three targets of this recommendation. First, eye care professionals need to be knowledgeable about the basics of public health and how eye and vision health relate to other measures of well-being and health. Ophthalmology residencies should include practical experiences in interdisciplinary settings, including community health centers. Optometry programs should include education in public health fundamentals and practical experiences working in primary care settings.

Second, other health care providers need to understand the importance of eye and vision health in maintaining the overall health of their patient populations and the role that eye care can play in identifying non-eye-related diseases and conditions. The training of primary care physicians should include developing competency at identifying vision impairment and the need for eye care as well as teaching them to be familiar with the underlying determinants of health, especially those that are risk factors for vision loss among vulnerable and at-risk populations.

Third, public health practitioners need to understand the basics of eye health and how it relates to programs that are eye and vision health specific; or how eye and vision health metrics can either complement or improve existing programs for related chronic diseases or health conditions. All public health programs should include modules on the vision care system and on the roles of other providers in that system. Training should emphasize the role of public health experts as coordinators and conveners of stakeholders in systems lacking integration. Research is needed to determine how best to utilize the eye and vision care, primary care, and public health workforces. Incentives and technologies to optimize workforce capacity should be identified and employed. In all of these efforts, patients and advocates should be involved to offer real-world patient-reported experiences and outcomes.

In addition to having basic knowledge about eye health and related risk and protective factors, health professional school students should be knowledgeable about population health approaches and about the roles and competencies of public health experts and vision rehabilitation therapists and other types of therapists in vision care. Training for vision rehabilitation and other vision therapists should include practical experiences working as part of an *interdisciplinary* rehabilitation team as well as instruction in the competencies and roles of physical and occupational therapists, orientation and mobility specialists, and optometrists and ophthalmologists.

As one potential enforcement mechanism, federal funding for training programs could be contingent upon these steps being taken and on the adoption and presentation of the curricula based on federal consensus guidelines.

ENHANCE PUBLIC HEALTH CAPACITIES TO SUPPORT VISION-RELATED ACTIVITIES

Eye and vision health is a critical part of population health and a valuable public health tool with which to assess the quality, effectiveness, and efficiencies of health care systems and population health programs and initiatives. Improving eye and vision health requires that comparable services, information, and healthy environments are accessible to all populations. Public health departments serve as key community conveners to coordinate responses that address multiple determinants of health and chronic conditions, such as vision impairment.

Integrating Eye and Vision Care

Population health approaches focus on the broad determinants of health, which include the social and environmental determinants of health across a lifespan, which in turn include (1) innate individual traits (e.g., age, sex, race, genetics); (2) individual behaviors; (3) social, family, and community networks; (4) living and working conditions (e.g., psychosocial factors, employment status and occupational factors, socioeconomic status, and health care services); and (5) broad social, economic, cultural, health, and environmental conditions and policies at the global, national, state, and local levels (e.g., economic inequality, urbanization, mobility, and cultural values) (IOM, 2003a). Responsibility for improving population health has never been the sole province of governmental public health departments. Governmental public health departments must work with and through other stakeholders, including other government agencies, the clinical care system, employers and businesses, media, nonprofit organizations, the education sector, and the community to reach established goals (IOM, 2003a, 2011b). Successful health promotion in eye and vision health will require innovative partnerships that engage in a variety of activities that advance different objectives within population health.

Integrating public health and local health care systems is an important strategy to improve community health (CDC, 2007). A well-functioning medical care system can expand access to appropriate eye and vision care services, allowing public health agencies to focus on preventive policies and action and assurance. Such preventive actions include linking people to needed care, assessing care quality, and promoting community support and policy and environmental conditions that maximize health (IOM, 2003a). Public health agencies and departments can also extend the reach of health care services through vision-specific programs. Unfortunately, there has been insufficient partnering to coordinate existing and emerging programs, policies, and quality improvement activities that either directly or indirectly affect eye and vision health.

<u>Recommendation 7</u>
State and local public health departments should partner with health care systems to align public health and clinical practice objectives, programs, and strategies about eye and vision health to:

- **Enhance community health needs assessments, surveys, health impact assessments, and quality improvement metrics;**
- **Identify and eliminate barriers within health care and public health systems to eye care, especially comprehensive eye exams, appropriate screenings, and follow-up services, and items and services intended to improve the functioning of individuals with vision impairment;**
- **Include public health and clinical expertise related to eye and vision health on oversight committees, advisory boards, expert panels, and staff, as appropriate;**
- **Encourage physicians and health professionals to ask and engage in discussions about eye and vision health as part of patients' regular office visits; and**

- **Incorporate eye health and chronic vision impairment into existing quality improvement, injury and infection control, and behavioral change programs related to comorbid chronic conditions, community health, and the elimination of health disparities.**

Opportunities to realize and support the integration of health care and public health systems can take many forms. Health care organizations and providers can benefit from public health expertise related to existing population health databases covering eye and vision health, assessment tools, existing community relationships, and existing knowledge and resources in order to incorporate eye and vision health into existing programs or extend vision services to populations in need of targeted preventative, clinical, or rehabilitative care. Public health departments can convene the partners and support the integration of the various capabilities around a shared vision and shared goals. Public health departments can also use the clinical expertise of health care workers to design better measures for vision surveillance, to conduct screenings, and to raise patient awareness of eye disease through counseling and health education. Federal guidelines may be a useful tactic for promoting harmonization among states and promoting a shared governance model to encourage long-term sustainability. Specific opportunities for effective collaboration include

- Local public health departments should identify populations at increased risk of developing eye disease and design vision screening initiatives targeting them for intervention. Ophthalmologists, optometrists, school nurses, and other health care professionals should ensure the quality of these efforts by performing screenings, referring patients for follow-up care, and educating patients on eye disease.
- Local public health departments should work to strengthen relations among primary care providers, eye care providers, health care professionals working in vision rehabilitation, social services, and other community health workers in order to improve the continuity, timeliness, and adequacy of eye care.
- Public health departments should lead the development and dissemination of health education materials that educate patients on making changes to lifestyle risk factors for eye disease, on health impacts, on the need for eye exams, and on treatments, and they should clarify best practices for clinicians.
- Ophthalmologists, optometrists, and primary care physicians should collaborate with biostatisticians and epidemiologists in public health departments on the identification of key indicators of eye and vision health and on the development of surveys and other surveillance tools that accurately measure these indicators.

- Health informaticians should aid health care organizations and public health departments in efforts to develop shared data systems that allow clinicians to tailor patient education and outreach to identified vision health risks and that allow epidemiologists to monitor changes in disease prevalence and adapt public health programs and policies to community needs.

Effective partnerships to advance eye and vision health will require a strong, effective governmental member at each locus of government (local, state, or federal). This is resource intensive and requires a long-term commitment of senior leadership and interest among nongovernmental partners to develop, implement, and evaluate the gains and efficiencies over time for different populations.

Enhancing State and Local Capacities

State health departments can make substantial contributions to national vision health efforts. First, their involvement in the planning process helps to develop realistic action plans and ensure that the appropriate high risk populations are targeted. State health departments provide an important link between federal and community programs, which can incorporate vision health strategies where appropriate. Second, state and local health departments are the logical, local conveners for collaborations between a variety of community stakeholders and surveillance efforts related to eye and vision health.

Advancing eye and vision health as a programmatic focus will require more than simply asking governmental public health agencies and departments to place greater emphasis on the topic. Governmental public health professionals are responsible for a wide range of activities and programs that face dwindling resources in the face of increasing demand. Unfortunately, current state and local public health agencies and departments struggle to meet state mandates and requirements in the face of declining public investment, limited political power, and competition (Jacobson et al., 2015). The result is that other, more traditional public health activities, such as surveillance, health promotion, and policy development (including tracking underlying social and environmental conditions as well as eye and vision health) do not receive adequate attention or resources (Brooks et al., 2009; Honoré and Schlechte, 2007; Jacobson et al., 2015).

Federal agencies charged with various responsibilities to promote public health are uniquely situated to provide the needed resources and expertise that will allow state and local health departments to incorporate eye and vision health as a programmatic focus. For example, in 2016, the CDC implemented a vision grant program, in partnership with state-based chronic disease programs and other clinical and nonclinical stakeholders "to engage in strategic initiatives or activities designed to improve vision and eye health" (NACDD, 2016). The current grant program will award three states an average of $25,000 toward the development of activities that (1) "achieve the overall goal of advancing vision loss and eye health as public health priorities"; (2) "implement a vision and eye health intervention that focuses" on characterizing the burden of eye disease or vision loss, promotes systems change, or implements interventions related to eye and vision health; and (3) focus on sustainability beyond the initial funding period (NACDD, 2016).

Unfortunately, public health strategies to promote eye and vision health are rarely supported as a categorical focus or even as part of chronic disease programs in most state and local health departments because of limitations in resources and shifting priorities. The programmatic emphasis in governmental public health departments typically complements national public health priority lists, which do not typically include eye and vision health or chronic vision impairment (e.g., CDC, 2015d). Moreover, the degree of flexibility in how state and local governments use federal grant funds varies (CBO, 2013). In the absence of increased funding for public health overall, establishing eye and vision health as a stand-alone programmatic focus will require additional and dedicated resources beyond those currently available as well as technical support from federal public health entities and established partners.

<u>Recommendation 8</u>
To build state and local public health capacity, the Centers for Disease Control and Prevention should prioritize and expand its vision grant program, in partnership with state-based chronic disease programs and other clinical and nonclinical stakeholders, to:

- **Design, implement, and evaluate programs for the primary prevention of conditions leading to visual impairment, including policies to reduce eye injuries;**
- **Develop and evaluate policies and systems that facilitate access to, and utilization of, patient-centered vision care and rehabilitation services, including integration and coordination among care providers; and**
- **Develop and evaluate initiatives to improve environments and socioeconomic conditions that underpin good eye and vision health and reduce eye injuries in communities.**

Grant opportunities offered to state health departments can be used in a variety of ways to support specific vision preservation activities in local health departments or other organizations or encourage these activities as part of a more comprehensive strategy in partnership with other groups. Some states are actively encouraging a systematic community health assessment and planning process to be completed on a regular basis, and they can offer guidance and tools in what to look for in the community, available data sources that can be consulted in the assessment, and metrics for ongoing evaluation and quality assurance related to eye and vision health. Again, this recommendation emphasizes the need for a coherent and comprehensive program to account for primary prevention activities, for access and utilization of health care services to reduce vision impairment and improve function following vision loss, and for a focus on establishing environments that can affect the eye and vision health of a broader population.

The prioritization and expansion of the CDC's vision grant program may require more than the provision of additional resources. Currently, VHI resides within the Division of Diabetes Translation (CDC, 2016). The committee has no opinion on the exact placement of VHI within the CDC. However, the organizational location should offer, for example, visibility, sufficient staffing, integration with other chronic disease activities, expertise in insurance coverage, surveillance, and policy and programmatic expertise. Furthermore, VHI should continue to integrate with other components of the CDC and work with state, local, and other stakeholders. This could enhance the capabilities to offer technical assistance, scientific bases for collaboration among stakeholders, aid in translating science into strategic activities, and advice on issues related to vision loss and vision impairment on a much larger scale than currently exists under VHI (CDC, 2015a).

PROMOTE COMMUNITY ACTIONS THAT ENCOURAGE EYE- AND VISION-HEALTHY ENVIRONMENTS

> Eye and vision health is affected by a wide range of health determinants within communities, including individual and collective behaviors, the built environment, social conditions, and the health care system. Populations should participate collectively in decision making about population health priorities, which affect and are affected by the eye and vision health of their communities.

Living with vision impairment or having a loved one with uncorrectable vision impairment, especially when it is severe, has the potential to affect many aspects of everyday life and has been associated with a diminished QOL, including independence (see Chapter 3). Vision loss has been associated with serious health comorbidities such as depression, anxiety, low self-esteem and insecurity, social isolation, stress, mental fatigue, cognitive decline and dementia, reduced mobility, falls, and mortality (see Chapter 3). The impact that vision loss has on function and QOL varies according to numerous factors, including the built environment, social support, access to health care and rehabilitation services, attitude, preferences, and socioeconomic factors. How these factors affect the occurrence, severity, and impact of vision loss differs for individuals and communities. This situation requires communities to engage in broad-based discussions with different stakeholders, including elected officials and public health departments, to determine how national level policies, data, and programs can be implemented at the local level.

Eye and vision health is a community issue—the needs, adequacy of resources, and priorities will vary based on population characteristics, cultures, and values. It is important that community stakeholders (businesses, advocacy organizations, neighborhood groups, local health and public health departments, religious organizations, professional organizations, school boards and faculty, parent support groups, health care providers, eye care providers, etc.) be actively consulted and engaged in options to translate and implement national goals into workable community action plans to reduce the burden of vision loss and the functioning of populations with vision impairment across different community settings.

Recommendation 9

Communities should work with state and local health departments to translate a broad national agenda to promote eye and vision health into well-defined actions. These actions should encourage policies and conditions that improve eye and vision health and foster environments to minimize the impact of vision impairment, considering the community's needs, resources, and cultural identity. These actions should:

- Improve eye and vision health awareness among different social groups within communities;
- Engage community organizations and groups to promote eye and vision health awareness in daily activities;
- Establish and enforce laws and policies intended to promote eye safety and the functioning of people with vision impairment;
- Identify the need for, and community-level barriers to, vision-related services and resources in their communities; and
- Adopt policies and create community networks that support the design of built environments and the establishment of social environments that promote eye and vision health and independent functioning.

A key role for the governmental public health departments is to act as conveners of the different stakeholders who then develop and implement action plans that may complement national initiatives and that reflect a community's needs and goals. Local health departments are a natural resource for communities (including, but not limited to, government agencies, elected officials, policy makers, local nonprofit organizations, community health centers, educators, religious organizations, employers, fraternal organizations, municipal sports leagues, and other stakeholder groups) to engage when exploring the needs and resources available to combat avoidable vision impairment and the impacts of vision loss in their communities. For example, health departments can play an important role in the built environment (i.e., the physical environment constructed by human activity) (e.g., Perdue et al., 2003). They are also uniquely positioned to bring together different stakeholders within communities to begin discussions about strategies to improve different community settings and environments (including the social, economic, and built environments) and how to measure the impact of community investment.

Communities must feel comfortable in expressing the values and goals that are most relevant to them, especially in the context of establishing local actions that respond to a national agenda. Depending on the characteristics of specific populations within those communities, some actions will be more or less relevant. For example, in communities with older populations, an emphasis on programs to improve the detection and treatment of age-related eye diseases and conditions may be more applicable. In communities with school-aged children and young adults, instituting visual acuity screenings and comprehensive eye examinations in schools and developing policies to promote wearing personal protective equipment may be more relevant.

Communities must also consider the broad range of factors that affect eye and vision health, including multiple determinants of health, when deciding not only what actions to take but also who should be involved in discussions that lead to decisions about priority actions. For example, strategies related to the built environment would benefit from input from local architecture firms and community planning experts, in addition to input from more traditional public health practitioners. Input could include identifying barriers and opportunities related to public awareness about the burden of poor eye and vision health; leveraging laws and policies designed to promote function; and utilizing resources drawn from a wide range of contributors (e.g., local religious organizations, nonprofit organizations, schools, workplaces, and sports leagues) to promote access to eye and vision services. It is important that these discussions be as broad and inclusive as possible and not to overlook the personal perspectives of those with vision impairment in order to promote the kind of change that will eventually lead to new social norms concerning eye and vision health.

Community collaborations with public health departments should provide a safe venue in which to promote shared experiences and expertise, create effective platforms for communication, and develop action plans and program or initiative evaluations that contribute to both local and national dialogues and collective action. Public health departments could produce materials and informational resources based on member input, which could be used to facilitate action in other neighboring communities. For example, action strategies targeting different stakeholders and community needs would be more effective if these strategies were part of a comprehensive plan to improve eye and vision health statewide.

RECOMMENDATIONS IN ACTION: EXAMPLES FOR IMPLEMENTATION

"As an approach, population health focuses on the interrelated conditions and factors that influence the health of populations over the life course, identifies systematic variations in their patterns of occurrence, and applies the resulting knowledge to develop and implement policies and actions to improve the health and well-being of those populations" (Public Health Agency of Canada, 2007). To this end, the committee's recommendations are visionary and are meant to set in motion a variety of broad-based actions that can contribute to the prioritization of eye and vision health at national, state, and local levels. This has the benefit of encouraging coordinated actions that can sustain a larger movement. But it also has drawbacks—most notably, it does not provide discrete, recommended actions for the range of stakeholders at every level and across every dimension of eye and vision health that are essential to the successful promotion of eye and vision health.

In Chapter 1, the committee proposed a model for action (see Figure 9-2), which suggested that the 10 essential health services of public health assessment, policy development, and assurance extended across four categories of prevention, including primordial, primary, secondary, and tertiary activities. The 10 services each are part of one of three core population health functions: assessment (i.e., monitoring communities to identify and characterize public health needs and priorities), policy development (i.e., the use of scientific evidence to guide the design and implementation of programs and policies to address public health issues), and assurance (i.e., policy development and enforcement, ensuring that health and public health systems have the resources to implement programs, and evaluating the health impacts of interventions) (CDC, 2007; IOM, 1988). In the context of eye and vision health and the committee's charge, these actions

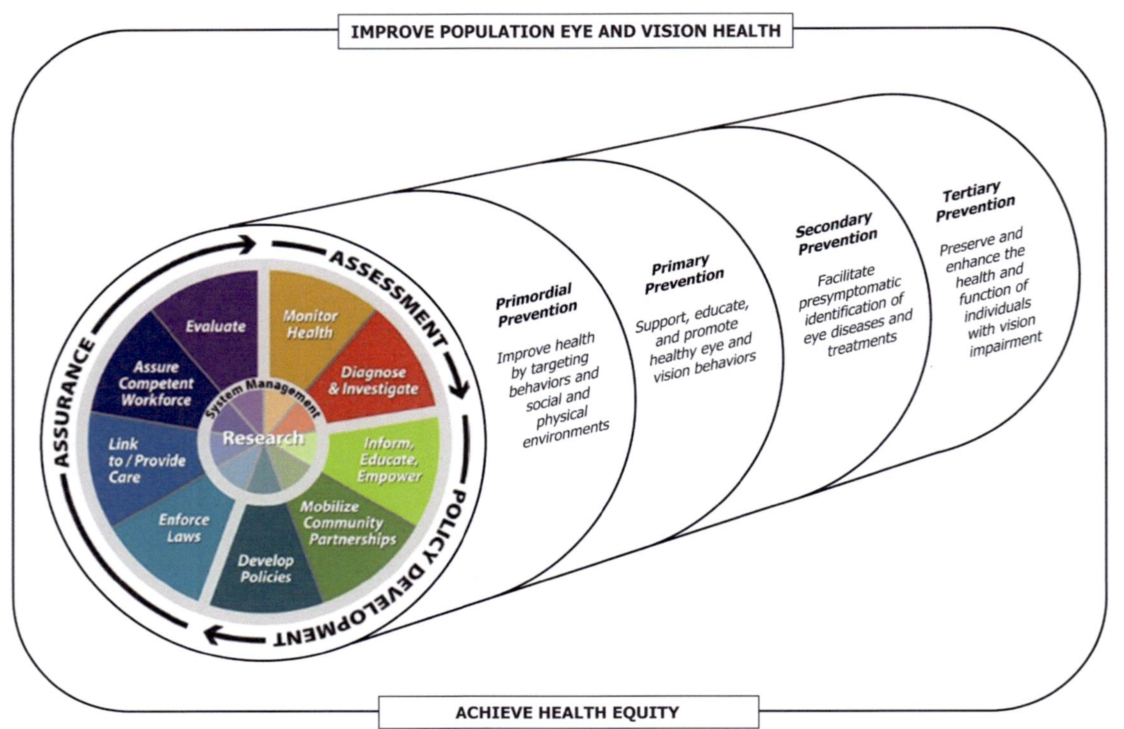

FIGURE 9-2 A conceptual framework to advance eye and vision health.
SOURCE: Adapted from CDC, 2014.

include short- and long-term strategies to address the overarching determinants of health (primordial prevention); efforts to support, educate, and promote healthy eye and vision behaviors (primary prevention); efforts to facilitate the pre-symptomatic identification of eye diseases and treatments (secondary prevention); and efforts to preserve and enhance the health and functioning of individuals with vision impairment (tertiary prevention).

The committee's recommendations are broad, intended to promote competencies and foundational evidence that can advance long-term improvements in eye and vision health in the United States. The challenges facing eye and vision health in the United States, particularly those associated with identified research gaps, the resources to establish eye and vision health as a public health programmatic focus, the formation of partnerships, and guidelines to inform the public about necessary services, will require a long-term commitment to promote competencies and foundational evidence that can guide specific action in the future.

To complement this approach, the committee also developed a stakeholder action table (see addendum to this chapter) to provide illustrative examples of activities that could logically flow from the committee's much broader recommendations. These actions are organized by key stakeholder groups, which include payers, professional groups, patient advocacy groups, state and local public health departments, private industry, community groups, and federal agencies, particularly the CDC and the National Institutes of Health. Within these groups, there are actions related to assessment, policy development, and assurance across the four stages of prevention: primordial, primary, secondary, and tertiary (see Figure 9-2); and many could easily be classified in other categories. The examples provided are not recommendations per se. Rather they are meant to stimulate discussion among stakeholders about the potential actions stakeholders can take by public health function and stages of prevention as part of a comprehensive and cohesive approach to improve eye and vision health and reduce health inequities in the United States.

CONCLUSION

Vision impairment is a significant public health problem that affects the health, economic well-being, and productivity of individuals, families, and society as a whole. The focus of population health approaches to eye and vision health should be on creating the conditions in which people can have the fullest capacity to see and that enable individuals to achieve their full potential. Despite evidence that vision impairment increases the risk of mortality and morbidity from other chronic conditions and related injuries and is associated with a reduced QOL, eye and vision health is not adequately recognized as a population health priority, so public health action has been extremely limited.

Achieving the twin goals of improving eye and vision health and increasing health equity will require action by a wide range of stakeholders at the national, state, and local levels. In the context of eye and vision health and the committee's charge, these actions will need to include short- and long-term strategies to address the overarching determinants of health (primordial prevention), as well as efforts to support, educate, and promote healthy eye and vision behaviors (primary prevention); to facilitate pre-symptomatic identification of eye diseases and treatments (secondary prevention); and to preserve and enhance the health and functioning of individuals with vision impairment (tertiary prevention).

To effectively promote eye and vision health and reduce vision impairment, sustained action across all stakeholders and levels of government will be necessary. It will require (1) better and constant surveillance; (2) policy, program, and funding incentives to stimulate and reinforce the adoption of best practices; (3) constant quality improvement experiments in all sectors in the area of vision health to discover and disseminate what works and what does not; (4) research to discover new means of prevention, rehabilitation, and treatment; (5) changes in personal and professional behavior and their surrounding systems so that they no longer reinforce current problems and instead constantly reinforce and reward making the right and best things the easiest things to do; (6) education and training for current and future workforces to improve behavior and practice; and (7) a change in political dynamics at the local, state, and federal levels to give priority once again to a broadened sense of "national and personal responsibility." Anchoring eye and vision health promotion in terms of prevention stages will allow the nation to reevaluate eye and vision health improvement as not only a valued outcome in and of itself, but also a strategy by which to achieve better health equity more broadly among populations.

REFERENCES

AAO (American Academy of Ophthalmology). 2012. Eye exams 101. http://www.aao.org/eye-health/tips-prevention/eye-exams-101 (accessed April 5, 2016).

———. 2014. Get screened at 40. http://www.aao.org/eye-health/tips-prevention/screening (accessed April 5, 2016).

———. 2015. *Policy statement: Frequency of ocular examinations.* San Francisco, CA: AAO.

AAPOS (American Association for Pediatric Ophthalmology and Strabismus). 2014. Vision screening recommendations. http://www.aapos.org/terms/conditions/131 (accessed April 6, 2016).

ACL (Administration for Community Living). n.d. Administration on Aging (AOA). http://www.aoa.gov (accessed April 5, 2016).

Alexander, Jr., R. L., N. A. Miller, M. F. Cotch, and R. Janiszewski. 2008. Factors that influence the receipt of eye care. *American Journal of Health Behavior* 32(5):547.

Anstev, E. H., C. A. MacGowan, and J. A. Allen. 2011. Five-year progress update on the Surgeon General's call to action to support breastfeeding. *Journal of Women's Health* 25(8):768–776.

AOA (American Academy of Ophthalmology). 2015. *Comprehensive adult eye and vision examination.* St. Louis, MO: AOA.

Bailey, R. N., R. W. Indian, X. Zhang, L. S. Geiss, M. R. Duenas, and J. B. Saaddine. 2006. Visual impairment and eye care among older adults—Five states, 2005. *Morbidity and Mortality Weekly Report* 55(49):1321–1325.

Berwick, D. M., T. W. Nolan, and J. Whittington. 2008. The triple aim: Care, health, and cost. *Health Affairs* 27(3):759–769.

Bray, J. E., L. Straney, B. Barger, and J. Finn. 2015. Effect of public awareness campaigns on calls to ambulance across Australia. *Stroke* 46(5):1377–1380.

Brooks, R. G., L. M. Beitsch, P. Street, and A. Chukmaitov. 2009. Aligning public health financing with essential public health service functions and national public health performance standards. *Journal of Public Health Management and Practice* 15(4):299–306.

Brouwers, M. C., M. E. Kho, G. P. Browman, J. S. Burgers, F. Cluzeau, G. Feder, B. Fervers, I. D. Graham, J. Grimshaw, S. E. Hanna, P. Littlejohns, J. Makarski, and L. Zitzelsberger. 2010. AGREE II: Advancing guideline development, reporting and evaluation in health care. *Canadian Medical Association Journal* 182(18):E839–E842.

CBO (Congressional Budget Office). 2013. *Federal grants to state and local governments.* Washington, DC: CBO.

CDC (Centers for Disease Control and Prevention). 2007. *Improving the nation's vision health: A coordinated public health approach.* Atlanta, GA: CDC.

———. 2009. Vision Health Initiative (VHI). http://www.cdc.gov/visionhealth/about/index.htm (accessed March 29, 2016).

———. 2015a. About us. http://www.cdc.gov/visionhealth/about/index.htm (accessed April 6, 2016).

———. 2015b. Establish a vision and eye health surveillance system for the nation (RFA-DP-15-004). http://www.cdc.gov/chronicdisease/about/foa/visioneyehealthsurveillance/index.htm (accessed April 5, 2016).

———. 2015c. National data. http://www.cdc.gov/visionhealth/data/national.htm (accessed May 26, 2016).

———. 2015d. Prevention status report. http://www.cdc.gov/psr/docs/psr-factsheet-2015.pdf (accessed June 30, 2016).

———. 2016. Vision Health Initiative (VHI). http://www.cdc.gov/visionhealth/home (accessed April 6, 2016).

Chou, C. F., C. E. Sherrod, X. Zhang, L. E. Barker, K. M. Bullard, J. E. Crews, and J. B. Saaddine. 2014. Barriers to eye care among people aged 40 years and older with diagnosed diabetes, 2006–2010. *Diabetes Care* 37(1):180–188.

CMS (Centers for Medicare & Medicaid Services). 2015. Preventive services chart. https.//www.cms.gov/Medicare/Prevention/PrevntionGenInfo/Downloads/MPS-QuickReferenceChart-1TextOnly.pdf (accessed April 6, 2016).

Cotter, S., L. Cyert, J. Miller, and G. Quinn, for the National Expert Panel to the National Center for Children's Vision and Eye Health. 2015. Vision screening for children 36 to <72 months: Recommended practices. *Optometry & Vision Science* 92(1):6–16.

DoD (U.S. Department of Defense). 2016. Vision center of excellence. http://vce.health.mil (accessed June 1, 2016).

DOL (U.S. Department of Labor). n.d. Americans with Disabilities Act. http://www.dol.gov/general/topic/disability/ada (accessed April 5, 2016).

ED (U.S. Department of Education). About ED. http://www2.ed.gov/about/landing.jhtml (accessed April 5, 2016).

Elam, A. R., and P. P. Lee. 2013. High-risk populations for vision loss and eye care underutilization: A review of the literature and ideas on moving forward. *Surveys of Ophthalmology* 58(4):348–358.

Hartmann, E., S. Block, and D. Wallace, for the National Expert Panel to the National Center for Children's Vision and Eye Health. 2015. Vision and eye health in children 36 to <72 months: Proposed data system. *Optometry & Vision Science* 92(1):24–30.

HHS (U.S. Department of Health and Human Services). 2015. Healthy People 2020 topics and objectives: Vision. http://www.healthypeople.gov/2020/topics-objectives/topic/vision (accessed October 7, 2015).

Honoré, P. A., and T. Schlechte. 2007. State public health agency expenditures: Categorizing and comparing to performance levels. *Journal of Public Health and Management Practice* 13(2):156–162.

HUD (U.S. Department of Housing and Urban Development). 2016. HUD's vision. http://portal.hud.gov/hudportal/HUD?src=/hudvision (accessed April 5, 2016).

Indian Health Service. 2008. American Academy of Ophthalmology joins Indian Health Service in treatment of diabetic retinopathy. May 27. http://www.ophthalmologyweb.com/1315-News/31690-American-Academy-Of-Ophthalmology-Joins-Indian-Health-Service-In-Treatment-Of-Diabetic-Retinopathy (accessed June 18, 2016).

IOM (Institute of Medicine). 1988. *The future of public health.* Washington, DC: National Academy Press.

———. 2003a. *The future of the public's health in the 21st century.* Washington, DC: The National Academies Press.

———. 2003b. *Unequal treatment: Confronting racial and ethnic disparities in health care.* Washington, DC: The National Academies Press.

———. 2011a. *Clinical practice guidelines we can trust.* Washington, DC: The National Academies Press.

———. 2011b. *For the public's health: The role of measurement in action and accountability.* Washington, DC: The National Academies Press.

Jacobson, P. D., J. Wasserman, H. W. Wu, and J. R. Lauer. 2015. Assessing enrepreneurship in governmental public health. *American Journal of Public Health* 105(S2):S318–S322.

Lam, N., and S. J. Leat. 2015. Reprint of: Barriers to accessing low-vision care: The patient's perspective. *Canadian Journal of Ophthalmology* 50(Suppl 1):S34–S39.

Mertz, E., and W. Mouradian. 2009. Addressing children's oral health in the new millennium: Trends in the dental workforce. *Academic Pediatrics* 9(6):433.

NACDD (National Association of Chronic Disease Directors). 2016. Vision and eye health initiative funding opportunity announcement (FOA #VI2015a). http://c.ymcdn.com/sites/www.chronicdisease.org/resource/resmgr/Vison_&_Eye_Health/Vision-EyeHealth_Initiative_.pdf (accessed July 8, 2016).

NEI/LCIF (National Eye Institute/Lions Club International Foundation). 2008. 2005 survey of public knowledge, attitudes, and practices related to eye health and disease. https://nei.nih.gov/kap (accessed October 7, 2015).

NEI/NIH (National Eye Institute/National Institutes of Health). 2004. Vision loss from eye diseases will increase as Americans age. https://nei.nih.gov/news/pressreleases/041204 (accessed October 7, 2015).

———. 2015. National Eye Health Education Program (NEHEP). https://nei.nih.gov/nehep/about (accessed June 18, 2016).

Office of Head Start. 2015. Head Start services. http://www.acf.hhs.gov/programs/ohs/about/head-start (accessed April 6, 2016).

Oto, M. A., O. Ergene, L. Tokgözoğlu, Z. Ongen, O. Kozan, M. Sahin, M. K. Erol, T. Tezel, and M. Ozkan. 2011. Impact of a mass media campaign to increase public awareness of hypertension. *Türk Kardiyoloji Derneği Arşivi* 39(5):355–364.

Perdue, W. C., L. A. Stone, and L. O. Gostin. 2003. The built environment and its relationship to the public's health: The legal framework. *American Journal of Public Health* 93(9):1390–1394.

Prevent Blindness. 2016. A lifetime of healthy vision. http://www.preventblindness.org (accessed April 5, 2016).

Public Health Agency of Canada. 2007. What is the population health approach? http://www.phac-aspc.gc.ca/ph-sp/approach-approche/index-eng.php (accessed April 5, 2016).

Research to Prevent Blindness. 2016. The catalyst for eye research. https://www.rpbusa.org/rpb/? (accessed March 29, 2016).

Saaddine, J. B., K. Venkat Narayan, and F. Vinicor. 2003. Vision loss: A public health problem? *Ophthalmology* 110(2):253–254.

Sabin, J. A., and A. G. Greenwald. 2012. The influence of implicit bias on treatment recommendations for 4 common pediatric conditions: Pain, urinary tract infection, attention deficit hyperactivity disorder, and asthma. *American Journal of Public Health* 102(5):988–995.

Scott, A. W., N. M. Bressler, S. Folkes, J. S. Wittenborn, J. Jorkavsky. 2016. Public attitudes about eye and vision health. *JAMA Ophthalmology* online: E1–E8.

Shah, M., D. Knoch, and E. Waxman. 2014. The state of ophthalmology medical student education in the United States and Canada, 2012 through 2013. *Ophthalmology* 121(6):1160–1163.

Thacker, S. B., and R. L. Berkelman. 1988. Public health surveillance in the United States. *Epidemiologic Reviews* 10:164–190.

U.S. Surgeon General. 2014. *The health consequences of smoking—50 years of progress: A report of the Surgeon General, 2014.* Rockville, MD: U.S. Department of Health and Human Services.

———. n.d. Surgeon General's calls to action. http://www.surgeongeneral.gov/library/calls (accessed April 5, 2016).

USDA (U.S. Department of Agriculture). 2015. Lowering risk of a major eye disease. https://agresearchmag.ars.usda.gov/2015/may/eye (accessed April 5, 2016).

USPSTF (U.S. Preventive Services Task Force). 2009. Final recommendation statement—Impaired visual acuity in older adults: Screening. https://www.uspreventiveservicestaskforce.org/Page/Document/RecommendationStatementFinal/impaired-visual-acuity-in-older-adults-screening1 (accessed September 1, 2016).

VA (U.S. Department of Veterans Affairs). VA vision care. http://explore.va.gov/health-care/vision (accessed April 5, 2016).

Varano, M., N. Eter, S. Winyard, K. U. Wittrup-Jensen, R. Navarro, and J. Heraghty. 2015. Current barriers to treatment for wet age-related macular degeneration (WAMD): Findings from the WAMD patient and caregiver survey. *Clinical Ophthalmology* 9:2243–2250.

Varma, R., T. S. Vajaranant, B. Burkemper, S. Wu, M. Torres, C. Hsu, F. Choudhury, and R. McKean-Cowdin. 2016. Visual impairment and blindness in adults in the United States: Demographic and geographic variations from 2015 to 2050. *JAMA Ophthalmology.* May 19 [Epub ahead of print].

West, S. K., and P. Lee. 2012. Vision surveillance in the United States: Has the time come? *American Journal of Ophthalmology* 154(6):S1–S2, e2.

WHO (World Health Organization). 2016. What is Vision 2020. http://www.who.int/blindness/partnerships/vision2020/en (accessed March 25, 2016).

Wittenborn, J., and D. Rein. 2013. *Cost of vision problems: The economic burden of vision loss and eye disorders in the United States.* Chicago, IL: NORC at the University of Chicago.

————. 2016 (unpublished). *The potential costs and benefits of treatment for undiagnosed eye disorders*. Paper prepared for the Committee on Public Health Approaches to Reduce Vision Impairment and Promote Eye Health. http://www.nationalacademies.org/hmd/~/media/Files/Report%20Files/2016/UndiagnosedEyeDisordersCommissionedPaper.pdf (accessed September 15, 2016).

Wittenborn, J. S., X. Zhang, C. W. Feagan, W. L. Crouse, S. Shrestha, A. R. Kemper, T. J. Hoerger, and J. B. Saaddine. 2013. The economic burden of vision loss and eye disorders among the United States population younger than 40 years. *Ophthalmology* 120(9):1728–1735.

Zambelli-Weiner, A., J. E. Crews, D. S. Friednman. 2012. Disparities in adult vision health in the United States. *American Journal of Ophthalmology* 154(Suppl):S23–S30, e1.

Zhang, X., M. F. Cotch, A. Ryskulova, S. A. Primo, P. Nair, C.-F. Chou, L. S. Geiss, L. Barker, A. F. Elliott, J. E. Crews, and J. B. Saaddine. 2012. Vision health disparities in the United States by race/ethnicity, education, and economic status: Findings from two nationally representative surveys. *American Journal of Ophthalmology* 154(6 Suppl):S53–S62, e51.

ADDENDUM

Stakeholder Action Table

		Primordial Prevention	Primary Prevention	Secondary Prevention	Tertiary Prevention
Payer	Assessment	Analyze payment policy for impacts on affordability and utilization of care (Rec 7)	Work with other payer organizations to track and compare process and health outcomes related to reimbursement policy on customer/beneficiary access to preliminary eye and vision care and appropriate follow-up care (Rec 9)	Fund demonstration projects to establish the effectiveness of coverage decisions related to regular eye screenings and examinations for Medicare and Medicare beneficiaries (Recs 4 and 5)	Fund research on cost-effectiveness of low vision therapies and devices at improving QOL and ameliorating functional disability; Assess payment policy for alignment of reimbursement with most cost-effective treatments (Recs 4 and 5)
	Policy Development	Create guidance committees charged with developing organizational goals and values that incorporate the eye and vision health of client populations (Rec 7)	Provide coverage and programs that encourage healthy behaviors (i.e., exercise, no smoking, protective lenses, blood pressure management) (Recs 8 and 9)	Expand Medicare and Medicaid coverage for routine eye exams and glasses (for Medicare; reduce/eliminate copays/deductibles for routine eye screenings and examinations, especially for the most at-risk populations) (Recs 5 and 9)	Develop coverage policies to cover low-vision rehabilitation devices in accordance with evidence-based guidelines (Rec 5)
	Assurance	Support value-based care and payment policies centered on improving patient outcomes (Recs 7 and 9)	Enforce policies that require training in, and utilization of, guideline-recommended vision screening by care	Implement quality-improvement processes to assure quality vision care particularly for high-risk beneficiaries and align with	Work with public health departments to implement quality-improvement processes to assure quality rehabilitation care for

continued

Stakeholder Action Table   Continued

		Primordial Prevention	Primary Prevention	Secondary Prevention	Tertiary Prevention
Professional Groups			providers as a condition of reimbursement (Recs 6 and 7)	incentive activities, such as pay for performance (Recs 6 and 7)	high-risk beneficiaries and align with existing laws, such as the ADA (Recs 7 and 9)
	Assessment	Support organizational agenda focused on assessment of care quality and need for a single set of eye and vision care guidelines (Rec 5)	Assess provider ability and willingness to provide patient counseling regarding links between eye disease and diabetes, smoking, ultraviolet radiation exposure, and other modifiable risk factors (Rec 7)	Assess provider knowledge and appropriate use of vision screening and comprehensive eye examination tools and techniques, as well as cultural competencies (Recs 5 and 6)	Assess provider knowledge of current treatments and available resources for vision impairment and how to educate patients (Rec 6)
	Policy Development	Establish partnerships to raise awareness about eye and vision health across a wide range of stakeholders, including group members; Establish common research agenda to advance eye and vison health as a population health priority, considering multiple determinants of health (Recs 2 and 4)	Develop evidence-based guidelines for vision care; advocate for patient-centric vision health policies; support eye and vision research; Educate the workforce about the link between eye and vision health and other measures of health (Recs 4, 5, and 6)	Advocate for payment policies related to eye and vision health, framing "vision impairment" as a chronic condition (Rec 5); Design and implement training programs to develop provider knowledge and use of vision screening and examination tools and techniques (Rec 6)	Educate health care and public health workers about services available (and needs/gaps) for people with low vision (Recs 6 and 7)
		Promote adoption of culturally appropriate health measures and	Support programs that provide incentives (e.g., discounts on continuing	Evaluate impact of training program on guideline-recommended	Evaluate impact of provider professional and post-professional training

Patient Advocacy Groups				
Assurance	integration of Culturally and Linguistically Appropriate Services (CLAS) standards to address needs of multicultural populations (Rec 6)	education units for high performers) to improve patient counseling about risk factors for vision loss (Recs 2 and 6)	vision screening and comprehensive eye examination rates as part of quality-improvement activities (Rec 7)	programs on provider adherence to standards of care and guidelines for rehabilitation services (Rec 7)
Assessment	Assess the social determinants of health that most affect specific patient populations, considering the interconnectedness of eye and vision health and other aspects of health (Rec 9)	Assess the specific eye and vision health needs within communities, especially in the context of other national, state, and local public health initiatives (Rec 9); Encourage constituents to participate in eye and vision health surveillance (Rec 3)	Petition government officials to fund actionable research on eye and vision health and behaviors to reduce the incidence and impact of vision loss (Recs 4 and 9)	Assess need for advocacy related to vision care quality and access and vision rehabilitation (Rec 9)
Policy Development	Allocate funding to mobilize partnerships with community groups, and other stakeholders; Develop organizational agendas that prioritize eye and vision health, including research on prevalence, risk and protective factors, and process and health outcomes (Recs 4 and 9)	Work with public health and health care systems to promote the messages of a coordinated public awareness campaign on eye and vision health; Establish a strong public health voice for eye health (Rec 2)	Collaborate with health departments and health providers to identify and refer at-risk individuals; work with diagnosed individuals to needed services (Rec 9)	Advocate for access to services, devices, and resources that promote independence for people with low vision. Lobby for policies that enable independence for blind/low vision people (Rec 9)

continued

Stakeholder Action Table   Continued

		Primordial Prevention	Primary Prevention	Secondary Prevention	Tertiary Prevention
Public Health Departments	Assurance	Incorporate eye health into health literacy programs and assure participation of at-risk populations; Support efforts to improve the social and environmental determinants of health (Rec 9)	Ensure that chronic disease prevention strategies and programs address particular needs for populations at risk for vision loss (Rec 9)	Provide disease-specific, culturally appropriate expertise, resources, and support for patients with early- and late-stage vision loss (Rec 2)	Through public-awareness advocacy efforts, ensure that vision rehabilitation and clinical care addresses need of at-risk populations (Recs 2 and 9)
	Assessment	Incorporate vision-related components into community health assessments; Establish surveillance systems for social and environmental determinants of health as well as risk factors for vision impairment (Recs 2 and 7)	Monitor occupational- and sports-related eye injuries; Assess ability of state and local health care and public health systems to implement public awareness campaigns and deliver preventive services for chronic disease, including vision loss (Recs 2, 6, and 7)	Establish surveillance systems that focus on or include metrics for eye health and care; Conduct research to identify risk factors for developing vision loss and insufficient access to needed preventive and prescriptive eye and vision care (Recs 2, 4 and 9)	Assess ability of clinical and public health systems to provide eyeglasses to vulnerable populations and coordinate multidisciplinary services involved in vision rehabilitation (Recs 7 and 9)
		Incorporate vision care as a strategic planning priority; Develop strategies for improving the built environment to enhance eye and vision health and	Implement public awareness campaigns about eye and vision health broadly, engaging a wide range of community stakeholders; Develop	Establish an advocacy platform for the inclusion of preventive eye care and corrective lenses in health insurance policies; Work with community	Develop policies that encourage provision of corrective lenses to school-age children and other populations where affordability is a barrier;

Policy Development	promote function following vision loss; Integrate eye and vision health into existing chronic disease and health-in-all-policies programs; Educate public health students and professionals about the ability to use eye and vision health as a tool to promote health equity (Recs 6, 7, and 9)	appropriate safety standards, regulations, and policies to reduce eye injuries; Serve as an integrator between clinical providers and community activities related to eye health and vision loss (Recs 7 and 9)	stakeholders to identify opportunities to implement policies that encourage vision screenings and appropriate comprehensive eye examinations in a variety of community settings (Recs 5, 7, and 9)	Develop programs to identify and support strategies that reduce the personal and societal burdens of low vision (Recs 7 and 9)
Assurance	Facilitate state- and local-level, interprofessional coordinating (e.g., chronic disease) committees to promote and facilitate communication, collaboration, and information sharing among providers across the continuum of care; Engage in efforts to establish valuation of community-based services (Recs 4 and 7)	Incorporate eye health into community health needs assessments and health impact assessments; Educate the workforce about the link between eye and vision health and other measures of health (Recs 6, 7, and 9)	Collaborate with eye care professionals, and general hospitals to evaluate impact of community interventions; Engage diverse community groups to expand access to appropriate vision screenings and comprehensive eye examinations (e.g., using telemedicine, smartphones, transportation services, and mobile offices) across a variety of community settings (Recs 7 and 9)	Lead collaborative of vision health stakeholders to maximize efficient use of available vision care and rehabilitation resources; Help enforce provisions of the ADA; Develop systems to track quality of vision care, particularly for at-risk populations and populations with severe vision impairment (Recs 4, 7, and 9)

continued

Stakeholder Action Table   Continued

		Primordial Prevention	Primary Prevention	Secondary Prevention	Tertiary Prevention
Private Industry	Assessment	Monitor the overall health of employees, including eye and vison health; Assess the ability of employees to access health care and vision care (Recs 3 and 9)	Track eye injury incidence and outcomes for employees; Support research to track and analyze risk factors for vision loss (Recs 3, 4, and 9)	Monitor employee vision screening and/or eye examination rates and assess the need for workplace-based eye care services (Recs 3 and 9)	Assess compliance with the ADA requirements; Assess the need for employer-offered vision insurance plans to improve health and productivity of individuals with vision impairment (Rec 9)
	Policy Development	Incorporate eye and vision health into existing or future health education and wellness programs; Encourage employee committees and resource groups to consider eye and vision health in the context of other organizational policies and programs; Offer vision insurance (Rec 9)	Require and provide safety glasses, and monitor their use; Set and monitor work standards to protect eye safety; Seek assistance from local public health departments to better understand the role of eye and vision health in promoting a healthy workforce (Recs 2 and 9)	Offer affordable at-work vision screenings and appropriate comprehensive eye examinations for employees; Provide expertise about preventing vision loss to other community stakeholders (Rec 9)	Remove barriers that impeded access, mobility, and function for individuals with severe vision impairment; Comply with the ADA regulations; Supply eyeglasses to at-risk populations, working with public health departments (Rec 9)
	Assurance	Ensure that the built environment complies with codes that promote general and eye and vision health; Develop committees responsible for developing evaluation standards and enforcement protocols for organizational policies related to vision health (Rec 9)	Monitor compliance with personal protection equipment requirements and participation in employee education on work-related eye injury prevention (Recs 2 and 9)	Assure that employer-sponsored health insurance includes comprehensive vision care (e.g., coverage for preventive examinations, eyeglasses, and rehabilitation services and equipment) (Rec 9)	Evaluate availability and adequacy of workplace-based low vision accommodations (Rec 9)

Community Groups					
	Assessment	Be an active participant in efforts to assess state of community vision health by helping identify what information is needed (Rec 9)	Assess opportunities to promote eye and vision health and educate at-risk groups about risks for vision loss in the general community and for at-risk groups within the community (Recs 2 and 9)	Be an active participant in discussions about key research and service delivery gaps to reduce vision impairment in communities (Rec 4)	Assess opportunities for improving access to vision rehabilitation services in the general community and for at-risk groups within the community (Rec 9)
	Policy Development	Work with local health departments, nonprofit organizations, and industry to better understand the relationship between eye and vision health, overall health, and underlying determinants of health; Advocate for needed public health resources to promote eye and vision health equity based on community needs (Recs 2 and 9)	Partner with eye and vision professional groups and public health departments to develop a single platform/resource that provides information about eye and vision health and related resources within specific communities (Rec 9)	Collaborate with community-based public health and clinical resources to identify and refer individuals with undiagnosed vision impairment; Identify opportunities for at-risk groups for vision screening and comprehensive eye examinations in the community (Recs 4 and 9)	Advocate for policies and programs that promote independence, function, and reduce injury in people with vision impairment; Advocate for and help guide programs that secure appropriate follow-up care in schools and workplaces for at-risk groups (Rec 9)
	Assurance	Work with local health departments to determine whether efforts to improve eye and vision health are improving health equity in communities, and vice versa (Recs 3 and 9)	Work with local health departments to determine whether vision loss prevention programs are reaching the right populations and have an impact (Recs 3 and 9)	Share successes and failures in reducing vision impairment for at-risk groups and promoting eye and vision health across the lifespan with other communities around the country (Rec 9)	Work with diagnosed individuals to secure needed services whether through transportation services, health system navigation, financial assistance, etc. (Rec 9)

continued

Stakeholder Action Table Continued

		Primordial Prevention	Primary Prevention	Secondary Prevention	Tertiary Prevention
HHS/CDC/ NIH	Assessment	Develop workgroup and conduct research to assess the effectiveness of economic, health care, and social policies at promoting social and environmental conditions supportive of good eye and vision health; Incorporate eye- and vision-related metrics into other chronic disease surveillance systems (Recs 3 and 4)	Implement surveillance system of eye and vision health; Assess gaps in public awareness about eye and vision health; Support the sustained inclusion of eye and vision health modules in existing public health surveillance programs; Integrate research on vision impairment and other chronic diseases (Recs 1, 3, and 4)	Conduct health services research concerning integration of eye care as well as mechanisms for better serving the at-risk population (Rec 4)	Fund and conduct research to assess disparities in the impact of vision impairment and contributing factors in communities; Fund research to understand the relationship between low vision and the downstream impact of vision loss (Rec 4)
	Policy Development	Support the inclusion of eye health components in existing health literacy campaigns; Label vision impairment as a chronic disease for federal program focus; Support and implement policies that identify and protect sustainable funding for research on social determinants of eye and vision health; Coordinate	Issue a Call to Action; Collaborate to implement a public awareness campaign targeting sensory deficits (e.g., vision and hearing); Fund research that targets the identification of risk factors for specific eye diseases and conditions and protective factors related to general eye health; Establish a formal working group to focus	Collaborate with private industry and other research centers to expand grant programs to facilitate public health capacities; Facilitate discussions with stakeholders about a single set of guidelines for eye and vision practice; Promote translational research to improve access to services through emerging technologies;	Support and implement policies that allocate funding for vision rehabilitation research; Collaborate with stakeholders to design and develop programs that promote awareness and access to services that improve vision impairment or improve quality of life (Recs 4 and 8)

	emphasis of eye and vision health across agencies, departments, and centers (Recs 2, 4, and 6)	on eye and vision health within and across different federal entities (Recs 1, 2, 3, and 4)	Fund research to improve sensitivity of screenings (Recs 4, 5, and 8)
Assurance	Create research positions, training programs, and grant opportunities to ensure development of a diverse, competent, and committed eye and vision health research workforce; Support programs that encourage cross-disciplinary training in eye and vision health and public health (Rec 6)	Collaborate with community groups and state and local public health departments to ensure the effectiveness of programs to promote public awareness of risk factors for eye disease and vision impairment (Rec 8)	Conduct research to evaluate and ensure the effectiveness and cost-effectiveness of preventive eye care services delivery programs, including community-based vision screening and eye examinations (Rec 4)	Require all grant recipients to evaluate the impact of interventions on process and health outcomes over time; Develop and implement a health services research program for rehabilitation including assessments of the cost and cost-effectiveness of treatment (Recs 4 and 8)

NOTE: ADA = Americans with Disabilities Act; CDC = Centers for Disease Control and Prevention; HHS = U.S. Department of Health and Human Services; NIH = National Institutes of Health; QOL = quality of life.

A

Committee Biographies

Steven M. Teutsch, M.D., M.P.H. (*Chair*), is an independent consultant, adjunct professor at the Fielding School of Public Health at the University of California, Los Angeles, senior fellow at the Public Health Institute, and senior fellow at the Schaeffer Center of the University of Southern California. Until 2014 he was the chief science officer of Los Angeles County Public Health, where he continued his work on evidence-based public health and policy. He had been in the outcomes research and management program at Merck since October 1997, where he was responsible for scientific leadership in developing evidence-based clinical management programs, conducting outcomes research studies, and improving outcomes measurement to enhance quality of care. Prior to joining Merck he was the director of the Division of Prevention Research and Analytic Methods (DPRAM) at the Centers for Disease Control and Prevention (CDC) where he was responsible for assessing the effectiveness, safety, and cost-effectiveness of disease and injury prevention strategies. DPRAM developed comparable methodology for studies of the effectiveness and economic impact of prevention programs, provided training in these methods, developed the CDC's capacity for conducting necessary studies, and provided technical assistance for conducting economic and decision analysis. The division also evaluated the impact of interventions in urban areas, developed the Guide to Community Preventive Services, and provided support for the CDC's analytic methods. He has served as a member of that task force and of the U.S. Preventive Services Task Force, which develops the Guide to Clinical Preventive Services, as well as on America's Health Information Community Personalized Health Care Workgroup and the Evaluation of

Genomic Applications in Prevention and Practice Workgroup. He chaired the Secretary's Advisory Committee on Genetics Health and Society and has served on and has chaired Institute of Medicine panels, Medicare's Evidence Development and Coverage Advisory Committee, and several subcommittees of the Secretary's Advisory Committee on Healthy People 2020. He received his undergraduate degree in biochemical sciences at Harvard University in 1970, an M.P.H. in epidemiology from the University of North Carolina School of Public Health in 1973, and his M.D. from Duke University School of Medicine in 1974.

Sandra S. Block, O.D., M.Ed., received her optometry degree in 1981 from the Illinois College of Optometry (ICO), after which she completed a pediatric residency at ICO. She has been on faculty at ICO since she completed her residency in 1982. In 1988, Dr. Block completed her master of education from National Louis University. She has been a consultant to the Special Olympics Lions Clubs International Opening Eyes program since 1995 and has been instrumental in developing the vision screening program that is now conducted globally. Dr. Block is an active member of the faculty, having served as the associate dean for academic affairs for 2 years and then as medical director of school-based vision clinics for the Illinois Eye Institute. Her interests lie in primary eye care for children of all ages, with a social focus on persons with disabilities, as well as the process of diagnosis and treatment of visually related learning problems. Dr. Block has been an active member of the American Academy of Optometry and American Optometric Association and sits on two committees for Prevent Blindness. She is a fellow and has achieved the level of diplomate in public health and environmental optometry at the American Academy of Optometry as well as a fellow in the College of Optometrists in Visual Development.

Anne L. Coleman, M.D., Ph.D., is the Fran and Ray Stark Professor of Ophthalmology in the Stein Eye Institute of the David Geffen School of Medicine at the University of California, Los Angeles (UCLA), as well as a professor of epidemiology in the UCLA Fielding School of Public Health. She is the director of the Stein Eye Institute Center for Community Outreach and Policy, UCLA Mobile Eye Clinic, and the vice-chair for academic affairs for the Department of Ophthalmology. Dr. Coleman received her medical degree from the Medical College of Virginia, completed her ophthalmology residency at the University of Illinois and her fellowship training in glaucoma at the Wilmer Eye Institute, Johns Hopkins University, and received a Ph.D. in epidemiology from UCLA. Dr. Coleman's research is focused on the diagnosis, treatment, gene–environment interactions, and the societal impact of glaucoma, cataracts, and age-related macular degeneration, including the study of lifestyle limitations imposed on patients with these eye diseases. With contributions to numerous studies and peer-reviewed journal articles and other publications, Dr. Coleman continues to serve as an investigator for a number of ongoing studies and clinical trials. A recent illustration of her research at the interface of ophthalmology and public health published in *JAMA* and summarized in *The New York Times* identified lower rates of hip fractures among elderly patients who had elective surgery to treat their cataracts. Dr. Coleman has been actively involved in national outreach programs in ophthalmology, as the prior chair of a 14-member committee of eye health experts overseeing the National Eye Health Educational Program's education programs and as the prior secretary of quality of care for the American Academy of Ophthalmology (AAO). She is the founding director of the AAO H. Dunbar Hoskins Center for Quality of Care and a member of the board of trustees of Helen Keller International and the St. John of Jerusalem Eye Hospital. She is a former at-large member of AAO's board of trustees, president of Women in Ophthalmology, and recipient of the Academy's Senior Achievement Award and Secretariat Award and is a consultant to the U.S. Food and Drug Administration Ophthalmic Devices Panel and a member of the Council of the American Ophthalmological Society. Since 2003 she has served as the executive editor of glaucoma for the *American Journal of Ophthalmology*.

Kevin Frick, Ph.D., was trained as a health economist. He received his Ph.D. in economics and health services organization and policy at the University of Michigan. Dr. Frick has been with Johns Hopkins University since 1996, spending more than 16 years at the Bloomberg School of Public Health before becoming the vice dean for education at the Carey Business School in April 2013. His research focuses on cost-effectiveness analysis in fields ranging from ophthalmology to nursing to cancer care. He has published more than 200 peer-reviewed journal articles, of which he is principal author on more than 60.

Karen Glanz, Ph.D., M.P.H., is the George A. Weiss University Professor, a professor of epidemiology in the Perelman School of Medicine, a professor of nursing in the School of Nursing, and the director of the University of Pennsylvania Prevention Research Center. She is a senior fellow of the Leonard Davis Institute on Health Economics, the Center for Public Health Initiatives, and the Penn Institute for Urban Research, and a distinguished fellow of the Annenberg Public Policy Center. She was previously at Emory University (2004–2009), the University of Hawaii (1993–2004), and Temple University.

Dr. Glanz is a globally influential public health scholar whose research, funded for more than $40 million over the past 15 years, focuses on cancer prevention and control, theories of health behavior, obesity and the built environment, social and health policy, and new health communication technologies. Her research and publications about understanding, measuring, and improving healthy food environments, has been widely recognized and replicated. She is a member of the U.S. Task Force on Community Preventive Services and has a long history of leading community-based health research and programs, and she currently serves in several related roles at the University of Pennsylvania. Her scholarly contributions consist of more than 400 journal articles and book chapters. Dr. Glanz is senior editor of *Health Behavior and Health Education: Theory, Research, and Practice*, a widely used text now in its fifth edition.

Dr. Glanz has been recognized with local and national awards for her work, including being elected to membership in the National Academy of Medicine in 2013. She was additionally named a fellow of the Society for Behavioral Medicine and received the Elizabeth Fries Health Education Award.

Lori Grover, O.D., Ph.D., FAAO, is an internationally recognized clinician and educator, and a national policy and program consultant, in the care of people with chronic vision impairment. She has specialized in the comprehensive clinical care of individuals with vision loss for more than 20 years. Dr. Grover is senior vice president for health policy at King Devick Technologies, Inc., and the former dean of the Pennsylvania College of Optometry at Salus University. Dr. Grover previously served as an associate professor in the College of Health Solutions, Nursing and Health Innovation and as the inaugural director of the Center for Translational Health Science at Arizona State University. She served on the medical staff in the Department of Ophthalmology of the Wilmer Eye Institute at the Johns Hopkins University School of Medicine from 2000 to 2012 and earned her Ph.D. in health services research and policy from the Johns Hopkins Bloomberg School of Public Health in 2012, including certificates in health economics and health informatics. She directed a national clinical research network while at the Wilmer Lions Vision Research and Rehabilitation Center for her research that examined medical and eye care access for people with chronic visual impairment, and established new metrics and policy strategies for evaluating access to health care in populations with chronic conditions. Her research interests include evidence-based multidisciplinary team models for care, clinical decision support and cost-effectiveness assessment, driving and third-party policies related to chronic vision loss, and collaborative interprofessional and translational discovery. Dr. Grover is a past executive committee chair of the American Optometric Association (AOA) Vision Rehabilitation Section, serves on the AOA Evidence Based Optometry Committee, and is an author of three AOA evidence-based clinical practice guidelines. She is a past member of the board of directors of the Association of Schools and Colleges of Optometry, and is chair-elect of the Professional Development and Education Committee of the Association for Research in Vision and Ophthalmology. She is a past council member of the Vision Care Section of the American Public Health Association, a distinguished practitioner of the National Academies of Practice, and a diplomate in public health and environmental vision of the American Academy of Optometry.

Eve Higginbotham, M.D., is the vice dean for diversity and inclusion at the Perelman School of Medicine at the University of Pennsylvania. Prior to joining Penn Medicine, Dr. Higginbotham held numerous academic leadership roles, including senior vice president and executive dean for Health Sciences at Howard University and dean and senior vice president for academic affairs at Morehouse School of Medicine in Atlanta. Most recently, she served as a visiting scholar for health equity at the Association of American Medical Colleges (AAMC) in Washington, DC. Dr. Higginbotham has a wide range of research interests, from ocular pharmacology to health disparities and policy, and has extensive experience conducting clinical trials, specifically the Ocular Hypertension Treatment Study, a multi-center, randomized trial that has significantly changed the care of ocular hypertensive patients. She earned her B.S. and M.S. in chemical engineering from the Massachusetts Institute of Technology and her medical degree from Harvard Medical School. She completed a glaucoma fellowship at the Massachusetts Eye and Ear Infirmary in Boston and is a board-certified ophthalmologist, with a subspecialty in glaucoma.

Peter D. Jacobson, J.D., M.P.H., is a professor of health law and policy and the director of the Center for Law, Ethics, and Health at the University of Michigan School of Public Health. He teaches courses on health law and public health policy. Before joining the University of Michigan, Mr. Jacobson was a senior behavioral scientist at the RAND Corporation in Santa Monica, California. In 1995 he received an investigator award in health policy research from the Robert Wood Johnson Foundation to examine the role of the courts in shaping health care policy. Mr. Jacobson's books include *Strangers in the Night: Law and Medicine in the Managed Care Era* (Oxford University Press, 2002) and *False Hope vs. Evidence-Based Medicine: The Story of a Failed Treatment for Breast Cancer* (co-authored; Oxford University Press, 2007). His most recent book is *Law and the Health System* (co-authored; Foundation Press, 2014). Mr. Jacobson is the associate editor for health law and public health at the *Journal of Health Politics, Policy, and Law,* and he is a member of the board of directors of Public Health Foundation Enterprises, Inc. From 2010 to 2012, Mr. Jacobson served as the president of the Public Health Law Association. Mr.

Jacobson's current research interests focus on the legal aspects of health care delivery and public health and public health systems. Mr. Jacobson's recent research includes projects on health departments' strategic adaptations to the new health care environment and public health entrepreneurship.

Edwin C. Marshall, O.D., M.S., M.P.H., is a professor emertius of optometry and public health at Indiana University (IU). Prior to this he was the vice president for diversity, equity and multicultural affairs at IU. Dr. Marshall has been the associate dean for academic affairs and student administration at the IU School of Optometry. Dr. Marshall was the founding chair of the Minority Health Advisory Committee of the Indiana State Department of Health and the vice chair of the Indiana Public Health Institute. He has served as the chair of the National Commission on Vision and Health, chair of the executive board and vice president (USA) of the American Public Health Association, and chair of *The Nation's Health* editorial advisory committee. He is a past president of the National Optometric Association, the Indiana Optometric Association, and the Indiana Public Health Association. He also has served on the Indiana Commission on Excellence in Health Care's Data and Quality Subcommittee, the Indiana Health Care Professional Development Commission, the Indiana Chronic Disease Advisory Council, the Benefits and Cost-Sharing Subcommittee of the Governor's Advisory Panel on the Indiana Children's Health Insurance Program, the board of directors of Bloomington Hospital and as a member of the Joint Commission on Accreditation of Healthcare Organization's Roundtable on Health Literacy and Patient Safety. Dr. Marshall currently serves as a member of the National Eye Health Education Program Planning Committee of the National Eye Institute, the Diversity Advisory Board of Transitions Optical, and the Indiana Interagency State Council on Black and Minority Health.

Christopher Maylahn, M.P.H., is a Dr.P.H. candidate in health policy at the State University of New York School of Public Health and holds a master's degree in public health from Yale University. His expertise is in the area of chronic disease epidemiology. He has more than 35 years of experience as a program research specialist with the New York State Department of Health, where he provides operational support for the New York state public health improvement plan. Mr. Maylahn has also worked with the Vermont Heart Association to develop a state hypertension control program and with the National Association of Chronic Disease Directors and the Council of State and Territorial Epidemiologists.

Mr. Maylahn's areas of research include system structure and performance, interorganizational relationships and partnerships, factors associated with sustainable public health partnerships for community health needs assessments, and practice-based research through the New York Public Health Practice-Based Research Network. Other foci of his work include cardiovascular diseases, diabetes, asthma, obesity, age-related eye diseases, and surveillance of epilepsy.

Mr. Maylahn's published work has addressed issues such as chronic disease public health services, factors affecting evidence-based decision making in local health departments, public health services and systems research, teaching evidence-based public health, older adult health surveillance, asthma, prostate cancer, and the behavioral risk factors for cardiovascular disease.

Joyal Mulheron, M.S., is the founder and executive director of EVERMORE, a nonprofit dedicated to supporting parents and families who have lost a child at any age and from any cause by building a holistic, evidence-based support system touching the lives of all of those who have been affected. She has worked in the nonprofit arena for nearly 15 years as an advisor to executive politicians and some of the nation's most respected public policy institutions. Her successes include establishing new nonprofit organizations, partnering with the private sector, philanthropic fundraising, management and reporting, evaluating organizational and program success, optimizing team talent for impact, budgeting, and organizational strategy.While Ms. Mulheron has spent most of her career advising politicians, both Republican and Democrat, and translating basic science into public policy, she has most enjoyed leading major efforts and initiatives for the National Governors Association; the National Academies of Sciences, Engineering, and Medicine; the American Cancer Society; and the Partnership for a Healthier America. In these efforts she has offered succinct policy recommendations and spearheaded teams in strategic planning, operations, and the implementation of deliverables under tight timeframes and budgets. She has managed a range of population health issues, including obesity, chronic disease, employee benefits, tobacco control, clinical trials, basic research, and genetics. Ms. Mulheron holds a master's degree in biotechnology from Johns Hopkins University as well as bachelor's degrees in both English and biochemistry from Virginia Tech. She has completed advanced studies in chemistry and World War II and minority literature.

Sharon Terry, M.A., is the president and chief executive officer of Genetic Alliance, a large network engaging individuals, families, and communities to transform health. She co-founded PXE International, a research advocacy organization for the genetic condition pseudoxanthoma elasticum (PXE), in response to the diagnosis of PXE in her two children in 1994. Ms. Terry co-discovered the *ABCC6* gene, patented it to ensure ethical stewardship in 2000, and assigned their rights to the foundation. She subsequently developed a diagnostic test and conducts clinical trials. She has a master's degree in theology and is the author of 140 peer-reviewed papers, 30 of which are clinical PXE studies.

In her focus at the forefront of consumer participation in genetics research, services, and policy, she serves in a leadership role on many of the major international and national organizations, including the Accelerating Medicines Partnership; the National Academies of Sciences, Engineering, and Medicine's Health and Medicine Division's Board on Health Sciences Policy; the National Academies Roundtable on Translating Genomic-Based Research for Health; the PubMed Central National Advisory Committee; the PhenX scientific advisory board; the Global Alliance for Genomics and Health; and the International Rare Disease Research Consortium executive committee. She is also the founding president of EspeRare Foundation of Geneva, Switzerland.

Ms. Terry is co-founder of the Genetic Alliance Registry and Biobank. She is on the editorial boards of several journals. She led the coalition that was instrumental in the passage of the Genetic Information Nondiscrimination Act. She received an honorary doctorate from Iona College for her work in community engagement in 2006, the Research!America Distinguished Organization Advocacy Award in 2009, and the Clinical Research Forum and Foundation's Annual Award for Leadership in Public Advocacy in 2011. She was named one of the U.S. Food and Drug Administration's "30 Heroes for the Thirtieth Anniversary of the Orphan Drug Act" in 2013. She is a co-inventor of the Platform for Engaging Everyone Responsibly (PEER). PEER received substantial funding awards from the Patient-Centered Outcomes Research Institute and the Robert Wood Johnson Foundation in 2014. Ms. Terry is an Ashoka Fellow.

Cheryl Ulmer, M.S., was a senior program officer and a study director for the Board on Health Care Services at the Institute of Medicine (IOM) from 2007 until her retirement in 2013. She most recently directed studies of the governance and financing of graduate medical education and of the development of an essential health benefit package under the Patient Protection and Affordable Care Act. She also served as the director of the projects Future Directions for the National Healthcare Quality and Disparities Reports and Race, Ethnicity, and Language Data and as the co-director of the Resident Duty Hours: Sleep, Supervision, and Safety project. With respect to the topic of the current report, she has personal experience with vision impairment. Before joining the IOM, she worked as an independent consultant on a wide-ranging set of health care issues, but with a primary focus on the delivery and content of health care services, disparities in health status and quality of care across populations, and options for financing and insurance. Previous consulting work for the IOM included research, writing, and editing services on the Pathways to Quality and the Consequences of Uninsurance series. Other illustrative independent consulting projects concluded in various reports, including *Serving Patients with Limited English Proficiency: Results of a Community Health Center Survey*; *Giving Back and Moving Forward*; *Finding a Future Through Service in Community Health Corps*; *Changing Lives Through Service to Medically Underserved Communities*; *Assessing Primary Care Content: Four Conditions Common in Community Health Center Practice—Hypertension, Diabetes, Otitis, Asthma*; *The Role of Behavioral Factors in Achieving National Health Outcomes*; and *Schools as Health Access Points for Underserved Children and Adolescents: Survey of School-Based Programs*. Ms. Ulmer has served as a senior associate with MDS Associates, a health care consulting firm, as well as in various positions within the U.S. Department of Health and Human Services, including in the Office of the Secretary, Assistant Secretary for Planning and Evaluation/Health; the Health Services Administration; the Health Resources Administration; Medicaid Services; and the National Institutes of Health. She has a master's degree from Georgetown University and a B.S. from Mary Washington College of the University of Virginia.

Rohit Varma, M.D., M.P.H., is the director of the University of Southern California (USC) Eye Institute, the chair of the Department of Ophthalmology, and a professor of ophthalmology and preventive medicine, and she holds the Grace and Emery Beardsley Chair in Ophthalmology. His primary research focuses on population studies of eye disease in children and aging populations. He is an expert on changes in the optic nerve in glaucoma and is also studying new imaging techniques for the early diagnosis of glaucomatous optic nerve damage. Dr. Varma is the principal investigator of multiple National Institutes of Health (NIH)-funded studies, including the Los Angeles Latino Eye Study (LALES), Multi-Ethnic Pediatric Eye Diseases Study (MEPEDS), African-American Eye Disease Study (AFEDS), and the Chinese American Eye Study (CHES). He also served as a principal investigator for studies on blindness and vision impairment for the World Health Organization.

Dr. Varma has published more than 227 papers in peer-reviewed journals, edited 2 books, and presented his research at national and international academic meetings. He served on the editorial board of *Ophthalmology*, the journal of the American Academy of Ophthalmology, and on the board of scientific counselors of the National Eye Institute, on the National Eye Health Education Program planning committee, and on the NIH anterior eye diseases study section.

Dr. Varma currently serves as the chair of the American Academy of Ophthalmology's Public Health Committee and as a member of the National Academies of Sciences, Engineering, and Medicine's Roundtable on the Promotion of Health Equity and the Elimination of Health Disparities. His honors and awards include the Research to Prevent Blindness Career Development and Sybil B. Harrington Scholar awards, the American Academy of Ophthalmology Senior Achievement Award, the Glaucoma Research Foundation President's Award, and the Association for Research in Vision and Opthamology Fellow Silver Award. He received his M.D. from the University of Delhi, India, and an M.P.H. from the Johns Hopkins Bloomberg School of Public Health.

Heather E. Whitson, M.D., M.H.S., performs research focused on improving care and health outcomes for people with multiple chronic conditions. In particular, she has interest and expertise related to the link between changes in the eye and brain (e.g., Why do cognitive and brain changes occur in the context of late-life vision loss? Is Alzheimer's disease associated with distinctive changes in the retina, and could such changes help diagnose Alzheimer's early in its course?). Dr. Whitson is also interested in improving care delivery systems and intervention programs to better serve medically complex patients. She has developed a novel rehabilitation model for people with co-existing cognitive deficits, and she is part of an interdisciplinary team seeking to improve peri-operative outcomes for frail or at-risk seniors who must undergo surgery.

B

Committee Meeting Agendas

MEETING 1 AGENDA

**Committee on Public Health Approaches
to Reduce Vision Impairment and Promote Eye Health**

Keck Center
500 Fifth Street, NW
Room 208
Washington, DC 20001

TUESDAY, MAY 19, 2015

10:30 – 10:45 a.m. **Welcome and Introductions**
Steven Teutsch, Committee Chair

10:45 a.m. – 12:15 p.m. **Discussion of the Charge to the Committee**
Perspectives from Study Sponsors:
- Centers for Disease Control and Prevention
  - *Jinan Saaddine*
- National Eye Institute
  - *Mary Frances Cotch*
- American Academy of Ophthalmology
  - *Michael Repka*
- American Academy of Optometry
  - *Lois Schoenbrun*
- American Optometric Association
  - *David Cockrell*
- Association for Research in Vision and Ophthalmology
  - *Iris M. Rush*

- National Alliance for Eye and Vision Research
  - *James Jorkasky*
- Prevent Blindness and National Center for Children's Vision and Eye Health
  - *Jeff Todd* and *Kira Baldonado*
- Research to Prevent Blindness
  - *Brian Hofland*

Committee Discussion with Study Sponsors

12:15 – 1:00 p.m.   **LUNCH**

1:00 – 2:15 p.m.   **Prevalence and Current Trends in Vision Impairment and Eye Health Across the Lifespan**

- *Sheila West*, Wilmer Eye Institute at the Johns Hopkins University
- *Susan Cotter*, Southern California College of Optometry at Marshall B. Ketchum University
- *Xinzhi Zhang*, National Institutes of Health

2:15 – 2:30 p.m.   **BREAK**

2:30 – 4:00 p.m.   **Lessons from the Past and Implications for Public Health Initiatives**

- *John Crews*, Centers for Disease Control and Prevention
- *Paul Lee*, University of Michigan

4:00 p.m.   **ADJOURN Open Session**

MEETING 2 AGENDA

Committee on Public Health Approaches to Reduce Vision Impairment and Promote Eye Health

Keck Center
500 Fifth Street, NW
Room 100
Washington, DC 20001

TUESDAY, JULY 28, 2015

8:10 – 8:20 a.m.	**Welcome and Opening Remarks** *Steven Teutsch*, Committee Chair

8:20 – 9:15 a.m.	**PANEL 1: DEVELOPING A PUBLIC HEALTH APPROACH: GOALS AND RESEARCH NEEDS**
	Moderator: *Steven Teutsch*, Committee Chair
	• **Broad Overview of the Public Health Approach**
	  ○ *Paul Jarris*, Association of State and Territorial Health Officials (ASTHO)
	• **Overview of Public Health Strategies to Improve Vision Health**
	  ○ *Alfred Sommer*, Johns Hopkins Bloomberg School of Public Health

9:15 – 10:45 a.m.	**PANEL 2: MODELS OF VISION CARE AND EXPANDING ACCESS**
	Moderator: *Anne Coleman*, Committee Member
	• **Lessons from International Models of Vision Care Delivery**
	  ○ *Hugh Taylor*, University of Melbourne
	• **Integrated Models of Care in Vision**
	  ○ *Paul Sternberg*, Vanderbilt University

> ○ *Andrea Thau*, State University of New York (SUNY) College of Optometry
- **Telemedicine and Bringing Primary Care Physicians into the Fold**
  - ○ *Jorge Cuadros*, University of California, Berkeley

10:45 – 11:00 a.m.	**BREAK**

11:00 a.m. – 12:30 p.m.   **PANEL 3: REVIEWING VISION CARE GUIDELINES: CURRENT EVIDENCE AND RESEARCH GAPS**

Moderator: *Karen Glanz*, Committee Member
- **The Centers for Disease Control and Prevention (CDC) Guide to Community Preventive Services**
  - ○ *Randy Elder*, Centers for Disease Control and Prevention
- **Review of Evidence-Based Guidelines for Eye Examinations and Treatment of Major Eye Diseases**
  - ○ *Paul Sternberg*, Vanderbilt University
  - ○ *Susan Primo*, Emory University
- **Guidelines and the E-Gap Project**
  - ○ *Kay Dickersin*, Johns Hopkins University Foundation, and Director, Cochrane Eyes and Vision Review Group

12:30 – 1:15 p.m.   **LUNCH**

1:15 – 2:30 p.m.   **PANEL 4: PREVENTION AND HEALTH PROMOTION INITIATIVES**

Moderator: *Edwin Marshall*, Committee Member
- **National Eye Institute (NEI) Health Education Program**
  - ○ *Neyal J. Ammary-Risch*, National Eye Health Education Program

- Ohio's Aging Eye Public–Private Partnership
  - ○ *Bonnie Kantor-Burman*, Ohio Department of Aging
- **Lessons Learned from Obesity Prevention and Related Promotion Initiatives**
  - ○ *William Dietz*, George Washington University

2:30 – 3:45 p.m. **PANEL 5: PERSPECTIVES ON POLICY AND SYSTEM CHANGE**
Moderator: *Eve Higginbotham*, Committee Member

- **Prevention, Treatment, and Rehabilitation: A Three-Pronged Approach to Optimizing Visual Health**
  - ○ *David Rein*, NORC at the University of Chicago
- **Understanding the Impact of the Patient Protection and Affordable Care Act (ACA)/Health Reform on Vision Coverage and Care Delivery**
  - ○ *Jeff Spahr*, Anthem, Inc.
- **Accomplishing Vision Health Policy Change: Barriers and Opportunities**
  - ○ *Mark Richert*, American Foundation for the Blind

3:45 – 4:00 p.m. **BREAK**

4:00 – 5:15 p.m. **PANEL 6: BUILDING COMMUNITY CAPACITY**
Moderator: *Joyal Mulheron*, Committee Member

- **Determining Priorities and How This Shapes Decisions About Public–Private Partnerships**
  - ○ *Matt Longjohn*, YMCA (via WebEx)

- **Using a Community Health Business Model to Engage Multi-Sectorial Partners**
  - *Donna Zimmerman*, HealthPartners (via WebEx)
- **Exploring Public Health Barriers and Opportunities in Eye Care: The Role of Community Health Centers**
  - *Susan Primo*, Emory University (via WebEx)
- **Building Community Capacity Through Informed Populations: Current Barriers and Needs**
  - *Anil Lewis*, Jernigan Institute at National Federation of the Blind

5:15 – 5:30 p.m.   **Public Comments**

5:30 – 5:35 p.m.   **Closing Remarks**
Steven Teutsch, Committee Chair

5:35 p.m.   **ADJOURN Open Session**

MEETING 3 AGENDA

Committee on Public Health Approaches to Reduce Vision Impairment and Promote Eye Health

Beckman Center of the National Academies
100 Academy Drive, Board Room
Irvine, CA 92617

THURSDAY, OCTOBER 29, 2015

10:00 – 10:05 a.m.	**Welcome and Opening Remarks** *Steven Teutsch*, Committee Chair
10:05 – 10:45 a.m.	**Innovative Approaches to Paying for Eye Care** Moderator: *Steven Teutsch*, Committee Chair • *Frank Sloan*, Duke University (via WebEx)
10:45 – 11:30 a.m.	**Building a Surveillance System for Vision** Moderator: *Steven Teutsch*, Committee Chair • *David Rein*, NORC at the University of Chicago (via WebEx)
11:30 a.m.	**ADJOURN Open Session**

C

Glossary

age-related macular degeneration (AMD)—A degenerative eye disease that causes damage to the macula. "Dry" AMD is caused by the breakdown of light-sensitive cells in the macula, where as neovascular or "wet" AMD is caused by fluid leaking from abnormal vessels under the retina, leading to blurred vision, dark areas or distortion in central field of vision, and loss of central vision (NEI, 2015a).

amblyopia—A neurological disorder in children, also referred to as "lazy eye," in which reduced vision in one or both eye occurs due to abnormal interaction or lack of a clear image (Barrett et al., 2013; Pascual et al., 2014).

anti-VEGF injection—"Anti-VEGF drugs are injected into the vitreous to block a protein called vascular endothelial growth factor (VEGF), which can stimulate abnormal blood vessels to grow and leak fluid. Blocking VEGF can reverse abnormal blood vessel growth and decrease fluid in the retina" (NEI, 2015d).

aphakia—The absence of the lens due to surgical removal, a wound or ulcer, or congenital anomaly (Anjum et al., 2010).

aqueous humor—"An optically clear, slightly alkaline liquid that occupies the anterior and posterior chambers of the eye. The aqueous humor . . . provides nutrients [and] oxygen to eye tissues that lack a direct blood supply . . . and removes their waste products. In addition, it provides an internal pressure, known as intraocular pressure, that keeps the eyeball properly formed" (Albert and Gamm, 2007).

aqueous shunt—A device that is used to reduce the intraocular pressure by draining the fluid from inside the eye to a small bleb behind the eyelid (Minckler et al., 2006).

astigmatism—A common refractive error that causes blurred or stretched vision. "An eye with astigmatism has a cornea that is curved more like a football, with some areas that are steeper or more rounded than others." As a result, the light is not refracted properly onto the retina and near and far vision become blurry (NEI, 2010c).

atropine—A topical medication used to induce dilation of the pupils to block the response to light and paralyze the accommodative reflex (Walsh and Hoyt, 2005, p. 770).

blind spot—"A zone of functional blindness all normally sighted people have in each eye, due to an absence of photoreceptors where the optic nerve passes through the surface of the retina" (Miller et al., 2015).

blindness—Total loss of sight (i.e., no light perception) (see Chapter 1).

cataract—Clouding or discoloration of the lens caused by the clumping of proteins (NEI, 2010f). Over time the cataracts may grow denser and cloud more of the lens, making it more difficult to see. Infants may be born with cataracts.

choroid—A primarily vascular structure lying between the sclera with the outer retina. Impairment of the flow of oxygen from choroid to retina may cause age-related macular degeneration (Nickla and Wallman, 2010).

chronic vision impairment—A vision impairment that is present and must be managed over the lifespan to maintain the activities of daily living (see Chapter 1).

color blindness—A defect in the perception of colors caused by genes that affect the sensitivity or loss of photo pigments found in cones. There are "three main kinds of color blindness, based on photo pigment defects in the three different kinds of cones that respond to blue, green, and red light. Red-green color blindness is the most common, followed by blue-yellow color blindness. A complete absence of color vision—total color blindness— is rare. Sometimes color blindness can be caused by physical or chemical damage to the eye, the optic nerve, or parts of the brain that process color information. Color vision can also decline with age, most often because of cataract" (NEI, 2015c).

community health needs assessment (CHNA)—Legislation imposed on all not-for-profit hospitals requiring such hospitals explicitly and publicly demonstrate community benefit by conducting a CHNA and adopting an implementation strategy to meet identified health needs, in order to maintain their tax-exempt status. This must be conducted every 3 years, with tax penalties imposed on hospitals that fail to comply (NICHSR, 2016).

comprehensive eye examination—A dilated eye examination that may include a series of assessments and procedures to evaluate the eyes and visual system, assess eye and vision health and related systemic health conditions, characterize the impact of disease or abnormal conditions on the function and status of the visual system, and provide treatment and follow-up options (see Chapter 1).

conjunctiva—"The mucous membrane that covers the front of the eye and the inside of the eyelids" (NEI, 2016b).

conjunctivitis—Also known as pink eye, the inflammation or infections of the conjunctiva, which lines the eyelid and covers the white part of the eyeball (NEI, 2015f).

contrast sensitivity—A measure of visual function related to how one sees objects that may not be outlined clearly or that do not stand out from their background. Contrast sensitivity is affected by situations "of low light, fog or glare, when the contrast between objects and their background often is reduced. Driving at night is an example of an activity that requires good contrast sensitivity for safety" (Heiting, 2016).

cornea—The transparent layer forming the front of the eye. It lies in front of the pupil, iris, and anterior chamber and its main function is to refract, or bend, light. The cornea shields the eye from germs, dust, and other harmful matter (UMN Eye Center, n.d.). The cornea is made up of cells and proteins and "unlike most tissues in the body . . . contains no blood vessels to nourish or protect it against infection. Instead, the cornea receives its nourishment from the tears and aqueous humor that fills the chamber behind it" (UMN Eye Center, n.d.).

corrective lens—A lens worn in front of the eye, usually to correct a refractive error. Examples of corrective lenses include glasses (which include lenses and frames) and contact lenses (see Chapter 1).

depth perception—Also known as binocular stereopsis, "the ability to perceive depth by combining images from the two eyes" (NEI, n.d.c).

diabetic retinopathy and diabetic macular edema—Two complications of diabetes that affect the eyes. Diabetic retinopathy is caused by damage to the blood vessels of the retina that leak fluid and/or hemorrhage and is progressive with diabetic macular edema leading to a build-up of fluid in the macula (NEI, 2015d). New blood vessels may also form either within the retina. Symptoms include seeing "floating" spots, blurred vision, and permanent vision loss (NEI, 2015d).

double vision—"A condition that causes people to see two images of an object. A variety of conditions cause diplopia, including strabismus, cranial nerve palsies, multiple sclerosis, myasthenia gravis, orbital injury, stroke, and intracranial tumor" (NEI, 2010h).

drusen—"Yellow deposits under the retina. Often found in people over age 60, drusen can be seen by an eye care professional during an eye exam in which the pupils are dilated. Drusen by themselves do not usually cause vision loss, but an increase in their size and/or number increases a person's risk of developing advanced AMD, which can cause serious vision loss" (NEI, 2001).

dry eye—"Dry eye occurs when the eye does not produce tears properly, or when the tears are not of the correct consistency and evaporate too quickly. In addition, inflammation of the surface of the eye may occur along with dry eye. If left untreated, this condition can lead to pain, ulcers, or scars on the cornea, and some loss of vision. However, permanent loss of vision from dry eye is uncommon. Dry eye can make it more difficult to perform some activities, such as using a computer or reading for an extended period of time, and it can decrease tolerance for dry environments, such as the air inside an airplane" (NEI, 2013b).

endophthalmitis—"[A] severe inflammation inside the eye caused by a bacterial or fungal infection. It is a rare complication of eye surgery, trauma, eye injections or bloodstream infections" (NEI, 2010f). Endophthalmitis can be caused by a preexisting infection in the bloodstream, or by a new infection originating from outside the body (CDC, 2015a).

eye and vision health—Creating the conditions where people can have the fullest capacity to see and that enable them to achieve their full potential (see Chapter 1).

eyestrain—Also known as asthenopia, eyestrain is a "condition arising from the efforts made by individuals to keep their eyes adjusted for seeing, . . . with emphasis on fixation, convergence, and control of the size of the pupil. . . . Discomfort [is] found to increase as the day progresses, being accompanied by the appearance of headache and fatigue, without refractive errors or changes in amplitude of accommodation, pupil size, phorias and fusional capacity" (NIOSH, 2015).

federally qualified health center (FQHC)—FQHCs are outpatient centers that are "receiving grants under Section 330 of the Public Health Service Act (PHS). FQHCs qualify for enhanced reimbursement from Medicare and Medicaid, as well as other benefits. FQHCs must serve an underserved area or population, offer a sliding fee scale, provide comprehensive services, have an ongoing quality assurance program, and have a governing board of directors" (HRSA, n.d.b).

fovea—Located at the center of the macula, the fovea is a small depression that contains the highest concentration of cones. These cones provide the sharpest daytime vision (NEI, 2009a).

functional vision loss—"A decrease in visual acuity or loss of visual field with no underlying physiologic or organic basis" (Chen and Chen, 2013).

glaucoma (open angle)—Loss of nerve tissue and axons in the optic nerve associated with elevated intraocular pressure above the level that the eye can tolerate, although normotensive glaucoma occurs in patients without elevated intraocular pressure (NEI, n.d.a).

halos—Circles appearing around lights (CDC, 2016). Halos are a common symptom of cataract (NEI, 2015b).

health impact assessment (HIA)—A "structured process that uses scientific data, professional expertise, and stakeholder input to identify and evaluate public-health consequences of proposals and suggests actions that could be taken to minimize adverse health impacts and optimize beneficial ones" (NRC, 2011, p. 3).

health literacy—The degree to which individuals have the capacity to obtain, process, and understand basic health information and services needed to make appropriate health decisions (see Chapter 4).

health professional shortage area—An area designated "by the HRSA as having shortages of primary medical care, dental or mental health providers. The area may be geographic (a county or service area), demographic (low income population) or institutional (comprehensive health center, federally qualified health center or other public facility)" (HRSA, n.d.a).

health risk assessment (HRA)—"A collection of health-related data a medical provider can use to evaluate the health status and the health risk of an individual. An HRA will identify health behaviors and risk factors known only to the patient (e.g., smoking, physical activity and nutritional habits) for which the medical provider can provide tailored feedback in an approach to reduce the risk factors as well as the potential inevitability of the disease to which they are related" (Staley et al., 2011, p. 2).

hyperopia—"Also known as farsightedness, [hyperopia] is a common type of refractive error where distant objects may be seen more clearly than objects that are near . . . it develops in eyes that focus images behind the retina instead of on the retina, which can result in blurred vision. This occurs when the eyeball is too short" (NEI, n.d.b).

intraocular lens (IOL)—A clear, plastic, artificial lens that often replaces the cloudy natural lens after cataract surgery. The IOL focuses light clearly, creating good vision (NEI, 2010a).

iris—"The colored part of the eye. It is located between the cornea and lens. The round, central opening of the iris is called the pupil. Very small muscles in the iris cause the pupil to get smaller and bigger to control how much light comes into the eye" (NLM, 2015a).

keratitis—"Inflammation of the cornea. . . . Infection is the most common cause of keratitis" (NEI, 2016b). Keratitis can be caused by infectious agents (bacteria, viruses, fungi, or parasites) or by noninfectious means (minor injury, wearing contact lenses too long) (NEI, 2016b).

keratoconjunctivitis—Inflammation of the cornea and conjunctiva (NEI, 2010g).

laser photocoagulation—A surgical technique that uses a laser to coagulate tissue. Laser photocoagulation is used primarily to treat retinopathy (NLM, 2016; Santos, 2015).

laser trabeculoplasty—The application of a laser surgery to burn areas of the trabecular meshwork, located near the base of the iris, to drain fluid (NEI, n.d.a). Laser trabeculoplasty is often used in the treatment of open-angle glaucoma.

legal blindness—A definition used by governments to determine eligibility for vocational training, rehabilitation, schooling, disability benefits, low vision devices, and tax exemption programs. Visual acuity of 20/200 or less in the better eye with the best possible correction and/or a visual field of 20 degrees or less (Social Security Act § 216(i)(1)(B)).

lens of eye—A structure that "focuses light rays onto the retina. The lens is transparent, and can be replaced if necessary. [The] lens deteriorates [with] age" (University of Michigan, 2015).

macula—A structure "made up of millions of light-sensing cells that provide sharp, central vision. It is the most sensitive part of the retina, which is located at the back of the eye" (NEI, 2015a).

macular edema—Swelling and thickening of the retina due to leaking of fluid from blood vessels within the macula. It can occur from damaged blood vessels in the nearby retina from diabetic retinopathy, after eye surgery, in association with age-related macular degeneration, or as a consequence of any inflammatory disease that affects the eye (NEI, 2015e).

myopia—"Also known as near sightedness, is a common type of refractive error where close objects appear clearly, but distant objects appear blurry. . . . In a myopic eye, the eyeball is usually too long from front to back. This causes light rays to focus at a point in front of the retina, rather than directly on its surface. This makes distant objects blurry" (NEI, 2016a).

night vision—"The ability to see in the dark" (Merriam-Webster, n.d.). Problems with night vision may be associated with cataracts, nearsightedness, drug use, birth defects, and retinis pigmentosa (NLM, 2014b).

onchocerciasis—Also known as African river blindness, a tropical skin disease caused by a parasitic worm, transmitted by the bite of black-flies that breed in fast-flowing rivers. The infection can cause blindness.

Onchocerciasis is the second most common cause of infectious blindness in the world (CDC, 2015b).

optic disk—A disk at the back of the eye where the optic nerve fibers connect the eye and the brain (NEI, n.d.d).

optic nerve—"The bundle of nerve fibers that connects the eye to the brain" (NEI, 2015d).

orthoptics or vision therapy—A program of eye exercises designed to help people with amblyopia, strabismus, eye teaming and fusion problems (Nash, 2013, pp. 385–389).

patching—Eye patching is used to cover the better-seeing eye in young patients with amblyopia to improve vision in the weaker eye (NEI, 2013a).

peripheral vision—Side vision; what is seen on the side by the eye when looking straight ahead (NEI, n.d.a).

presbyopia—A condition resulting in the inability to focus up close. "The eye is not able to focus light directly onto the retina due to the hardening of the natural lens" (NEI, 2010d).

pseudophakia—An eye in which the natural lens has been removed and an artificial intraocular lens has been implanted, usually after cataract surgery (NEI, 2010b).

refractive error—Irregular shape of cornea, lens, or eyeball prevents light from focusing properly on the retina, causing blurred vision (NEI, 2010i). "The most common types of refractive errors are myopia, hyperopia, presbyopia, and astigmatism" (NEI, 2010e).

retina—A structure that "detects light and converts it to signals sent through the optic nerve to the brain" (NEI, 2015d).

retinal detachment—An injury of the eye in which the retina "is lifted or pulled from its normal position" (NEI, 2009b). The three types of retinal detachment are rhegmatogenous, tractional, and exudative. Retinal detachment can result in permanent vision loss if not treated promptly (NEI, 2009b).

sclera—"The white outer coating of the eye. It is tough, fibrous tissue that extends from the cornea (the clear front section of the eye) to the optic nerve at the back of the eye. The sclera gives the eyeball its white color" (NLM, 2015b).

strabismus—A condition in which there is a misalignment of the eyes, such that one eye constantly or intermittently turns in (esotropia), out (exotropia), up, or down as the other eye looks straight ahead (Hatt and Gnanaraj, 2013).

trabeculectomy—A surgical procedure used to treat the intraocular pressure associated with glaucoma. During a trabeculectomy "a small piece of tissue is removed to create a new channel for the fluid to drain from the eye. This fluid will drain between the eye tissues layers and create a blister-like filtration bleb" (NEI, n.d.a).

trachoma—"An eye infection that is more common in the rural areas of developing countries. The bacteria Chlamydia trachomatis causes trachoma. People can spread the bacteria by touching infected clothing or skin. Repeated trachoma infections can cause scars inside the eyelids. The scar tissue inside the eyelids causes the eyelashes turn in—a condition known as trichiasis. This causes the lashes to constantly rub and irritate the cornea. This can eventually lead to severe vision loss and blindness. If antibiotics are used early to clear up the infection, it can prevent long-term damage" (NLM, 2011).

traumatic brain injury (TBI)—"A form of acquired brain injury [that] occurs when a sudden trauma causes damage to the brain" (NINDS, 2016).

uveitis—"A group of inflammatory diseases that produces swelling and destroys eye tissue. These diseases can slightly reduce vision or lead to severe vision loss. . . . Uveitis is not limited to the uvea. These diseases also affect the lens, retina, optic nerve, and vitreous, producing reduced vision or blindness" (NEI, 2011).

vision impairment—A measure of the type and severity of clinical or functional limitation of one or both eyes or visual information processing structures in the brain (see Chapter 1).

vision loss—The process by which physiological changes or structural, neurological, or acquired damage to the structure or function of one or both eyes or visual information processing structures in the brain occurs, resulting in vision impairment (see Chapter 1).

vision rehabilitation—A medical rehabilitation aimed at restoring functional ability, independence and quality of life in an individual who has lost visual function through illness or injury (see Chapter 7).

vision screening—A tool that allows for the possible identification, but not diagnosis, of eye disease (see Chapter 1).

visual acuity—A number that indicates the sharpness or clarity of vision, measured by the ability to discern objects at a given distance according to a fixed standard (see Chapter 1).

visual field—The total area an individual can see off to the side without moving the eye (see Chapter 1).

visual fixation—Maintaining a visual gaze on an object (Martinez-Conde et al., 2004).

vitrectomy—"The surgical removal of the vitreous gel in the center of the eye. . . . A clear salt solution is gently pumped into the eye . . . to maintain eye pressure during surgery and to replace the removed vitreous" (NEI, 2015d).

vitreous body—The clear colorless transparent jelly that fills the eyeball behind the lens and in front of the retina at the back of the eye. The vitreous body consists mostly of water and remains stagnant (NEI, 2009c).

REFERENCES

Albert, D. M., and D. M. Gamm. 2007. Aqueous humour. https://www.britannica.com/science/aqueous-humor (accessed June 28, 2016).

Anjum, I., H. Eiberg, S. M. Baig, N. Tommerup, and L. Hansen. 2010. A mutation in the FOXE3 gene causes congenital primary aphakia in an autosomal recessive consanguineous Pakistani family. *Molecular Vision* 16:549–555.

Barrett, B. T., A. Bradley, and T. R. Candy. 2013. The relationship between anisometropia and amblyopia. *Progress in Retinal and Eye Research* 36:120–158.

CDC (Centers for Disease Control and Prevention). 2015a. Fungal eye infection statistics. http://www.cdc.gov/fungal/diseases/fungal-eye-infections/statistics.html (accessed June 30, 2016).

———. 2015b. Parasites—onchocerciasis (also known as river blindness). http://www.cdc.gov/parasites/onchocerciasis (accessed July 1, 2016).

———. 2016. Keep an eye on your vision health. http://www.cdc.gov/features/healthyvision (accessed July 5, 2016).

Chen, J. J., and Y. Chen. 2013. Functional visual loss. http://www.eyerounds.org/cases/165-functional-visual-loss.htm (accessed July 5, 2016).

Heiting, G. 2016. Contrast sensitivity testing. http://www.allaboutvision.com/eye-exam/contrast-sensitivity.htm (accessed June 28, 2016).

HRSA (Health Resources and Services Administration). n.d.a. Health professional shortage areas (HPSAs) definition. http://nhsc.hrsa.gov/ambassadors/hpsadefinition.html (accessed June 30, 2016).

———. n.d.b. What are federally qualified health centers (FQHCs)? http://www.hrsa.gov/health it/toolbox/RuralHealthITtoolbox/Introduction/qualified.html (accessed June 29, 2016).

Martinez-Conde, S., S. L. Macknik, and D. H. Hubel. 2004. The role of fixational eye movements in visual perception. *Nature Reviews Neuroscience* 5(3):229–240.

Merriam-Webster. n.d. Night vision. http://www.merriam-webster.com/dictionary/night%20 vision (accessed July 1, 2016).

Miller, P. A., G. Wallis, P. J. Bex, and D. H. Arnold. 2015. Reducing the size of the human physiological blind spot through training. *Current Biology* 25(17):R747–R748.

Minckler, D. S., S. S. Vedula, T. J. Li, M. C. Mathew, R. S. Ayyala, and B. A. Francis. 2006. Aqueous shunts for glaucoma. *Cochrane Database of Systematic Reviews* (2):Cd004918.

Nash, J. K. 2013. Vision therapy as a complementary procedure during neurotherapy. In *Clinical neurotherapy: Application of techniques for treatment*, edited by D. S. Cantor and J. R. Evans. London, UK: Academic Press.

NEI (National Eye Institute). 2001. Antioxidant vitamins and zinc reduce risk of vision loss from age-related macular degeneration. https://nei.nih.gov/news/pressreleases/101201 (accessed June 30, 2016).

———. 2009a. Facts about histoplasmosis. https://nei.nih.gov/health/histoplasmosis/histoplasmosis (accessed June 30, 2016).

———. 2009b. Facts about retinal detachment. https://nei.nih.gov/health/retinaldetach/retinaldetach (accessed July 1, 2016).

———. 2009c. Facts about vitreous detachment. https://nei.nih.gov/health/vitreous/vitreous (accessed July 1, 2016).

———. 2010a. Cataract | intraocular lens (IOL). https://answers.nei.nih.gov/app/answers/detail/a_id/2353/~/cataract-%7C-intraocular-lens-%28iol%29 (accessed July 1, 2016).

———. 2010b. Cataract | pseudophakia. https://answers.nei.nih.gov/app/answers/detail/a_id/2357/~/cataract-%7C-pseudophakia (accessed July 1, 2016).

———. 2010c. Facts about astigmatism. https://nei.nih.gov/health/errors/astigmatism (accessed June 30, 2016).

———. 2010d. Facts about presbyopia. https://nei.nih.gov/health/errors/presbyopia (accessed July 1, 2016).

———. 2010e. Facts about refractive errors. https://nei.nih.gov/health/errors/errors (accessed July 1, 2016).

———. 2010f. Inflammation | endophthalmitis. https://answers.nei.nih.gov/app/answers/detail/a_id/2445/~/inflammation-%7C-endophthalmitis (accessed June 30, 2016).

———. 2010g. Inflammation | phlyctenular keratoconjunctivitis. https://answers.nei.nih.gov/app/answers/detail/a_id/2456/~/inflammation-%7C-phlyctenular-keratoconjunctivitis (accessed July 1, 2016).

———. 2010h. Visual processing | double vision (diplopia). https://answers.nei.nih.gov/app/answers/detail/a_id/2756/~/visual-processing-%7C-double-vision-%28diplopia%29 (accessed June 30, 2016).

———. 2011. Facts about uveitis. https://nei.nih.gov/health/uveitis/uveitis (accessed July 1, 2016).

———. 2013a. Extended daily eye patching effective at treating stubborn amblyopia in children. https://nei.nih.gov/news/briefs/eye_patching (accessed July 1, 2016).

———. 2013b. Facts about dry eye. https://nei.nih.gov/health/dryeye/dryeye (accessed June 30, 2016).

———. 2015a. Facts about age-related macular degeneration. https://nei.nih.gov/health/macular degen/armd_facts (accessed July 1, 2016).

————. 2015b. Facts about cataracts. https://nei.nih.gov/health/cataract/cataract_facts (accessed June 30, 2016).

————. 2015c. Facts about color blindness. https://nei.nih.gov/health/color_blindness/facts_about (accessed June 28, 2016).

————. 2015d. Facts about diabetic eye disease. https://nei.nih.gov/health/diabetic/retinopathy (accessed June 28, 2016).

————. 2015e. Facts about macular edema. https://nei.nih.gov/health/macular-edema/fact_sheet (accessed July 1, 2016).

————. 2015f. Facts about pink eye. https://nei.nih.gov/health/pinkeye/pink_facts (accessed June 28, 2016).

————. 2016a. Facts about myopia. https://nei.nih.gov/health/errors/myopia (accessed July 1, 2016).

————. 2016b. Facts about the cornea and corneal disease. https://nei.nih.gov/health/cornealdisease (accessed June 20, 2016).

————. n.d.a. Facts about glaucoma. https://nei.nih.gov/health/glaucoma/glaucoma_facts (accessed July 1, 2016).

————. n.d.b. Facts about hyperopia. https://nei.nih.gov/health/errors/hyperopia (accessed July 1, 2016).

————. n.d.c. Vision. https://nei.nih.gov/intramural/lsr/vision (accessed June 30, 2016).

————. n.d.d. What is a comprehensive dilated eye exam? https://nei.nih.gov/healthyeyes/eyeexam (accessed July 1, 2016).

NICHSR (National Information Center on Health Services Research and Health Care Technology). 2016. Community benefit / community health needs assessment. https://www.nlm.nih.gov/hsrinfo/community_benefit.html (accessed June 28, 2016).

Nickla, D. L., and J. Wallman. 2010. The multifunctional choroid. *Progress in Retinal and Eye Research* 29(2):144–168.

NINDS (National Institute of Neurological Disorders and Stroke). 2016. NINDS traumatic brain injury information page. http://www.ninds.nih.gov/disorders/tbi/tbi.htm (accessed July 1, 2016).

NIOSH (National Institute for Occupational Safety and Health). 2015. Ocular discomfort and other symptoms of eyestrain at low levels of illumination. http://www.cdc.gov/niosh/nioshtic-2/00168704.html (accessed July 1, 2016).

NLM (U.S. National Library of Medicine). 2011. Inflammation | trachoma. https://answers.nei.nih.gov/app/answers/detail/a_id/2834/kw/Trachoma (accessed July 1, 2016).

————. 2014a. Strabismus. https://www.nlm.nih.gov/medlineplus/ency/article/001004.htm (accessed July 1, 2015).

————. 2014b. Vision—night blindness. https://www.nlm.nih.gov/medlineplus/ency/article/003039.htm (accessed July 1, 2016).

————. 2015a. Iris. https://www.nlm.nih.gov/medlineplus/ency/article/002386.htm (accessed July 1, 2016).

————. 2015b. Sclera. https://www.nlm.nih.gov/medlineplus/ency/article/002295.htm (accessed July 1, 2016).

————. 2016. Laser photocoagulation—eye. https://www.nlm.nih.gov/medlineplus/ency/article/007664.htm (accessed July 1, 2016).

NRC (National Research Council). 2011. *Improving health in the United States: The role of health impact assessment.* Washington, DC: The National Academies Press.

Pascual, M., J. Huang, M. G. Maguire, M. T. Kulp, G. E. Quinn, E. Ciner, L. A. Cyert, D. Orel-Bixler, B. Moore, and G. S. Ying. 2014. Risk factors for amblyopia in the vision in preschoolers study. *Ophthalmology* 121(3):622–629, e621.

Santos, E. M. G. 2015. Retinal photocoagulation. http://emedicine.medscape.com/article/1844294-overview (accessed July 1, 2016).

Staley, P., P. Stange, and C. Richards. 2011. *Interim guidance for health risk assessments and their modes of provision for medicare beneficiaries*. Atlanta, GA: Centers for Disease Control and Prevention.

UMN Eye Center (University of New Mexico Eye Center). n.d. Facts about the cornea and corneal disease. http://hospitals.unm.edu/eyes/conditions/cornea_disease.html (accessed June 29, 2016).

University of Michigan. 2015. The eye. http://kellogg.umich.edu/patientcare/conditions/anatomy.html (accessed July 1, 2016).

Walsh, F. B., and W. F. Hoyt. 2005. *Walsh and Hoyt's clinical neuro-ophthalmology*, edited by N. R. Miller, N. J. Newman, V. Biousse and J. Kerrison. Vol. 1. Philadelphia, PA, Baltimore, MD: Lippincott Williams & Wilkins.

D

Examples of Federal Entities Involved in Advancing Eye Health and Safety

Federal Entity	Mission	Examples of Activities Related to Eye Health
Administration for Children and Families (ACF)	The entity within HHS responsible for overseeing federal programs that promotes "the economic and social well-being of children, families, individuals, and communities" (ACF, n.d.).	The Office of Head Start promotes the Head Start and Early Head Start programs to support "comprehensive development of children from birth to age 5" (ACF, 2015b). The programs include early learning, health screening and follow-up, nutrition, social services, and services for children with disabilities (ACF, 2015a,b). Vision impairment and blindness are addressed in the eligibility criteria because they adversely affect learning outcomes (ACF, 2015a).
Administration on Aging	"Promotes the well-being of older individuals by providing services and programs designed to help them live independently in their homes and communities" (AoA, 2015a).	Provides home and community services to older persons, including programs related to "transportation, adult day care, caregiver supports, [and] health promotion programs" (AoA, 2015a). "Manages health, prevention, and wellness programs for older adults. This includes behavioral health information, chronic disease self-management education programs, diabetes self-management, disease prevention and health promotion services, falls prevention programs . . . nutrition services, and oral health promotion" (AoA, 2015a).

continued

Federal Entity	Mission	Examples of Activities Related to Eye Health
		Advocates for changes at the local, state and national levels that will improve care and quality of life "for residents of nursing homes, board and care homes, assisted living facilities and similar adult care facilities" (AoA, 2015b).
Centers for Disease Control and Prevention (CDC)	Aims to ensure public health through the control and prevention of safety and security threats (CDC, 2014).	The CDC's Division of Diabetes Translation contains a Vision Health Initiative that aims to optimize opportunities for addressing vision as a public health challenge (CDC, 2015a). CDC is currently funding an effort to advance the surveillance of vision health (CDC, 2015b). The CDC's National Institute for Occupational Safety and Health supports programs promoting safe and healthy working conditions. The research programs are divided by industry sector (CDC, 2015c).
Centers for Medicare & Medicaid Services (CMS)	Provides government funded health insurance to more than 100 million Americans through programs such as Medicare, Medicaid, and the Children's Health Insurance Program (CHIP) (CMS, 2016a).	Covers diagnosis, evaluation, and treatment of eye diseases and some vision costs, primarily if poor vision is the result of another illness or injury. Relevant programs include • Center for Medicare & Medicaid Innovation conducts demonstration projects for potential program changes on the systemic and individual coverage determination level. These include projects aimed at home health pay, electronic health records, care management for high-cost beneficiaries, and low vision rehabilitation, among others (CMS, 2016c). • The early and periodic screening, diagnostic, and treatment (EPSDT) benefit for children, which provides at minimum coverage of the "diagnosis and treatment for defects in vision, including eyeglasses" (CMS, 2016b).
Health Resources and Services Administration (HRSA)	Aims to achieve health equity and universal access to care by training	HRSA provides programs targeted specifically at people who live in isolated areas and/or are economically or medically vulnerable (HRSA, 2016).

Federal Entity	Mission	Examples of Activities Related to Eye Health
	health workers, researching important health care topics, and providing education to the public (HRSA, 2016).	Relevant programs include (but are not limited to): • The National Health Service Corps, provides primary health care in underserved communities through incentivizing providers with loan repayment options (National Health Service Corps, 2016). • Bright Futures, which provides guidelines for the health supervision of children and adolescents and guides coverage of services managed by the EPSDT (AAP, 2016). • Federally qualified health centers (FQHCs) is a designation given to primary care service sites in underserved areas that provide a range of services to those who otherwise might lack access (HRSA, n.d.). Preventive services provided include glaucoma screening, diabetes screening, and the annual wellness visit (CMS, 2015).
Indian Health Service (IHS)	Provides "health services to American Indians and Alaska Natives" (IHS, 2016).	The IHS provides eye care on or near reservations. The services provided are for the most part by physicians and optometrists. Services include eye health promotion, eye exams, treatments, and prescription ophthalmic devices (IHS, 2016, n.d.).
National Institutes of Health (NIH)	A biomedical research facility responsible for biomedical and health-related research (NIH, n.d.).	The National Eye Institute (NEI) supports research as it pertains to improving knowledge about how the visual system works in health and disease, and pioneers advances in the prevention, management, and treatment of eye health (NEI, 2015). The NEI's National Eye Health Education Program increases awareness among health care professionals and the public about preserving eye health (NEHEP, n.d.). Other institutes often fund vision-related research endeavors. These may include (among others):

continued

Federal Entity	Mission	Examples of Activities Related to Eye Health
		• National Institute on Aging • National Institute of Neurological Disorders and Stroke • National Institute of Diabetes and Digestive and Kidney Diseases • *Eunice Kennedy Shriver* National Institute of Child Health and Human Development
Office of Disease Prevention and Health Promotion	Sets "national health goals and objectives and supporting programs, services, and education activities" (ODPHP, 2016a).	Oversees Healthy People 2020, which includes vision-specific goals and recommendations (ODPHP, 2016b).
U.S. Department of Agriculture (USDA)	Responsible for developing and executing government policy on farming, agriculture, forestry, and food (USDA, 2016).	Researchers at the USDA promote eye health through studies that link eye disease to diet. For example, recently two age-related eye disease studies found that the use of a supplement containing vitamins C and E, lutein/zeaxanthin, and zinc delays progression to advanced age-related macular degeneration (AMD) (USDA, 2015).
U.S. Department of Defense (DoD)	"To provide the military forces needed to deter war and to protect the security" of the United States (DoD, 2015).	The DoD's Defense Health Agency is an "integrated combat support agency that enables the Army, Navy, and Air Force medical services to provide a medically ready force" through the provision of health services generally through the TRICARE Health Plan (DHA, 2016). The DoD Vision Center of Excellence leads programs related to "improv[ing] vision health, optimiz[ing] readiness, and enhanc[ing] quality of life for Service members and Veterans" (VCE, 2016). Some of the activities include • Implementing a vision registry surveillance system that collects eye injury and vision dysfunction data from the DoD and the VA. • Promoting research for evidence-based prevention, diagnosis, mitigation, treatment, and rehabilitation. • Training the Tactical Combat Casualty Care workforce to improve care readiness for eye trauma and vision impairment.

Federal Entity	Mission	Examples of Activities Related to Eye Health
		• Expanding vision health education across involved parties (patients, families, clinicians). • Promoting "Shields Save Sight" campaign to advocate for protective eyewear. • Enhancing coordination of injured and visually impaired service members through the military health care system (VCE, 2016).
U.S. Department of Education (ED)	Fosters "educational excellence and ensuring equal access" to education (ED, 2016a).	Among other activities, houses the Office of Special Education and Rehabilitative Services (ED, 2016b), as well as the Helen Keller National Center, which provides services on a national basis to individuals who are deaf-blind, their families, and service providers (ED, 2014).
U.S. Department of Housing and Urban Development (HUD)	"Create strong, sustainable, inclusive communities and quality affordable homes for all" (HUD, 2016c).	Supports programs that "promote homeownership, support community development, and increase access to affordable housing, free from discrimination" (HUD, 2016b). The HUD's Office of Fair Housing and Equal Opportunity has information resources aimed at people with disabilities, housing providers, and building design professionals to disseminate regulations and policies aimed at shaping a built environment suitable for those with disabilities (HUD, 2016a).
U.S. Department of Labor (DOL)	Responsible "to foster, promote, and develop the welfare of the wage earners, job seekers, and retirees of the United States; improve working conditions; advance opportunities for profitable employment; and assure work-related benefits and rights" (DOL, n.d.b).	The Occupational Safety and Health Administration (OSHA) holds employers accountable, raises awareness about eye injury, and enforces eye safety in the workplace though the use of eye and face protective tools such as goggles and eye wash stations (DOL, n.d.a). The Office of Disability Employment Policy (ODEP) provides assistance on the basic requirements of the Americans with Disabilities Act (ADA) (DOL, 2016).

continued

Federal Entity	Mission	Examples of Activities Related to Eye Health
U.S. Department of Transportation (DOT)	Ensures a safe and effective transportation system. The DOT creates and enforces regulations on roads, railways, and seaways and in the skies (DOT, n.d.).	Ensures that all drivers meet a certain standard of vision through mandatory vision exams, though there are state-by-state variations in vision requirements; for example, some states require all licensed drivers to have at least 20/40 vision with or without glasses or contacts, normal peripheral vision, and the ability to recognize colors on traffic signs and signals (FMCSA, n.d.). The DOT enforces regulations governing transit under the ADA. These regulations are meant to ensure a user-friendly built environment for transportation services, and include designing accessible public transportation services and maintaining communication features such as fire alarms and signs (U.S. Access Board, 2006).
U.S. Department of Veterans Affairs (VA)	Provides patient care and federally funded benefits to veterans and their families (VA, 2015a).	VA patients who are visually impaired can apply for vision benefits "including clinical examinations, vision-enhancing devices, and specialized training in the use of innovative vision technology" (VA, 2016). Diagnosis, evaluation, and treatment are covered in those with eye diseases or injuries (VA, 2015b).
U.S. Environmental Protection Agency (EPA)	"Protects human health and the environment" through science-based policies and enforcement (EPA, 2015b).	Responsible for the classification, regulation, and labeling of eye irritants, such as pesticides and cleaning supplies, that if put in the eye can lead to vision loss and blindness (EPA, 2015a).
U.S. Food and Drug Administration (FDA)	Ensures the safety of drugs, biologics, devices, food, tobacco, and cosmetic products (FDA, 2015).	Provides regulation for pharmaceuticals and devices, such as contact lenses, intraocular lenses, and LASIK surgery on the public market (FDA, 2016).

REFERENCES

AAP (American Academy of Pediatrics). 2016. *About.* https://brightfutures.aap.org/about/Pages/About.aspx (accessed April 6, 2016).

ACF (Administration for Children and Families). 2015a. § 1308.13 eligibility criteria: Visual impairment including blindness. http://eclkc.ohs.acf.hhs.gov/hslc/standards/hspps/1308/1308.13%20%20Eligibility%20criteria_%20Visual%20impairment%20including%20blindness..htm (accessed April 6, 2016).

———. 2015b. Head Start services. http://www.acf.hhs.gov/ohs/about (accessed April 6, 2016).

———. n.d. Administration for Children & Families. https://www.acf.hhs.gov (accessed April 6, 2016).

AoA (Administration on Aging). 2015a. Administration on Aging (AOA). http://www.aoa.gov/ (accessed April 6, 2016).

———. 2015b. AOA programs. http://www.aoa.acl.gov/AoA_Programs/Elder_Rights/Ombudsman/index.aspx (accessed Ausgut 22, 2016).

CDC (Centers for Disease Control and Prevention). 2014. Mission, role and pledge. http://www.cdc.gov/about/organization/mission.htm (accessed August 22, 2016).

———. 2015a. About us. http://www.cdc.gov/visionhealth/about/index.htm (accessed April 6, 2016).

———. 2015b. Establish a vision and eye health surveillance system for the nation (RFA-DP-15-004). http://www.cdc.gov/chronicdisease/about/foa/visioneyehealthsurveillance/index.htm (accessed August, 22, 2016).

———. 2015c. NIOSH programs. http://www.cdc.gov/niosh/programs.html (accessed April 6, 2016).

CMS (Centers for Medicare & Medicaid Services). 2015. Preventive services chart. https://www.cms.gov/Medicare/Prevention/PrevntionGenInfo/Downloads/MPS-QuickReferenceChart-1TextOnly.pdf (accessed April 6, 2016).

———. 2016a. Centers for Medicare & Medicaid Services. https://www.cms.gov (accessed April 6, 2016).

———. 2016b. Early and periodic screening, diagnostic, and treatment. https://www.medicaid.gov/Medicaid-CHIP-Program-Information/By-Topics/Benefits/Early-and-Periodic-Screening-Diagnostic-and-Treatment.html (accessed April 6, 2016).

———. 2016c. Medicare demonstrations. https://innovation.cms.gov/Medicare-Demonstrations (accessed April 6, 2016).

DHA (Defense Health Agency). 2016. Defense Health Agency. http://www.health.mil/dha (accessed April 6, 2016).

DoD (U.S. Department of Defense). 2015. About the Department of Defense (DOD). http://www.defense.gov/About-DoD (accessed April 6, 2016).

DOL (U.S. Department of Labor). 2016. Disability employment policy resources by topic. https://www.dol.gov/odep/topics/ADA.htm (accessed April 11, 2016).

———. n.d.a. Occupational Safety and Health Administration. https://www.osha.gov/SLTC/etools/eyeandface/employer/requirements.html (accessed August 22, 2016).

———. n.d.b. Our mission. https://www.dol.gov/opa/aboutdol/mission.htm (accessed August 22, 2016).

DOT (U.S. Department of Transportation). n.d. About us. https://www.transportation.gov/about (accessed August 22, 2016).

ED (U.S. Department of Education). 2014. Helen Keller National Center. http://www2.ed.gov/programs/helenkeller/index.html (accessed August 28, 2016).

———. 2016a. About ED. http://www2.ed.gov/about/landing.jhtml (accessed April 6, 2016).

————. 2016b. Office of Special Education and Rahabilitative Services. http://www2.ed.gov/about/offices/list/osers/index.html (accessed August 28, 2016).

EPA (U.S. Environmental Protection Agency). 2015a. Alternate testing framework for classification of eye irritation potential of EPA-regulated pesticide products. https://www.epa.gov/pesticide-registration/alternate-testing-framework-classification-eye-irritation-potential-epa (accessed April 6, 2016).

————. 2015b. Our mission and what we do. https://www.epa.gov/aboutepa/our-mission-and-what-we-do (accessed July 14, 2016).

FDA (U.S. Food and Drug Administration). 2015. What we do. http://www.fda.gov/AboutFDA/WhatWeDo/ (accessed August 22, 2016).

————. 2016. Medical devices. http://www.fda.gov/MedicalDevices/default.htm (accessed April 6, 2016).

FMCSA (Federal Motor Carrier Safety Administration). n.d. Part 391 qualifications of drivers and longer combination vehicle (LCV) driver instructors. https://www.fmcsa.dot.gov/regulations/title49/section/391.41 (accessed August 22, 2016).

HRSA (Health Resources and Services Administration). 2016. About HRSA. http://www.hrsa.gov/about/index.html (accessed July 14, 2016).

————. n.d. What are Federally qualified health centers (FQHCs)?. http://www.hrsa.gov/healthit/toolbox/RuralHealthITtoolbox/Introduction/qualified.html (accessed August 22, 2016).

HUD (U.S. Department of Housing and Urban Development). 2016a. Fair housing and equal opportunity. http://portal.hud.gov/hudportal/HUD?src=/program_offices/fair_housing_equal_opp (accessed April 6, 2016).

————. 2016b. HUD's vision. http://portal.hud.gov/hudportal/HUD?src=/hudvision (accessed April 6, 2016).

————. 2016c. Mission. http://portal.hud.gov/hudportal/HUD?src=/about/mission (accessed April 6, 2016).

IHS (Indian Health Service). 2016. Agency overview. https://www.ihs.gov/aboutihs/overview (accessed January 14, 2016).

————. n.d. Indian health manual. https://www.ihs.gov/ihm/index.cfm?module=dsp_ihm_pc_p3c9#3-9.2 (accessed July 14, 2016).

National Health Service Corps. 2016. The National Health Service Corps. http://www.nhsc.hrsa.gov (accessed April 6, 2016).

NEHEP (National Eye Health Education Program). n.d. NEHEP programs. https://nei.nih.gov/nehep (accessed August 22, 2016).

NEI (National Eye Institute). 2015. NEI's research progress. https://nei.nih.gov/about/mission (accessed April 6, 2016).

NIH (National Insitutues of Health). n.d. Impact of NIH research. https://www.nih.gov/about-nih/what-we-do/impact-nih-research (accessed August 22, 2016).

ODPHP (Office of Disease Prevention and Health Promotion). 2016a. About ODPHP. http://health.gov/about-us (accessed July 14, 2016).

————. 2016b. Vision. https://www.healthypeople.gov/2020/topics-objectives/topic/vision/objectives (accessed April 6, 2016).

U.S. Access Board. 2006. ADA standards for transportation facilities. https://www.access-board.gov/guidelines-and-standards/transportation/facilities/about-the-ada-standards-for-transportation-facilities/ada-standards-for-transportation-facilities-single-file#a10 (accessed April 6, 2016).

USDA (U.S. Department of Agriculture). 2015. Lowering risk of a major eye disease. https://agresearchmag.ars.usda.gov/2015/may/eye (accessed April 6, 2016)

————. 2016. About the U.S. Department of Agriculture. http://www.usda.gov/wps/portal/usda/usdahome?navid=ABOUT_USDA (accessed April 6, 2016).

VA (U.S. Department of Veterans Affairs). 2015a. About VA. http://www.va.gov/about_va/mission.asp (accessed August 22, 2016).

———. 2015b. Chapter 1 health care benefits. http://www.va.gov/opa/publications/benefits_book/benefits_chap01.asp (accessed August 22, 2016).

———. 2016. VA vision care. http://explore.va.gov/health-care/vision (accessed April 6, 2106).

VCE (Vision Center of Excellence). 2016. About us. http://vce.health.mil/About-Us (accessed April 6, 2016).

E

Examples of Recommended Eye Protection for Recreational Sports

Sport	Eye Protection
Baseball	Polycarbonate face guard or other certified safe protection attached to the helmet for batting and base running; sports goggles with polycarbonate lenses[a] for fielding
Basketball	Sports goggles with polycarbonate lenses[a]
Bicycling (LER)[b]	Sturdy street-wear frames with polycarbonate or CR-39 lenses
Boxing	None is available
Fencing	Full-face cage
Field hockey (both sexes)	Goalie: full-face mask; all others: sports goggles with polycarbonate lenses[a]
Football	Polycarbonate shield on helmet
Full-contact martial arts	Not allowed
Handball	Sports goggles with polycarbonate lenses[a]
Ice hockey	Helmet and full-face protection
Lacrosse (female)	Should at least wear sports goggles with polycarbonate lenses and have option to wear helmet and full-face protection
Lacrosse (male)	Helmet and full-face protection required
Racquetball	Sports goggles with polycarbonate lenses[a]
Soccer	Sports goggles with polycarbonate lenses[a]
Softball	Polycarbonate face guard on a helmet for batting and base running; sports goggles with polycarbonate lenses[a] for fielding
Squash	Sports goggles with polycarbonate lenses[a] (U.S. Squash, 2016)
Street hockey	Sports goggles with polycarbonate lenses[a]; goalie: full face cage[c]
Swimming and pool sports	Swim goggles recommended
Tennis: singles	Sturdy street-wear frames with polycarbonate lenses
Track and field (LER)[a]	Sturdy street-wear frames with polycarbonate or CR-39 lenses

continued

Sport	Eye Protection
Water polo	Swim goggles with polycarbonate lenses[a]
Wrestling	None is available

NOTE: [a] Goggles without lenses are not effective.

[b] For sports in which face masks or helmets with eye protection are worn, functionally one-eyed athletes and those with previous eye trauma or surgery for whom their ophthalmologists recommend eye protection must also wear sports goggles with polycarbonate lenses to ensure protection.

[c] A street hockey ball can penetrate into a molded goalie mask and injure an eye.

LER = low eye risk.

SOURCES: Reproduced with permission from AAP, 2004.

REFERENCES

AAP (American Academy of Pediatrics). 2004. The National Eye Institute. Finding the right eye protection. *Pediatrics* 113(3):619–622. https://nei.nih.gov/sports/findingprotection (accessed September 23, 2015).

U.S. Squash. 2016. Protective eyewear. https://www.ussquash.com/officiate/protective-eyewear (accessed May 18, 2016).

F

Eye and Vision Care Professionals and Education

Profession	Definition	Education and Training Requirements (all)	Examples of Professional Responsibilities
Ophthalmologist	An allopathic (M.D.) or osteopathic (D.O.) medical physician who specializes in the medical and surgical treatment of ophthalmic disorders (AAPOS, 2011).	• 4 years of medical school (same education as primary care physicians, pediatricians, surgeons, etc.) (required). • Medical licensure examination by the U.S. Medical Licensure Examination by the Federation of State Medical Boards and the National Board of Medical Examiners. • 1 year of internal medicine or surgery residency (same as surgeons and other medically trained physicians) (required). • 3 years of ophthalmology residency with required volumes of surgical procedures performed and patient examinations (required).	• Provide the full spectrum of eye care, ranging from primary care to the surgical care of patients with complex ophthalmic disorders in all 50 states. • "Diagnoses and treat all eye diseases, [and] perform eye surgery" (AAO, 2013). • "Prescribe and fit eyeglasses and contact lenses to correct [additional] vision problems" (AAO, 2013). • Conduct scientific research on the causes and cures for eye diseases and vision disorders (AAPOS, 2011). • May specialize in a specific area of medical or surgical eye care, such as glaucoma,

continued

Profession	Definition	Education and Training Requirements (all)	Examples of Professional Responsibilities
		• Board certification by the American Board of Ophthalmology of American Board of Medical Specialties. • Eligible for Federal Drug Enforcement Agency license. • State licensure (AAO, 2011).	cornea and external disease, low vision, neuro-ophthalmology, plastic surgery, or pediatrics, among others (AAO, 2013).
Optometrist	A doctor of optometry (O.D.) who provides primary care of the eye and visual system (AAO, 2013).	• 4 years of optometry school (required). • Optometric licensure examination by the National Board of Examiners in Optometry (NBEO) (National Board of Examiners of Optometry, 2016). • Additional board certification by the American Board of Optometry and/or NBEO board certification (optional). • Some optometrists complete an optional residency in a specific area of practice (e.g., pediatric optometry, vision therapy and rehabilitation, etc.) (ORMatch, 2016). • State licensure.	• Examine, diagnose, treat, and manage diseases, injuries, and disorders of the visual system and the eye (AOA, 2012). • Prescribe medications and, as needed, low vision rehabilitation, vision therapies, and can, in two states, perform certain surgical procedures (AOA, 2012). • Prescribe and fit eyeglasses and contact lenses to correct vision problems. • Conduct scientific research on vision and the visual system.
Orthopist	Accredited professional (C.O.) who generally works under ophthalmologists or neuro-ophthalmologists and focuses on the examination and treatment of eye movements abnormalities (AAPOS, 2016).	• 2 years of training and clinical work at a program accredited by American Association of Certified Orthoptists (AOC). • National certification from AOC (AAPOS, 2016).	• Liaison between the ophthalmologist and patient (AACO, 2015). • Assist with patient evaluation, formation of a differential diagnosis, and subsequent patient care (AACO, 2015). Engage in clinical research and the teaching of medical students, orthoptic students, and residents (AACO, 2015; AAPOS, 2016).

Profession	Definition	Education and Training Requirements (all)	Examples of Professional Responsibilities
Optician	A technician who designs, fits, and dispenses corrective lenses for the correction of a person's vision (AAPOS, 2011).	• Formal job training program, certificate program, or associate's degree. Associate's degree programs are accredited by the Commission on Opticianry (OAA, 2016). • Certification by American Board of Opticianry (optional). • Certification by National Contact Lens Examiners (optional). • State licensure required in 23 states (OAA, 2016). States may also require a state written exam, state practical exam, or certification exam.	• Uses prescriptions supplied by ophthalmologists or optometrists to fit eyeglasses, contact lenses, and other eyewear (AAPOS, 2011). • Do not diagnose or treat eye diseases.
Neuro-ophthalmologists	Allopathic or osteopathic physicians who complete residencies in either neurology or ophthalmology and a sub-specialty (AAO, 2013).	• In addition to the requirements for an ophthalmologist or neurologist, neuro-ophthalmologists must complete a fellowship. Fellowships approved by the Association of University Professors of Ophthalmology Fellowship Compliance Committee must be at least 12 months long, in addition to other requirements (FCC, 2013).	• Specialists in visual problems that relate to the nervous system, usually by way of injury from "trauma, inflammation, strokes, tumors, toxicities, and infections" (Weill Cornell Medical College, n.d.).
Low Vision Therapist	Develops and conducts vision functional assessment tests of everyday tasks for those with low vision (AHRQ, 2004).	• Bachelor's degree with emphasis on vision rehabilitation or bachelor's degree with proof of basic competency in all core areas. Certification from Academy for Certification of Vision Rehabilitation & Education Professionals (ACVREP) (AHRQ, 2004).	• Work under the direction of an ophthalmologist or optometrist to provide clinical low vision evaluation, assist with treatment plans, and provide instruction for use of adaptive equipment (ACVREP, 2015).

continued

Profession	Definition	Education and Training Requirements (all)	Examples of Professional Responsibilities
Low Vision Occupational Therapists	An occupational therapy practitioner who helps people with low vision to function at the highest possible level (AOTA, 2011).	• Master's degree from a program accredited by the Accreditation Council for Occupational Therapy Education. • National Board for Certification in Occupational Therapy certification (AOTA, 2016). • State license. • Specialty certification in low vision occupational therapy from the American Occupational Therapy Association (optional) (AOTA, 2011).	• Work with individuals with disabilities or medical conditions to help develop skills needed for independent, daily function (BLS, 2015). • For vision impairment, occupational therapists focus on the promotion of independence and participation in valued activities (AOTA, 2011) through task or environmental modification, education about use of adaptive devices and assistive technology, and assistance using remaining vision (AOTA, 2011). • May specialize in areas of practice such as environmental modifications or pediatrics upon certification (AOTA, 2016).
Orientation and Mobility Specialist	Professional responsible for evaluating mobility capacity and teaching patients how to get oriented and navigate through their environments (AHRQ, 2004).	• "Bachelor's degree . . . with emphasis in orientation and mobility" or bachelor's degree and completion of an orientation and mobility certification preparation program (AHRQ, 2004, p. 163). • ACVREP certified orientation and mobility specialist certificate.	• Assist visually impaired individuals to use remaining vision and senses to determine their orientation and position and negotiate safe movement (ACVREP, 2014a).
Vision Rehabilitation Therapist	Professional responsible for evaluating functional capabilities and teaching behavioral and environmental adaptations to overcome vision disabilities. (AHRQ, 2004).	• Bachelor's degree with emphasis in vision rehabilitation therapy or bachelor's degree with post-secondary education demonstrating knowledge of ACVREP vision rehabilitation therapist knowledge domain areas (ACVREP, 2014b). • Certification from ACVREP.	• Develop individualized rehabilitation plans and teach visually impaired individuals how to use compensatory skills and assistive technology in an effort to enhance opportunities for career and educational development and independent living (ACVREP, 2014b).

REFERENCES

AACO (American Association of Certified Orthoptists). 2015. Qualifications and training. http://orthoptics.org/become-an-orthoptist/qualifications-training (accessed January 11, 2016).

AAO (American Academy of Ophthalmology). 2011. Differences in education between optometrists and ophthalmologists. http://www.aao.org/about/policies/differences-education-optometrists-ophthalmologists (accessed March 29, 2016).

———. 2013. What is an ophthalmologist? http://www.aao.org/eye-health/tips-prevention/what-is-ophthalmologist (accessed January 12, 2016).

AAPOS (American Association for Pediatric Ophthalmology and Strabismus). 2011. Difference between an ophthalmologist, optometrist and optician. http://www.aapos.org/terms/conditions/132 (accessed January 12, 2016).

———. 2016. Orthoptist/orthoptics. http://www.aapos.org/terms/conditions/85 (accessed January 12, 2016).

ACVREP (Academy for Certification of Vision Rehabilitation & Education Professionals). 2014a. *Orientation and mobility specialist certification handbook.* Tucson, AZ: Academy for Certification of Vision Rehabilitation and Education Professionals.

———. 2014b. *Vision rehabilitation therapist certification handbook.* Tucson, AZ: Academy for the Certification of Vision Rehabilitation and Education Professionals.

———. 2015. Certified low vision therapist (CLVT) handbook, section 2—Scope of practice for low vision therapists. https://www.acvrep.org/ascerteon/control/certifications/clvt-scope (accessed January 12, 2016).

AHRQ (Agency for Healthcare Research and Quality). 2004. *Vision rehabilitation for elderly individuals with low vision or blindness.* Rockville, MD: Agency for Healthcare Research and Quality. https://www.cms.gov/Medicare/Coverage/InfoExchange/downloads/rtcvisionrehab.pdf (accessed June 29, 2016).

AOA (American Optometric Association). 2012. What is a doctor of optometry? http://www.aoa.org/about-the-aoa/what-is-a-doctor-of-optometry?sso=y (accessed January 12, 2016).

AOTA (American Occupational Therapy Association). 2011. Occupational therapy services for persons with visual impairment. https://www.aota.org/-/media/Corporate/Files/AboutOT/Professionals/WhatIsOT/PA/Facts/Low%20Vision%20fact%20sheet.pdf (accessed June 29, 2016).

———. 2016. FAQ on OT education and career planning. http://www.aota.org/education-careers/considering-ot-career/faqs/planning.aspx (accessed January 12, 2016).

BLS (Bureau of Labor Statistics). 2015. Occupational therapists. http://www.bls.gov/ooh/healthcare/occupational-therapists.htm (accessed January 12, 2016).

FCC (Fellowship Compliance Committee of the Association of University Professors of Ophthalmology). 2013. Program requirements for fellowship education in neuro-ophthalmology. http://www.aupo.org/subspecialties/neuro/neuro_guidelines.pdf (accessed June 29, 2016).

National Board of Examiners of Optometry. 2016. Welcome to the NBEO website. http://www.optometry.org/president.cfm (accessed March 29, 2016).

OAA (Opticians Association of America). 2016. Becoming an optician. http://www.oaa.org/opticianry-defined/becoming-an-optician (accessed January 12, 2016).

ORMatch. 2016. List of participating programs. https://www.natmatch.com/ormatch/instdirp/aboutproglist.html (accessed April 8, 2016).

Weill Cornell Medical College. n.d. Neuro-ophthalmology. http://weillcornelleye.org/services/neuro.html (accessed April 8, 2016).

G

Medicaid Vision Coverage by State

TABLE G-1 Medicaid Vision Coverage by State

State	Eligible population[a]	Vision benefits covered for children (defined as <21 with exceptions as noted) In addition to the early and periodic screening, diagnostic, and treatment (EPSDT) services for beneficiaries under the age of 21 (with exceptions, as noted); this table lists additional services or stipulations listed by each state's Medicaid program	Vision benefits covered for adults (in addition to the basic services covered by Medicaid in all states per Medicaid guidelines, e.g., emergency eye treatment as a result of injury. Prosthetic eyes are covered in all states but for >21 in Mississippi and Texas)	Copay required?[b]
Alabama[c]	Children under age 19 and pregnant woman up to 146% of federal poverty level (FPL) (Alabama Medicaid Agency, 2014). "Children up to 312% of FPL qualify for CHIP (Children's Health Insurance Program); parents up to 13% of FPL; elderly and disabled individuals with certain medical conditions and income levels" (Norris, 2016a).	Medicaid pays for eye examinations and glasses once every calendar year. Additional covered services may be available if medically necessary (Alabama Medicaid Agency, 2013).	Medicaid pays for eye exams and eyeglasses once every 3 calendar years. Contact lenses may be provided only under certain conditions and when approved ahead of time (Alabama Medicaid Agency, 2013).	$1.30–$3.90 per optometric visit (Alabama Medicaid Agency, 2013).
Alaska[d]	Children up to age 19 are eligible if the family income is up to 203% of FPL,	Between ages 3 and 21, vision screening by an optometrist or an	Medicaid "will cover one vision examination per calendar year by an optometrist or an ophthalmologist to	"$3 for each visit to a health care provider or

	177% of FPL if the child is covered by other insurance. Pregnant women with family income are eligible up to 200% of FPL (Alaska Department of Health and Social Services, 2016). "As of September 1, 2015, other adults with family income up to 138% of FPL; blind or disabled individuals who qualify for Alaska Adult Public Assistance" (Norris, 2015a).	ophthalmologist covered in yearly well child exams, as are referrals to vision specialists. Additional vision exams covered if medically necessary. If glasses are required, "Medicaid will pay for one pair of Medicaid-approved glasses per calendar year" (Alaska Department of Health and Social Services, 2012). One additional pair of eyeglasses covered if medically necessary. Any subsequent eyeglasses covered with prior authorization based upon medical justification submitted by provider. Vision therapy services covered (Alaska Department of Health and Social Services, 2012, 2013).	determine if glasses are required and for treatment of diseases of the eye. Medicaid will pay for one pair of Medicaid-approved glasses per calendar year. One company makes all of the eyeglasses for Medicaid. The same eye doctor that gives you a prescription can order your glasses. If you want different frames or a feature that is not covered, you will need to pay the entire cost of the glasses yourself. The amount that Medicaid would have paid cannot be applied to the cost of other glasses. Additional vision coverage may be authorized if medically necessary" (Alaska Department of Health and Social Services, 2012).	clinic" (Alaska Department of Health and Social Services, 2012).
Arizona[e]	Children under age 1 with family income capped at 147% of FPL. Children ages 1 to 5 with income up to 141% of FPL, and aged 6 to 19 with income up to 133% of FPL (AHCCCS, 2016a). Pregnant women	Vision exams and glasses are covered for children under age 21 (AHCCCS, 2016b,d). Beyond the minimum ESPDT requirement, if/when other procedures or tests are medically indicated, the	"Treatment of medical conditions of the eye, excluding eye examinations for prescriptive lenses and the provision of prescriptive lenses, is covered" (AHCCCS, 2016b, pp. 310–314). "Vision examinations and the provision of prescriptive lenses are covered . . . for	

continued

TABLE G-1 Continued

	are eligible with family income up to 156% of FPL; parents and caretakers are eligible up to 106% of FPL; adults under age 65 whose children have coverage are eligible with family income up to 133% of FPL (AHCCCS, 2016a).	physician is obligated to perform them (AHCCCS, 2016c).	adult members when medically necessary following cataract removal" (AHCCCS, 2016b). "Cataract removal is a covered service for all eligible members. Cataract removal is a covered service when the cataract is visible by exam, ophthalmoscope, or slit lamp, and any of the following apply: (1) visual acuity that cannot be corrected by lenses to better than 20/70 and is reasonably attributable to cataract; (2) in the presence of complete inability to see posterior chamber, vision is confirmed by potential acuity meter reading; or (3) for FFS members, who have corrected visual acuity between 20/50 and 20/70, a second opinion by an ophthalmologist to demonstrate medical necessity may be required" (AHCCCS, 2016b, pp. 310–314). "Other cases that may require medically necessary ophthalmic services include, but are not limited to: (1) phacogenic glaucoma and (2) phacogenic uveitis" (AHCCCS, 2016b, pp. 310–315).	
Arkansas	"Children from 0 to 18 years with incomes up to 211% of FPL; pregnant women with incomes up to 209% of FPL; parents	One exam and pair of glasses, if necessary, every 12 months. Contact lenses, if medically necessary, are covered but require	One visual examination and one pair of glasses are available to all eligible adult Medicaid beneficiaries every 12 months; lens replacement as medically necessary with prior authorization (and must fit	$2 dispensing fee for prescription eyeglasses for patients ages 21 and older

State	Eligible Population	Coverage	Citation
	with incomes up to 133% of FPL; non-elderly adults with household incomes up to 133% of FPL; certain elderly and disabled individuals" (Norris, 2016b).	authorization. Vision therapy developmental testing is covered, with prior authorization (ARMedicaid, n.d.). minimum change criteria); tinted lenses only available for post-op cataract or albino patients (ARMedicaid, n.d.). "A total of twelve (12) office visits allowed per state fiscal year for any combination of the following: certified nurse midwife, nurse practitioner, physician, medical services provided by a dentist, medical services furnished by an optometrist and Rural Health Clinics" (Arkansas Department of Human Services, 2012, p. 7).	(Arkansas Department of Human Services, 2012; ARMedicaid, n.d.; Kaiser Family Foundation, 2012a).
California[f]	"Children from birth through age 18 with family income levels up to 266% of FPL; pregnant women with incomes up to 213% of FPL; and nonelderly adults—with or without dependent children—with incomes up to 138% of FPL" (Norris, 2015b).	Children "are eligible for a routine eye exam every 24 months, which checks the health of the eyes and tests for an eyeglass prescription. Only members under 21 years old . . . receive coverage for eyeglasses (frames and lenses)" (CDHCS, 2016a). "All Medi-Cal members are eligible for a routine eye exam every 24 months, which checks the health of the eyes and tests for an eyeglass prescription . . . residents of a nursing home receive coverage for eyeglasses (frames and lenses)" (CDHCS, 2016a). This is limited to one pair of glasses every 2 years. For lost or broken glasses, an interim pair will be covered once in 2 years. "Contact lens testing may be covered if the use of eyeglasses is not possible due to eye disease or condition. Low-vision testing is available for those with vision impairment that is not correctable by standard glasses, contact lenses, medicine	Some members have a $1 copay, others have no copay (CDHCS, 2016b; HPSM, 2016; Kaiser Family Foundation, 2012b).

continued

TABLE G-1 Continued

			or surgery and that interferes with a person's ability to perform everyday activities (e.g., age-related macular degeneration)" (CDHCS, 2016a). "All Medi-Cal members are eligible for a routine eye exam every 24 months, which checks the health of the eyes and tests for an eyeglass prescription . . . residents of a nursing home receive coverage for eyeglasses (frames and lenses)" (CDHCS, 2016a). This is limited to one pair of glasses every 2 years. For lost or broken glasses, an interim pair will be covered once in 2 years.	
Colorado[g]	"Children 0–18 with family incomes up to 142% of FPL; children with family incomes up to 260% of FPL qualify for Child Health Plan Plus (CHP+); pregnant women with family income up to 195% of FPL; pregnant women with family income up to 260% of FPL qualify for CHP+; non-elderly adults	Children's vision benefits include medically necessary exams and eyewear. Contacts are allowed only if eyeglasses do not correct the refraction error. Future policy may allow orthoptic/pleoptic vision training for children with a diagnosis of convergence insufficiency (Colorado Medical Assistance Program, 2015).	"Adult vision care benefit includes medically necessary eye exams, glasses, and contact lenses only after surgery" (COHCPF, 2016). Does not include orthotic or eye training therapy (COHCPF, 2016).	$2 per visit. Children under 19 and pregnant women do not have copayment (COHCPF, 2016).

| **Connecticut**[b] | with family income up to 138% of FPL; some individuals who are elderly or disabled" (Norris, 2015c). "HUSKY A: Children ages 0–18 with incomes up to 196% FPL; pregnant women with incomes up to 258% FPL; parents of dependent children with incomes up to 155% of FPL (for parents who were already enrolled in HUSKY prior to August 2015 and who have earned income from a job, the household income limit will continue to be 201% of FPL until August 1, 2016).

HUSKY B: Children up to 318% of FPL.

HUSKY C/MED-Connect: Aged, blind, and disabled beneficiaries who meet income and asset criteria.

HUSKY D: Childless adults with incomes up to 138% of FPL" (Anderson, 2015a). | "Vision care is a covered service that can be done by ophthalmologists, optometrists, and opticians. . . . Eye exams are covered" (Husky Health Connecticut, 2015, p. 16). | "Vision care is a covered service that can be done by ophthalmologists, optometrists, and opticians. . . . Eye exams are covered. For members who are age 21 or older, one (1) pair of eyeglasses will be covered every 2 years. If there has been a serious change in vision and the member needs a new prescription for eyeglasses, they will be covered. No exception will be made for eyeglasses that are lost, stolen, or broken" (Husky Health Connecticut, 2015, p. 16). Special lenses may be covered when specific criteria are met, lenses are considered necessary, and a prior authorization is submitted. | No copay for HUSKY A, C, and D. $15 copay for HUSKY B (Husky Health Connecticut, 2016). |

continued

TABLE G-1 Continued

Delaware[i]	"Children birth to 1 year with family income up to 212% of FPL; children 1–5 years with family income up to 142% of FPL; children 6–18 with family income up to 133% of FPL; pregnant women with family income up to 212% of FPL; parents with family income up to 138% of FPL; childless, non-elderly adults with family income up to 138% of FPL; elderly and disabled individuals with special requirements and who meet certain income limits. Children 1–18 up to 212% of FPL are covered through the Healthy Children" (Anderson, 2015b).	Lenses and frames covered when medically necessary. The Delaware Medical Assistance Program (DMAP) will cover the replacement of damaged lenses and/or repair broken frames. The DMAP may cover contact lenses to correct a medical condition if the medical condition is not correctable with eyeglasses. This service must be prior authorized (DMAP, n.d.).	Routine eye care and glasses are not covered except for aphakic or bandage lenses necessary after cataract surgery. Examination limited to the diagnosis and treatment of medical conditions (DMAP, 2016).	None
District of Columbia[i]	"Children 0–18 with incomes up to 319% of FPL; pregnant women with incomes up to 319% of FPL; parents with dependent children with incomes up to 216% of FPL; other non-elderly adults with incomes up to 210% of FPL" (Anderson, 2015c).	One pair of eyeglasses covered every year. A minimum diopter correction is required. Repairs or replacements covered if medically necessary (DHCF, 2016).	If medically necessary, DC Medicaid pays for 1 pair of glasses every 2 years. A minimum diopter correction is required (DHCF, 2012, 2016).	$2/dispensing service for glasses (Kaiser Family Foundation, 2012a).

| Florida | "Children up to 1 year old with family income up to 206% of FPL; children 1–5 with family income up to 140% of FPL; children 6–18 with family income up to 133% of FPL; pregnant women with family income up to 191% of FPL; young adults 19–20 with family income up to 30% of FPL; adults with dependents with family income up to 30% of FPL. People who qualify for Supplemental Security Income automatically qualify for Medicaid" (Norris, 2015d). | Eyeglasses are limited to two pairs of glasses per enrollee (under age 21) per year. Contact lenses are limited to "when the recipient has a documented medical condition where eyeglasses would not provide any benefit for their visual impairment" (Florida Agency for Health Care Administration, 2015, p. 3). Other services for enrollees under age 21 covered if approved and medically necessary (Florida Agency for Health Care Administration, 2015). | Eyeglasses are limited to one frame per enrollee every 2 years and two lenses per enrollee per year (Florida Agency for Health Care Administration, 2015). "Contact lenses are limited to Enrollees who have unilateral aphakia or bilateral aphakia" (Florida Agency for Health Care Administration, n.d., p. 6).

Polycarbonate or thermoplastic lenses covered for safety, or when medically necessary. Metal frames are covered when medically necessary. Eyeglass repair is covered except for when cost exceeds that of new eyeglasses (Florida Agency for Health Care Administration, 2015). "Only elements of the frames or lenses that are damaged beyond repair may be replaced" (Florida Agency for Health Care Administration, 2015, p. 3). | $2/visit for optometrist visits (Kaiser Family Foundation, 2012b). |
| Georgia[k] | "Children up to age 1 with family income up to 205% of FPL; children 1–5 with family income up to 149% of FPL; children 6–18 with family income up to 133% of FPL; pregnant women with family income up to 220% of FPL; parents with family income up to 35% of FPL; individuals who are elderly, blind, or disabled" (Anderson, 2015d). | Eye exams and eyeglasses are covered once per year. Second exams covered with prior approval, second glasses covered with minimum diopter change. Polycarbonate lenses covered if medically necessary. Contact lenses covered with prior approval. Replacement of broken glasses covered with prior approval. Replacement | Eyeglass coverage is limited to nursing facility residents with physician referral. Adults are not eligible for eyeglasses, refractions, dispensing fees, and other refractive services. Members can receive medical diagnostic and treatment services for ocular disease. Vision therapy is covered with prior approval (Georgia DCH, 2016). | $0.50–$3/ optometrist visit (Georgia DCH, 2016; Kaiser Family Foundation, 2012b). |

continued

TABLE G-1 Continued

		of lost eyeglasses not covered. New lenses must improve visual acuity by at least one line on a standard acuity chart. Vision therapy covered with prior approval (Children's Vision Georgia, 2013; Georgia DCH, 2016).		
Hawaii[l]	"Children with family income levels up to 308% of FPL. Pregnant women with family income up to 191% of FPL. Adults with family income up to 133% of FPL" (Norris, 2015e).	Eyeglasses and a routine eye exam by an optometrist are covered once every 12 months for those age 20 and under. More frequent exams covered if medically necessary with prior authorization (Hawaii Department of Health, 2011a).	Eyeglasses and a routine eye exam by an optometrist are covered once every 24 months. More frequent exams covered if medically necessary with prior authorization. Prescription lenses and cataract removal covered for all members (Hawaii Department of Health, 2011a). Non-covered services include "tinted lenses (except in the case of aphakia); contact lenses for cosmetic purposes; bifocal contact lenses; oversized lenses; blended or progressive bifocal lenses; tinted or absorptive lenses (except for aphakia, albinism, glaucoma, medical photophobia); trifocal lenses (except as a specific job requirement); spare glasses" (Hawaii Department of Health, 2011b, p. 3)	
Idaho	"Children ages 0–5 with family income up to 142% of FPL. Children ages 6–18 and pregnant women with	One eye examination during any 12-month period by a physician or optometrist to determine need for glasses.	Services necessary to treat or monitor a chronic condition, such as diabetes, that may damage the eye; and acute conditions that if left untreated may cause permanent	"$3.65/visit, up to 5% of income/ year across all services"

	family income up to 133% of FPL. Parents with family income up to 124% of FPL . . . additional eligibility criteria for individuals who are aged or disabled" (Noris, 2016c).	Following a diagnosis, eyeglasses are covered, one pair every 4 years except if there is documentation of a major visual change (Idaho Department of Health and Welfare, 2009). "Scratch resistant coating is required for all plastic and polycarbonate lenses" (Idaho Department of Health and Welfare, 2009). Tinted lenses only covered with a diagnosis of albinism or other extreme medical condition. Contact lenses covered in extreme conditions when eyeglasses are not medically sufficient. Replacement of broken or lost frames is not covered (Idaho Department of Health and Welfare, 2009).	or chronic damage to the eye (Idaho Department of Health and Welfare, 2009).	(Kaiser Family Foundation, 2012b).
Illinois	"Children ages 0–18 with family income levels up to 142% of FPL. Pregnant women with family income up to 208% of FPL. Adults with family income up to 133% of FPL" (Anderson, 2016).	"One routine eye exam each year. . . . One pair of [eye]glasses every year for members under age 21. Medically necessary contact lenses. Replacement glasses [covered] for members aged 19 and 20 as needed" (Aetna, 2016).	"Diagnosis and treatment of medical conditions of the eye (may be provided by an optometrist operating within the scope of his or her license)" (Illinois Department of HFS, 2009, p. 38). One pair of glasses covered every 2 years (Illinois Department of HFS, 2012). "Replacement lenses [covered] for members ages 21 and older, when medically necessary. One	$3.65/visit to an optometrist (Kaiser Family Foundation, 2012b).

continued

TABLE G-1 Continued

Indiana[m]	"Children up to 1 year with household income up to 208% of FPL. Children ages 1–18 with household income up to 158% of FPL. Pregnant women with household income up to 208% of FPL. Adults with incomes up to 138% of FPL can enroll in HIP 2.0" (Norris, 2015f).	"One routine vision care examination and refraction for members 20 years old and younger, per rolling calendar year" unless more frequent care is medically necessary (IHCP, 2016). Coverage for eyeglasses, including frames and lenses, is limited to a maximum of one pair per year except when a specified minimum prescription change makes additional coverage medically necessary or the member's lenses and/or frames are lost, stolen, or broken beyond repair (IHCP, 2016). Tinted and polycarbonate lenses covered when medically necessary (IHCP, 2016).	replacement pair of [eye]glasses each year if the first pair of [eye]glasses is lost or broken beyond repair" (Aetna, 2016). One routine eye exam covered each year (Aetna, 2016; Illinois Department of HFS, 2012). The standard Medicaid plan is limited to one vision examination and refraction every 2 years for members ages 21 and older, unless more frequent care is medically necessary (IHCP, 2016). Coverage for eyeglasses, including frames and lenses, is limited to a maximum of one pair every 5 years. Exceptions are when a specified minimum prescription change makes additional coverage medically necessary or the member's lenses and/or frames are lost, stolen, or broken beyond repair (IHCP, 2016). Tinted and polycarbonate lenses covered when medically necessary (IHCP, 2016).	
Iowa[n]	"Children up to age 1 with family income up to 375% of FPL. Children ages	Eye exams covered once every 12 months and more often if there are complaints	Eye exams covered once every 12 months and more often if there are complaints or symptoms of eye disease or injury.	$2/day for optometrist or optician services

	1–18 with family income up to 167% of FPL; children with family income up to 302% of FPL may qualify for the Hawk-I program. Pregnant women with family income up to 375% of FPL. Adults with family income up to 133% of FPL" (Norris, 2016d).	or symptoms of eye disease or injury. Contact lenses covered following cataract surgery or other extreme conditions when vision cannot be corrected with glasses. New frames covered three times for children up to 1, four times for children 1–3. One time every 12 months for children ages 4 to 7. Once every 24 months after the age of 8. Repairs and replacement frames are covered with no limit. Vision therapy covered when medically necessary. Polycarbonate lenses and safety frames covered for children through 7 years and when medically necessary (Iowa Department of Human Services, 2014).	Glasses covered once every 24 months. Contact lenses covered following cataract surgery or other extreme conditions when vision cannot be corrected with glasses. Replacement of lost or damaged glasses is covered once every 12 months except when member has mental or physical disability. Vision therapy covered when medically necessary. Polycarbonate lenses and safety frames covered when medically necessary (Iowa Department of Human Services, 2014).	(Kaiser Family Foundation, 2012a,b).
Kansas	"Children up to age 1 with family income up to 166% of FPL. Children ages 1–5 with family income up to 149% of FPL. Children ages 6–18 with family income up to 133% of FPL; children with family income up to		Prescription drugs, medical care by doctors, and eyewear coverage are included for most people (KanCare, 2012). "One complete eye exam covered every 4 years . . . however a total of two eye exams are covered per month to detect	$2/date of service for glasses; $2/date of service for visits (Kaiser Family Foundation, 2012a,b).

continued

TABLE G-1 Continued

	242% of FPL are eligible for CHIP. [Additional eligibility guidelines for] individuals who are elderly or disabled" (Norris, 2015g).		and/or follow medical conditions. . . . Refraction is not included in a basic eye exam" (KHPA, 2010, p. 8-3). Eyeglasses are covered with certain limitations, polycarbonate lenses are covered when considered medically necessary. Contact lenses are covered upon approval through a prior authorization (KHPA, 2010). Kansas provides Medicaid coverage through three managed care organizations (MCOs), all of which cover eyeglasses. One of the MCOs (United Healthcare) has more expansive benefits, stating coverage for a "better choice of eyeglass frames . . . replacement if glasses are lost or stolen" and possibly contact lenses for some members (KanCare, 2016).	
Kentucky[o]	"Children up to age 1 with family income up to 195% of FPL. Children ages 1–18 with family income up to 159% of FPL; children with family income up to 213% of FPL are eligible for the Kentucky Children's Health Insurance Program. Pregnant women with family income up to 195% of FPL. Adults with income up to 133% of FPL"	New patient eye exams limited to one every 3 years, established patient eye exams limited to one every 12 months. Physician office visits limited to two every 12 months per diagnosis. Eyeglasses covered up to $200 for Global Choice members and up to $400 for Family Choice, Comprehensive Choice and Optimum Choice members.	New patient eye exams limited to one every 3 years, established patient eye exams limited to one every 12 months. Physician office visits limited to two every 12 months per diagnosis. Eyeglasses are not covered. Contact lenses are not covered (Kentucky CHFS, 2007).	$3/visit for adults, $0/visits for children (Commonwealth of Kentucky, n.d.).

| Louisiana[p] | (Norris, 2015h). Workers with disabilities up to 250% of FPL (Kentucky CHFS, 2015). "Children ages 0–18 with household income up to 212% of FPL; kids with family income between 212% and 250% of FPL are eligible for the Louisiana Children's Health Insurance Program. Pregnant women with household income up to 133% of FPL. Parents with dependent children with household income up to 19% of FPL. . . . [There are other qualifications for] those who receive SSI or who are elderly, blind, or disabled" (Norris, 2016e). | Tinted lenses covered with diagnosis of photophobia. Contact lenses not covered (Kentucky CHFS, 2007). "Examinations and treatment of eye conditions, including examinations for vision correction [and] refraction error. Regular eyeglasses are covered when they meet a certain minimum strength requirement. Medically necessary specialty eyewear and contact lenses can be covered with prior authorization. Contact lenses are covered if they are the only means for restoring vision. Other related services may be covered if medically necessary" (Louisiana Medicaid, 2016, p. 18). | "Examinations and treatment of eye conditions such as infections and cataracts are covered" (Louisiana Medicaid, 2016, p. 18). If the recipient has both Medicare and Medicaid, some vision-related services may be covered. "The recipient should contact Medicare for more information since Medicare would be the primary payer. . . . Non-covered services include routine eye examinations for vision correction . . . [and] refraction error [as well as] eyeglasses" (Louisiana Medicaid, 2016, p. 18). | Medicaid may pick up a calculated portion of the payment as a Medicare crossover claim.[p] |
| Maine | "Children up to 1 year old with household income up to 191% of FPL. Children ages 1–18 with household income up to 157% of FPL; children with family income up to 208% of FPL qualify for the Children's Health | One annual routine eye exam covered (Maine DHHS, 2012). "Contact lenses [are covered] only for treatment of ocular pathology, or for cases in which acuity is not correctable to 20/70 with | One routine eye exam covered every 3 rolling calendar years, unless specific medical diagnoses warrant more frequent examination (Maine DHHS, 2012). Contact lenses not covered. "One pair of eyeglasses per lifetime is covered when the power is equal to or greater than 10.00 diopters" (Maine DHHS, 2012, p. 5). | $0.50–$2/ day of service for glasses; up to $20/month if service is provided by an optician (Kaiser Family |

continued

TABLE G-1 Continued

	Insurance Program; 19- and 20-year-olds with household income up to 156% of FPL; pregnant women with household income up to 209% of FPL; parents and other caretakers with household income up to 100 percent of FPL" (Anderson, 2015e).	ophthalmic lenses, but can be improved to 20/70 or better with contact lenses" (Maine DHHS, 2012, p. 4). Eyeglasses covered when the refractive error in at least one eye meets a minimum requirement, with prior authorization. Replacement frames and repairs covered (Maine DHHS, 2012). Glasses must be purchased through the state contractor. Tint, photochromatic, or ultraviolet (UV) lenses covered when medically necessary. Orthoptic therapy covered with prior authorization when medically necessary (Maine DHHS, 2012).	Replacement frames and repairs covered. Glasses must be purchased through the state contractor. Tint, photochromatic, or UV lenses covered when medically necessary. Orthoptic therapy covered with prior authorization when medically necessary (Maine DHHS, 2012).	Foundation, 2012a). Visits may require a copay between $0.50 and $3 per visit, up to $30 per month (Kaiser Family Foundation, 2012b).
Maryland[q]	"Children ages 0–21 with household income up to 317% of FPL. Pregnant women with household income up to 250% of FPL. Adults with household income up to 133% of FPL. Aged, blind, or disabled individuals" (Anderson, 2014).	One pair of glasses covered every year if medically necessary. Replacement eyeglasses covered. One eye exam covered every year (Maryland DHMH, 2014).	Eye examination covered every 2 years. Glasses are not covered (Maryland DHMH, n.d.).	

| Massachusetts | "Children up to 1 year with household income up to 200% of FPL. Children ages 1–18 with household income up to 150% of FPL. Pregnant women with household income up to 200% of FPL. Adults with household income up to 133% of FPL" (Anderson, 2015f). | Comprehensive eye exams covered once every 12 months. More often if medically necessary. One pair of eyeglasses covered. New pair covered with a specific change in prescription. Replacement glasses covered, but only covered within the first 12 months with prior authorization. Eyeglass repairs covered. Tinted lenses and contact lenses covered if medically necessary (MassHealth, 2008). | Comprehensive eye exams covered once every 24 months. More often if medically necessary. Replacement glasses covered, but only covered within the first 12 months with prior authorization. Eyeglass repairs covered after the first 12 months. Tinted lenses and contacts covered if medically necessary (MassHealth, 2008). | |
| Michigan[r] | "Children up to 1 year with household income up to 195% of FPL. Children ages 1–18 with household income up to 160% of FPL; children with household income up to 212% of FPL qualify for MICHILD (low-cost health insurance for kids). Pregnant women with household income up to 195% of FPL. Adults with household income up to 133% of FPL" (Anderson, | "Corrective lenses and/or frames are covered if determined to be medically necessary by a licensed optometrist or ophthalmologist. Determination of medical necessity is based on specific diopter criteria and/or concurrent complicating medical conditions. . . . Two pairs of replacement eyeglasses or contact lenses in a year for recipients | One eye exam is covered every 24 months to determine the prescription for corrective lenses. Vision therapy is covered for limited clinical conditions (MDHHS, 2016, p. 25). "Corrective lenses and/or frames are covered if determined to be medically necessary by a licensed optometrist or ophthalmologist. Determination of medical necessity is based on specific diopter criteria and/or concurrent complicating medical conditions. . . . One pair of replacement eyeglasses or contact lenses in a year for recipients age 21 and over" is covered | $2/date of service for glasses; $2/visit (Kaiser Family Foundation, 2012a,b). |

continued

TABLE G-1 Continued

	2015g). Aged, blind, or disabled individuals are also eligible (State of Michigan, 2016).	under age 21. Prior authorization is required for eyeglasses that exceed the replacement limits" (MDHHS, 2016, p. 25).	without prior authorization (MDHHS, 2016, p. 25). "Prior authorization is required for eyeglasses that exceed the replacement limits" (MDHHS, 2016, p. 25).	
Minnesota	"Children up to 1 year with household income up to 283% of FPL. Children ages 1–18 with household income up to 275% of FPL. Pregnant women with household income up to 278% of FPL. Adults with household income up to 138% of FPL; adults with income between 138% and 200% of FPL qualify for MNCare" (Norris, 2015i).	"Deluxe eyeglass frames . . . for children" (Minnesota DHS, 2016). "Visual therapy for amblyopia is limited to children under 10 years old. If improvement is not noted after four sessions, the recipient must be referred to an appropriate professional (for example, neurologist or ophthalmologist) for further evaluation" (Minnesota DHS, 2016).	Eye exams are covered without copay; eyeglasses are covered without cost sharing, limited to one pair every 2 years unless lost, broken, or stolen (Minnesota DHS, 2013). Tinted, UV, polarized and photochromatic lenses covered if medically necessary (Minnesota DHS, 2016). Contact lenses covered with medically necessary diagnosis or with prior authorization (Minnesota DHS, 2016).	$3/optician visit, or $25/ pair of glasses (Kaiser Family Foundation, 2012a). Higher copay is for beneficiaries in "Group B"; parents and caretakers with income up to 215% of FPL. $3/visit required for a non-preventive service (Kaiser Family Foundation, 2012b).
Mississippi	"Parents with dependent children are eligible with household incomes up to 22% of FPL. Children are eligible for Medicaid	"2 pairs of eyeglasses per year [for] EPSDT-eligible beneficiaries. Eligible for more services if medically necessary" (Mississippi	"One complete pair of eyeglasses per 5 years. . . . This includes eyeglass lenses and frames. Repairs and replacements not covered. . . . Tinted, photochromatic or UV protected lenses [covered] when	$3/pair of eyeglasses; $3/ visit, limited to 12 per year (Mississippi

	or CHIP with household incomes up to 209% of FPL, and pregnant women are eligible with household incomes up to 194% of FPL" (Norris, 2015j).	Division of Medicaid, 2016).	medically necessary" (Mississippi Division of Medicaid, 2014, p. 7). One eye examination by optometrist or ophthalmologist every 5 years. Contact lenses provided for specific disease or injury (Mississippi Division of Medicaid, 2014).	Division of Medicaid, 2016).
Missouri	"Parents with dependent children are eligible with household incomes up to 18% of FPL. Children are eligible for Medicaid or CHIP with household incomes up to 300% of FPL, and pregnant women are eligible with household incomes up to 196% of FPL" (Healthinsurance.org, 2015a).	One eye exam covered per year (MO HealthNet, 2016). Frames covered once every 24 months. Lenses covered if medically necessary or required for school performance once every 2 years. Photochromatic, tinted, and polycarbonate lenses covered when medically necessary. Replacement of broken or lost frames and/or lenses covered when glasses are necessary for school with prior approval. Orthoptic and/or pleoptic training covered when medically necessary (MO HealthNet, 2016).	One eye exam allowed per 2 years, allowed every year for the blind, pregnant women, and nursing home residents (MO HealthNet, 2016). Frames covered once every 24 months. Lenses covered if medically necessary once every 2 years. Photochromatic, tinted, and polycarbonate lenses covered when medically necessary. Replacement frames not covered unless significant change in diopter. Orthoptic and/or pleoptic training covered when medically necessary (MO HealthNet, 2016).	$0.50–$3/service for glasses or visit (Kaiser Family Foundation, 2012a,b).
Montana[s]	"Parents 50–138% of FPL and childless adults with incomes up to 138% of FPL" (Kaiser Family	Eye exams are covered. One exam per year, unless medically necessary. Glasses providers must show	One eye exam every 12 months unless vision changes significantly, or for treatment of eye disease (Montana DPHHS, 2016). Glasses providers	$3/service for the Healthy Montana Kids/ CHIP program members.

continued

TABLE G-1 Continued

	Foundation, 2015, p. 3). Pregnant women with incomes up to 157% of FPL; children are eligible for Medicaid or CHIP with incomes up to 261% of FPL (Norris, 2016f).	special frames approved by Medicaid, which are covered, with a 24-month warranty. Most add-ons, including photo-grey lenses, are not covered (Montana DPHHS, 2013).	must show special frames approved by Medicaid, which are covered, with a 24-month warranty. One pair of glasses covered every 365 days, but most add-ons, including photo-grey lenses, are not covered (Montana DPHHS, 2013, 2016).	Effective June 1, 2016, $4/service for Medicaid program including the expansion-HELP program (Montana DPHHS, 2016).
Nebraska[t]	Parents with dependent children are eligible with income up to 58% of poverty. Pregnant women with income up to 194% of poverty (Nebraska DHHS, 2016). Children 0–1 with income up to 162% of poverty, ages 1–5 up to 145% of poverty, ages 6–18 up to 133% of poverty (Nebraska DHHS, 2016). CHIP is up to 213% of poverty (Nebraska DHHS, 2016). Adults that meet criteria for the aged, blind, and disabled with income up to 100% of the poverty level.	Eye exams covered annually. More frequent eye exams covered if medically necessary. Vision therapy covered when medically necessary (NMAP, 2003).	"Eye examinations to determine the need for glasses, the purchase of glasses, and necessary repairs. . . . Eye exams for adults 21 years and older are limited to one every 24 months. . . . Eyeglasses including lenses and frames are covered when required for medical reasons" (Nebraska Medicaid Program, 2014). Repairs covered when less costly then new frames. Contact lenses covered when medically necessary. Vision therapy training covered when medically necessary. Polycarbonate, tint, and UV frames covered when medically necessary. (NMAP, 2003).	$2/pair of glasses or visit (Kaiser Family Foundation, 2012a,b).
Nevada[u]	"The aged, blind, and disabled. Also, coverage is available if your household	"Vision screenings as referred by any appropriate health, developmental, or	"Refractive examinations performed by an optometrist or ophthalmologist are covered for Medicaid recipients of all ages	None

	income is up to 138% of poverty (about $16,105 for a single person). For pregnant women, income can be up to 160% of FPL, and children are eligible for CHIP with household income up to 200% of poverty" (Norris, 2015k).	educational professional after a Healthy Kids Screening Exam. Optometrists and ophthalmologists may perform such exams without prior authorization upon request or identification of medical need. "Medical Need" may be identified as any ophthalmological examination performed to diagnose, treat, or follow any ophthalmological condition that has been identified. . . . Glasses may be provided at any interval without prior authorization for EPSDT recipients, as long as there is a change in refractive status from the most recent exam, or for broken or lost glasses" (DHCFP, 2015, p. 7).	once every 12 months. Any exceptions require prior authorization" (DHCFP, 2015, p. 7). Lenses are covered with prior authorization. Vision therapy covered with prior authorization (DHCFP, 2015).
New Hampshire[v]	Adults with household incomes up to 133% of poverty, and pregnant women with incomes up to 196% of poverty. Children age 1–18 are eligible for Medicaid with a household	Same as adults except that replacement of lost glasses is covered once in a lifetime (New Hampshire Medicaid, 1994, 2013).	Fee-for-service (FFS) as well as via two separate MCOs, which offer the same coverage as FFS. One MCO (NH Health Families) offers a vision credit if someone opts for frames outside of standard benefits (New Hampshire Medicaid Care Management, 2015).

continued

TABLE G-1 Continued

	income up to 196% FPL. Children aged 0–18 are eligible for CHIP with household incomes >196% FPL and up to 318% of poverty. In addition, individuals are covered on the basis of being elderly, blind, or disabled (Norris, 2016g).		"One complete eye exam [covered] every 12 months to determine the need for glasses. When certain prescription requirements are met, one pair of single vision glasses; or one pair bifocal glasses or one pair each reading and distance glasses. Replacement glasses only when vision changes of 1/2 diopter or more occur in each eye. One repair of glasses per year— replacement of broken parts only" (New Hampshire Medicaid Client Services, 2014, p. 1). "Contact lenses [are covered] for ocular pathology in cases where visual acuity is not correctable to 20/70 or better without contact lenses, or when required to correct aphakia or to treat corneal disease" (New Hampshire Medicaid, 2013, p. 4). Transition lenses covered for recipients with ocular albinism (New Hampshire Medicaid, 2013). Trifocal lenses for work. Eye exams covered "to diagnose and monitor medical conditions of the eye" (New Hampshire Medicaid, 2013, p. 4).	
New Jersey	"The aged, blind, and disabled. Also, adults with income up to 138% of poverty, and pregnant women with income up to 200% of poverty. Children are eligible for Medicaid or CHIP with income up to	"Age 18 and under . . . replacement eyeglasses or contact lenses annually if prescription changes. . . . Replacement eyeglasses or contact lenses may be dispensed more frequently if significant vision changes	"[Age] 60 and older—Replacement eyeglasses or contact lenses annually if prescription changes. Age 19 to 59— Replacement eyeglasses or contact lenses every two years if prescription changes. Replacement eyeglasses or contact lenses may be dispensed more frequently if significant vision changes occur. Contact	$5.00 per office visit for Plan C and Plan D members (New Jersey DMAHS, 2004).

	350% of poverty (Norris, 2014a).	occur. Contact lens exams and fittings are covered only when deemed medically necessary over glasses. . . . Cover[age applies to] one routine eye exam per year" (Horizon NJ Health, 2014, p. 21).	lens exams and fittings are covered only when deemed medically necessary over glasses. . . . Cover[age applies to] one routine eye exam per year" (Horizon NJ Health, 2014, p. 21) "Members with diabetes can have an eye exam every year, which should include a dilated retinal eye exam" (Horizon NJ Health, 2014, p. 17).	
New Mexico[w]	"The aged, blind, and disabled. Also, adults with income up to 138% of poverty. Pregnant women are eligible for pregnancy-related coverage with household income up to 250% of poverty. Children are eligible for CHIP with income up to 240% of poverty (ages 7–18) or 300% of poverty (ages 0–6)" (Norris, 2015l).	Limited to one routine eye exam per year unless otherwise medically necessary. One frame and one set of corrective lenses covered per year; "more frequently when an ophthalmologist or optometrist recommends a change in prescription due to a medical condition" (NMAC, 2010). Polycarbonate lenses are covered. New lenses covered for diopter changes to plus or minus 0.75 or with the diagnosis of certain medical conditions; if the lenses cannot fit into the existing frames, frames will be replaced as well.	Limited to one routine vision exam every 36 months. One frame and set of corrective lenses covered every 36 months; "more frequently when an ophthalmologist or optometrist recommends a change in prescription due to a medical condition" (NMAC, 2010). Polycarbonate lenses covered for recipients with certain medical conditions, "with monocular vision . . . [or with] high-activity physical jobs" (NMAC, 2010). New lenses covered for diopter changes to plus or minus 0.75 or with the diagnosis of certain medical conditions. Contact lenses covered with prior authorization. Lost or broken eyeglasses covered with documentation on the recipient's visual examination record (NMAC, 2010). Medicaid expansion recipients are not covered for eye exams to correct refract error or eyeglasses. Eye exams only	Visit copay ranges from $0 to $7 (Kaiser Family Foundation, 2012b).

continued

TABLE G-1 Continued

		Contact lenses covered with prior authorization (NMAC, 2010). Lost or broken eyeglasses covered with documentation on the recipient's visual examination record (NMAC, 2010).	covered to detect a disease of the eye or when part of a wellness exam. Eyeglasses only covered following cataracts removal surgery.	
New York[x]	Adults with incomes up to 138% poverty level. Pregnant women and infants to age 1 with income up to 223% of poverty level. Separate CHIP is available in New York for all children with income up to 400% of poverty level (Norris, 2015m).	"Polycarbonate lenses covered if needed for safety reasons; medical documentation is not necessary in this case" (New York State Medicaid Program, 2013, p. 10).	Optometric eye exam covered every 2 years, Covered more often if medically necessary. Glasses are covered when the initial correction or change in correction is at least .50 diopter (New York State Medicaid Program, 2013). Eyeglass lenses may be changed more frequently than every 2 years when medically necessary. Contact lenses covered when medically necessary. Orthoptic training may be covered with prior authorization (New York State Medicaid Program, 2013). "The maximum time period for which approval of a treatment plan will be granted is 6 months. At the end of the 6 month approved period, it is necessary to reapply for prior approval and supply information that details the progress made, the anticipated treatment plan, and the prognosis" (New York State Medicaid Program, 2013, p. 13).	None (New York State Medicaid Program, 2013).

| North Carolina | "The aged, blind, and disabled. Also, parents with dependent children are eligible for Medicaid with a household income up to 45 percent of poverty level, and children are eligible for Medicaid or CHIP with incomes up to 211% of poverty; maternity-related coverage is available for pregnant women with incomes up to 196% of poverty" (Norris, 2015n). | Eligible for routine eye exams once per year. Eligible for eyeglasses once per year with prior approval. Eligible for contact lenses if medically necessary with prior approval (NC DMA, 2015b). | Routine eye exams and eyeglasses are not covered for adults (Kaiser Family Foundation, 2012a; NC DMA, 2015a). Pregnant women can request an eye exam if medically necessary due to complications of pregnancy (NC DMA, 2015b).

"General ophthalmological services are covered for . . . patients when the level of service includes several routine optometric/ophthalmologic examination techniques that are integrated with the diagnostic evaluation" and are deemed medically necessary, and "not in excess of the beneficiary's needs" (NC DMA, 2015a, p. 3). | $3/visit (Kaiser Family Foundation, 2012b). |
| North Dakota[y] | "The aged, blind, and disabled as well as all adults are eligible with household incomes up to 133% of poverty, and pregnant women with incomes up to 147% of poverty. Children are eligible for Medicaid or CHIP with household incomes up to 170% of poverty (Norris, 2015o). | Covers one eye exam and refraction every 365 days for beneficiaries under age 20 (NDDHS, 2011). Exceptions made when medically necessary. Eye glasses covered once every 365 days (NDDHS, 2011). More often if medically necessary with prior authorization. Photochromic, tinted, UV, slab-off, and Fresnel prism lenses covered if medically necessary with prior | Covers one eye exam and refraction every 2 years. Exceptions made when medically necessary, or for adult diabetic clients (NDDHS, 2011). Eyeglasses covered once every 2 years. More often if medically necessary with prior authorization. Photochromic, certain tints, UV, slab-off, and Fresnel prism lenses covered if medically necessary with prior authorization (NDDHS, 2011). Some hard contact lenses covered for the correction of certain conditions. Replacement lenses and frames covered after 24 months (NDDHS, 2010). "An exception to the replacement limitation may be made | $2/visit (Kaiser Family Foundation, 2012b). |

continued

TABLE G-1 Continued

			authorization (NDDHS, 2011). Replacement lenses and frames covered within the 12-month warranty with prior authorization. Contact lenses provided when medically necessary (NDDHS, 2011).	if new eyeglasses are required for a significant change in correction and the eyeglasses are prior approved" (NDDHS, 2010).
Ohio	"Adults are eligible with incomes up to 133% of FPL. Children are eligible with incomes up to 206% of FPL, and pregnant women are eligible with incomes up to 200% of FPL" (Norris, 2015p).	"One exam and pair of eyeglasses covered every 12 months (individuals younger than age 21)" (ODM, n.d.).	Adults ages 60 and older are eligible for "one eye exam and one pair or eyeglasses every 12 months" (ODM, n.d.). Adults between 21 and 59 are eligible for "one eye exam and one pair of eyeglasses every 24 months" (ODM, n.d.). Glaucoma screenings covered. Contact lenses covered with prior authorization. Medical and surgical services covered when medically necessary (ODM, n.d.).	$2/refractive exam and $1/ for dispensing eyeglasses (ODM, n.d.).
Oklahoma	The aged, blind, and disabled are eligible. "Children under age 19 with income up to 210% of the poverty level, parents with income up to 46% of poverty, pregnant women with income up to 185% of the poverty level . . . includes pregnant women related to CHIP (134–185%)."[z] "Insure Oklahoma helps cover the	"Payment will be made for children with lenses, frames, low vision aids and certain tints when medically necessary including to protect children with monocular vision. Coverage includes one set of lenses and frames per year. Any glasses beyond this limit must be prior authorized and determined to be medically necessary" (OHCA, 2015).	Coverage for medical services necessary for the diagnosis and treatment of illness or injury (OHCA, 2015). "There is no provision for routine eye exams, examinations for the purpose of prescribing glasses or visual aids, determination of refractive state, treatment of refractive errors, or purchase of lenses, frames, or visual aids" (OHCA, 2015).	$4/visit (OHCA, 2014).

	cost of private insurance for adults working for small employers, benefits for low income adults that are self-employed and adults receiving unemployment benefits."[z]	"Eye examinations are covered when medically necessary. Determination of the refractive state is covered when medically necessary" (OHCA, 2015).		
Oregon[aa]	"The aged, blind, and disabled. Also, coverage is available if household income does not exceed 133% of poverty (135% for pregnant women and infants). CHIP is available for children with household incomes up to 300% of poverty" (Norris, 2016h).	Eye exams and glasses covered. Contact lenses not covered (OHP, n.d.).	Eye exams covered for pregnant women. For nonpregnant adults eye exams covered for eye conditions "except for disorders of refraction and accommodation (e.g. nearsightedness, farsightedness, astigmatism). Diagnostic services are still covered" (OHP, n.d.). Glasses covered for pregnant adults and other adults when medically necessary due to conditions such as aphakia or after cataracts surgery. Contact lenses not covered (OHP, n.d.).	Beneficiary may be responsible for a $3 copay per visit (Kaiser Family Foundation, 2012b).
Pennsylvania[bb]	"Adults with income up to 138 percent of FPL are eligible for Medicaid. Children in households with incomes up to 319% of FPL are eligible for Medicaid or CHIP" (Norris, 2015q).	Two frames and four lenses covered per calendar year. Additional eyeglasses or contact lenses may be approved if medically necessary.	Two vision exams covered per calendar year. With fee-for-service, eyeglasses or contact lenses covered only with a diagnosis of aphakia. Eyeglasses may be covered without diagnoses for adults enrolled in a managed care plan.	$0.65–$3.80/ service for glasses or visit (Kaiser Family Foundation, 2012a,b).
Rhode Island[cc]	"The aged, blind, and disabled. Also, adults with income up to 133% of poverty, pregnant women	Covered as medically necessary with no other limits (State of Rhode Island, 2016).	Eye exams, eyeglasses (lenses, frames, and dispensing fee) and contact lenses (with prior authorization) covered once every 24 months for beneficiaries ages 21 and older	None (State of Rhode Island, 2016).

continued

TABLE G-1 Continued

	with income up to 253% of poverty, and children with incomes up to 261% of poverty" (Norris, 2015r).		(State of Rhode Island, 2016). Office visits covered for diagnosis and treatment when medically necessary. "The RI Medicaid program does not pay for a spare pair of eyeglasses; information provided over the telephone; cancelled office visits or appointments not kept; lost or stolen frames or lenses. The Medicaid program will not pay for any procedures or services that are unproved, experimental or research in nature. Services which are not medically necessary to treat the patient's condition, or are not directly related to the patient's diagnosis, symptoms or medical history are not reimbursable" (State of Rhode Island, 2016).	
South Carolina[dd]	"The aged, blind, and disabled. Also children with household incomes up to 208% of FPL; working parents with dependent children with household incomes up to 89% of FPL; jobless parents with dependent children with household incomes up to 50% of FPL; pregnant women with household incomes up to 194% of FPL" (Norris, 2015s).	One comprehensive eye exam and one complete set of glasses covered once a year (South Carolina Health Connections, 2016). All lenses must be polycarbonate. Repairs covered as necessary. Replacements covered once per year. Contact lenses covered when medically necessary (South Carolina Health Connections, 2016). Orthotic and pleoptic	"Routine vision services for beneficiaries 21 and over are non-covered services. Routine vision services are defined as services related to refractive care: routine eye exams, refractions, corrective lenses, and glasses. Services related to disease of the eye are covered for an example glaucoma, conjunctivitis and cataracts" (South Carolina Health Connections, 2016, p. 2-198). "Adults can get an eye exam every year and a pair of glasses following cataract surgery" (South Carolina Healthy Connections, 2008, p. 15).	$3.30 per optometrist visit for adults over age 21 (South Carolina Healthy Connections, 2015).

		training not covered (South Carolina Healthy Connections, 2016).		
South Dakota	"Pregnant women with household incomes up to 133% of FPL; children with household incomes up to 204% of FPL (for CHIP); parents with dependent children are eligible with incomes up to 58% of FPL" (Norris, 2015t).	Medicaid will pay for vision examinations; "annual examinations must be 12 months apart after age three" (SD DSS, 2015, p. 3).	"Covers exam, glasses and frames. Contact lenses are covered only when necessary for the correction of certain conditions. Replacement eyeglasses covered if 15 months have passed and a lens change is medically necessary" (SD DSS, 2015, p. 19). Optometrists and opticians may be seen without a referral; ophthalmology appointments require a referral (SD DSS, 2015).	"$2 for each procedure, lens, frame, exam, and repair service" (SD DSS, 2015, p. 14).
Tennessee[ee]	Parents with dependent children are eligible for Medicaid coverage with household incomes up to 103% of poverty (Brooks et al., 2015). "Children are eligible for Medicaid or CHIP with household incomes up to 250% of poverty, and pregnant women are eligible with incomes up to 195% of poverty" (Norris, 2015u).	"[For beneficiaries] under age 21: Preventive, diagnostic, and treatment services (including eyeglasses) [are] covered" (TennCare, 2014, p. 19).	"Vision services are limited to medical evaluation and management of abnormal conditions and disorders of the eye. The first pair of cataract glasses or contact lens/lenses following cataract surgery are covered" (TennCare, 2015, p. 5).	
Texas[ff]	"The aged, blind, and disabled. Also, parents with dependent children are eligible with household incomes up to 15% of FPL. Children are eligible for	Children's Medicaid covers eye exams and eyeglasses (Texas HHSC, 2014).	"One examination of the eyes by refraction may be provided to each eligible recipient every 24 months. This limit does not apply to diagnostic or other treatment of the eye for medical conditions" (Texas Medicaid, 2015).	

continued

TABLE G-1 Continued

	Medicaid or CHIP with household incomes up to 201% of FPL, and pregnant women are eligible with household incomes up to 198% of FPL" (Norris, 2015v).		"Non-prosthetic eyewear includes contact lenses and eyeglasses (lenses and frames) [and] . . . is a benefit when the eyewear is medically necessary to correct defects in vision. This eyewear is covered once every 24 months unless the recipient experiences a visual acuity change measured in diopters or axis changes. . . . Contact lenses require prior authorization by the commission or its designee. . . . Prior authorization decisions are based on the provider's written documentation supporting the need for contact lenses as the only means of correcting the vision defect" (Texas Medicaid, 2015). Replacement eyewear is not covered (Texas Medicaid, 2015).	
Utah[gg]	"Coverage is available for pregnant women with incomes up to 139% of poverty, children with incomes up to 200% of poverty, and parents with incomes up to 51% of poverty. Utah's guidelines also provide for other groups to obtain coverage depending on circumstances" (Norris, 2015w).	"Eyeglasses services, including lenses and frames" are covered by Utah Medicaid under EPSDT (Utah Department of Health, 2015, p. 2).	Medicaid covers one eye exam each year. Additional eye exams can be done when medically necessary (Utah Department of Health, 2015). Corrective lenses and frames covered once every 2 years when medically necessary (e.g., changes in prescription). Damaged lens or frame repair covered as long as not due to member neglect or abuse once every 12 months (Utah Department of Health, 2015). Replacement glasses covered with change of 0.75 in diopter or when disease or damage to eye makes it medically necessary (Utah Department of Health,	No copay for the annual eye exam if done by optometrist. $3 copayment for visits to the ophthalmologist (Utah Department of Health, 2016).

			2015). Contact lenses covered when medically necessary (Utah Department of Health, 2015).	
Vermont[bh]	Adults with incomes up to 133% of FPL are eligible for Medicaid. Children with household incomes up to 312% of FPL, and pregnant women with incomes up to 208% of FPL (CMS, 2014).	"One comprehensive eye exam and one intermediate eye exam are covered within the 24 month limit or more than two intermediate eye exams within a 2 year period" (DVHA, 2016a, p. 2). Beneficiaries under the age of 6 are allowed one new pair of eyeglasses every year, when medically necessary, whereas beneficiaries ages 6 and older and under 21 are eligible for new glasses every 2 years without prior approval (DVHA, 2012). Lenses are polycarbonate (DVHA, 2015). Replacement glasses covered within a 24-month period, and certain special lenses covered with prior authorization (DVHA, 2016a).	"Refraction and eye exams [are covered] when provided by an enrolled ophthalmologist or optometrist. Routine eye exams with the following limitations: one comprehensive eye exam and one intermediate eye exam are covered within a 2-year period, or two intermediate eye exams within a 2-year period. Diagnostic testing [is covered]. Non-eyewear aids to vision (such as closed circuit television) when the beneficiary is legally blind and when providing the aid to vision will foster independence by improving at least one activity of daily living" are covered with prior authorization (DVHA, 2012, p. 102). Eyeglasses, lenses, and contact lenses are not covered (DVHA, 2016a).	No copay for members under 21 (DVHA, 2016b).
Virginia[ii]	"The aged, blind, and disabled. Also, parents with dependent children	Eyeglasses and their repair are covered. Tinted lenses covered when medically	Eye examinations are covered once every 2 years. More frequent eye exams covered if medically necessary. Repair of frames	$1 copay for beneficiaries over age 21 for

continued

TABLE G-1 Continued

	are eligible with household incomes up to 49% of FPL. . . . Children are eligible for Medicaid or CHIP with household incomes up to 200% of FPL" (Healthinsurance.org, 2015b). Pregnant women are eligible with household incomes up to 200% of FPL for FAMIS MOMS (Cover Virginia, n.d.).	justified. Contact lenses not covered unless medically necessary. Eye exercises covered when medically necessary. Written documentation of need required after six sessions of orthoptic trainings (DMAS, 2012).	limited to once every 12 months. Repairs covered more often if medically justified (DMAS, 2012).	eye examinations and non-emergency vision analysis (DMAS, 2012).
Washington[ii]	The aged, blind, and disabled. Also, adults with incomes up to 133% of FPL; children with household incomes up to 210% of FPL are eligible for no-premium Medicaid; children with household incomes 260% to 312% of FPL eligible (with premium); pregnant women with incomes up to 193% of FPL (Washington Apple Health, 2016c).	Vision hardware is covered for beneficiaries under age 20, including, vision therapy, eyeglasses (frames, lenses, and repairs) with a minimum prescription required, contact lenses (and backup glasses every 2 years), and replacement lenses with minimum required refractive change (Washington Apple Health, 2016b). Eye exam covered for asymptomatic clients once every 12 months (Washington Apple Health, 2016a).	Eye exams covered for asymptomatic clients once every 24 months (Washington Apple Health, 2016a). Orthotics, vision therapy, cataract surgery, strabismus surgery, blepharoplasty surgery, and implantable miniature telescope are covered services (Washington Apple Health, 2016a).	

State	Eligibility	Coverage (children)	Coverage (adults)	Copay
West Virginia[kk]	"The aged, blind, and disabled. Also, adults with incomes up to 138% of FPL; children with household incomes up to 300% of FPL are eligible for CHIP; pregnant women with incomes up to 158% of FPL" (Norris, 2016i).	Exams to prescribe eyeglasses or contact lenses including fitting, adjusting, or replacement are covered (West Virginia BMS, 2015). Frames are covered, as are replacements when the frames cannot be used or repaired. Contacts covered when medically necessary for a given condition. Orthoptics/pleoptic training is covered for children under age 10 when medically necessary (West Virginia BMS, 2015).	One comprehensive eye exam is covered per calendar year with prior authorization from utilization management vendor for medical necessity (West Virginia BMS, 2015). Addition diagnostic evaluations may be reimbursed if there is a documented, justifiable need. Glasses coverage is limited to beneficiaries post-cataract operation (within 60 days of surgery) (West Virginia BMS, 2015). Repair/replacement glasses not covered. Contact lenses covered with diagnosis of keratoconus or aphakia (West Virginia BMS, 2015).	None
Wisconsin[ll]	"The aged, blind, and disabled. Also, children and pregnant women with incomes up to 300% of poverty; other adults with incomes up to 100% of poverty" (Norris, 2014b).	Coverage same as for adults.	One comprehensive ophthalmologic exam covered once per year (ForwardHealth, 2016). One low vision exam is covered once per year with prior authorization (ForwardHealth, 2016). Cataract surgery covered when medically necessary. Contact lenses covered with prior authorization if medically necessary. Contact lenses covered without prior authorization with diagnosis of aphakia or keratoconus. Contact lens replacements covered once per year. Eyeglasses covered once per year. Minor repairs covered. Replacements for lost or damaged glasses covered once per year. Any addition replacements require prior approval (ForwardHealth, 2016).	$0.50–$3 for glasses or exams, depending on the specific service (Kaiser Family Foundation, 2012a,b).

continued

TABLE G-1 Continued

| Wyoming[mm] | "Pregnant women and children are eligible with household incomes up to 154% of poverty (children are eligible for CHIP with household incomes up to 200% of poverty). Parents with dependent children are eligible with household incomes up to 56% of poverty" (Norris, 2015x). | "Comprehensive services including eyeglasses for clients under the age of 21, with limits, covered when provided by an ophthalmologist, optometrist or optician" once per year (Wyoming Department of Health, 2011, p. 15). Eye exams covered when medically necessary to determine visual acuity or treat eye disease or injury. Replacement of lenses and frames allowed once. Contact lenses covered if medically necessary with prior authorization. Vision therapy covered without prior authorization. (Wyoming Department of Health, 2016). | Glasses and contact lenses not covered (Wyoming Department of Health, 2011). Eye exams are only covered for the treatment of eye disease or eye injury. Medical treatment is covered for beneficiaries who are either at risk for eye disease due to chronic illness or otherwise, or with eye injuries (Wyoming Department of Health, n.d.). | None. |

NOTE: Footnotes indicate that a state representative has verified the accuracy of the information.

[a] For Medicaid benefits in general, includes the 5 percent federal poverty level disregard, unless otherwise excluded by the state representative.

[b] Many states require a pharmacy copay (not enumerated here), which presumably would apply to prescription eye medications including various drops. Individual prescription copay are not always listed for each state but are typically <$3. Copays in general often do not apply for beneficiaries under age 18 (or, sometimes, 21), pregnant women, or patients in long-term care programs/nursing facility residents.

[c] Personal communication, R. Rawls, Alabama Medicaid Agency, May 24, 2016.

[d] Personal communication, S. Dunkin, Alaska Division of Health Care Services, March 23, 2016.

[e] Personal communication, L. Raymond, Arizona Health Care Cost Containment System, May 10, 2016.

[f] Personal communication, H. Hendrix, Jr., California Department of Health Care Services, May 24, 2016.
[g] Personal communication, E. Freudenthal, Colorado Department of Health Care Policy & Financing, May 10, 2016.
[h] Personal communication, E. Atwerebour, Connecticut Division of Health Services—Medical Policy, April 5, 2016.
[i] Personal communication, K. Mahoney, Delaware Division of Medicaid and Medical Assistance, May 8, 2016.
[j] Personal communication, C. Bishop, District of Columbia Department of Health Care Finance, May 11, 2016.
[k] Personal communication, A. Russell, Georgia Department of Community Health, May 19, 2016.
[l] Personal communication, C. Toma, Hawaii Medicaid, March 28, 2016.
[m] Personal communication, M. Cook, Indiana Family and Social Services Administration, March 29, 2016.
[n] Personal communication, A. L. McCoy, Iowa Department of Human Services, May 31, 2016.
[o] Personal communication, S. Robinson, Kentucky Cabinet for Health Services, May 9, 2016.
[p] Personal communication, L. Gonzales, Louisiana Department of Health and Hospitals, April 20, 2016.
[q] Personal communication, M. Lehner, Maryland Acute Care Administration, May 13, 2016.
[r] Personal communication, E. Emerson, Michigan Department of Health and Human Services, May 10, 2016.
[s] Personal communication, D. Preshinger, Montana Department of Public Health & Human Services, April 11, 2016.
[t] Personal communication, J. Swenson, Nebraska Department of Health & Human Services, May 12, 2016.
[u] Personal communication, J. Osalvo, Nevada Division of Health Care Financing and Policy, May 9, 2016.
[v] Personal communication, D. Peterson, New Hampshire Department of Health and Human Services, June 1, 2016.
[w] Personal communication, K. Armijo, New Mexico Human Services Department, May 13, 2016.
[x] Personal communication, M. J. O'Brien, New York State Department of Health, May 13, 2016.
[y] Personal communication, T. Solberg, North Dakota Department of Human Services, May 10, 2016.
[z] Personal communication, M. Triplet, The Oklahoma Health Care Authority, May 13, 2016.
[aa] Personal communication, A. Robbins, Oregon Health Authority, May 24, 2016.
[bb] Personal communication, R. V. Foster, Pennsylvania Department of Human Services, May 20, 2016.
[cc] Personal communication, S. O'Connell, Rhode Island Executive Office of Health & Human Services, March 25, 2016.
[dd] Personal communication, V. Williams, South Carolina Health Connections, May 20, 2016.
[ee] Personal communication, A. Butler, Division of Health Care Finance & Administration, March 23, 2016.
[ff] Personal communication, J. Seyller, Texas Health & Human Services, March 28, 2016.
[gg] Personal communication, K. Young, Utah Department of Health, May 31, 2016.
[hh] Personal communication, D. Fuoco, Vermont Agency of Human Services, May 27, 2016.
[ii] Personal communication, B. McCormick, Virginia Department of Medical Assistance Services, May 11, 2016.
[jj] Personal communication, A. McKoy, Washington Health Care Authority, March 28, 2016.
[kk] Personal communication, R. D. Ernest Jr., West Virginia Bureau for Medical Services, May 11, 2016.
[ll] Personal Communication, S. Thomas, Wisconsin Department of Health Services, May 25, 2016.
[mm] Personal Communication, A. Burton, Wyoming Medicaid, May 17, 2016.

REFERENCES

Aetna. 2016. Vision benefits. https://www.aetnabetterhealth.com/illinois/members/icp/vision (accessed May 19, 2016).

AHCCCS (Arizona Health Care Cost Containment System). 2016a. *AHCCCS eligibility requirements February 1, 2016.* https://www.azahcccs.gov/Members/Downloads/Eligibility Requirements.pdf (accessed April 12, 2016).

———. 2016b. *Chapter 300 medical policy for AHCCCS covered services.* Phoenix: AHCCCS. https://www.azahcccs.gov/shared/Downloads/MedicalPolicyManual/Chap300.pdf (accessed June 30, 2016).

———. 2016c. *Chapter 400 medical policy for maternal and child health.* Phoenix: AHCCCS. https://www.azahcccs.gov/shared/Downloads/MedicalPolicyManual/Chap400.pdf (accessed June 30, 2016).

———. 2016d. Covered medical services. https://azahcccs.gov/Members/AlreadyCovered/coveredservices.html (accessed April 8, 2016).

Alabama Medicaid Agency. 2013. *Your guide to Alabama Medicaid.* Montgomery: Alabama Medicaid Agency. http://216.226.177.83/documents/4.0_Programs/4.2_Covered_Services/4.2_Your_Guide_to_Medicaid_12-13.pdf (accessed June 30, 2016).

———. 2014. *Medicaid eligibility handout.* Montgomery: Alabama Medicaid Agency. http://medicaid.alabama.gov/documents/3.0_Apply/3.1_General_Info/3.1_MAGI_Medicaid_Eligibility_Handout_3-1-16.pdf (accessed June 30, 2016).

Alaska Department of Health and Social Services. 2012. *Alaska Medicaid recipient services.* Anchorage: Alaska Department of Health and Social Services. http://dhss.alaska.gov/dhcs/Documents/PDF/Recipient-Handbook.pdf (accessed June 30, 2016).

———. 2013. Vision services, policies, and procedures. In *Alaska medical assistrance provider billing manual.* Anchorage: Alaska Department of Health and Social Services. http://manuals.medicaidalaska.com/vision/vision.htm (accessed June 30, 2016).

———. 2016. *MAGI Medicaid income eligibility standards—FPL based.* Anchorage: Alaska Department of Health and Social Services. http://dpaweb.hss.state.ak.us/POLICY/PDF/Medicaid_standards.pdf (accessed June 30, 2016).

Anderson, C. 2014. Maryland Medicaid. https://www.healthinsurance.org/maryland-medicaid (accessed July 10, 2016).

———. 2015a. Connecticut Medicaid. https://www.healthinsurance.org/connecticut-medicaid (accessed July 10, 2016).

———. 2015b. Delaware Medicaid. https://www.healthinsurance.org/delaware-medicaid (accessed July 10, 2016).

———. 2015c. District of Columbia Medicaid. https://www.healthinsurance.org/dc-medicaid (accessed July 10, 2016).

———. 2015d. Georgia Medicaid. https://www.healthinsurance.org/georgia-medicaid (accessed July 10, 2016).

———. 2015e. Maine Medicaid. https://www.healthinsurance.org/maine-medicaid (accessed July 10, 2016).

———. 2015f. Massachusetts Medicaid. https://www.healthinsurance.org/massachusetts-medicaid (accessed July 10, 2016).

———. 2015g. Michigan Medicaid. https://www.healthinsurance.org/michigan-medicaid (accessed July 10, 2016).

———. 2016. Illinois Medicaid. https://www.healthinsurance.org/illinois-medicaid/ (accessed July 10, 2016).

Arkansas Department of Human Services. 2012. *Arkansas Medicaid program overview sfy 2012.* Little Rock, AR: Division of Medical Services. http://humanservices.arkansas.gov/dms/DMS%20Public/Medicaid_Program_Overview_SFY2012.pdf (accessed June 30, 2016).

ARMedicaid. n.d. *Medicaid vision program coverage.* Little Rock: Arkansas Department of Human Services. https://static.ark.org/eeuploads/hbe/PediatricVision_Benchmark_Plan. pdf (accessed June 30, 2016).

Brooks, T., J. Touschner, S. Artiga, J. Stephens, and A. Gates. 2015. *Modern era Medicaid: Findings from a 50-state survey of eligibility, enrollment, renewal, and cost-sharing policies in Medicaid and CHIP as of January 2015.* Menlo Park, CA: The Henry J. Kaiser Family Foundation.

CDHCS (California Department of Health Care Services). 2016a. *Medi-Cal benefits.* http://www.coveredca.com/medi-cal/benefits/ (accessed March 8, 2016).

———. 2016b. Medi-Cal eligibility and Covered California: Frequently asked questions. http://www.dhcs.ca.gov/services/medi-cal/eligibility/Pages/Medi-CalFAQs2014a.aspx (accessed April 8, 2016).

Children's Vision Georgia. 2013. *Georgia Medicaid and PeachCare vision benefits for children.* Atlanta: Children's Vision Georgia. http://www.childrensvisiongeorgia.org/cvg/wp-content/uploads/2014/12/CVG-GA-Medicaid-and-PeachCare-Vision-Benefits-for-Children-Table-1.29.13.pdf (accessed June 30, 2016).

CMS (Centers for Medicare & Medicaid Services). 2014. *State Medicaid and CHIP income eligibility standards.* Baltimore, MD: CMS. https://www.medicaid.gov/medicaid-chip-program-information/program-information/downloads/medicaid-and-chip-eligibility-levels-table.pdf (accessed June 30, 2016).

COHCPF (Colorado Department of Health Care Planning and Financing). 2016. Colorado Medicaid: Benefits & services overview. https://www.colorado.gov/hcpf/colorado-medicaid-benefits-services-overview (accessed April 8, 2016).

Colorado Medical Assistance Program. 2015. *Vision care and eyewear manual.* Denver: Colorado Department of Health Care Policy & Financing. https://www.colorado.gov/pacific/sites/default/files/CMS1500_VisionEyewear_6.pdf (accessed June 30, 2016).

Commonwealth of Kentucky. n.d. *Kentucky medical member handbook.* Frankfort: Kentucky Department of Medicaid Services. http://kidshealth.ky.gov/en/kchip/costs.htm (accessed June 30, 2016).

Cover Virginia. n.d. Am I eligible? http://www.coverva.org/button_eligibility.cfm (accessed May 12, 2016).

DHCF (Department of Health Care Finance). 2012. *D.C. Medicaid fee-for-service member handbook.* Washington: Government of the District of Columbia. http://dhcf.dc.gov/sites/default/files/dc/sites/dhcf/publication/attachments/DHCF%20FFS%20Medicaid%20Version%2013_red.pdf (accessed June 30, 2016).

———. 2016. *Optometry services notice of final rulemaking.* Washington: Government of the District of Columbia. http://dhcf.dc.gov/sites/default/files/dc/sites/dhcf/publication/attachments/Optometry%20Services%20Notice%20of%20Final%20Rulemaking.pdf (accessed June 30, 2016).

DHCFP (Department of Health Care Financing and Policy). 2015. *Medicaid services manual.* Carson City: Nevada Department of Health and Human Services. http://dhcfp.nv.gov/uploadedFiles/dhcfpnvgov/content/Resources/AdminSupport/Manuals/MSM/C1100/MSM_1100_15-10-01.pdf (accessed June 30, 2016).

DMAP (Delaware Medical Assistance Program). 2016. *General policy manual.* New Castle: Delaware Health and Social Services. http://www.dmap.state.de.us/downloads/manuals/General.Policy.Manual.20150714.pdf (accessed June 30, 2016).

———. n.d. *Optician services.* New Castle: Delaware Health and Social Services. http://www.dmap.state.de.us/downloads/manuals/optician.provider.specific.pdf (accessed June 30, 2016).

DMAS (Department of Medical Assistance Services). 2012. Covered services and limitations. Richmond: Virginia Medicaid. https://www.ecm.virginiamedicaid.dmas.virginia.gov/WorkplaceXT/getContent?vsId={1472F4F9-6938-403F-BE93-76BF912A374F}&impersonate=true&objectType=document&id={7D859539-B064-4F1F-B168-D63EE45A0437}&objectStoreName=VAPRODOS1 (accessed June 30, 2016).

DVHA (Department of Vermont Health Access). 2012. Medicaid covered services rules. Waterbury: Vermont Agency of Human Services. http://humanservices.vermont.gov/online-rules/dvha/medicaid-covered-services-7100-7700-1/view (accessed April 8, 2016).

———. 2015. Vermont Medicaid eyeglass–program: Frequently asked questions. Waterbury: Vermont Agency of Human Services. https://vtmedicaid.com/Information/VTFAQVision07012015.pdf (accessed April 8, 2016).

———. 2016a. *The Department of Vermont Health Access medical policy.* Waterbury: Vermont Agency of Human Services. http://dvha.vermont.gov/for-providers/vision042516.pdf (accessed May 31, 2016).

———. 2016b. *Provider manual.* Waterbury: Vermont Agency of Human Services. http://vtmedicaid.com/assets/manuals/VTMedicaidProviderManual.pdf (accessed May 31, 2016).

Florida Agency for Health Care Administration. n.d. *Covered services.* Tallahassee: Florida Department of Children and Families. http://www.betterhealthflorida.com/pdf/PT_CoveredServices.pdf (accessed April 8, 2016).

———. 2015. *Florida Medicaid visual aid services coverage policy.* Tallahasse: Florida Department of Children and Families.

ForwardHealth. 2016. *Covered and noncovered services: Covered services and requirements.* Madison: Wisconsin Department of Health Services. https://www.forwardhealth.wi.gov/WIPortal/Subsystem/KW/Display.aspx?ia=1&p=1&sa=64&s=2&c=61 (accessed May 26, 2016).

Georgia DCH (Department of Community Health). 2016. *Policies and procedures for vison care services.* Atlanta, GA: Georgia DCH. https://www.mmis.georgia.gov/portal/Portals/0/StaticContent/Public/ALL/HANDBOOKS/Vision%20Care%20Manual%20April%20 2016%20%20V1%2010-05-2016%20223805.pdf (accessed May 19, 2016).

Hawaii Department of Health. 2011a. Chapter 20: Eye examinations/vision and hearing. In *Hawaii Medicaid provider manual.* Honolulu: Hawaii Department of Health. http://www.med-quest.us/PDFs/Provider%20Manual/PMChp2011.pdf (accessed May 18, 2016).

———. 2011b. *Provider manual: Appendix 1 services and items not covered by the Hawaii Medicaid program.* Honolulu: Haiwaii Department of Health. http://www.med-quest.us/PDFs/Appendix01/A50toA54ServicesandItemsNotCovered.pdf (accessed April 8, 2016).

Healthinsurance.org. 2015a. Missouri Medicaid. https://www.healthinsurance.org/missouri-medicaid (accessed July 10, 2016).

———. 2015b. Virginia Medicaid. https://www.healthinsurance.org/virginia-medicaid (accessed July 10, 2016).

Horizon NJ Health. 2014. *Member handbook.* West Trenton: Horizon Blue Cross Blue Shield of New Jersey. https://www.horizonnjhealth.com/sites/default/files/Member_Handbook_1_0.pdf (accessed July 18, 2016).

HPSM (Health Plan of San Mateo). 2016. Medi-Cal benefits & costs. https://www.hpsm.org/members/medi-cal/costs.aspx (accessed April 8, 2016).

Husky Health Connecticut. 2015. *Husky health program member handbook: Husky A, Husky C, Husky D.* Hartford: Connecticut Department of Social Services. http://www.huskyhealthct.org/members/member_postings/member_benefits/HUSKY_A-C-D-Handbook_9-15.pdf (accessed April 8, 2016).

———. 2016. Husky health prior authorization requirements grid vision. http://www.huskyhealthct.org/providers/provider_postings/benefits_grids/Vision_Grid.pdf (accessed April 8, 2016).

Idaho Department of Health and Welfare. 2009. *Administrative rule, 16.03.09, Medicaid Basic Plan Benefits.* Caldwell: Idaho Department of Health and Welfare. http://adminrules. idaho.gov/rules/current/16/0309.pdf (accessed April 12, 2016).

IHCP (Indiana Health Coverage Programs). 2016. *Vision services.* Indianapolis: Indiana Family & Social Services. http://provider.indianamedicaid.com/media/155592/vision%20 services.pdf (accessed April 8, 2016).

Illinois Department of HFS (Healthcare and Family Services). 2009. *Handbook for providers of medical services, Chapter 100: General policy and procedures.* Chicago: Illinois Department of HFS. http://www.hfs.illinois.gov/assets/100.pdf (accessed April 8, 2016).

———. 2012. Change to adult eyeglasses benefit effective July 1, 2012. Chicago: Illinois Department of HFS. http://www.illinois.gov/hfs/MedicalProviders/notices/Pages/ prn120630g.aspx (accessed April 12, 2016).

Iowa Department of Human Services. 2014. *Optometrist and optician services provider manual.* Des Moines: Iowa Department of Human Services. http://dhs.iowa.gov/sites/ default/files/Optomet.pdf (accessed May 19, 2016).

Kaiser Family Foundation. 2012a. Medicaid benefits: Eyeglasses. http://kff.org/medicaid/state-indicator/eyeglasses (accessed March 8, 2016).

———. 2012b. Medicaid benefits: Optometrist services. http://kff.org/medicaid/state-indicator/ optometrist-services (accessed March 8, 2016).

KanCare. 2012. *Basic eligibility requirements.* Topeka: Kansas Department of Health and Environment. http://www.kancare.ks.gov/download/factsheets/Fact_Sheet_Medical_ Coverage_Basic_Eligibility_Requirements.pdf (accessed April 8, 2016).

———. 2016. Medicaid for Kansas. http://www.kancare.ks.gov/health_plan_info.htm (accessed April 8, 2016).

Kentucky CHFS (Cabinet for Health and Family Services). 2007. *Kentucky Medicaid vision program manual.* Frankfort: Kentucky Department of Medicaid Services. http://chfs. ky.gov/nr/rdonlyres/eb814317-97a7-444f-a993-cbf8843f21db/0/visionman0616082.pdf (accessed April 8, 2016).

———. 2015. Programs and services. http://www.chfs.ky.gov/dms/services.htm (accessed April 13, 2016).

KHPA (Kansas Health Policy Authority). 2010. *Kansas Medical Assistance Program provider manual: Vision.* Topeka: KHPA. https://www.kmap-state-ks.us/Documents/Content/ Provider%20Manuals/VISION_%2012272010_10153.pdf (accessed May 19, 2016).

Louisiana Medicaid. 2016. *Medicaid services chart.* Baton Rouge: Louisiana Department of Health & Hospitals. http://new.dhh.louisiana.gov/assets/docs/Making_Medicaid_Better/ Medicaid_Services_Chart.pdf (accessed April 8, 2016).

Maine DHHS (Department of Health and Human Services). 2012. Section 75: Vision services. In *Chapter 101: MaineCare benefits manual.* Augusta: Maine DHHS. Pp. 10–144. http:// www.maine.gov/sos/cec/rules/10/144/ch101/c2s075.docx (May 19, 2016).

Maryland DHMH (Department of Health and Mental Hygiene). 2014. *04 covered services.* Baltimore: Maryland DHMH.

———. n.d. Medicaid eligibility and benefits. https://mmcp.dhmh.maryland.gov/Pages/ Medicaid-Eligibility-and-Benefits.aspx (accessed April 8, 2016).

MassHealth. 2008. *Vision care manual.* Quincy: Commonwealth of Massachusetts Executive Office of Health and Human Services. http://www.mass.gov/eohhs/docs/masshealth/regs-provider/regs-visioncare.pdf (accessed May 19, 2016).

MDHHS (Michigan Department of Health and Human Services). 2016. *Medcaid state plan.* Lansing: MDHHS. http://www.mdch.state.mi.us/dch-medicaid/manuals/ MichiganStatePlan/MichiganStatePlan.pdf (April 14, 2016).

Minnesota DHS (Department of Health Services). 2013. *Minnesota health care programs (MHCP)—Medical Assistance (MA)—Fee-for-service (FFS)*. St Paul: Minnesota DHS. http://www.dhs.state.mn.us/main/idcplg?IdcService=GET_FILE&RevisionSelectionMethod=LatestReleased&Rendition=Primary&allowInterrupt=1&noSaveAs=1&dDocName=dhs16_174311 (accessed April 14, 2016).

———. 2016. Eyeglass and vision care. http://www.dhs.state.mn.us/main/idcplg?IdcService=GET_DYNAMIC_CONVERSION&RevisionSelectionMethod=LatestReleased&dDocName=id_008954#cs (accessed May 19, 2016).

Mississippi Division of Medicaid. 2014. *Administrative code*. Jackson: Mississippi Division of Medicaid. https://www.medicaid.ms.gov/wp-content/uploads/2014/01/Admin-Code-Part-217.pdf (accessed April 8, 2016).

———. 2016. *Vision comparison chart*. Jackson: Mississippi Division of Medicaid.

MO HealthNet. 2016. *Optical manual*. Jefferson City, MO: MO HealthNet. http://manuals.momed.com/collections/collection_opt/print.pdf (accessed May 19, 2016).

Montana DPHHS (Department of Public Health and Human Services). 2013. *Member guide: Montana Medicaid and Healthy Montana Kids Plus*. Helena: Montana DPHHS. http://dphhs.mt.gov/Portals/85/hrd/documents/memberguide.pdf (accessed April 8, 2016).

———. 2016. *Before the Department of Public Health and Human Services of the state of Montana*. Helena: Montana DPHHS. https://dphhs.mt.gov/Portals/85/rules/37-737pro-arm.pdf (accessed May 26, 2016).

NC DMA (North Carolina Division of Medical Assistance). 2015a. *General ophthalmological services*. Raleigh: North Carolina Health and Human Services. https://ncdma.s3.amazonaws.com/s3fs-public/documents/files/1T1.pdf (accessed July 19, 2016).

———. 2015b. *Routine eye examination and visual aids*. Raleigh: North Carolina Health and Human Services. https://www2.ncdhhs.gov/dma/mp/6A.pdf (accessed June 30, 2016).

NDDHS (North Dakota Department of Human Services). 2010. Medicaid general information. https://www.nd.gov/dhs/services/medicalserv/medicaid/covered.html (accessed April 8, 2016).

———. 2011. *Provider manual for optometric and eyeglass services*. Bismarck: NDDHS. http://www.nd.gov/dhs/services/medicalserv/medicaid/docs/optometric-manual.pdf (accessed July 19, 2016).

Nebraska DHHS (Department of Health & Human Services). 2016. *Medicaid eligibility*. Lincoln: Nebraska DHHS.

Nebraska Medicaid Program. 2014. Services covered by Medicaid. http://dhhs.ne.gov/medicaid/Pages/med_medserv.aspx (accessed April 8, 2016).

New Hampshire Medicaid. 1994. Chapter He-W 500: Medical Assistance. http://www.gencourt.state.nh.us/rules/state_agencies/he-w500.html (accessed June 3, 2016).

———. 2013. *Vision provider manual, volume II*. Concord: New Hampshire Department of Health and Human Services. https://nhmmis.nh.gov/portals/wps/wcm/connect/0a16230040ce67c6ab9dff3e8fa48611/NH+Medicaid+Final+Vision+Provider+Billing+Manual+20130401.pdf?MOD=AJPERES (accessed May 23, 2016).

New Hampshire Medicaid Care Management. 2015. *Meet your health plans*. Concord: New Hampshire Department of Health and Human Services. http://www.dhhs.nh.gov/ombp/caremgt/documents/dcs-1060-mcm-sbs.pdf (accessed April 8, 2016).

New Hampshire Medicaid Client Services. 2014. *Recipient information about: Recipient responsibilities, transportation, service limits, co-payments, non-covered services, prescription drugs, prior authorization*. Concord: New Hampshire Department of Health and Human Services. http://www.dhhs.nh.gov/ombp/medicaid/documents/med77l.pdf (accessed April 8, 2016).

New Jersey DMAHS (Division of Medical Assistance and Health Services). 2004. *Chapter 49 administration manual*. Trenton: New Jersey Department of Human Services.

New York State Medicaid Program. 2013. *Vision care manual policy guidelines.* Albany: New York State Medicaid Program. https://www.emedny.org/ProviderManuals/VisionCare/ PDFS/VisionCare_Policy_Guidelines.pdf (accessed May 23, 2016).

NMAC (New Mexico Administrative Code). 2010. *New Mexico register.* Santa Fe: Commission of Public Records, Administrative Law Division. http://164.64.110.239/nmregister/ xxi/xxi09/8.310.6amend.htm (accessed May 23, 2016).

NMAP (Nebraska Medical Assistance Program). 2003. *Manual letter # 59-2003 and support manual.* Lincoln: Nebraska Department of Health & Human Services. http://www.sos. ne.gov/rules-and-regs/regsearch/Rules/Health_and_Human_Services_System/Title-471/ Chapter-24.pdf (accessed May 20, 2016).

Norris, L. 2014a. New Jersey Medicaid. https://www.healthinsurance.org/new-jersey-medicaid (accessed July 10, 2016).

———. 2014b. Wisconsin Medicaid. https://www.healthinsurance.org/wisconsin-medicaid (accessed July 10, 2016).

———. 2015a. Alaska Medicaid. https://www.healthinsurance.org/alaska-medicaid (accessed July 10, 2016).

———. 2015b. California Medicaid. https://www.healthinsurance.org/california-medicaid (accessed July 10, 2016).

———. 2015c. Colorado Medicaid. https://www.healthinsurance.org/colorado-medicaid (accessed July 10, 2016).

———. 2015d. Florida Medicaid. https://www.healthinsurance.org/florida-medicaid (accessed July 10, 2016).

———. 2015e. Hawaii Medicaid. https://www.healthinsurance.org/hawaii-medicaid (accessed July 10, 2016).

———. 2015f. Indiana Medicaid. https://www.healthinsurance.org/indiana-medicaid (accessed July 10, 2016).

———. 2015g. Kansas Medicaid. https://www.healthinsurance.org/kansas-medicaid (accessed July 10, 2016).

———. 2015h. Kentucky Medicaid. https://www.healthinsurance.org/kentucky-medicaid (accessed July 10, 2016).

———. 2015i. Minnesota Medicaid. https://www.healthinsurance.org/minnesota-medicaid (accessed July 10, 2016).

———. 2015j. Mississippi Medicaid. https://www.healthinsurance.org/mississippi-medicaid (accessed July 10, 2016).

———. 2015k. Nevada Medicaid. https://www.healthinsurance.org/nevada-medicaid (accessed July 10, 2016).

———. 2015l. New Mexico Medicaid. https://www.healthinsurance.org/new-mexico-medicaid (accessed July 10, 2016).

———. 2015m. New York Medicaid. https://www.healthinsurance.org/new-york-medicaid (accessed July 10, 2016).

———. 2015n. North Carolina Medicaid. https://www.healthinsurance.org/north-carolina-medicaid (accessed July 10, 2016).

———. 2015o. North Dakota Medicaid. https://www.healthinsurance.org/north-dakota-medicaid (accessed July 10, 2016).

———. 2015p. Ohio Medicaid. https://www.healthinsurance.org/ohio-medicaid (accessed July 10, 2016).

———. 2015q. Pennsylvania Medicaid. https://www.healthinsurance.org/pennsylvania-medicaid (accessed July 10, 2016).

———. 2015r. Rhode Island Medicaid. https://www.healthinsurance.org/rhode-island-medicaid (accessed July 10, 2016).

———. 2015s. South Carolina Medicaid. https://www.healthinsurance.org/south-carolina-medicaid (accessed July 10, 2016).

———. 2015t. South Dakota Medicaid. https://www.healthinsurance.org/north-dakota-medicaid (accessed July 10, 2016).

———. 2015u. Tennessee Medicaid. https://www.healthinsurance.org/tennessee-medicaid (accessed July 10, 2016).

———. 2015v. Texas Medicaid. https://www.healthinsurance.org/texas-medicaid (accessed July 10, 2016).

———. 2015w. Utah Medicaid. https://www.healthinsurance.org/utah-medicaid (accessed July 10, 2016).

———. 2015x. Wyoming Medicaid. https://www.healthinsurance.org/wyoming-medicaid (accessed July 10, 2016).

———. 2016a. Alabama Medicaid. https://www.healthinsurance.org/alabama-medicaid (accessed July 10, 2016).

———. 2016b. Arkansas Medicaid. https://www.healthinsurance.org/arkansas-medicaid (accessed July 10, 2016).

———. 2016c. Idaho Medicaid. https://www.healthinsurance.org/idaho-medicaid (accessed July 10, 2016).

———. 2016d. Iowa Medicaid. https://www.healthinsurance.org/iowa-medicaid (accessed July 10, 2016).

———. 2016e. Louisiana Medicaid. https://www.healthinsurance.org/louisiana-medicaid (accessed July 10, 2016).

———. 2016f. Montana Medicaid. https://www.healthinsurance.org/montana-medicaid (accessed July 10, 2016).

———. 2016g. New Hampshire Medicaid. https://www.healthinsurance.org/new-hampshire-medicaid (accessed July 10, 2016).

———. 2016h. Oregon Medicaid. https://www.healthinsurance.org/oregon-medicaid (accessed July 10, 2016).

———. 2016i. West Virginia Medicaid. https://www.healthinsurance.org/west-virginia-medicaid (accessed July 10, 2016).

ODM (Ohio Department of Medicaid). n.d. Ohio Medicaid covered services. http://medicaid.ohio.gov/FOROHIOANS/CoveredServices.aspx#671251-medical-and-surgical-vision-services (accessed April 8, 2016).

OHCA (Ohio Health Care Association). 2014. Re: Changes in co-pays for SoonerCare members. Oklahoma City: State of Oklahoma. https://www.okhca.org/WorkArea/linkit.aspx?LinkIdentifier=id&ItemID=16024&libID=15007 (accessed July 19, 2016).

———. 2015. Title 317. Oklahoma health care authority chapter 30. Medical providers-fee for service. Oklahoma City: Oklahoma Medicaid Agency.

OHP (Oregon Health Plan). n.d. Oregon health plan benefits frequently asked questions. http://www.oregon.gov/oha/healthplan/Pages/benefits-faq.aspx (accessed April 8, 2016).

SD DSS (South Dakota Department of Social Services). 2015. *South Dakota Medicaid recipient handbook*. Pierre: SD DSS. https://dss.sd.gov/formsandpubs/docs/MEDSRVCS/MedicalAssistanceRecipientHdbk.pdf (accessed April 8, 2016).

South Carolina Healthy Connections. 2008. *South Carolina Healthy Connections Medicaid program*. Columbia: South Carolina Department of Health and Human Services. https://www.scdhhs.gov/internet/pdf/Medicaid%20Handbook.pdf (accessed April 8, 2016).

———. 2015. Appendix 3 copayment schedule. Columbia: South Carolina Department of Health and Human Services. https://www.scdhhs.gov/internet/pdf/manuals/Appendix%203.pdf (accessed May 20, 2016).

————. 2016. *Physicians provider manual.* Columbia: South Carolina Department of Health and Human Services. https://www.scdhhs.gov/internet/pdf/manuals/Physicians/Section%202.pdf (accessed May 20, 2016).

State of Michigan. 2016. Health care programs eligibility. http://www.michigan.gov/mdhhs/0,5885,7-339-71547_4860-35199--,00.html (accessed April 14, 2016).

State of Rhode Island. 2016. Vision coverage guidelines. http://www.eohhs.ri.gov/Providers Partners/ProviderManualsGuidelines/MedicaidProviderManual/Vision/VisionCoverage Policy.aspx (accessed April 8, 2016).

TennCare. 2014. TennCare quick guide. Nashville, TN: Division of Health Care Finance & Administration. https://www.tn.gov/assets/entities/tenncare/attachments/quickguide.pdf (accessed July 19, 2016).

————. 2015. TennCare benefit package. Nashville, TN: Division of Health Care Finance & Administration. https://www.tn.gov/assets/entities/tenncare/attachments/benefitpackages.pdf (accessed April 8, 2016).

Texas HHSC (Health and Human Services Commission). 2014. What's covered. https://chip medicaid.org/en/Benefits (accessed July 19, 2016).

Texas Medicaid. 2015. Texas administrative code. http://texreg.sos.state.tx.us/public/readtac$ext.TacPage?sl=R&app=9&p_dir=&p_rloc=&p_tloc=&p_ploc=&pg=1&p_tac=&ti=1&pt=15&ch=354&rl=1015 (accessed April 8, 2016).

Utah Department of Health. 2015. Section 2: Vision care services. Salt Lake City: Utah Division of Medicaid and Health Financing. https://medicaid.utah.gov/Documents/manuals/pdfs/Medicaid%20Provider%20Manuals/Vision%20Care%20Services/Vision7-15.pdf (accessed May 23, 2016).

————. 2016. *Medicaid member guide.* Salt Lake City: Utah Department of Health. https://health.utah.gov/umb/forms/pdf/Medicaid_Member_Guide.pdf (accessed April 8, 2016).

Washington Apple Health. 2016a. *Physician-related services/health care professional services provider guide.* Olympia: Washington State Health Care Authority. http://www.hca.wa.gov/medicaid/billing/Documents/guides/physician-related_services_mpg.pdf (accessed April 8, 2016).

————. 2016b. *Vision hardware for clients age 20 and younger: Provider guide.* Olympia: Washington State Health Care Authority. http://www.hca.wa.gov/medicaid/billing/documents/guides/vision_hardware_for_kids_bi.pdf (accessed April 8, 2016).

————. 2016c. *Washington Apple health income and resource standards.* Olympia: Washington State Health Care Authority. http://www.hca.wa.gov/medicaid/eligibility/Documents/incomestandards.pdf (accessed April 8, 2016).

West Virginia BMS (Bureau for Medical Services). 2015. *Chapter 525 vision services.* Charleston: West Virginia Department of Health and Human Resources. http://www.dhhr.wv.gov/bms/Provider/Documents/Manuals/Chapter_525_Vision_Services.pdf (accessed April 8, 2016).

Wyoming Department of Health. 2011. *Medicaid handbook.* Cheyenne: Wyoming Department of Health. http://wyequalitycare.acs-inc.com/manuals/Client_Handbook_08.25.11.pdf (accessed April 8, 2016).

————. 2016. *CMS 1500 ICD-10.* Cheyenne: Wyoming Department of Health. http://wyequalitycare.acs-inc.com/manuals/Manual_CMS1500_4_1_16_final.pdf (accessed May 17, 2016).

————. n.d. *Wyoming Medicaid rules.* Cheyenne: Wyoming Department of Health. http://soswy.state.wy.us/Rules/RULES/6252.pdf (accessed April 8, 2016).